GLOBAL
SPINAL ALIGNMENT
Principles, Pathologies, and Procedures

GLOBAL
SPINAL ALIGNMENT
Principles, Pathologies, and Procedures

EDITED BY

Regis W. Haid, Jr., MD, FAANS
Medical Director, Atlanta Brain and Spine Care;
Piedmont Spine Center and Neuroscience Service Line,
Piedmont Atlanta Hospital, Atlanta, Georgia

Frank J. Schwab, MD
Chief of Spinal Deformity, Department of Orthopedic Surgery,
New York University Langone Medical Center,
New York, New York

Christopher I. Shaffrey, MD
John A. Jane Professor,
Departments of Neurosurgery and Orthopaedic Surgery,
University of Virginia, Charlottesville, Virginia

Jim A. Youssef, MD
Senior Partner and Founder, Spine Colorado,
Durango Orthopedic Associates, PC;
Medical Director, Spine Center of Excellence,
Mercy Regional Medical Center, Durango, Colorado

Quality Medical Publishing, Inc.
ST. LOUIS, MISSOURI
2015

Printed in United States of America

This book presents current scientific information and opinion pertinent to medical professionals. It does not provide advice concerning specific diagnosis and treatment of individual cases and is not intended for use by the layperson. Medical knowledge is constantly changing. As new information becomes available, changes in treatment, procedures, equipment, and the use of drugs become necessary. The editors/authors/contributors and the publisher have, as far as it is possible, taken care to ensure that the information given in this text is accurate and up to date. However, readers are strongly advised to confirm that the information, especially with regard to drug usage, complies with the latest legislation and standards of practice. The authors and publisher will not be responsible for any errors or liable for actions taken as a result of information or opinions expressed in this book.

The publishers have made every effort to trace the copyright holders for borrowed material. If they have inadvertently overlooked any, they will be pleased to make the necessary arrangements at the first opportunity.

EDITORIAL DIRECTOR   Michelle Berger
EDITOR   Amy Debrecht
PROJECT MANAGER   Makalah Boyer
MEDICAL ILLUSTRATIONS   Amanda Tomasikiewicz Good
COVER ILLUSTRATION   William M. Winn

Quality Medical Publishing, Inc.
2248 Welsch Industrial Court
St. Louis, Missouri 63146
Telephone: 1-800-348-7808
Web site: *http://www.qmp.com*

LIBRARY OF CONGRESS CATALOGING-IN-PUBLICATION DATA

Global spinal alignment : principles, pathologies, and procedures / edited
by Regis W. Haid, Jr., Christopher I. Shaffrey, Jim A. Youssef, Frank J.
Schwab.
    p. ; cm.
  Includes bibliographical references and index.
  ISBN 978-1-57626-484-3 (hardcover)
  I. Haid, Regis W., editor. II. Shaffrey, Christopher I., editor. III.
Youssef, Jim A., editor. IV. Schwab, Frank J., editor.
  [DNLM: 1. Spinal Diseases--pathology. 2. Spinal Diseases--surgery. 3.
Orthopedic Procedures--methods. 4. Spine--pathology. 5. Surgical
Procedures, Minimally Invasive--methods. WE 725]
  RD768
  617.4'71--dc23
                                        2014027130

**To those in our professional careers
who have mentored, influenced, and inspired us.
We thank you.**

Dr. Paul Cooper
Dr. Volker Sonntag
Dr. Michael MacMillan
Dr. G. Robert Nugent
R.W.H

Dr. Jean-Pierre Farcy
Dr. Jean Dubousset
Dr. Thomas Errico
Dr. Virginie Lafage
F.J.S.

Dr. John Jane
Dr. Richard Whitehill
Dr. David Cahill
Dr. Donald Chan
Dr. Gwo-Jaw Wang
Dr. H. Richard Winn
C.I.S.

Dr. Daniel Benson
Dr. Robert McLain
Dr. Luiz Pimenta
Dr. Philip Bernini
Dr. William Abdu
Dr. James Murphy
J.A.Y.

Contributors

Khaled Aboushaala, MD
Orthopedic Surgeon, Department of Orthopedics, Rush University Medical Center, Chicago, Illinois

Junyoung Ahn, BS
Research Coordinator, Department of Orthopedics, Rush University Medical Center, Chicago, Illinois

Todd J. Albert, MD
Surgeon-in-Chief and Medical Director, Korein-Wilson Professor of Orthopaedic Surgery, Department of Orthopaedic Surgery, Hospital for Special Surgery; Chair, Department of Orthopaedic Surgery, Weill Cornell Medical College, New York, New York

Nabeel S. Alshafai, MD, FRCS(C), FEANS
Neurosurgeon and Spine Fellow, Division of Neurosurgery, Toronto Western Hospital, University of Toronto, Toronto, Ontario, Canada

Christopher P. Ames, MD
Professor, Department of Neurological Surgery, University of California, San Francisco, San Francisco, California

D. Greg Anderson, MD
Professor, Department of Orthopaedic and Neurological Surgery, Thomas Jefferson University, Philadelphia, Pennsylvania

Prokopis Annis, MD
Instructor—Spine, Department of Orthopaedics, University of Utah, Salt Lake City, Utah

Navid R. Arandi, BS
Research Fellow, San Diego Center for Spinal Disorders, San Diego, California

Paul M. Arnold, MD, FACS
Professor of Neurosurgery and Vice-Chairman for Research, Department of Neurosurgery; Director, Spinal Cord Injury Center, The University of Kansas Medical Center, Kansas City, Kansas

Christopher D. Baggott, MD
Neurosurgical Resident, Department of Neurological Surgery, University of Wisconsin, Madison, Madison, Wisconsin

Daniel A. Baluch, MD
Resident, Department of Orthopaedic Surgery and Rehabilitation, Loyola University Medical Center, Maywood, Illinois

John C. Barr, MD
Department of Neurosurgery, Vanderbilt Medical Center, Nashville, Tennessee

Rahul Basho, MD
Director of Spine Surgery, Department of Orthopedic Surgery, Hannibal Regional Hospital; Midwest Orthopedic Specialists, Hannibal, Missouri

Sharath Bellary, MD, MEng
Research Fellow, Department of Orthopedic Surgery, Northwestern University, Chicago, Illinois

David M. Benglis, Jr., MD
Atlanta Brain and Spine Care, Atlanta, Georgia

Sigurd Berven, MD
Professor, Department of Orthopaedic Surgery, University of California, San Francisco, San Francisco, California

Shay Bess, MD
Department of Orthopaedic Surgery, Rocky Mountain Hospital for Children/Presbyterian St. Luke's Medical Center, Denver, Colorado

Anthony J. Boniello, BS
Clinical Research Fellow, Department of Orthopaedic Surgery, New York University Langone Medical Center, New York, New York

Darrel S. Brodke, MD
Professor and Vice-Chair, Department of Orthopaedics, University of Utah, Salt Lake City, Utah

Jaysson T. Brooks, MD
Resident Physician, Department of Orthopaedic Surgery,
The Johns Hopkins University School of Medicine, Baltimore,
Maryland

Leah Yacat Carreon, MD, MSc
Clinical Research Director, Norton Leatherman Spine Center,
Louisville, Kentucky

Vincent Challier, MD
Research Fellow, Department of Orthopaedic Surgery,
New York University Langone Medical Center, New York,
New York; Department of Orthopedics, Hôpital Pellegrin,
Bordeaux, France

Joseph S. Cheng, MD, MS, FAACS, FAANS
Director, Neurosurgery Spine Program, Department of
Neurosurgery, Vanderbilt University, Nashville, Tennessee

Michael R. Conti Mica, MD
Resident Physician, Department of Orthopaedic Surgery,
Stritch School of Medicine, Loyola University Chicago,
Chicago, Illinois

Vedat Deviren, MD
Professor, Clinical Orthopaedic, Department of Orthopaedic
Surgery, University of California, San Francisco, San Fran-
cisco, California

Bassel Diebo, MD
Research Fellow, Department of Orthopaedic Surgery,
New York University Langone Medical Center, New York,
New York

Jean Dubousset, MD
Professor, Pediatric Orthopedics, Académie Nationale de
Médicine, Paris, France

Rachel Eve Ebner, MS
Research Assistant, Spine Colorado, Durango Orthopedic
Associates, P.C., Durango, Colorado

Islam M. Elboghdady
Medical Student, Research Assistant, Department of Ortho-
pedics, Midwest Orthopedics at Rush, Rush Medical College,
Chicago, Illinois

Jean-Pierre Farcy, MD
Director, Balance Research Foundation, New York, New York

Michael G. Fehlings, MD, PhD, FRCS (C)
Division of Neurosurgery, Toronto Western Hospital, University Health Network, Toronto, Ontario, Canada

Emmanuelle Ferrero, MD
Research Fellow, Department of Orthopaedic Surgery,
New York University Langone Medical Center, New York,
New York; Resident, Department of Orthopedic Surgery,
Robert Debre Hôpital, Paris, France

Ricardo B.V. Fontes, MD, PhD
Chief Resident, Department of Neurosurgery, Rush University Medical Center, Chicago, Illinois

Vance Fredrickson, MD
Resident Physician, Department of Neurological Surgery,
University of Wisconsin, Madison, Madison, Wisconsin

Elizabeth A. Friis, PhD
Associate Professor, Department of Mechanical Engineering,
University of Kansas, Lawrence, Kansas

Kai-Ming Fu, MD, PhD
Assistant Professor, Department of Neurological Surgery,
Weill Cornell Medical College, New York, New York

Haruki Funao, MD
Department of Orthopaedic Surgery, The Johns Hopkins
University, Baltimore, Maryland

Zoher Ghogawala, MD, FACS
Charles A. Fager Chairman, Department of Neurosurgery,
Lahey Hospital and Medical Center, Burlington, Massachu-
setts; Associate Professor of Neurosurgery, Department of
Neurosurgery, Tufts University School of Medicine, Boston,
Massachusetts

Steven D. Glassman, MD
Professor, Department of Orthopaedic Surgery, University
of Louisville School of Medicine; Norton Leatherman Spine
Center, Louisville, Kentucky

Yakov Gologorsky, MD
Assistant Clinical Professor, Department of Neurosurgery,
Mount Sinai Hospital, New York, New York

Randall B. Graham, MD
Resident Physician, Department of Neurological Surgery,
Northwestern University, Chicago, Illinois

Michael W. Groff, MD
Director of Spinal Neurosurgery, Department of Neurosurgery, Brigham and Women's Hospital, Boston, Massachusetts

Jeffrey L. Gum, MD
Adult and Pediatric Spine Surgeon, Norton Leatherman Spine
Center, Louisville, Kentucky

Munish Chandra Gupta, MD
Professor and Vice-Chair, Department of Orthopaedic Surgery, Co-Director, Spine Center, University of California, Davis, Sacramento, California

Regis W. Haid, Jr., MD, FAANS
Medical Director, Atlanta Brain and Spine Care; Piedmont Spine Center and Neuroscience Service Line, Piedmont Atlanta Hospital, Atlanta, Georgia

James S. Harrop, MD, FACS
Professor of Neurological Surgery, Chief, Division of Spine and Peripheral Neurosurgery, Department of Neurosurgery, Thomas Jefferson University, Philadelphia, Pennsylvania

Robert A. Hart, MD
Professor, Department of Orthopaedics and Rehabilitation, Oregon Health and Science University, Portland, Oregon

Sohaib Z. Hashmi, MD
Resident Physician, Department of Orthopaedic Surgery, Northwestern University Feinberg School of Medicine, Chicago, Illinois

Hamid Hassanzadeh, MD
Assistant Professor, Department of Orthopaedic Surgery, University of Virginia, Charlottesville, Virginia

Kenneth A. Hood, DO
Resident, Department of Orthopaedic Surgery, Riverside County Regional Medical Center, Moreno Valley, California

Richard Hostin, MD
Chief of Orthopedics, Department of Orthopedic Surgery, Baylor Regional Medical Center at Plano; Medical Director, Baylor Scoliosis Center, Plano, Texas

Clifford M. Houseman, DO
Clinical Spine Instructor, Department of Neurosurgery, Vanderbilt University Medical Center, Nashville, Tennessee

R. Mark Hoyle, MD, FACS
General and Vascular Surgeon, Methodist Hospital for Surgery, Addison, Texas

Wellington K. Hsu, MD
Clifford C. Raisbeck Distinguished Professor of Orthopaedic Surgery, Director of Research, Department of Orthopaedic Surgery, Northwestern University Feinberg School of Medicine, Chicago, Illinois

Alice Jane Hughes, BS
Medical Student, Thomas Jefferson University Hospital, Department of Orthopaedic Surgery, Rothman Institute, Philadelphia, Pennsylvania

Megan M. Jack, MD, PhD
Resident Physician, Department of Neurosurgery, The University of Kansas Medical Center, Kansas City, Kansas

Charles I. Jones III, MD, MS
Resident Physician, Department of Orthopaedic Surgery, University of Arkansas for Medical Sciences, Little Rock, Arkansas

Isaac O. Karikari, MD
Assistant Professor, Department of Neurosurgery, Duke University Medical Center, Durham, North Carolina

Satoshi A. Kawaguchi, MD
Instructor, Department of Orthopaedics and Rehabilitation, Oregon Health and Science University, Portland, Oregon

Khaled M. Kebaish, MD
Department of Orthopaedic Surgery, The Johns Hopkins University, Baltimore, Maryland

John Paul Kelleher, MD
Neurosurgery Spine Fellow, Department of Neurosurgery, University of Virginia, Charlottesville, Virginia

Randall P. Kirby, MD, FACS
Vascular and General Surgeon, Department of Surgery, Baylor University Medical Center, Dallas, Texas

Eric Otto Klineberg, MD
Associate Professor, Department of Orthopaedic Surgery, University of California, Davis, Sacramento, California

John D. Koerner, MD
Department of Orthopaedic Surgery, Thomas Jefferson University and Rothman Institute, Philadelphia, Pennsylvania

Tyler R. Koski, MD
Associate Professor, Department of Neurological Surgery, Northwestern University Feinberg School of Medicine, Chicago, Illinois

Charles Kuntz IV, MD
Professor and Vice Chairman, Department of Neurosurgery, Mayfield Clinic, University of Cincinnati, Cincinnati, Ohio

Hubert Labelle, MD
Head of Orthopedics, Department of Surgery, University of Montreal; Orthopedic Surgeon, Department of Surgery, Sainte-Justine Mother-Child University Hospital, Montreal, Quebec, Canada

Virginie Lafage, PhD
Director of Spine Research, Department of Orthopaedic Surgery, New York University Langone Medical Center, New York, New York

Anthony C.W. Lau, MD, PhD
Division of Neurosurgery, University of Toronto, Toronto,
Ontario, Canada

Hai V. Le, MD
Resident, Department of Orthopedic Surgery, Harvard
Combined Orthopedic Residency Program (HCORP),
Boston, Massachusetts

Lawrence G. Lenke, MD
The Jerome J. Gilden Distinguished Professor of Orthopae-
dic Surgery; Professor of Neurological Surgery; Chief, Spine
Surgery; Co-Director, Pediatric/Adult Spinal Deformity
Service; Director, Advanced Deformity Fellowship (ADF),
Department of Orthopaedic Surgery, Washington University
School of Medicine, St. Louis, Missouri

Yiping Li, MD
Neurosurgery Resident, Department of Neurosurgery,
University of Wisconsin Hospitals and Clinics, Madison,
Wisconsin

Adam Lindsay, MS
Medical Student, Drexel University College of Medicine, Philadelphia, Pennsylvania

Shian Liu, BS
Research Fellow, Department of Orthopaedic Surgery,
New York University Langone Medical Center, New York,
New York

Philip K. Louie, MD
Resident Physician, Department of Orthopaedic Surgery,
Rush University, Chicago, Illinois

Jean-Marc Mac-Thiong, MD, PhD
Associate Professor, Department of Surgery, University of
Montreal; Department of Surgery, Sainte-Justine Mother-
Child University Hospital; Department of Surgery, Hôpital du
Sacre-Coeur de Montreal, Montreal, Quebec, Canada

Erin M. Mannen, BS
Graduate Researcher and Doctoral Candidate, Mechanical
Engineering, The University of Kansas, Lawrence, Kansas

Daniel M. Mazzaferro, BA, MBA
Medical Student, Drexel University College of Medicine;
Research Volunteer, Rothman Institute, Philadelphia, Penn-
sylvania

Richard E. McCarthy, MD
Professor, Department of Orthopaedics and Neurosur-
gery, University of Arkansas for Medical Sciences; Professor,
Department of Orthopaedics and Neurosurgery, Arkansas
Children's Hospital, Little Rock, Arkansas

Matthew McDonnell, MD
Spine Surgery Fellow, Department of Orthopaedic Surgery,
Thomas Jefferson University and Rothman Institute, Philadel-
phia, Pennsylvania

Firoz Miyanji, MD, FRCS (C)
Pediatric Orthopedic Surgeon, BC Children's Hospital;
Clinical Assistant Professor, Department of Orthopedics,
University of British Columbia, Vancouver, British Columbia,
Canada

Sergey Mlyavykh, MD, PhD
Chief of Spine Surgery and Neurological Surgery, Department of Neurosurgery, Nizhny Novgorod Research Institute
of Traumatology and Orthopedics, Nizhny Novgorod, Russia

Nelson Moussazadeh, MD
Resident Physician, Department of Neurological Surgery,
New York–Presbyterian Hospital/Weill Cornell Medical
Center, New York, New York

Elisa R. Mullikin, BA
Physician Assistant Student, Physician Assistant Studies,
University of the Sciences in Philadelphia, Philadelphia,
Pennsylvania

Praveen V. Mummaneni, MD
Professor and Vice Chairman of Neurological Surgery,
Department of Neurological Surgery, University of Califor-
nia, San Francisco, San Francisco, California

Gregory M. Mundis, Jr., MD
Medical Director, Pediatric and Adult Spinal Deformity, San
Diego Center for Spinal Disorders; Co-Director, San Diego
Spine Fellowship, San Diego, California

Abbas Naqvi, BS
Research Coordinator, Department of Orthopaedic Surgery,
Rush University Medical Center, Chicago, Illinois

Ngoc-Lam Nguyen, MD
Resident Physician, Department of Orthopaedic Surgery and
Rehabilitation, Loyola University Medical Center, Maywood,
Illinois

Michael F. O'Brien, MD
Southwest Scoliosis Institute; Medical Director of Research,
Baylor Scoliosis Center, Plano, Texas

Taemin Oh, BA
Predoctoral Clinical Research Fellow, Department of Neuro-
logical Surgery, Northwestern University Feinberg School of
Medicine, Chicago, Illinois; Medical Student, Department of
Neurological Surgery, University of California, Los Angeles,
School of Medicine, Los Angeles, California

Douglas G. Orndorff, MD
Orthopedic Surgeon, Spine Colorado, Durango Orthopedics, Durango, Colorado

Stefan Parent, MD, PhD, FRCS
Associate Professor, Department of Surgery, Director, Pediatric and Adult Spine Fellowship, University of Montreal; Orthopedic Surgeon, Department of Surgery, Sainte-Justine Mother-Child University Hospital, Montreal, Quebec, Canada

Michael S. Park, MD
Resident Physician, Department of Neurosurgery and Brain Repair, Morsani College of Medicine, University of South Florida, Tampa, Florida

Alpesh A. Patel, MD, FACS
Director, Orthopaedic Spine Surgery, Co-Director, Northwestern Spine Center, Associate Professor, Department of Orthopaedic Surgery, Northwestern University Feinberg School of Medicine, Chicago, Illinois

Murat Pekmezci, MD
Assistant Clinical Professor, Department of Orthopedic Surgery, University of California, San Francisco, San Francisco, California

Mark D. Peterson, MD
Medical Director, Spine Institute, Providence Medford Medical Center, Medford, Oregon

Luiz Pimenta, MD, PhD
Medical Director, Instituto de Patologia da Coluna, São Paulo, SP Brazil; Assistant Professor, Department of Neurosurgery, University of California, San Diego, San Diego, California

David W. Polly, Jr., MD
Professor and Chief of Spine Surgery, Department of Orthopaedic Surgery, University of Minnesota, Minneapolis, Minnesota

Laura Ellen Prado, MSN, NP
Nurse Practitioner, Atlanta Brain and Spine Care, Atlanta, Georgia

Themistocles S. Protopsaltis, MD
Assistant Professor, Department of Orthopaedics, Spine Division, New York University Langone Hospital for Joint Diseases; Director, Bellevue Hospital Orthopaedic Spine Service, New York, New York

Daniel K. Resnick, MD, MS
Professor and Vice Chairman, Department of Neurological Surgery, University of Wisconsin, Madison, Madison, Wisconsin

Rajiv Saigal, MD, PhD
Chief Resident, Department of Neurological Surgery, University of California, San Francisco, San Francisco, California

Jason W. Savage, MD
Assistant Professor, Department of Orthopaedic Surgery, Northwestern University, Chicago, Illinois

Justin K. Scheer, BS
Predoctoral Clinical Research Fellow, Department of Neurological Surgery, Northwestern University Feinberg School of Medicine, Chicago, Illinois; Medical Student, University of California, San Diego School of Medicine, La Jolla, California

Paul J. Schmitt, MD
Resident Physician, Department of Neurosurgery, University of Virginia Health System, Charlottesville, Virginia

Frank J. Schwab, MD
Chief of Spinal Deformity, Department of Orthopedic Surgery, New York University Langone Medical Center, New York, New York

Daniel M. Sciubba, MD
Associate Professor of Neurosurgery, Oncology, and Orthopaedic Surgery; Director of Research, Department of Neurosurgery, The Johns Hopkins University, Baltimore, Maryland

Morgan Scott, MS
Research Coordinator, Department of Research, Spine Colorado, Durango, Colorado

Christopher I. Shaffrey, MD
John A. Jane Professor, Departments of Neurosurgery and Orthopaedic Surgery, University of Virginia, Charlottesville, Virginia

Kern Singh, MD
Associate Professor, Department of Orthopaedic Surgery, Rush University Medical Center, Chicago, Illinois

Koopong Siribumrungwong, MD
Clinical Instructor, Spine Unit, Department of Orthopaedic Surgery, Faculty of Medicine, Prince of Songkla University, Hadyai, Songkla, Thailand

Justin S. Smith, MD, PhD
Associate Professor, Department of Neurosurgery, University of Virginia, Charlottesville, Virginia

Kyle A. Smith, MD
Resident Physician, Department of Neurosurgery, The University of Kansas Medical Center, Kansas City, Kansas

William D. Smith, MD
Chief of Neurosurgery, Department of Neurosurgery, University Medical Center of Southern Nevada, Las Vegas, Nevada

Kevin Sonn, MD
Research Fellow, Department of Orthopaedic Surgery, Northwestern University Feinberg School of Medicine, Chicago, Illinois

Paul D. Sponseller, MD, MBA
Professor and Head, Division of Pediatric Orthopedics, Johns Hopkins Bloomberg Children's Center, Baltimore, Maryland

Vincent C. Traynelis, MD
Professor, Department of Neurosurgery, Rush University Medical Center, Chicago, Illinois

Cliff B. Tribus, MD
Professor, Department of Orthopedics and Rehabilitation, University of Wisconsin, Madison, Madison, Wisconsin

Juan S. Uribe, MD
Associate Professor, Department of Neurosurgery, University of South Florida, Tampa, Florida

Alexander R. Vaccaro, MD, PhD
Everett and Marion Gordon Professor of Orthopaedic Surgery and Professor of Neurosurgery, Thomas Jefferson University and Rothman Institute, Philadelphia, Pennsylvania

Rishi Wadhwa, MD
Clinical Instructor, Department of Neurological Surgery, University of California, San Francisco, San Francisco, California

Jeffrey C. Wang, MD
Chief, Orthopaedic Spine Service; Professor of Orthopaedic Surgery and Neurosurgery, Department of Orthopaedic Surgery and Neurosurgery, University of Southern California Spine Center, Los Angeles, California

Michael Y. Wang, MD
Professor, Department of Neurological Surgery and Rehabilitative Medicine, University of Miami Miller School of Medicine, Miami, Florida

Robert G. Whitmore, MD
Department of Neurosurgery, Lahey Hospital and Medical Center, Burlington, Massachusetts; Assistant Professor, Department of Neurosurgery, Tufts University School of Medicine, Boston, Massachusetts

Cyrus C. Wong, MD
Neurological Surgery Resident Physician, Department of Neurological Surgery, Vanderbilt University Medical Center, Nashville, Tennessee

Jim A. Youssef, MD
Senior Partner and Founder, Spine Colorado, Durango Orthopedic Associates, PC; Medical Director, Spine Center of Excellence, Mercy Regional Medical Center, Durango, Colorado

Alp Yurter, BS
Department of Neurosurgery, The Johns Hopkins University School of Medicine, Baltimore, Maryland

Patricia L. Zadnik, BA
Department of Neurosurgery, The Johns Hopkins University School of Medicine, Baltimore, Maryland

Foreword

The field of spinal surgery continues to expand the horizons of care for patients afflicted with pain and deformity. Treatment of spinal deformity and malalignment has significantly progressed since the pioneering work of Harrington, Moe, Winter, and others for the correction of scoliotic deformities. Surgical options have expanded from the early posterior hook-rod construct to polyaxial pedicle screws and circumferential procedures. Over the past decade, our understanding of spinal alignment, from the pelvis to the cranium, has also evolved.

Global Spinal Alignment: Principles, Pathologies, and Procedures, edited by Drs. Regis W. Haid, Jr., Frank J. Schwab, Christopher I. Shaffrey, and Jim A. Youssef, gives clinicians a single resource to more fully understand and treat patients with spinal malalignment. A distinguished author list, including orthopaedic surgeons, neurosurgeons, radiologists, engineers, and basic scientists, have contributed to the text.

Beginning with goals and basic principles, the text is richly illustrated with clear, concise radiographs and figures. Surgical indications, techniques, and outcome measures are fully described for a variety of degenerative, acquired, and iatrogenic deformities. Recent advances in the field of bone healing and fusion are covered in an up-to-date section. Finally, the most recent developments in the field of minimally invasive surgery are also described.

This textbook is an important contribution to advance our knowledge in treating patients with spinal deformity. *Global Spinal Alignment: Principles, Pathologies, and Procedures* will be a vital resource for younger clinicians to more experienced surgeons to assist in the care of deformity and a welcome addition to the body of spinal literature.

Jeffrey S. Fischgrund, MD
President, Lumbar Spine Research Society; Professor and Chairman,
Department of Orthopaedics, William Beaumont Hospital,
Royal Oak, Michigan

On behalf of the Scoliosis Research Society, I would like to commend the authors and editors of *Global Spinal Alignment: Principles, Pathologies, and Procedures* for this important contribution to the spinal surgery literature. For many years, the members of the SRS have recognized the critical role of spinal balance in the evaluation and management of spinal deformity patients. In this outstanding textbook, the state of the art is conveyed by many of the authors responsible for the development of our present understanding. The book includes an introductory chapter from Dr. Jean Dubousset, whose innovative ideas underlie so many of our current concepts regarding spinal balance and alignment. In addition to a thorough review of basic principles, the text addresses specifics of anatomic and radiographic characteristics, as well as their implications for surgical treatment.

Beyond examining the work that has been done to date, *Global Spinal Alignment* also reflects on potential future applications of this critical concept. Increasingly, it is becoming clear that the need to consider global alignment, well accepted for spinal deformity patients, applies equally in the management of lumbar and cervical degenerative disorders. One of the unique aspects of this text is an in-depth review of spinal alignment as it pertains to regions of the spine for which the role of spinal balance and alignment is less fully understood.

To paraphrase one of our insightful young members: All spine surgeons are deformity surgeons. Some create deformity and others manage deformity. This comprehensive review of our existing knowledge regarding global spinal alignment will undoubtedly help to move surgeons into the latter category. I recommend *Global Spinal Alignment: Principles, Pathologies, and Procedures* as a valuable resource for experienced spine surgeons as well as residents and fellows with an interest in spinal surgery.

Steven D. Glassman, MD
Professor, Department of Orthopaedic Surgery, University of Louisville School of Medicine;
Norton Leatherman Spine Center, Louisville, Kentucky

During my neurosurgical training, there were two indications for surgery that covered most of the spine patients that we operated on. The first was neurologic compression, and the second was structural instability. Historically, we have always known that spinal balance must be respected to create an environment conducive to a successful fusion, and so, to the extent that spinal balance was considered, it was in the service of achieving structural stability. Neurosurgery at that time was vaguely aware of scoliosis surgery and the work done there to correct deformity. More recently, however, the thought leaders in spinal surgery, both orthopedic and neurosurgical, have helped us to understand that spinal balance is an important determinate of clinical outcome in its own right.

In the current era, optimizing spinal balance and correcting deformity has been shown to play an important, perhaps the most important, role in the domains of not only scoliosis but also degenerative disease, tumor, and trauma. This book provides both a solid introduction to these important concepts, and a rich discussion for those ready for a deeper understanding. The chapters are written by the thought leaders that have led the charge toward a fuller understanding of the spine. The book is organized in a logical sequence with the *why* being fully explained before diving into *the what*. The chapters are well written and easily accessible. The subject is covered fully with discussion ranging from vertebral column resection to minimally invasive surgery and from clinical outcome measures to the role of biologics in fusion. At the same time, the book is filled with practical advice that surgeons can employ in the operating room.

The aspects of spinal surgery that make it such an engaging area to work in, is the rapid advancement of both the technique and scientific foundation. This book will make a useful addition to the library of residents interested in spine care, busy practitioners, and academic faculty alike, who share a desire to remain abreast of one of the most important concepts to sweep through our field. The importance being placed on global spinal balance in contemporary clinical care represents nothing less than a genuine paradigm change. This book provides a full understanding of the concepts and the opportunity to apply them successfully in clinical practice.

Michael W. Groff, MD
Past Chairman, AANS/CNS Section on Disorders of the Spine and Peripheral Nerve, Director of Spinal Neurosurgery, Department of Neurosurgery, Brigham and Women's Hospital, Boston, Massachusetts

When asked to write this foreword for *Global Spinal Alignment: Principles, Pathologies, and Procedures*, I was flattered and confused. I was flattered, because over the years I have worked closely with two of the editors, Drs. Haid and Shaffrey. I have developed the greatest respect for their intellect, experience, and commitment to improving the field of spinal surgery. I don't know Dr. Youssef nearly so well, but I do remember him as an orthopedic surgery resident at Dartmouth, while I was there on the Neurosurgery faculty. Even then, it was easy to tell that he had a great career ahead of him. I regret to say that I know Dr. Schwab only by his outstanding reputation and the excellence of this text. Of course I was flattered to be asked to write the foreword for a book with such luminary editors. I was, however, also confused by this request. I can claim no expertise in complex spinal surgery or its associated principles and pathologies and felt woefully inadequate to comment on the work. However, I think I can see the method in the madness of the request for a foreword from someone so ill prepared to be a knowledgeable critic.

It has been nearly 30 years since I finished my neurosurgery residency. During that time, there have been dramatic changes in spinal surgery. The comprehensive goals of spinal surgery during my training were to decompress the neural elements and prevent spinal instability. This simplistic approach is long gone. Because of the work of the editors of this text and others who have been pioneers in the field of deformity surgery, we now know that surgery that corrects neural impingement and spinal instability, but creates poor coronal or sagittal alignment, usually produces a less than satisfactory result for our patients. The mechanical disadvantage that comes with poor global alignment means that patients must compensate for the anatomic deformation by increased energy expenditure, muscle contraction, and limitation of activity, resulting in an unacceptable functional health status outcome for patients after surgery. Those already immersed in the field of complex spine surgery understand all of this. Perhaps it takes an outsider like me to really appreciate the scope of what the editors have created. This outstanding book addresses the entire range of issues that need to be considered and understood if we hope to achieve the excellent functional outcomes patients expect after complex spine surgery.

The editors have succeeded in creating a text that will be useful for residents in training, spinal surgery fellows, and expert practitioners in complex spine surgery. To accomplish this, the editors have recruited the thought leaders in spinal anatomy, pathology, radiology, biomechanics, and surgery to create a broad-ranging text on the multifaceted topic of global spinal alignment. They have also organized the text in a way that takes the reader from basic goals and principles, through the anatomic, radiographic, biologic, and surgical factors that need to be considered when treating patients with spinal deformity. In addition, the biomechanics of spinal deformity and the effects of spinal instrumentation, host factor biologic variation, and the use of biologic materials on the outcomes from surgery are thoroughly reviewed. Following this extensive review of underlying principles, numerous chapters address specific conditions requiring treatment. Expert authors discuss these conditions and the various surgical techniques that can be employed to produce a successful outcome.

I believe this book will become the definitive text on global spinal alignment. The editors should be congratulated on producing such an outstanding contribution to the medical and surgical literature on spine disease and its treatment.

Robert E. Harbaugh, MD, FAANS, FACS, FAHA
President, American Association of Neurological Surgeons; Director, Institute of Neurosciences; Distinguished Professor and Chair, Department of Neurosurgery, The Pennsylvania State University, Milton S. Hershey Medical Center, Hershey, Pennsylvania

Preface

*"Learn from yesterday, live for today, hope for tomorrow.
The important thing is not to stop questioning."*
—ALBERT EINSTEIN

Spine surgery is a rapidly evolving field of medicine. The established principles, surgical techniques, and expanding indications are in constant evolution. Technological advances, coupled with minimally disruptive surgical approaches and evidence-based treatment, can offer improved and more predictable outcomes. Global spinal alignment has emerged over the past decade as a critical concept in understanding the impact of pathology and treatment such as spinal fusion. Through substantial contributions from forward-thinking researchers who recognized the impact of sagittal alignment on human function, we have become more aware of a need to compile the latest information on this subject. The treatment of any spinal pathology must include consideration of the complexity of spinopelvic alignment. This is of particular importance in the setting of spinal fusion, where significant, immediate, but also downstream effects on global spinal alignment occur.

Global Spinal Alignment: Principles, Pathologies, and Procedures aims to provide an up-to-date review of the surgical considerations, indications, and techniques in open and MIS approaches, from both a basic science and clinical perspective. Emphasis has been placed on emerging information and relevance, as it relates to global spinal alignment. The editors recognized the need for such a textbook, given the exploding advancements in outcomes modeling and spinal instrumentation, and the expanding indications to implement MIS approaches for treating various spinal pathologies. We have all experienced situations in which our inability to recognize the impact of a simple spinal fusion has created the need to offer a more involved, secondary procedure, based on the limited success of the index procedure. A need for a greater understanding of this impact spurred our interest in compiling this comprehensive summary of a global spinal alignment textbook. We have attempted to identify the pertinent topics related to this subject and the leading contributors for each topic.

This book is written for practicing spine surgeons and those in spine fellowship training seeking a profession dedicated to spine surgery. It is our hope that as we learn from our past experiences and growing outcomes data, we embrace new technology on more certain footing. It is critical that we offer greater value through the care we deliver to patients through innovation and solid principles. We are faced with the need to address limitations of current technologies and iatrogenic failures, and this demands that we improve our approaches in index procedures and leverage our understanding, research, and technology to provide guidance, sustainability, and reproducibility through our surgical interventions.

This book is organized in eight comprehensive parts. Beginning with the goals and basic principles of spinal alignment, the most up-to-date information on anatomic, radiographic, and clinical outcomes of treating spinal deformity is outlined. A special chapter dedicated to the distinction between spinal balance and spinal alignment provides an important distinction of these concepts and an understanding of how neurodegenerative and myelopathic conditions contribute to clinical presentation. Part II is a compilation of the anatomic, radiographic, and surgical considerations of global alignment. Taking an anthropomorphic approach to the sagittal curvatures of the spine and the relation of each to the adjacent region is the intent of this section. Part III is dedicated to the biomechanical considerations of spinal deformity and the effects of spinal instrumentation on treating such pathologies. Part IV takes into consideration the most important aspect of any spinal fusion, the biologic considerations, and the site-specific challenges of obtaining a solid arthrodesis. Unfortunately, the evidence supporting many currently used osteobiologics is limited. Contributing authors provide clarity on specific biologics and their efficacy in promoting arthrodesis in specific host environments. This section also addresses considerations related to biomaterials and the effects of treating spinal deformity with spinal instrumentation.

Part V brings to light the impact of isolated considerations of surgical spinal fusions on global spinal alignment. This section introduces the concept that every spinal fusion influences spinal alignment. By focusing on specific spinal pathologies such as degenerative disc disease, the contributing authors provide guidance on how to manage such indications with the least untoward effect on overall spinal alignment. Part VI is dedicated to scoliosis and the specific considerations in treating idiopathic, congenital, and neuromuscular causes of scoliosis and the treatment of Scheuermann's kyphosis. This section provides detail on spinal alignment in specific deformities, from planning to technical execution. Part VII provides insight on the latest techniques for revision strategies for surgical management of spinal deformity. Finally, the last part is dedicated to minimally invasive surgical management of spinal deformities, implementation of the latest techniques, and evidence for such surgical approaches. Less invasive techniques are certain to expand within spinal surgery. Such techniques have demonstrated benefits with regard to blood loss, length of hospital stay, and postoperative narcotic needs. However, such approaches require a greater understanding of their impact on global spinal alignment, where concerns over restoration of the sagittal plane have come to light.

We are hopeful you will find this book a valuable resource and a reliable reference for understanding the latest in surgical principles and advances in treating spinal pathologies, with an emphasis on the consideration for global spinal alignment. Although we have come to realize the need to pay attention to spinopelvic parameters in treating spinal deformity, there remains an unrecognized need for a deeper understanding of global alignment. This book aims to provide this understanding through new concepts in planning and surgical technologies. We intended to provide a stage for spinal surgeons to share specific research, experiences, clinical outcomes, and unique strategies for coping with specific spinal pathologies.

We recognize and acknowledge the contributions of the pioneers of spinal surgery in creating this book. Without their endless efforts toward understanding the importance of sagittal spinal curvatures, global decompensation, implications of pelvic parameters, and the long-term effects of spinal arthrodesis, we would be at a loss in understanding global spinal alignment. Our goal is to complement and contribute to the substantial research data and knowledge through a collaborative effort of the contributing authors on this subject.

Regis W. Haid, Jr., MD, FAANS
Frank J. Schwab, MD
Christopher I. Shaffrey, MD
Jim A. Youssef, MD

Contents

Part III
Biomechanics of Spinal Deformity and Effects of Spinal Instrumentation

Part IV
Biologic Considerations of Spinal Fusion in Spinal Deformity

Part V
Isolated Considerations of Global Spinal Alignment

Part VI
Specific Considerations for Operative Management of Spinal Deformity

Part VII
Revision Strategies for Surgical Management of Spinal Deformity

Part VIII
Minimally Invasive Surgery:
Considerations for Management of Spinal Deformity

GLOBAL
SPINAL ALIGNMENT
Principles, Pathologies, and Procedures

PART I

Goals and Basic Principles

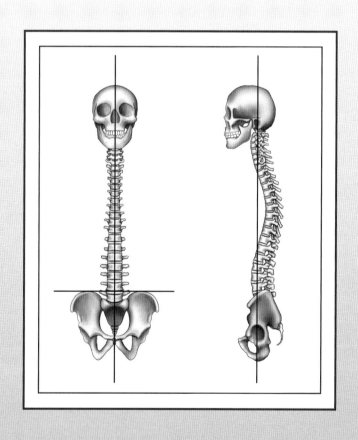

1

Spinal Alignment
Versus Spinal Balance

Jean Dubousset ▪ *Vincent Challier* ▪ *Jean-Pierre Farcy*
Frank J. Schwab ▪ *Virginie Lafage*

The distinction between alignment and balance is evident to engineers, physiologists, and choreographers but not to most surgeons. At many spinal and surgical scientific conferences, the word *imbalance* is used in conjunction with the projection of pictures, radiographs, and three-dimensional reconstructions that show the static alignment of the body or the skeleton in a standing position. Confusion occurs because these images are referred to as demonstrating balance; however, balance is not static but dynamic, and it can only be evaluated when the body and the skeleton are in motion.

Although it had not yet been formalized, this concept was the premise for the description of the *pelvic vertebrae,* which was introduced in 1972; it was also the foundation for the idea that the body's chain of balance works like a reverse pendulum and for the concept of a *cone of economy,* which was published as early as 1975 and which assumed that the standing posture involved minimal muscle consumption.[1]

In light of recent scientific developments, the objectives of this chapter are to clarify the distinction between balance and alignment and to introduce the concept of *stability within movement,* which is a continuous process that defines balance.

ACQUISITION OF LOCOMOTION

To appreciate the meaning of balance, one must consider the acquisition of posture and gait across the evolution of *Homo sapiens* and during the lifespan of human growth.

ANTHROPOLOGY

The development of bipedalism and erect posture has been studied by anthropologists for centuries. The anthropologic nomenclature addresses these features: *Pithecanthropus erectus* (1.6 million years BC; named by Eugène Dubois in 1894) "stood" and walked on his feet most of the time. The development of this bipedal feature from apes to humans intrigued many paleoanthropologists in their research, because the first hominid descended from the dichotomy between great apes and humans.[2-6] Bipedalism, which evolved intermittently and later exclusively, produced deep modifications of the skeleton's morphology.[7] The pelvic vertebrae, which are the keystones of equilibrium, hold a special place in this evolution. Progressive remodeling via the widening and retroversion[8] of the pelvic ring allows the acquisition of an erect posture. These modifications have driven the spinopelvic transformation from a primitive C-shape to the modern

S-shape, with its cervical, thoracic, and lumbar curves. With this advancement in bipedal equilibrium came improved means of hunting, carrying food, using tools, and parenting.[9] Whether *P. erectus* came from the trees or the savannah,[10-13] the human ancestor progressively evolved with the liberation of the head and hands.[14,15] This slow transformation, which science postulates occurred over the course of 7 million years, is analogous to the acquisition of gait and posture from early childhood to adulthood.

Human Locomotion

Self-sustained gait in humans is typically acquired between 11 and 15 months of age,[16] and it is based on a stable reference frame. Maintenance of postural alignment requires that the center of the body mass be kept over the supporting base.[17] Conversely, locomotor balance is a more complex task that involves achieving a compromise between the forward momentum of the body during gait, which is a highly destabilizing force, and the need to maintain the lateral stability of the body.[18] This quest for equilibrium is based on two functional principles that are common to children and adults: the reference frame and the gradual mastery of the body's joints.

- The reference frame for the organization of balance control[19] involves the head, shoulders, trunk, and pelvis. At the beginning, the head and upper limbs try to "reach the object." These movements are driven by a child's sensory curiosity, and they force mobilization of the body. During this period, the recruitment of control descends from head to toe. Then, during the acquisition of posture, the control is ascending. Pelvic locking of the lumbosacral and femoroacetabular joints allows a child to stand up. Control ascends and descends from the pelvis. From about 6 years of age, control includes anticipatory processes and becomes predominantly descending in response to stimuli from the environment.
- Gradual mastery of the degrees of freedom of the body joints[20-22] is also called *locking*. This behavior can stabilize globally or joint by joint. At first, locking occurs globally. As the neuromuscular circuits mature, control sharpens and becomes segmental.

Impact on Musculoskeletal System Development

Gait and posture acquisition has consequences for the development of the musculoskeletal system. Jean-Baptiste de Lamarck,[23] who is considered the father of modern physiology, postulated that the consistent use of an organ causes that organ to develop further with regard to its shape and function. For example, the pelvis will progressively transform in response to the effects of musculoligamentous groups during the development of balance.[24] Comparisons of the human adult pelvis with the neonatal pelvis and the early hominid pelvis reveal that pelvic incidence and sacral slope increase during growth, with an increased correlation between the two that may be linked to load and gravity.[25] A relationship between the evolution of the pelvic parameters and the spinal curves during the evolution of humans has been found, with a posterior pelvic shift trend and a progressive increase in lumbar lordosis; this can be seen by comparing modern humans with specimen STS 14 *Australopithecus africanus* from 2.8 million years BC (pelvic incidence 47 to 54 degrees; lumbar lordosis 41 degrees).[26] Thus the ontogenic acquisition of standing posture and gait during normal human growth reflects, in a small way, the phylogenic evolution of mankind.[25]

POSTURAL CONTROL

Balance depends on multisensory control of posture. Although vision has a significant influence on standing balance, humans are able to maintain balance in the dark or with closed eyes[27]; however, there is a degree of sway with this sensory deprivation. Light active touch that is insufficient to provide mechanical stabilization reduces sway to affect only those with active vision.[28-31]

Biologic Function

Balance is also a biologic function that is fundamental to human physiology, and it is based on two fundamental principles: the signal and the feedback loop. The signal can be electrical, piezoelectrical, caloric, chemical, hormonal, or molecular. The feedback loop responds to the signal and completes the biologic cycles that occur as part of metabolism as well as immunologic, cardiologic, and orthopedic processes. The balance *engine* is realized by sensory inputs, centers of integration and modulation, and muscular effectors.

Neurosensorial

Postural control is a continuous multisensorial process during which the central nervous system analyzes several afferent sensory inputs from the vestibular, visual, and proprioceptive systems and then responds through muscular effectors (Fig. 1-1).

- The vestibular system has both sensory and motor characteristics.[32] As a sensory system, the semicircular canals of the vestibular system detect the angular acceleration and velocity of the head; the otoliths sense the linear acceleration of the head, including gravitational acceleration. As a motor system, the vestibulospinal system projects all over the spine from the cervical level to the lumbar level, and it is related to postural stability.[33]

- The visual system is uniquely positioned to provide information about the static and dynamic features of the near and far environments. It is the only sensory system that can provide information about distant inanimate features. Visual input plays a major role in the avoidance of obstacles[34] and the regulation of dynamic stability.[35] The cortex processes input from the retina by means of the geniculate nucleus and then parcels the data to various surrounding cortical areas. Retinal inputs are also processed subcortically by the superior colliculus, which responds to novel stimuli in the visual field.[36] Other subcortical fibers go to the hippocampus, which has been implicated in cognitive spatial mapping and memory, thereby building a library of experiences that are useful for anticipating certain events and making the necessary gait adjustments.[37]

- The term *proprioception* refers to the sense of position and motion of one's body parts. Several classes of receptors from the muscles, joints, skin, and cardiovascular system contribute to the proprioceptive system.[38-41] Receptors abound on the skin, tendons, ligaments, capsules, and bones, and transmitters permeate the peripheral nerves and the spinal cord tracts. Input travels up to the modulators through the spinal cord itself; it terminates in the cortical areas of the brain, where it is analyzed and stored. Output goes from the central nervous system back to the muscles, tendons, bones, joints, and skin through a system of neurotransmitters and via the intricate neuronal anatomy.[42]

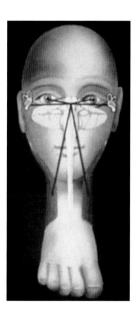

Fig. 1-1 Sensory inputs and oculo-motor control. (Courtesy of Patrice Tran Ba Huy, MD.)

It is interesting to examine how the central nervous system handles all of these different inputs and integrates them for self-orientation. In 2000 Jeka et al[43] discussed the concept of a *sensory fusion process.* This involves three behavioral categories that result from combining different sensory signals in the nervous system: (1) enhancement, (2) degradation, and (3) averaging. When signals from different sensory sources share the same spatial and temporal characteristics, the combination of the signals enhances the behavioral response. When one source is different from the others, its gain decreases through the process of degradation. When all sources show different spatial and temporal characteristics, averaging is the behavioral result of the multisensory integration that the nervous system uses to deal with discrepant sensory signals by creating equality among the sensory inputs.

In 2006 Maurer et al[44] proposed the concept of *sensory reweighting effects,* which suggests that the combination of simple sensory summations and detection thresholds results in a sensory reweighting that is related to the amplitudes, frequencies, and conditions of various stimuli. By means of this multisensory control of posture, the whole body interacts with the environment in a complex and dynamic way to maintain an erect posture with the head over the pelvis.

ALIGNMENT

In an attempt to bridge the gap between balance and alignment, several authors have investigated the combination of force plate and radiographic data.[45-47] In 2006 Schwab et al[48] published the first study of age-related changes in alignment parameters along with the investigation of the gravity line location. This study revealed a significant posterior pelvic shift in relation to the feet with advancing age. These findings supported the cone of economy concept, which assumes that the pelvis is a crucial regulator of sagittal alignment.

Alignment is related to the relative disposition of the body segments. In the static condition, full-length 36-inch radiography cassettes are the most common items used to quantify alignment. Sagittal spinopelvic alignment is now recognized as a key element of patient assessment. The chain of correlation from the head to the feet has been established,[49] thereby bringing to light the necessity of dissociate parameters intrinsic to pathology that result from compensatory mechanisms. More recently, correlations between sagittal alignment parameters and patient-reported outcomes have demonstrated the clinical relevance of sagittal malalignment.[50-56] The key concepts of spinopelvic alignment are detailed later in this book.

BALANCE, ALIGNMENT, AND PATIENT EVALUATION

As described previously, balance depends on numerous factors, including the vestibular, ocular, proprioceptive, and cerebral systems; sagittal alignment is related to the relative location of anatomic structures at a given point in time. Although they are different, these two concepts reflect a similar goal of stability.

In the context of surgical procedures, alignment alone is not sufficient to achieve balance. Ignoring the reality of balance's multiple mechanisms can lead to disappointing functional results despite apparent excellent realignment after surgery. Preoperative planning relies mostly on static radiographs, which do not show a patient's capacity to compensate passively. Ideal preoperative assessment should involve a thorough examination of alignment and balance conjointly.

From a theoretical point of view, this exercise requires a combination of motion analysis, full-body radiographic evaluation[57] (with the EOS 2D/3D imaging), force plate acquisition, and of course a neurosensorial evaluation that includes inputs, integration, modulation, and cognition.

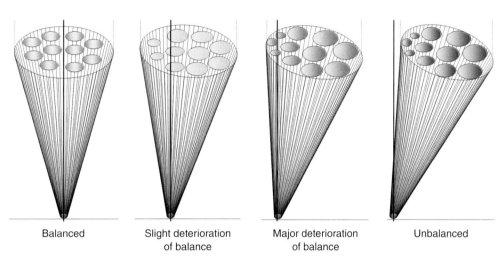

| Balanced | Slight deterioration of balance | Major deterioration of balance | Unbalanced |

Fig. 1-2 Progressive three-dimensional loss of balance with an associated increase in energy expenditure.

This multidisciplinary approach can provide pertinent findings related to the posture and mobility of the spinal segments, the pelvis, and the lower limbs. Such an effort will confirm the predominant roles of the pelvis and lower limbs as compensatory mechanisms. Longitudinal evaluation of the three-dimensional cone of balance with regard to age-related changes could provide an indication of the optimal time for correction before deterioration reaches a point of no return (Fig. 1-2). Unfortunately, sophisticated laboratory tools have limited use in the regular clinical setting, and objective, simple, and reproducible functional measurements are needed.

From a pragmatic point of view, this can be achieved in the clinical setting with the use of a chronometer by compiling the outcomes of the following four simple tests:
1. Speed and ease of rising from a seated position, walking 5 feet forward and backward, and then returning to a seated position
2. Speed and ease of climbing up and down three stairs
3. Speed and ease of squatting up and down (probably the most discriminate test but not always possible for elderly people)
4. Speed and ease of walking while speaking on the telephone (double task)

CONCLUSION

Alignment and balance are not interchangeable terms, but they are also not opposites. In fact, they are complementary components of the upright posture of humans. Alignment must be assessed in three dimensions and from head to foot to encompass the entire chain of segments. Good alignment is preferable to obtain good balance, but it alone is not sufficient. It is necessary to have sufficient amplitude of passive joint motion, especially as it applies to compensation and the acceptable neurologic loop of perception, integration, modulation, action, and cognition. The problem of balance deterioration with aging in the normal population is an important one for society; this concern is one of the key objectives tackled by both the Balance Research Foundation *(www.balancefoundation.org),* and the French Academy of Medicine *(www.academie-medecine.fr).* This research will hopefully allow us, as a scientific community, to prevent and treat the failure of balance associated with aging.

REFERENCES

1. Dubousset J. Three-dimensional analysis of the scoliotic deformity. In Weinstein S, ed. The Pediatric Spine: Principles and Practices. New York: Raven Press, 1994.
2. Johanson D, Taieb M. Plio-Pleistocene hominid discoveries in Hadar, Ethiopia. Nature 260:293-297, 1976.
3. White T, Suwa G, Asfaw B. Australopithecus ramidus, a new species of early hominid from Aramis, Ethiopia. Nature 375:88, 1995.
4. Senut B, Pickford M, Gommery D, et al. First hominid from the Miocene (Lukeino Formation, Kenya). Comptes Rendus de l'Académie des Sciences–Series IIA. Earth Planet Sci 332:137-144, 2001.
5. Brunet M, Guy F, Pilbeam D, et al. A new hominid from the Upper Miocene of Chad, Central Africa. Nature 418:145-151, 2002.
6. Haile-Selassie Y, Saylor BZ, Deino A, et al. A new hominin foot from Ethiopia shows multiple Pliocene bipedal adaptations. Nature 483:565-569, 2012.
7. Schmitt D. Insights into the evolution of human bipedalism from experimental studies of humans and other primates. J Exp Biol 206:1437-1448, 2003.
8. Berge C. Heterochronic processes in human evolution: an ontogenetic analysis of the hominid pelvis. Am J Phys Anthropol 105:441-459, 1998.
9. Lovejoy CO. The origin of man. Science 211:341-350, 1981.
10. Richmond BG, Begun DR, Strait DS. Origin of human bipedalism: the knuckle-walking hypothesis revisited. Am J Phys Anthropol 105:70-105, 2001.
11. Lovejoy CO. The natural history of human gait and posture. Part 3. The knee. Gait Posture 25:325-341, 2007.
12. Lovejoy CO. The natural history of human gait and posture. Part 2. Hip and thigh. Gait Posture 21:113-124, 2005.
13. Lovejoy CO. The natural history of human gait and posture. Part 1. Spine and pelvis. Gait Posture 21:95-112, 2005.
14. Le Huec JC, Aunoble S, Philippe L, et al. Pelvic parameters: origin and significance. Eur Spine J 20(Suppl 5):564-571, 2011.
15. O'Connell CA, DeSilva JM. Mojokerto revisited: evidence for an intermediate pattern of brain growth in Homo erectus. J Hum Evol 65:156-161, 2013.
16. Malina RM. Biosocial correlates of motor development during infancy and early childhood. In Greene LS, Johnston FE, eds. Social and Biological Predictors of Nutritional Status, Physical Growth, and Neurological Development. New York: Academic Press, 1980.
17. Massion J. Postural changes accompanying voluntary movements. Normal and pathological aspects. Hum Neurobiol 2:261-267, 1984.
18. Assaiante C, Amblard B. An ontogenetic model for the sensorimotor organization of balance control in humans. Hum Move Sci 14:13-43, 1995.
19. Assaiante C, Chabrol B. [Developmental and locomotor disorders in children] Rev Neurol 166:149-157, 2010.
20. Nashner LM, McCollum G. The organization of human postural movements: a formal basis and experimental synthesis. Behav Brain Sci 8:135-150, 1985.
21. Horak FB, Nashner LM. Central programming of postural movements: adaptation to altered support-surface configurations. J Neurophysiol 55:1369-1381, 1986.
22. Rietdyk S, Patla AE, Winter D, et al. NACOB presentation CSB New Investigator Award. Balance recovery from medio-lateral perturbations of the upper body during standing. North American Congress on Biomechanics. J Biomech 32:1149-1158, 1999.
23. de Lamarck JB. [Philosophie zoologique: ou exposition des considérations relatives à l'histoire naturelle des animaux] Paris: Dentu et L'Auteur, 1809.
24. Mangione P, Gomez D, Senegas J. Study of the course of the incidence angle during growth. Eur Spine J 6:163-167, 1997.
25. Tardieu C, Bonneau N, Hecquet J, et al. How is sagittal balance acquired during bipedal gait acquisition? Comparison of neonatal and adult pelves in three dimensions. Evolutionary implications. J Hum Evol 65:209-222, 2013.
26. Been E, Gómez-Olivencia A, Kramer PA. Lumbar lordosis of extinct hominins. Am J Phys Anthropol 147:64-77, 2012.
27. Soechting JF, Berthoz A. Dynamic role of vision in the control of posture in man. Exp Brain Res 36:551-561, 1979.
28. Jeka JJ, Lackner JR. Fingertip contact influences human postural control. Exp Brain Res 100:495-502, 1994.
29. Clapp S, Wing AM. Light touch contribution to balance in normal bipedal stance. Exp Brain Res 125:521-524, 1999.

30. Riley MA, Wong S, Mitra S, et al. Common effects of touch and vision on postural parameters. Exp Brain Res 117:165-170, 1997.
31. Rogers MW, Wardman DL, Lord SR, et al. Passive tactile sensory input improves stability during standing. Exp Brain Res 136:514-522, 2001.
32. Horak FB, Shupert CL, Dietz V, et al. Vestibular and somatosensory contributions to responses to head and body displacements in stance. Exp Brain Res 100:93-106, 1994.
33. Kushiro K, Bai R, Kitajima N, et al. Properties and axonal trajectories of posterior semicircular canal nerve-activated vestibulospinal neurons. Exp Brain Res 191:257-264, 2008.
34. Patla AE, Prentice SD, Robinson C, et al. Visual control of locomotion: strategies for changing direction and for going over obstacles. J Exp Psychol Hum Percept Perform 17:603-634, 1991.
35. Patla AE, Vickers JN. How far ahead do we look when required to step on specific locations in the travel path during locomotion? Exp Brain Res 148:133-138, 2003.
36. Stein B, Meredith M. The Merging of the Senses. Representation of the sensory space in the superior colliculus. Cambridge, MA: MIT Press, 1993.
37. Patla AE. Understanding the roles of vision in the control of human locomotion. Gait Posture 5:54-69, 1997.
38. Jola C, Davis A, Haggard P. Proprioceptive integration and body representation: insights into dancers' expertise. Exp Brain Res 213:257-265, 2011.
39. Ferrell WR, Smith A. Position sense at the proximal interphalangeal joint of the human index finger. J Physiol 399:49-61, 1988.
40. Pleger B, Villringer A. The human somatosensory system: from perception to decision making. Prog Neurobiol 103:76-97, 2013.
41. Vaitl D, Mittelstaedt H, Saborowski R, et al. Shifts in blood volume alter the perception of posture: further evidence for somatic graviception. Int J Psychophysiol 44:1-11, 2002.
42. Saint-Côme C, Acker GR, Strand FL. Peptide influences on the development and regeneration of motor performance. Peptides 3:439-449, 1982.
43. Jeka J, Oie KS, Kiemel T. Multisensory information for human postural control: integrating touch and vision. Exp Brain Res 134:107-125, 2000.
44. Maurer C, Mergner T, Peterka RJ. Multisensory control of human upright stance. Exp Brain Res 171:231-250, 2006.
45. Vaz G, Roussouly P, Berthonnaud E, et al. Sagittal morphology and equilibrium of pelvis and spine. Eur Spine J 11:80-87, 2001.
46. Gangnet N, Pomero V, Dumas R, et al. Variability of the spine and pelvis location with respect to the gravity line: a three-dimensional stereoradiographic study using a force platform. Surg Radiol Anat 25:424-433, 2003.
47. El Fegoun AB, Schwab F, Gamez L, et al. Center of gravity and radiographic posture analysis: a preliminary review of adult volunteers and adult patients affected by scoliosis. Spine 30:1535-1540, 2005.
48. Schwab F, Lafage V, Boyce R, et al. Gravity line analysis in adult volunteers: age-related correlation with spinal parameters, pelvic parameters, and foot position. Spine 31:E959-E967, 2006.
49. Ames CP, Blondel B, Scheer JK, et al. Cervical radiographical alignment: comprehensive assessment techniques and potential importance in cervical myelopathy. Spine 38(22 Suppl 1):S149-S160, 2013.
50. Lafage V, Schwab F, Patel A, et al. Pelvic tilt and truncal inclination: two key radiographic parameters in the setting of adults with spinal deformity. Spine 34:E599-E606, 2009.
51. Djurasovic M, Glassman SD. Correlation of radiographic and clinical findings in spinal deformities. Neurosurg Clin North Am 18:223-227, 2007.
52. Glassman SD, Berven S, Bridwell K, et al. Correlation of radiographic parameters and clinical symptoms in adult scoliosis. Spine 30:682-688, 2005.
53. Glassman SD, Bridwell K, Dimar JR, et al. The impact of positive sagittal balance in adult spinal deformity. Spine 30:2024-2029, 2005.
54. Jackson RP, Simmons EH, Stripinis D. Coronal and sagittal plane spinal deformities correlating with back pain and pulmonary function in adult idiopathic scoliosis. Spine 14:1391-1397, 1989.
55. Schwab FJ, Blondel B, Bess S, et al. Radiographical spinopelvic parameters and disability in the setting of adult spinal deformity: a prospective multicenter analysis. Spine 38:E803-E812, 2013.
56. Schwab FJ, Smith VA, Biserni M, et al. Adult scoliosis: a quantitative radiographic and clinical analysis. Spine 27:387-392, 2002.
57. Dubousset J, Charpak G, Dorion I, et al. [A new 2D and 3D imaging approach to musculoskeletal physiology and pathology with low-dose radiation and the standing position: the EOS system] Bull Acad Natl Med 189:287-297; discussion 297-300, 2005.

2

Spinal Anatomy and Parameters of Normal Spinal Alignment: Stratification by Age

Charles Kuntz IV

Neutral upright spinal alignment (NUSA) in asymptomatic individuals is defined as a position that involves standing with the knees and hips comfortably extended, the shoulders neutral or flexed, the neck neutral, and the gaze horizontal. The ability to maintain NUSA is intrinsic to the human condition, because the species is in part defined by its ability to comfortably stand in a neutral upright position for long periods of time. Many spinal procedures are performed to return the patient to asymptomatic NUSA.

Despite wide variations in the "normal" regional spinal alignment of asymptomatic individuals, global NUSA from the occiput to the pelvis in asymptomatic individuals is maintained in a relatively narrow range to preserve a horizontal gaze and the balance of the spine over the pelvis and femoral heads. As alignment changes in one region of the spine in asymptomatic individuals, compensatory changes occur in adjacent regional axial skeletal alignment to maintain global spinal alignment. In the coronal plane, the pelvis is relatively fixed so that as regional spinal scoliosis develops, compensatory scoliotic curves (rotations in the opposite direction) develop above and below the main scoliosis to maintain neutral coronal global spinal alignment (Figs. 2-1 and 2-2 and Table 2-1).

In the sagittal plane, the pelvis may rotate on the femoral heads so that as regional spinal kyphosis develops, the pelvis rotates posteriorly on the femoral heads, and compensatory lordotic spinal changes develop above and below the main kyphosis to maintain neutral sagittal global spinal alignment. Also in the sagittal plane, as regional spinal lordosis develops, the pelvis may rotate anteriorly on the femoral heads, and compensatory kyphotic spinal changes may develop above and below the main lordosis to maintain neutral global spinal alignment (Figs. 2-3 and 2-4 and Table 2-2).

The human spine is a complex organ that has four major functions: (1) to support the head, the upper extremities, and the torso, (2) to protect the spinal cord and the nerve roots, (3) to control complex axial skeletal movements, and (4) to transmit the body's weight to the hips by articulating with the pelvis. In asymptomatic adults and in patients standing in a neutral upright position, the spine and pelvis maintain comfortable rotational alignment in such a way that despite the wide variation in "normal" regional spinal curves, global spinal alignment is maintained in a narrower range to preserve a horizontal gaze and the balance of the spine over the pelvis and the femoral heads.

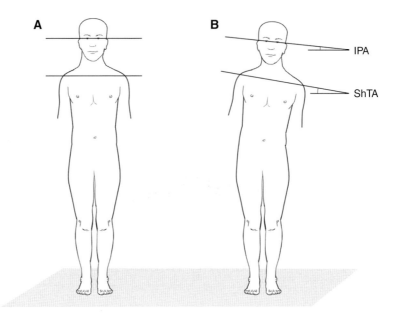

Fig. 2-1 The clinical measurement of the interpupillary angle *(IPA)* and the shoulder tilt angle *(ShTA)*. **A,** Normal IPA and ShTA. **B,** IPA and ShTA with a coronal plane deformity. (With permission from the Mayfield Clinic.)

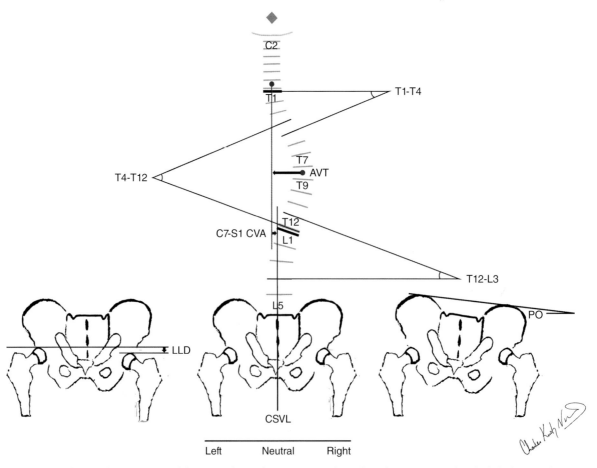

Fig. 2-2 AP radiographic imaging of the spine from the occiput to the pelvis shows regional and global neutral upright coronal spinal alignment. Radiographic coronal spinal angles and displacements from the occiput to the pelvis are depicted. (With permission from the Mayfield Clinic.)

Table 2-1   CKIV Neutral Upright Coronal Spinal Alignment Guide: Asymptomatic Individuals

	Mean Neutral Values (1 SD)		
	Adolescent (10 to 18 years old)	Adult (>18 years old)	Geriatric (>60 years old)
Regional Spinal Alignment (degrees)			
Occipitocervical junction angle O-C2 apex		—	
Cervical angle C2-3 disc to C6-7 disc apex		—	
Cervicothoracic junction angles C7-T1 apex		—	
Proximal thoracic angle T1-2 disc to T5 apex	<15*	<20*	<25-30*
Main thoracic angle T5-6 disc to T11-12 disc apex	<15*	<20*	<25-30
Thoracolumbar angle T12-L1 apex	<15*	<20*	<25-30
Lumbar angle L1-2 disc to L4-5 disc apex	<15*	<20*	<25-30
Lumbosacral junction angle L5-S1 apex		—	
Shoulder tilt angle (ShTA)		1 (2)	
Angle of trunk inclination (ATI)		—	
Apical vertebral translation (AVT) (mm)		—	
Apical vertebral rotation (AVR)		<5-10*	
Pelvic Alignment			
Pelvic obliquity (PO) angle (ShTA)		<8*	
Leg-length discrepancy (LLD) (mm)		6 (4)	
Global Spinal Alignment			
Head tilt angle (degrees) Interpupillary angle (IPA)		0 (1)	
Coronal spinal balance (mm) Thoracic trunk to S1 coronal vertical axis (CVA)		—	
C7-S1 coronal vertical axis (CVA)		+4 (12)	

With permission from the Mayfield Clinic.
Pooled estimates of the mean and variances of the neutral upright coronal spinal angles and displacements from the occiput to the pelvis. Assuming a normal distribution for coronal spinal angles and displacements in the population, the mean ± 1 SD includes approximately 68% of the population, the mean ± 2 SD includes approximately 95% of the population, and the mean ± 2.5 SD includes approximately 98.5% of the population. For empty data cells, there were few or no reproducible data.[1,2]
*Approximately 98.5% of asymptomatic individuals have coronal curves that are smaller than the estimated angle.

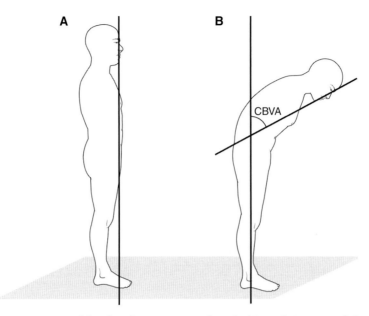

Fig. 2-3   The clinical measurement of the chin-brow to vertical angle *(CBVA)*. **A,** Normal CBVA. **B,** CBVA with a sagittal plane deformity. (With permission from the Mayfield Clinic.)

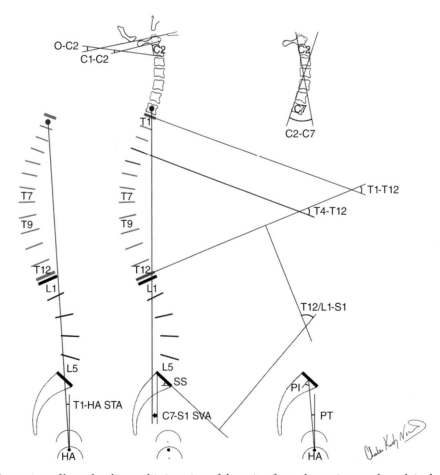

Fig. 2-4   This illustration of lateral radiographic imaging of the spine from the occiput to the pelvis shows regional and global neutral upright sagittal spinal alignment. Radiographic sagittal spinal angles and displacements from the occiput to the pelvis are depicted. (With permission from the Mayfield Clinic.)

Table 2-2 CKIV Neutral Upright Sagittal Spinal Alignment Guide: Asymptomatic Individuals

	Mean Neutral Values (1 SD)		
	Adolescent (10 to 18 years old)	**Adult** (>18 years old)	**Geriatric** (>60 years old)
Regional Spinal Alignment (degrees)			
Occipitocervical junction angles			
O-C2	−17 (9)	−14 (7)	−12 (6)
C1-2	−28 (9)	−29 (7)	−26 (8)
Cervical lordosis			
C2-7	−12 (11)	−17 (14)	−20 (13)
Cervicothoracic junction angles			
C6-T2		—	
Total thoracic kyphosis			
T1-12		+45 (10)	+53 (12)
Proximal thoracic kyphosis			
T1-5		+14 (8)	+15 (8)
Main thoracic kyphosis			
T4-12	+38(10)	+41 (11)	+49 (14)
Thoracolumbar junction angle			
T10-L2	+3 (10)	+6 (8)	
Total lumbosacral lordosis			
T12/L1-S1	−61 (11)	−62 (11)	−60 (14)
Lumbar lordosis			
L1-5		−44 (11)	
Lumbosacral junction angles			
L4-S1		—	
L4-5	−18 (6)	−17 (5)	−18 (9)
L5-S1	−25 (6)	−24 (6)	−23 (9)
Pelvic alignment			
Pelvic incidence (PI)	+49 (11)	+54 (10)	+60 (15)
Pelvic tilt (PT)	+8 (8)	+13 (6)	+18 (9)
Sacral slope (SS)	+41 (8)	+41 (8)	+42 (10)
Global Spinal Alignment			
Chin-brow to vertical angle			
CBVA		−1 (3)	
Sagittal spinal balance			
C7-S1 sagittal vertical axis (SVA) (mm)	−5 (42)	0 (24)	+40 (37)
T1 to hip axis sagittal tilt angle (STA)		−1 (3)	
T9 to hip axis sagittal tilt angle (STA)		−11 (3)	

With permission from the Mayfield Clinic.
Pooled estimates of the mean and variances of the neutral upright sagittal spinal angles and displacements from the occiput to the pelvis. Assuming a normal distribution for sagittal spinal angles and displacements in the population, the mean ± 1 SD includes approximately 68% of the population, the mean ± 2 SD includes approximately 95% of the population, and the mean ± 2.5 SD includes approximately 98.5% of the population. For empty data cells, there were few or no reproducible data.[1,2]

The spine is composed of regions with distinct alignment and biomechanical properties that contribute to global alignment. Because the treatment of many patients with spinal disorders is directed at restoration of normal alignment, spinal deformity needs to be defined in relation to NUSA in asymptomatic individuals. The analysis of spinal alignment involves both clinical and radiographic evaluation. Although there are myriad angles and displacements for the measurement of spinal alignment, the analysis presented in this chapter will offer a systematic approach to analyzing regional and global spinal alignment from the occiput to the pelvis.

As evidenced by the literature and my own experience, it is important to recognize four critical components when treating spinal alignment problems:
- Achieving satisfactory neural element decompression
- Maintaining or restoring global spinal alignment to neutral
- Maintaining or restoring pelvic alignment to neutral
- Maintaining or restoring regional spinal alignment to neutral

CLINICAL AND RADIOGRAPHIC EVALUATION OF SPINAL ALIGNMENT

For the evaluation of a spinal deformity, the following measurements and imaging studies are essential:
- Clinical measurements are performed and facilitated with photographs with the patient in a neutral upright position (standing with the knees and hips comfortably extended and the shoulders and neck neutral) and then in a forward-bending position (standing with the feet together, the knees comfortably extended, the hips and spine flexed, and the arms dependent, with the fingers and palms opposed).
- Occipitocervical and cervical angles and displacements are measured using standard standing AP and lateral cervical spine radiographs, with the patient in a neutral upright position (standing with the knees and hips comfortably extended and the shoulders and neck neutral).
- Thoracic, lumbar, sacral, and pelvic angles and displacements, including spinal balance, are measured with standard standing AP and lateral long cassette radiographs that show the patient in a neutral upright standing position (standing with the knees and hips comfortably extended, the shoulders neutral or flexed [flexed for lateral radiographs], and the neck neutral).
- Side-bending (supine) and flexion-extension (standing) radiographs are obtained when appropriate for the evaluation of the flexibility of a deformity curve.

All upright imaging is performed while the patient is barefoot. For patients with increased or decreased numbers of thoracic or lumbar vertebrae, the anomalous vertebrae are included in the appropriate alignment and biomechanical zones. Leg-length discrepancy of less than 2 cm is ignored unless it significantly contributes to the spinal deformity. When the leg-length discrepancy is more than 2 cm, an appropriately thick lift is placed under the shorter leg.

Coronal Alignment Angles and Displacements

By convention, coronal angles have a positive (+) value. Scoliotic curves are named for their convexity to the right or left. Coronal angulation of the head, shoulders, or pelvis is named for the elevated side: *right* indicates that the right side is up, and *left* means that the left side is up.

Regional Spinal Alignment

The shoulder tilt angle is defined as the angle subtended by a horizontal reference line and a line drawn through the right and left coracoid processes. Trunk asymmetry (distortion of the torso) is measured using a scoliometer, with the patient in a forward-bend position (standing with the feet together, the knees comfortably extended, the hips and spine flexed, and the arms dependent, with the fingers and palms opposed). The angle of trunk inclination is the angle created between a horizontal reference line and the plane across the back at the greatest elevation of a rib or lumbar prominence. In contrast with radiographic measurements, the shoulder tilt angle and the angle of trunk inclination are clinical measurements of the effects of a regional spinal deformity on trunk symmetry.

Occipitocervical (O-C2) curves are defined as having an apex from the occiput to C2; a coronal occipital reference line and the caudal end vertebra are defined for the measurement of the Cobb angle.[3] Cervical coronal curves are defined as having an apex from the C2-3 disc to the C6-7 disc and measured by the Cobb method from the end vertebrae.[3] The cervicothoracic junction angles are defined from C7 to T1. Cervicothoracic coronal curves are defined as having an apex from C7 to T1 and measured by the Cobb method from the end vertebrae.[3]

Proximal thoracic (T1-2 to T5), main thoracic (T5-6 to T11-12), thoracolumbar (T12-L1), lumbar (L1-2 to L4-5), and lumbosacral (L5-S1) coronal curves are defined as having an apex in the above regions or zones and measured by the Cobb method from the end vertebrae.[3] The end vertebrae for all coronal curves are defined as the most cephalad and caudad vertebrae that maximally tilt into the concavity of the curve. The end vertebrae define the ends of the scoliotic curve. The cephalad end vertebra is the first vertebra in the cephalad direction from a curve apex with a *superior* surface that is tilted maximally toward the concavity of the curve. The caudad end vertebra is the first vertebra in the caudad direction from a curve apex with an *inferior* surface that is tilted maximally toward the concavity of the curve. The apical vertebra or disc of a curve is defined as the most horizontal and laterally deviated vertebra or disc of the curve.[4] Apical vertebral translation is defined as the horizontal distance measured from the C7 plumb line to the center of the apical vertebral body or disc for proximal thoracic and main thoracic curves and from the central sacral vertical line (CSVL) to the center of the apical vertebral body or disc for thoracolumbar and lumbar curves.[4] The CSVL is defined as a vertical reference line drawn through the center of the S1 endplate. Apical vertebral rotation is defined by the Nash-Moe classification system.[4,5] Because apical vertebral rotation is determined with the use of AP radiographs, it is included with the coronal alignment. Lateral olisthesis is defined by using a modified Meyerding classification system.[4,6] For lumbosacral coronal curves, the apical vertebra or disc is defined from L5 to S1; the cephalad end vertebra and a horizontal reference line are defined for the measurement of the Cobb angle.[3] (With radiographs that show the patient in a supine, side-bending position, the horizontal reference line may be reconstructed from the standing radiographs.)

Pelvic Alignment

Pelvic alignment and morphology are defined by the pelvic obliquity and the leg-length discrepancy. Pelvic obliquity is defined most frequently as the angle subtended by a horizontal reference line and a line drawn tangential to the top of the crests of the ilium or the base of the sulci of the S1 ala. Pelvic obliquity may result from an intrinsic sacropelvic deformity, a leg-length discrepancy, or a combination of both. Leg-length discrepancy is defined as the vertical distance measured between horizontal lines drawn tangential to the top of the right and left femoral heads.

Global Spinal Alignment

Head tilt is defined by the interpupillary angle, which is defined as the angle subtended by a horizontal reference line and the interpupillary line. The interpupillary line is defined by a line drawn though the center of the right and left pupils. In contrast with radiographic measurements, the interpupillary angle is a clinical measurement of the total coronal deformity of the spine and its effect on the horizontal gaze.

Coronal spinal balance is defined from the center of C7 and the midpoint of the thoracic trunk to the sacrum. The C7-S1 coronal vertical axis (CVA) is defined as the horizontal distance from a vertical plumb line centered in the middle of the C7 vertebral body to the CSVL. The C7-S1 CVA has a (+) value when the vertical plumb line is to the right of the CSVL and a (−) value when the vertical plumb line is to the left of the CSVL. The CVA of the thoracic trunk to S1 (TT-S1 CVA) is defined as the horizontal distance measured from a vertical plumb line centered at the midpoint of the thorax to the CSVL; this is also known as the *thoracic trunk shift*. The TT-S1 CVA is measured at the midpoint between the rib cage on the left and the rib cage on the right at the level of the main thoracic apical vertebra; if there is no main thoracic apical vertebra, then the TT-S1 CVA is measured at the level of T9. The TT-S1 CVA has a (+) value when the vertical plumb line is to the right of the CSVL and a (−) value when the vertical plumb line is to the left of the CSVL.

Sagittal Alignment Angles and Displacements

By convention, kyphosis has a (+) value, and lordosis has a (−) value.

Regional Spinal Alignment

Occipitocervical junction angles are defined from the occiput to C2. The O-C2 angle is defined as the angle subtended by the McGregor line and a line drawn parallel to the inferior endplate of C2. The McGregor line is drawn from the posterosuperior aspect of the hard palate to the most caudal point on the midline of the occipital curve.[7] The C1-2 angle is defined as the angle subtended by a line drawn parallel to the inferior aspect of C1 and a line drawn parallel to the inferior endplate of C2.

Cervical lordosis angles are defined from C2 to C7. The C2-7 angle is defined as the angle subtended by a line drawn parallel to the posterior border of the C2 vertebral body and a line drawn parallel to the posterior border of the C7 vertebral body. Cervicothoracic junction angles are defined from C6 to T2 and measured by the Cobb method.[3] The C6-T2 angle is measured from the superior endplate of C6 to the inferior endplate of T2.

Thoracic kyphosis angles are defined from T1 to T12 and measured using the Cobb method.[3] Total thoracic kyphosis is measured from the superior endplate of T1 to the inferior endplate of T12. The proximal thoracic kyphosis is measured from the superior endplate of T1 to the inferior endplate of T5. The main thoracic kyphosis is measured from the superior endplate of T4 to the inferior endplate of T12. Thoracolumbar junction angles are defined from T10 to L2 and measured with the Cobb method.[3] The T10-L2 angle is measured from the superior endplate of T10 to the inferior endplate of L2.

Lumbosacral lordosis angles are defined from T12-L1 to S1 and measured using the Cobb method.[3] Total lumbosacral lordosis is measured from either the inferior endplate of T12 or the superior endplate of L1 to the superior endplate of S1. Lumbar lordosis is measured from the superior endplate of L1 to the inferior endplate of L5. Lumbosacral junctional angles are measured from L4 to S1 and measured with the Cobb method.[3] The L4-S1 angle is measured from the superior endplate of L4 to the superior endplate of S1. The L4-5 angle is measured from the superior endplate of L4 to the superior endplate of L5. The L5-S1 angle is measured from the superior endplate of L5 to the superior endplate of S1. Anterior and posterior olistheses are defined by using a modified Meyerding classification system.[4,6]

Pelvic Alignment

Pelvic morphology and rotation are defined by the pelvic incidence (PI), the pelvic tilt (PT), and the sacral slope (SS). The PI is a constant value that is unaffected by body posture, and it is defined as an angle subtended by a line drawn from the hip axis to the midpoint of the sacral endplate and a line perpendicular to the center of the sacral endplate.[8] The hip axis (HA) is defined as the midpoint between the approximate centers of both femoral heads. As the PI increases, lumbosacral lordosis must increase to maintain balanced sagittal global spinal alignment. In contrast with the PI, the SS and the PT are posturally dependent values that change with the rotation of the pelvis on the HA. The SS is defined as the angle subtended by a horizontal reference line and the sacral endplate. The PT is defined as the angle subtended by a vertical reference line through the HA and a line drawn from the midpoint of the sacral endplate to the HA. The PT has a ($+$) value when the midpoint of the sacrum is posterior to the vertical reference line and a ($-$) value when the midpoint of the sacrum is anterior to the vertical reference line. Geometrically these pelvic angles produce the following equation: $PI = SS + PT$.[8] The pelvis rotates on the HA to help maintain balanced sagittal global spinal alignment.

Global Spinal Alignment

The chin-brow to vertical angle is defined as the angle subtended by a vertical reference line and a line drawn parallel to the chin and the brow, with the neck in a neutral or fixed position and the knees and hips extended. In contrast with the radiographic measurements, the chin-brow to vertical angle is a clinical measurement of the total sagittal deformity of the spine and its effect on the horizontal gaze.

Sagittal spinal balance is defined from C7, T1, and T9 to the sacrum or the HA. The C7-S1 sagittal vertical axis is defined as the horizontal distance measured from a vertical plumb line centered in the middle of the C7 vertebral body to the posterosuperior corner of the S1 endplate. The C7-S1 sagittal vertical axis has a ($+$) value when the vertical plumb line is anterior to the sacral reference point and a ($-$) value when the vertical plumb line is posterior to the sacral reference point. The T1-HA sagittal tilt angle (STA) is defined as the angle subtended by a vertical reference line through the HA and a line drawn from the midpoint of the T1 vertebral body to the HA. The T9-HA STA is defined as the angle subtended by a vertical reference line through the HA and a line drawn from the midpoint of the T9 vertebral body to the HA. The T1-HA STA and the T9-HA STA have ($+$) values when the T1 or T9 midpoint is anterior to the HA vertical reference line and ($-$) values when the T1 or T9 midpoint is posterior to the HA vertical reference line.

CONCLUSION

The spine needs to be evaluated in its entirety from the occiput to the pelvis before a treatment plan can be formulated. The axial skeleton is composed of spinal regions with distinct alignment and biomechanical properties that contribute to global spinal alignment. Although regional curves vary widely from the occiput to the pelvis in asymptomatic individuals, global spinal alignment is maintained in a much narrower range for the maintenance of the horizontal gaze and for the balance of the spine over the pelvis and the femoral heads. Spinal deformity is defined as a deviation from normal spinal alignment. The four critical components for the correction of spinal alignment problems are as follows:
- Satisfactory neural element decompression
- Maintenance or restoration of global spinal alignment to neutral
- Maintenance or restoration of pelvic alignment to neutral
- Maintenance or restoration of regional spinal alignment to neutral

REFERENCES

1. Kuntz C, Levin LS, Ondra SL, et al. Neutral upright sagittal spinal alignment from the occiput to the pelvis in asymptomatic adults: a review and resynthesis of the literature. J Neurosurg Spine 6:104-112, 2007.
2. Kuntz C, Shaffrey CI, Ondra SL, et al. Spinal deformity: a new classification derived from neutral upright spinal alignment measurements in asymptomatic juvenile, adolescent, adult, and geriatric individuals. Neurosurgery 63:25-39, 2008.
3. Cobb JR. Outline for the study of scoliosis. In Edwards JW, ed. Instructional Course Lectures. Ann Arbor: American Academy of Orthopaedic Surgeons, 1948.
4. O'Brien MF, Kuklo TR, Blanke KM, et al. Radiographic Measurement Manual. Memphis: Medtronic Sofamor Danek, 2004.
5. Nash CL, Moe JH. A study of vertebral rotation. J Bone Joint Surg Am 51:223-229, 1969.
6. Meyerding HW. Spondylolisthesis. J Bone Joint Surg Am 13:39-48, 1931.
7. McGregor M. The significance of certain measurements of the skull in the diagnosis of basilar impression. Br J Radiol 21:171-181, 1948.
8. Legaye J, Duval-Beaupere G, Hecquet J, et al. Pelvic incidence: a fundamental pelvic parameter for three-dimensional regulation of spinal sagittal curves. Eur Spine J 7:99-103, 1998.

3

Radiographic Evaluation of Spinal Alignment

Taemin Oh ▪ *Justin K. Scheer* ▪ *Virginie Lafage*
Themistocles S. Protopsaltis ▪ *Christopher P. Ames*

The term *adult spinal deformity* (ASD) encompasses a broad range of pathologies that result in axial, coronal, or sagittal malalignment of the spine. ASD can be derived from an idiopathic, degenerative, or iatrogenic etiology, and it is particularly prevalent in the elderly population. Clinically, patients with ASD face an increased risk for pain or disability; these conditions consequently impair patients' activities of daily living and diminish their health-related quality of life (HRQOL).[1,2]

Historically, the treatment of ASD has primarily focused on scoliosis correction and the prevention of scoliotic curve progression; however, sagittal plane deformities and global spinal alignment have been implicated in affecting patient outcomes such as pain and disability, and this has underscored the necessity of restoring spinal balance beyond the site of primary deformity. As a result, emphasis is now being placed on reestablishing physiologic lumbar lordosis (LL), thoracic kyphosis, and the C7 plumb line (sagittal vertical axis [SVA]). The spinopelvic relationship has also emerged as another important consideration. Given that the pelvis acts as an intercalary unit between the spine and the lower extremities,[3,4] the position of the pelvis plays a critical role in the maintenance of upright sitting and standing postures. Failure to account for pelvic alignment when treating ASD increases the risk for spinal malalignment, decompensation, and treatment failure.

Even fewer studies have directly evaluated cervical alignment and HRQOL or the influence of segmental, regional, and global balance on outcomes after cervical surgery. Malalignment of the cervical spine can be debilitating, and it may induce adverse effects on the overall functioning and HRQOL of the patient. The cervical spine plays a pivotal role in influencing subjacent global spinal alignment and pelvic tilt (PT) as compensatory changes occur to maintain the horizontal gaze. Currently the indications for surgery to correct cervical alignment are not well defined, and there is no set standard that addresses the amount of correction to be achieved. Classifications of cervical deformity have yet to be fully established, and treatment options need to be defined and clarified.

The proper management of ASD includes the clinical and radiographic evaluation of both preoperative spinal alignment and postoperative correction of malalignment. The recent implementation of normative radiographic parameters for the evaluation of spinal deformity has changed the diagnosis and surgical management of ASD. Quantitative markers for alignment have facilitated the critical appraisal of preoperative deformity and helped establish some of the thresholds for correction required to maintain proper standing balance and improve function. In clinical practice, these parameters have also been associated with outcomes such as disability,[5] pain,[6] and HRQOL.[5] The use of radiographic parameters has also helped to illustrate the dynamic reciprocal changes induced by deformity and deformity correction.[7]

Radiographic evaluation facilitates assessment and treatment planning. In this chapter, we will highlight the most relevant radiographic parameters and discuss their measurement and interpretation.

THE FUNDAMENTALS OF RADIOGRAPHIC EVALUATION OF THE SPINE

CONVENTIONAL RADIOGRAPHY

Conventional standing radiographs offer a first-line assessment of spinal deformity on multiple planes. The initial imaging workup involves posteroanterior (PA) and lateral long-cassette 36-inch standing radiographs to provide an overview of coronal and sagittal alignment, respectively. All patients should be instructed to face straight ahead (if PA; Fig. 3-1, *left*) or to the right (if lateral; Fig. 3-1, *right*) in relation to the radiographic film and to stand upright, with the feet placed at shoulder width and with full leg extension. Bending at the knees should be discouraged. The elbows should be flexed to 45 degrees, and patients should be asked to rest their fingertips on their clavicles to maximize visualization of the spinal deformity (see Fig. 3-1, *right*). To achieve proper magnification and minimize distortion, the ideal distance between the patient and the film is a minimum of 6 feet.[8,9] Visualization of the craniocervical junction and the femoral heads is required to facilitate the global assessment of the spine.

Standard conventions for assessing films are as follows. On a PA film, the patient's right corresponds to the right side of the image. On a lateral film, the patient is always facing toward the right side of the scan. Linear displacements to the right or left as visualized on the radiograph are noted as positive or negative displacement, respectively. Angular displacements are noted as positive or negative if they are clockwise (kyphosis) or counterclockwise (lordosis), respectively.[8] Additional scans (flexion, extension) can be requisitioned to assess the full magnitude and severity of the deformity, and standard 11 × 17-inch radiographs may offer a more focused view of specific regional deformity.[8]

Radiographs created when the patient is seated in a chair allow for the evaluation of spinal alignment when the spine is in a more relaxed position (Fig. 3-2). This technique may be used for patients with sagittal malalignment; patients with this condition compensate through pelvic retroversion and with thoracic hypokyphosis. Seated radiographs allow for the possible prediction of thoracic reciprocal change (relaxation of the thoracic hypokyphosis) after surgical correction of the sagittal malalignment.

THREE-DIMENSIONAL EOS IMAGING

As compared with standard radiographs, which provide single planar images, the EOS system is an imaging modality that offers a three-dimensional configuration of the spine by concurrently imaging the PA and lateral spine from the skull to the feet.[10] Patients enter the EOS imaging device, which is an enclosure that is 2.7 m tall with a base of 2 m². They can then be instructed to adopt a seated or weight-bearing standing stance as they would for standard radiography. One limitation of EOS imaging may be its longer acquisition time, which may result in movement artifacts generated by the patient; however, patients can be stabilized with the use of devices placed into the EOS system, or they can be instructed to stand against one of the walls of the EOS system if only a single plane of imaging is required. There are several potential benefits of this system: (1) the entire body can be imaged at once, thereby obviating the need for taking and joining multiple images, (2) images can be reformatted into three-dimensional configurations with semiautomatic contouring of the individual vertebrae, (3) the radiation dose that is delivered is lower by a factor of 10 than that associated with standard radiography, and (4) all points of alignment compensation are concurrently visualized.[11] Recently published studies have demonstrated that the results of the EOS system are highly accurate, reproducible, and precise for the measurement of spinal curvature and that the system itself can be reliably compared with computed tomography scanning.[12-15]

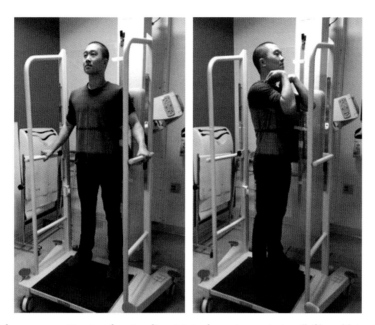

Fig. 3-1 Examples of proper positioning for standing 36-inch posteroanterior *(left)* and lateral *(right)* radiographs.

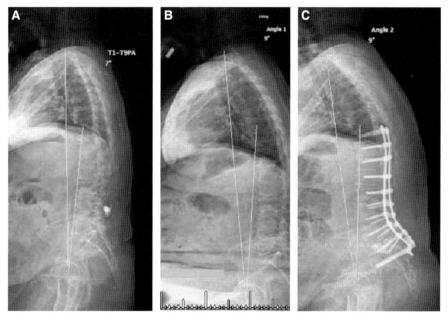

Fig. 3-2 Example of the use of seated radiographs for the radiographic evaluation of sagittal malalignment. Patients with sagittal malalignment compensate with pelvic retroversion and thoracic hypokyphosis. Seated radiographs allow for the possible prediction of thoracic reciprocal change (relaxation of the thoracic hypokyphosis) after surgical correction of the sagittal malalignment. **A,** Standing lateral 36-inch radiograph with the T1-9 pelvic angle measured at 7 degrees. **B,** Preoperative seated radiograph demonstrating relaxation of the thoracic hypokyphosis, with the T1-9 pelvic angle increased to 9 degrees. **C,** Postoperative standing lateral radiograph showing the T1-9 pelvic angle at 9 degrees.

RADIOGRAPHIC EVALUATION OF GLOBAL SPINE ALIGNMENT

CORONAL ALIGNMENT

The coronal alignment (CA) of the spine is determined with PA radiographs, and it is defined as the horizontal distance between a plumb line dropped from the C7 centroid and a plumb line dropped from the central sacral vertical line[16] (Fig. 3-3). Baseline values are set at zero to reflect the physiologic alignment of C7 vertically and centrally over the sacrum; this is also referred to as the *C7–central sacral vertical line offset*. Negative and positive values for CA represent left and right spinal malalignment, respectively. The postoperative goal for correction is to achieve an offset of less than 4 cm,[2] because coronal malalignment of more than 4 cm has been shown in some studies to be significantly associated with more pain and worse function.[17]

CORONAL AND SAGITTAL CURVATURE

The descriptive terms *coronal curvature* and *sagittal curvature* are used to identify the type of deformity present on imaging scans. Both curvatures are categorized according to the location of the curve's apex, which is the vertebral body or disc that demonstrates the greatest displacement from the midline with minimal angulation. For example, apices for thoracic, thoracolumbar, and lumbar deformities must occur between the T2 body and the T12 disc, between the T12 and L1 vertebral bodies, and at the level of or distal to the L1 body and the L2 disc, respectively. Patients with ASD can present with multiple curves, the largest of which is called the *main curve*. For patients with scoliosis, curves are additionally classified with respect to their convexity: a right convex curve represents dextroscoliosis, whereas a left convex curve represents levoscoliosis.[8,9]

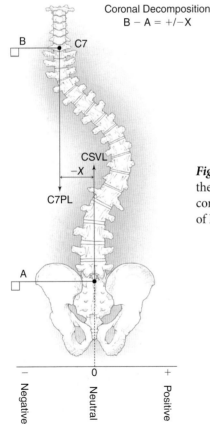

Fig. 3-3   The distance between the C7 plumb line *(C7PL)* and the central sacral vertical line *(CSVL)* defines the amount of coronal plane decompensation in centimeters *(−X)*. (Courtesy of K.X. Probst/Xavier Studio, 2012; with permission.)

SAGITTAL VERTICAL AXIS

The SVA is a measure of global spinal alignment in the sagittal plane. The SVA can be measured as the distance from either the C2 (C2 SVA) or C7 (C7 SVA) plumb line to the posterosuperior aspect of the sacrum[16] (S1; Fig. 3-4, *A*, and Fig. 3-5, *A*). Although C2 and C7 serve as markers for head positioning and S1 marks the positioning of the feet, it is important to note that these offer an incomplete assessment of the global spine, because they do not fully account for cervical or pelvic alignment.[18] The gravity line, which is measured from the center of gravity (COG) of the head, has been proposed as an additional method for the assessment of global sagittal alignment (COG SVA) (see Fig. 3-5, *A*).[19-25] This method involves drawing a plumb line from the COG of the head instead of from C2 or C7. On lateral radiographs, the COG of the head can be approximated by using the anterior portion of the external auditory canal as the initial point for the plumb line.[26]

Positive SVA values indicate that the plumb line falls anterior to S1, whereas negative SVA values indicate the converse.[16] Greater sagittal malalignment as noted by larger SVAs, particularly in the positive direction, has been associated with worse functional outcomes, greater pain, and worse HRQOL.[17,27] In patients without cervical deformities, the SVA is usually less than 5 cm.[18] As with measures of CA, the postoperative benchmark is to attain an SVA of less than 4 to 5 cm.[16,28] When this occurs, the plumb line becomes more closely aligned posterior to the femoral heads and thus prevents patients from feeling as though they are leaning forward.[28]

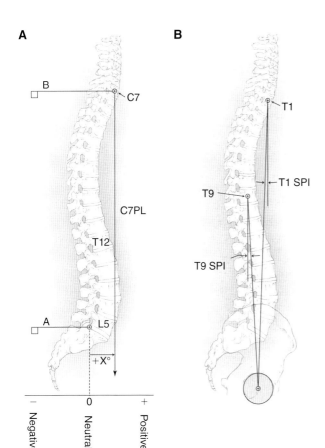

Fig. 3-4 Measurement parameters for spinal sagittal alignment. **A,** The sagittal vertebral axis is measured as the distance from the posterosuperior corner of the sacrum to a vertical plumb line dropped from the C7 centroid *(+X°)*. **B,** Spinopelvic inclination *(SPI)* is a global angular measurement of sagittal alignment. It is the angle formed by a line drawn from the femoral heads to the T1 or T9 centroid and the vertical plumb line. Because this is an angle rather than a length measurement, it is not subject to magnification variability in a radiograph. (Courtesy of K.X. Probst/Xavier Studio, 2012; with permission.)

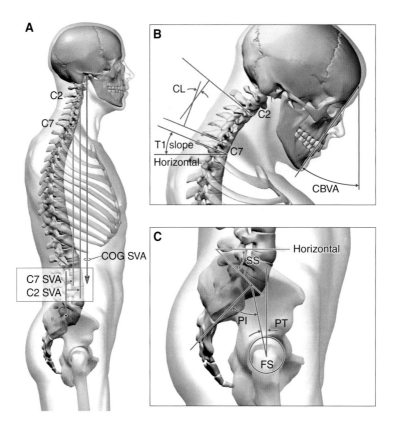

Fig. 3-5   **A-C,** The spine functions as a global unit so that cervical alignment parameters influence and are influenced by parameters in the lower regions. (*CBVA,* Chin-brow vertical angle; *CL,* cervical lordosis; *COG,* center of gravity; *FS,* femoral shaft; *PI,* pelvic incidence; *PT,* pelvic tilt; *SS,* sacral slope; *SVA,* sagittal vertical axis.) (Courtesy of K.X. Probst/Xavier Studio, 2012; with permission.)

Spinopelvic Inclination

Spinopelvic inclination (SPI), which can be measured from either T1 (T1 SPI) or T9 (T9 SPI), offers an alternative measurement of global sagittal alignment. A single line is drawn from the posterosuperior aspect of the sacrum to the centroid of the T1 vertebral body, and a vertical plumb line is dropped from the T1 centroid (see Fig. 3-4, *B*). For T9 SPI, the T9 vertebral body is used as the reference point (see Fig. 3-4, *B*). The angle formed by the intersection of these two lines represents the SPI. A value of zero is considered neutral for both T1 SPI and T9 SPI.[9] In contrast with the SVA, T1 SPI and T9 SPI are angular measurements and are thus not as susceptible to measurement error caused by limited magnification.[16] Lafage et al[27] demonstrated that T1 SPI may be a better correlative predictor of HRQOL than either SVA or T9 SPI. Postoperative targets for T1 SPI are less than 0 degrees.[28]

T1 Pelvic Angle

The T1 pelvic angle (TPA) is a novel angular measure that includes both pelvic retroversion and SVA and thus provides a better assessment of true sagittal deformity, especially in cases of flatback with pelvic retroversion. It is measured as the angle subtended from two lines drawn from the femoral heads, one of which ends at the T1 centroid and the other which ends at the midpoint of the sacral endplate. The TPA accounts for both the SVA and PT, and it correlates with HRQOL measures such as the Oswestry Disability Index, the Scoliosis Research Society questionnaire, and the Short Form-36 Physical Component Summary. Postoperative correction recommendations for TPA are less than 14 degrees.[29]

RADIOGRAPHIC EVALUATION OF CERVICAL SPINE ALIGNMENT

CERVICAL COBB ANGLE

The Cobb angle is a measure of coronal or sagittal alignment that helps with the determination of segmental lordosis or kyphosis. It is frequently ascertained by employing the four-line method, and the caudal and rostral vertebral bodies used as endpoints determine which spinal segments are being measured. By convention, kyphosis is noted by negative Cobb angles, whereas lordosis is noted by positive Cobb angles. Cobb angle measurements generally have an error range of 3 to 5 degrees, so only changes of more than 5 degrees between consecutive films can be categorized as true changes.[9]

The cervical Cobb angle is used to determine and quantify cervical lordosis (CL) or kyphosis, and it is frequently measured from either C1-7 or C2-7.[30] The first line is drawn parallel to the superior endplate of C1 or C2 (based on whether C1-7 or C2-7 is measured) or from the anterior tubercle of the vertebral body to the posterior aspect of the corresponding spinous process. The second line is drawn parallel to the inferior endplate of C7. Two perpendicular lines are subsequently extended from each of these lines, and the angle at which these lines intersect represents the Cobb angle (Fig. 3-6; see Fig. 3-5, B). Although there is some evidence to suggest that Cobb angles may not be as accurate as other methods (such as the Harrison posterior tangent method[30]), they are by and large still considered the gold standard for the measurement of lordosis.[31,32] It is very important that patients look straight ahead when the imaging occurs; cervical alignment measurements may be artificially increased or decreased if the patients do not maintain a horizontal gaze as best they can. For a patient who cannot achieve a complete horizontal gaze, it is best to standardize the location of his or her gaze for reproducibility and comparison with prior films. For patients without cervical spinal deformity, the mean CL is approximately −40 degrees, with the bulk of the lordosis concentrated at C1-2.[33] When deformities are present, they most often occur on the sagittal plane.[34-36]

If a patient's regional cervical radiographs indicate cervical hyperlordosis, full 36-inch films should be ordered. The hyperlordosis may be a compensatory mechanism for sagittal malalignment, and it may spontaneously correct after the correction of the sagittal malalignment. Smith et al[37] evaluated 75 patients who underwent lumbar pedicle subtraction osteotomy for global sagittal malalignment and found reciprocal changes in CL. The hyperlordosis had spontaneously corrected after lumbar pedicle subtraction osteotomy.

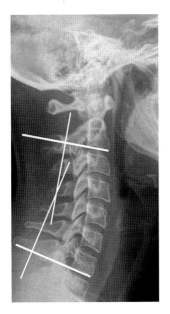

Fig. 3-6 This sagittal radiograph demonstrates the four-line method for the measurement of cervical Cobb angles. This method includes drawing a line either parallel to the inferior endplate of C2 or extending from the anterior tubercle of C1 to the posterior margin of the spinous process; another line is then drawn parallel to the inferior endplate of C7. Perpendicular lines are drawn from each of these two lines, and the angle that is subtended between the crossings of the perpendicular lines is the cervical curvature angle.

CERVICAL SAGITTAL VERTICAL AXIS

The cervical SVA represents the distance from the plumb line of the centroid of C2/dens to the posterior superior margin of C7 (Figs. 3-7 and 3-8). This measure of cervical sagittal alignment is also known as the *C2-7 SVA;* it is perhaps a more comprehensive marker for global alignment than the cervical sagittal Cobb angle, because it is often dependent on the alignment of the thoracolumbar spine as well as the lumbar spine.[38-42] Larger C2-7 SVAs have been shown to correlate with worse HRQOL.[5]

THORACIC INLET ANGLE, TILT, AND T1 SLOPE

The thoracic inlet angle, tilt, and T1 slope are measures of sagittal alignment on lateral radiographs. The thoracic inlet angle is the angle formed between a line drawn perpendicular to the midpoint of the T1 endplate and a line drawn from the midpoint of the superior endplate of T1 to the upper aspect of the sternum (Fig. 3-9). Tilt can be measured as neck, cervical, or cranial tilt. Neck tilt is the angle subtended from a

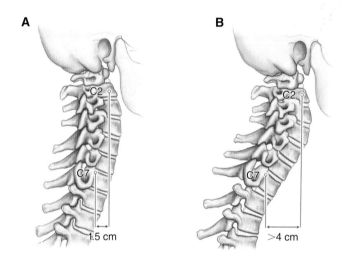

Fig. 3-7   **A,** This drawing of normal cervical lordosis highlights a small difference between the C2 and C7 plumb lines. **B,** A drawing of cervical sagittal malalignment highlights a large difference between the C2 and C7 plumb lines.

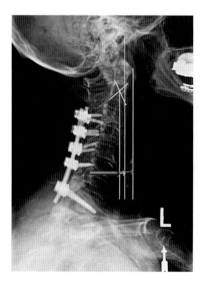

Fig. 3-8   A visual representation of the technique used to measure the cervical sagittal vertical axis (SVA). The *green arrow* represents the C1-7 SVA (the distance between the plumb line dropped from the anterior tubercle of C1 and the posterosuperior corner of C7), the *red arrow* represents the C2-7 SVA (the distance between the plumb line dropped from the centroid of C2 and the posterosuperior corner of C7), and the *yellow arrow* represents the center of gravity–C7 SVA (the distance between the plumb line dropped from the anterior margin of the external auditory canal and the posterosuperior corner of C7).

vertical plumb line from the upper aspect of the sternum and a line drawn from the upper aspect of the sternum to the midpoint of the T1 superior endplate. Cervical tilt is the angle subtended from one line perpendicular to the midpoint of the T1 superior endplate and another that connects the same midpoint to the tip of the dens. Cranial tilt is measured in a similar fashion but with the first line being a vertical plumb line from the midpoint of the T1 endplate. T1 slope is measured as the angle between a horizontal reference line and a line drawn parallel to the superior endplate of T1[43] (Fig. 3-10).

These parameters are interrelated as illustrated by the following equation[43]:

$$\text{Thoracic inlet angle} = \text{T1 slope} + \text{Neck tilt}$$

Neck tilt is typically around 44 degrees, and it is maintained as such to reduce the amount of work expended by the neck muscles to sustain horizontal gaze. A small thoracic inlet angle translates to a small T1 slope,[43] which subsequently results in less CL needed to maintain the balance of the head over the body. Alternatively, larger thoracic inlet angles result in larger T1 slopes and greater CL for compensation.[44]

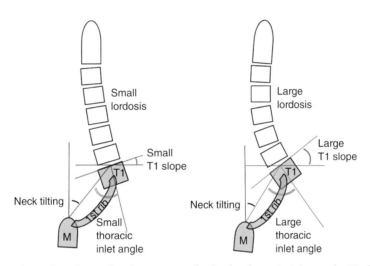

Fig. 3-9 These images show the relationship between neck tilt, the thoracic inlet angle, T1 slope, and cervical lordosis. A small thoracic inlet angle yields a low T1 slope so that less cervical lordosis is required to balance the head over the thoracic inlet and the trunk. Conversely, a large thoracic inlet angle yields a greater T1 slope so that a greater magnitude of cervical lordosis is required to balance the head over the thoracic inlet and the trunk.

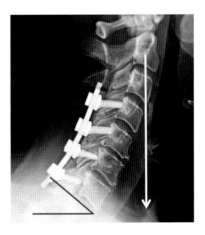

Fig. 3-10 This lateral radiograph demonstrates the angle of T1 slope and its relationship to the cervical sagittal vertical axis.

RADIOGRAPHIC EVALUATION OF THORACIC AND THORACOLUMBAR SPINE ALIGNMENT

Thoracic and Thoracolumbar Cobb Angles

Thoracic kyphosis (TK) is measured as the Cobb angle that is subtended from lines drawn parallel to the superior endplate of T2 and the inferior endplate of T12[16] (Fig. 3-11, *A*). Alternatively, T5-12 can also serve as the endplates for measurement.[16] Normal aging results in increased TK. Thoracolumbar kyphosis is determined by measuring the Cobb angle between T10 and L2[16] (Fig. 3-11, *B*).

RADIOGRAPHIC EVALUATION OF SPINOPELVIC ALIGNMENT

Pelvic Incidence

The pelvic incidence (PI) is a fixed sagittal parameter that is measured as the angle subtended between two lines: one drawn from the center of the femoral heads to the midpoint of the sacral endplate and another drawn perpendicular to the sacral endplate[16,45] (Fig. 3-12; see Fig. 3-5, *C*). If the femoral heads do not align, the midpoint of the bicoxofemoral axis can be used as a surrogate endpoint.[9]

The PI illustrates the relationship between the sacrum and the acetabulum. Normal values for PI range between 45 and 55 degrees, with an average of approximately 53 degrees.[4,9,36] Given the constant nature of this morphologic parameter after puberty, patients with deformities largely have PI values that are similar to those of normal subjects.[45]

PI is closely related to other radiographic parameters of the pelvis, and these relationships bear implications for global alignment. A large PI (for example, more than 60 degrees) results in greater LL to compensate for the increased vertical alignment of the sacrum. A smaller PI (for example, less than 45 degrees) in turn results in greater horizontal alignment of the sacrum and thus is associated with decreased sacral slope (SS) and lower LL.[46] To reflect these significant interdependent relationships, PI can be calculated with the following equation[45]:

$$PI = SS + PT$$

The mismatch between PI and LL (PI-LL) is another metric that is used to assess spinopelvic alignment. It is represented by the following equation[28,47]:

$$PI = LL + 9 \text{ degrees } (\pm 9 \text{ degrees})$$

Pelvic Tilt

PT is measured as the angle between a vertical plumb line drawn from the femoral heads and another drawn from the midpoint of the sacral endplate to the femoral heads[16,45] (Fig. 3-13; see Fig. 3-5, *C*). Mean normative PT values generally lie somewhere between 10 and 15 degrees,[45,47,48] but they can also range from −2 to 30 degrees in normal patients without deformity.[46] High PT values represent reciprocal compensatory changes induced by sagittal malalignment (age-induced arthritis, loss of lordosis, increased kyphosis), thereby leading to hyperextension and retroversion of the hip in an attempt to maintain an upright posture and gait.[9,16,27] However, high PT values are generally incompatible with efficient ambulation; such values strongly correlate with walking disability and translate into increased pain and functional disability.[27] Postoperative correction thresholds aim for a PT target of less than 20 degrees to reestablish an "extension reserve" for walking.[28]

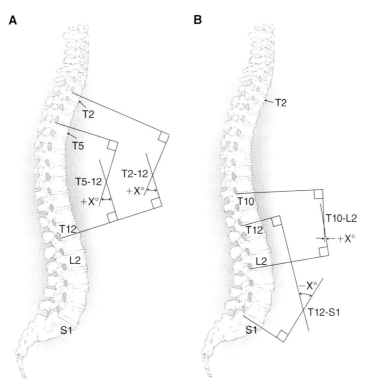

Fig. 3-11 **A,** This diagram shows the method for measuring thoracic kyphosis *(+X°)*. Typically thoracic kyphosis is measured from T5-12, because often the T2 endplate is difficult to visualize. **B,** This diagram shows the method for measuring lumbar lordosis. Lumbar lordosis is generally measured from T12 to S1 *(−X°),* and thoracolumbar alignment is measured from T10 to L2 *(+X°)*. (Courtesy of K.X. Probst/Xavier Studio, 2012; with permission.)

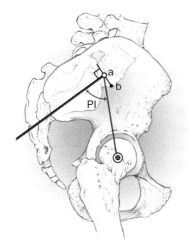

Fig. 3-12 This diagram demonstrates the measurement of the pelvic incidence *(PI)*. It is measured as the angle subtended between two lines: one drawn from the center of the femoral heads to the midpoint of the sacral endplate *(a)* and another drawn perpendicular to a line drawn across the sacral endplate *(b)*. (Courtesy of K.X. Probst/Xavier Studio, 2012; with permission.)

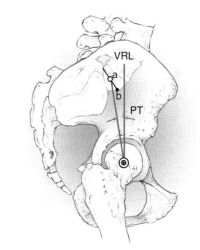

Fig. 3-13 This diagram demonstrates the measurement of the pelvic tilt *(PT)*. (*VRL,* Vertical reference line; *a* = center of sacral endplate; *b* = line drawn across the sacral endplate.) (Courtesy of K.X. Probst/Xavier Studio, 2012; with permission.)

Sacral Slope

SS is defined as the angle between a horizontal reference line that extends from the posterosuperior aspect of the sacrum and a parallel line that extends from the sacral endplate[16] (Fig. 3-14; see Fig. 3-5, C). Normal slope averages 30 to 40 degrees.[21,28,45-48] When the sacrum demonstrates greater horizontal alignment, the SS is high; a low SS denotes greater vertical alignment of the sacrum.[45]

Lumbar Cobb Angle

LL is determined as the Cobb angle created between two parallel lines that extend from the superior endplates of L1 and S1 or T12 and S1[16] (see Fig. 3-11, B). LL helps to maintain upright posture, and normal values average 60 degrees.[48] A loss of LL (for example, to less than 40 degrees) is often a consequence of normal aging.[18] It results in flat-back syndrome,[41] and it correlates with pain and functional disability.[27]

Pelvic Incidence and Lumbar Lordosis Mismatch

There exists a mathematical relationship in which LL may be predicted on the basis of PI by the following equation[47]:

$$LL = PI \pm 9 \text{ degrees}$$

As discussed previously, PI is a fixed morphologic parameter, so a patient in whom there is a loss of LL (someone with flat-back deformity) will have a mismatch between PI and LL that can be described by the mathematical difference between the two radiographic measurements (PI-LL). Values of more than 9 degrees may lead to disability.[47] Schwab et al[49] recently reported correlations between radiographic parameters (both coronal and sagittal) and HRQOL among 492 patients with spinal deformities. Of the many parameters assessed, PI-LL, SVA, and PT had the highest correlations with disability.[49] Patients with flat-back deformity usually have global sagittal malalignment that is characterized by a C7 SVA of more than 5 cm. However, there also exists a subset of patients with flat-back deformity that have normal global sagittal alignment (C7 SVA of less than 5 cm). Smith et al[50] recently investigated the HRQOL outcomes in these two different patient populations after surgical correction. The authors found that patients with PI-LL mismatch and normal global sagittal alignment had improvements in HRQOL outcomes that were similar to the patients with both PI-LL mismatch and global sagittal malalignment. Although it is known that the correction of global sagittal malalignment results in improved HRQOL, the evaluation of sagittal spinal malalignment should include PI-LL mismatch in addition to C7 SVA. Patients may not have global sagittal malalignment but instead functional disability as a result of a high PI-LL mismatch and thus benefit from surgical correction. As evidenced by the Smith et al study,[50] a PI-LL mismatch in the setting of normal global sagittal malalignment may be considered a primary surgical indication.

Pelvic Obliquity

Pelvic obliquity offers an assessment of coronal plane pelvic deformity that may be the result of a leg-length discrepancy from congenital or acquired conditions (hip or knee osteoarthritis, prior arthroplasty) or from primary sacropelvic deformity. It is measured as the angle formed by the intersection of a line drawn between the pelvic coronal reference line and a horizontal reference line. The pelvic coronal reference line is measured as a line drawn between the ala of the sacrum[16] (Fig. 3-15). Pelvic obliquity quantifies leg-length discrepancies, and it is becoming an increasingly important parameter to consider during surgical planning.[16]

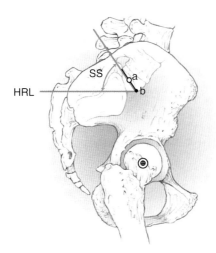

Fig. 3-14   This diagram demonstrates the measurement of the sacral slope *(SS)*. (*HRL,* Horizontal reference line; *a* = center of sacral endplate; *b* = line drawn across the sacral endplate.) (Courtesy of K.X. Probst/Xavier Studio, 2012; with permission.)

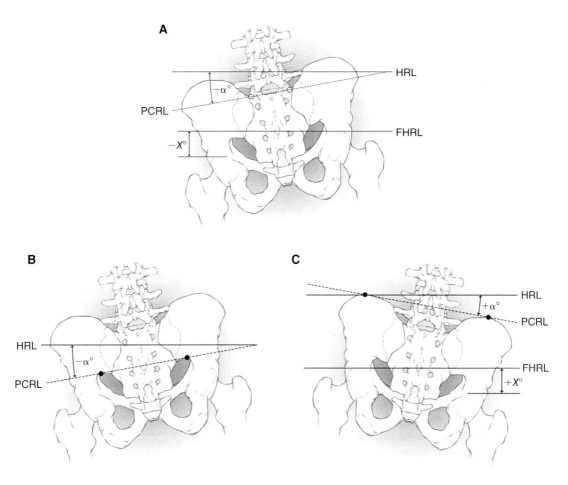

Fig. 3-15   These diagrams demonstrate the measurement of pelvic obliquity and leg length discrepancy. Pelvic is obliquity (± alpha) can be quantified by measuring the angle formed between a horizontal reference line (HRL) and the pelvic coronal reference line (PCRL). The PCRL can be drawn from three different pelvic landmarks, which include **A,** the two superior points of the sacral ala, **B,** the two superior points of the greater sciatic notch, or **C,** the two superior points of the iliac crests. The leg length discrepancy (± *X*) can be measured as distance between a horizontal reference line at the superior edge of the femoral head on the right and left side (FHRL) and the superior aspect of the femoral head (**A** and **C**). (*FHRL,* Femoral horizontal reference line; *HRL,* horizontal reference line; *PCRL,* pelvic coronal reference line.) (Courtesy of K.X. Probst/Xavier Studio, 2012; with permission.)

The lumbar spine may have a compensatory coronal curve in response to the pelvic obliquity to balance the spine. Whether the pelvic obliquity is primary or secondary, correction strategies must take that obliquity into account, because there may be adverse postoperative alignment failures. If the correction of a lumbar coronal curve does not account for the primary driver of the pelvic obliquity, coronal decompensation of the lumbar correction may occur[16] (Fig. 3-16). If the pelvic obliquity is secondary (attempting to compensate) for the spinal scoliotic curve, then the curve-correction strategies must be of sufficient magnitude to allow the pelvis to relax in the coronal plane[16] (Fig. 3-17) so that postoperative lumbar alignment is maintained.

All patients should be evaluated clinically and radiographically for leg-length discrepancies. If such a discrepancy is identified, it should be reevaluated after the patient is fitted with a shoe lift to assess how the spine and pelvis respond to correction[16] (Fig. 3-18). Patients with a flexible curve secondary to a pelvic obliquity due to a leg-length discrepancy may respond well to the addition of a shoe lift only, or they may choose to undergo the surgical treatment of the leg-length discrepancy.

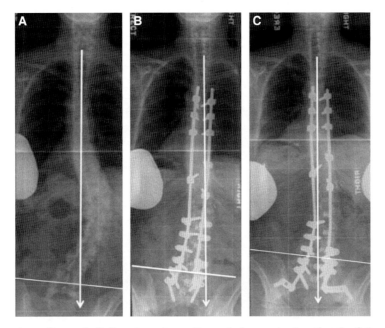

Fig. 3-16 **A,** Preoperative radiograph. **B,** Postoperative radiograph demonstrating that the failure to note a leg-length discrepancy led to further coronal decompensation with correction of the scoliosis. Further decompensation to the right was noted in this patient after curve correction. **C,** Postoperative radiograph after a second surgery showing that some of the curve correction was removed and that the instrumentation was extended to the pelvis. Note that the pelvic obliquity that resulted from a leg-length discrepancy was not significantly addressed. (From Ames CP, Smith JS, Scheer JK, et al. Impact of spinopelvic alignment on decision making in deformity surgery in adults: a review. J Neurosurg Spine 16:547-564, 2012.)

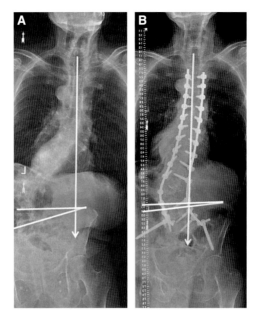

Fig. 3-17 Pelvic obliquity may be compensatory with severe curves in an attempt to maintain balance. In these cases, correction of the scoliosis results in a rebalancing of the spine and a spontaneous reciprocal decrease in pelvic obliquity. **A,** Preoperative radiograph displaying severe scoliosis and high pelvic obliquity. **B,** Postoperative radiograph showing coronal correction and a decrease in pelvic obliquity. (From Ames CP, Smith JS, Scheer JK, et al. Impact of spinopelvic alignment on decision making in deformity surgery in adults: a review. J Neurosurg Spine 16:547-564, 2012.)

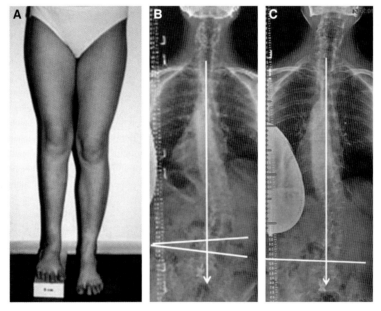

Fig. 3-18 A patient with pelvic obliquity as demonstrated by standing radiographs should be assessed for a leg-length discrepancy and the radiographs repeated with the patient wearing a shoe lift that approximates the discrepancy to assess its effect on the spinal curve. **A,** Clinical assessment of leg-length discrepancy. **B,** Standing anteroposterior radiograph without a shoe lift. **C,** Standing anteroposterior radiograph with the addition of a shoe lift to the side with the short leg. Note the partial correction of the scoliosis. The coronal alignment shifted back slightly to the left of neutral. Despite the curve correction that occurred with the shoe lift, the patient's back pain continued, and she elected to undergo surgery for her symptoms. (From Ames CP, Smith JS, Scheer JK, et al. Impact of spinopelvic alignment on decision making in deformity surgery in adults: a review. J Neurosurg Spine 16:547-564, 2012.)

If the spinal curve is rigid, the addition of a shoe lift will not correct the curve. In this case, there are two options: (1) correct the curve perpendicular to the oblique pelvis and ignore the pelvic obliquity or (2) correct the spine to a level pelvis if the leg-length correction is planned (for example, with a future hip replacement) or if the patient tolerates a shoe lift[16] (Fig. 3-19).

Close attention to the preoperative side of malalignment will determine the magnitude of the curve corrections possible while maintaining standing global coronal balance[16] (Fig. 3-20). Often the fractional curve may allow rebalancing of the spine via small angular coronal corrections at the lumbosacral junction[16] (Fig. 3-21). The comparison of preoperative prone and standing films may assist the surgeon with estimating the anticipated difference in alignment that is likely to be seen on the operative table and therefore the likely magnitude of optimal curve correction. Preoperative bending films will also assist the surgeon with determining how much correction may occur if a curve is not included in the fusion. Intraoperative full-cassette films should be obtained and interpreted with an understanding of the patient's baseline pelvic malalignment. These images are obtained by placing the long cassette on a film holder lateral to the patient and by placing the long film plate on a stool underneath a radiolucent table for anteroposterior assessment. In general the global sagittal plane is more accurately assessed than the global coronal plane; leg-length discrepancies, which mainly affect the coronal plane, are not easily assessed until the patient stands during the early postoperative period. Early postoperative standing films are thus recommended to allow further coronal adjustments if needed, because it is often difficult to predict how the spines of patients with complex curve patterns and pelvic obliquity will be corrected when the patient is standing.

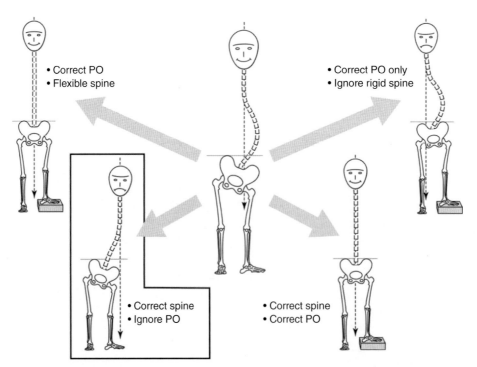

Fig. 3-19   A general algorithm for the treatment of patients with scoliosis, coronal malalignment, and pelvic obliquity. In patients with pelvic obliquity in which the spine is flexible and aligned, full correction of the curve may lead to significant coronal decompensation, because the scoliotic curve may be compensatory. In some of these patients, the addition of a shoe lift will allow the flexible spine to relax, and this may improve alignment and deformity-related symptoms. If the spine is rigid, which is more common in adults, a shoe lift may be poorly tolerated and may not be effective for rebalancing the spine. These patients may require incomplete curve corrections and sometimes a shoe lift as well, depending on the final standing alignment. (*PO,* Pelvic obliquity.) (Courtesy of K.X. Probst/Xavier Studio, 2012; with permission.)

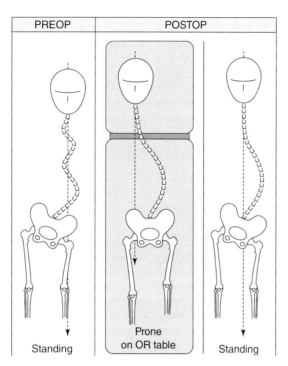

Fig. 3-20 With complex curve patterns, the coronal correction strategy must take into account the alignment shift that will likely occur when the patient is standing to determine how much curve correction is possible in each direction. This often involves shifting the patient's coronal plumb slightly off to the side opposite the short leg. (*OR,* Operating room.) (Courtesy of K.X. Probst/Xavier Studio, 2012; with permission.)

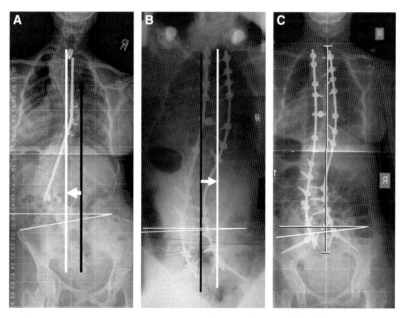

Fig. 3-21 **A,** This standing anteroposterior preoperative radiograph shows that the patient was initially off to the left (the side of the short leg). **B,** The intraoperative correction strategy was designed to shift the intraoperative plumb a few centimeters to the right. **C,** When the pelvic obliquity returned during standing, this resulted in a well-aligned spine in the coronal plane. (*White line,* C7 plum line; *black line,* central sacral vertical line.) (From Ames CP, Smith JS, Scheer JK, et al. Impact of spinopelvic alignment on decision making in deformity surgery in adults: a review. J Neurosurg Spine 16:547-564, 2012.)

CONCLUSION

As summarized in Table 3-1, both regional and global spinal malalignment can be ascertained with the use of standard radiography. The assessment of radiographic parameters is an important tool for both preoperative diagnosis and surgical planning for patients with ASD. These parameters may be used to elucidate several undercharacterized but important relationships that are present in the spine. For example, the pelvis plays a critical role in upright balanced sitting and standing postures, but spinopelvic parameters have traditionally been neglected during the evaluation of spinal deformities.

Table 3-1   Radiographic Parameters in the Evaluation of Spinal Deformity

Radiographic Parameter	Alignment	Measurement
Coronal alignment	Coronal	Horizontal distance between: • C7 centroid vertical plumb line • S1 centroid vertical plumb line (central sacral vertical line)
Spinal curvature	Coronal or sagittal	Classified by the apex of maximal displacement and minimal angulation: • Thoracic deformity: apex between T2 body and T12 disc • Thoracolumbar deformity: apex between T12 and L1 bodies • Lumbar deformity: apex at or distal to L1 body and L2 disc
Sagittal vertical axis	Sagittal	Horizontal distance between: • C2 or C7 centroid vertical plumb line • Vertical plumb line from posterosuperior aspect of S1
T1 spinopelvic inclination	Sagittal	Angle subtended from: • T1 centroid vertical plumb line • Line extended from posterosuperior aspect of S1 to T1 centroid
T9 spinopelvic inclination	Sagittal	Angle subtended from: • T9 centroid vertical plumb line • Line extended from posterosuperior aspect of S1 to T9 centroid
T1 pelvic angle	Sagittal	Angle subtended from: • Line extended from femoral heads to T1 centroid • Line extended from femoral heads to midpoint of sacral endplate
Cervical Cobb angle	Coronal or sagittal	Angle subtended from: • Line extended parallel to superior endplate of C2 • Line extended parallel to inferior endplate of C7 Note: C1 can also serve as the rostral vertebral body for measurement.
Cervical sagittal vertical axis	Sagittal	Horizontal distance between: • C2 centroid/dens vertical plumb line • Vertical plumb line from posterosuperior margin of C7

Radiographic Parameter	Alignment	Measurement
Thoracic inlet angle	Sagittal	Angle subtended from: • Line extended perpendicular to midpoint of superior endplate of T1 • Line extended from midpoint of superior endplate of T1 to upper aspect of sternum
Neck tilt	Sagittal	Angle subtended from: • Line extended from midpoint of superior endplate of T1 to upper aspect of sternum • Vertical plumb line
Cranial tilt	Sagittal	Angle subtended from: • Line extended from midpoint of superior endplate of T1 to tip of dens • Vertical plumb line
Cervical tilt	Sagittal	Angle subtended from: • Line extended from midpoint of superior endplate of T1 to tip of dens • Line extended perpendicular to midpoint of superior endplate of T1
T1 slope	Sagittal	Angle subtended from: • Line extended parallel to superior endplate of T1 • Horizontal reference line
Thoracic Cobb angle	Coronal or sagittal	Angle subtended from: • Line extended parallel to superior endplate of T2 • Line extended parallel to inferior endplate of T12 Note: Cobb angles can also be measured in similar fashion from T5-12.
Thoracolumbar Cobb angle	Coronal or sagittal	Angle subtended from: • Line extended parallel to superior endplate of T10 • Line extended parallel to inferior endplate of L2
Pelvic obliquity	Coronal	Angle subtended from: • Horizontal reference line • Line extended between sacral ala
Pelvic incidence	Sagittal	Angle subtended from: • Line extended from center of femoral heads to midpoint of sacral endplate • Line extended perpendicular to sacral endplate
Pelvic tilt	Sagittal	Angle subtended from: • Vertical plumb line from femoral heads • Line extended from midpoint of sacral endplate to femoral heads
Sacral slope	Sagittal	Angle subtended from: • Horizontal reference line from posterosuperior aspect of S1 • Line extended parallel to sacral endplate
Lumbar Cobb angle	Coronal or sagittal	Angle subtended from: • Line extended parallel to superior endplate of L1 • Line extended parallel to superior endplate of S1

Recent data have demonstrated that the failure to account for pelvic alignment when treating ASD increases the risk for residual deformity and treatment failure. Pelvic alignment parameters (including PI, PT, SS, and pelvic obliquity) must be evaluated by treating physicians at the same time that more traditional measures (including SVA, LL, TK, and regional scoliotic curves) are assessed. Particular attention must be paid to PT, which is a dynamic pelvic parameter that reflects pelvic retroversion. Increased PT implies residual postoperative spinal deformity, and this will negatively affect postoperative function and outcomes.

Pelvic obliquity and its associated causes must also be accounted for in strategies for coronal plane correction. The correction of the lumbar curve in the setting of pelvic obliquity may generate postoperative coronal decompensation. If the pelvic obliquity is the result of a compensatory mechanism for the spinal coronal malalignment, then the correction of the spine may restore pelvic CA. If the spine is flexible, a shoe lift may yield a considerable amount of spinal coronal correction. However, if the spine is rigid, then surgery is likely necessary in conjunction with a shoe insert. Intraoperative full-cassette radiographs should be used to evaluate the CA and to account for the patient's pelvic obliquity.

Radiographic parameters also contribute greatly to the understanding of cervical deformity and correction. The sagittal alignment of the cervical spine is becoming a very important parameter; it will continue to be so during the next few years, because the same concepts used to successfully characterize the effect of thoracolumbar alignment on outcomes can be applied to the cervical spine. The cervical spine is complex, and the surgical management of cervical disease remains a significant challenge. An understanding of cervical alignment, biomechanics, and the normative data for cervical alignment is necessary for the management of complex cervical pathology. The major parameters used to assess cervical spine alignment include Cobb angles for sagittal curvature and the gravity line (COG of the head) or the C2 plumb line for SVA. Newer parameters include the thoracic inlet angle, cervical tilt, neck tilt, and cranial tilt. It has been shown that these parameters affect the alignment of the cervical spine, and the relationships among these factors provide a foundation for future investigation as well as for the surgical planning of cervical fusions. It is critical to remain cognizant of the fact that spinal regions are not independent of one another. CL depends on both TK and LL. CL can be considered an adaptive spinal parameter in that it can change in relation to other spinal segments as a means of keeping the head over the pelvis and maintaining the horizontal gaze. In a patient with global sagittal malalignment, CL increases as a compensatory mechanism.

The T1 slope also plays a role in CL, and patients can alter their T1 slope through compensatory mechanisms such as retroverting the pelvis, thoracic hypokyphosis, and lumbar hyperlordosis. Patients who develop cervicothoracic deformities after thoracolumbar fusions (for example, patients with proximal junctional kyphosis) cannot rely on thoracic and lumbar compensatory mechanisms, but they do rely on pelvic retroversion to improve the horizontal gaze. Unlike T1 slope, T1 incidence is independent of the pelvis and thus can be a better predictor of the magnitude of cervical deformity correction necessary for optimal balance. These concepts are in their early stages, and future studies that correlate them with HRQOL will expand the current understanding of cervical alignment and deformity surgery. Further investigation of the cervical spine in other areas is much needed as well. Those subjects deserving of particular attention are the relationships between the various cervical alignment parameters and HRQOL, cervical deformity and osteotomy classification, and more standardized indications for surgery.

In summary, conceptualizing these parameters as independent entities and in relation to each other will continue to shape and improve the quality of care being delivered to patients with ASD. As the implementation of these parameters becomes more popular, the field of spinal deformity correction will move forward and optimize the likelihood of the achievement of satisfactory surgical and patient outcomes.

REFERENCES

1. Schwab F, Dubey A, Pagala M, et al. Adult scoliosis: a health assessment analysis by SF-36. Spine 28:602-606, 2003.

2. Smith JS, Fu KM, Urban P, et al. Neurological symptoms and deficits in adults with scoliosis who present to a surgical clinic: incidence and association with the choice of operative versus nonoperative management. J Neurosurg Spine 9:326-331, 2008.

3. Dubousset J. Importance de la vertèbre pelvienne dans l'équilibre rachidien. Application à la chirurgie de la colonne vertébrale chez l'enfant et l'adolescent. In Villeneuve P, ed. Pied Équilibre et Rachis. Paris: Frison-Roche, 1998.

4. Dubousset J. Reflections of an orthopaedic surgeon on patient care and research into the condition of scoliosis. J Pediatr Orthop 31(1 Suppl):S1-S8, 2011.

5. Tang JA, Scheer JK, Smith JS, et al. The impact of standing regional cervical sagittal alignment on outcomes in posterior cervical fusion surgery. Neurosurgery 71:662-669; discussion 669, 2012.

6. McAviney J, Schulz D, Bock R, et al. Determining the relationship between cervical lordosis and neck complaints. J Manipulative Physiol Ther 28:187-193, 2005.

7. Ames CP, Blondel B, Scheer JK, et al. Cervical radiographical alignment: comprehensive assessment techniques and potential importance in cervical myelopathy. Spine 38:149-160, 2013.

8. Angevine PD, Kaiser MG. Radiographic measurement techniques. Neurosurgery 63:40-45, 2008.

9. Smith JS, Shaffrey CI, Fu KM, et al. Clinical and radiographic evaluation of the adult spinal deformity patient. Neurosurg Clin N Am 24:143-156, 2013.

10. Wade R, Yang H, McKenna C, et al. A systematic review of the clinical effectiveness of EOS 2D/3D X-ray imaging system. Eur Spine J 22:296-304, 2013.

11. Wybier M, Bossard P. Musculoskeletal imaging in progress: the EOS imaging system. Joint Bone Spine 80:238-243, 2013.

12. Al-Aubaidi Z, Lebel D, Oudjhane K, et al. Three-dimensional imaging of the spine using the EOS system: is it reliable? A comparative study using computed tomography imaging. J Pediatr Orthop B 22:409-412, 2013.

13. Lazennec JY, Brusson A, Rousseau MA. Hip-spine relations and sagittal balance clinical consequences. Eur Spine J 20(Suppl 5):686-698, 2011.

14. Obeid I, Hauger O, Aunoble S, et al. Global analysis of sagittal spinal alignment in major deformities: correlation between lack of lumbar lordosis and flexion of the knee. Eur Spine J 20(Suppl 5):681-685, 2011.

15. Somoskeoy S, Tunyogi-Csapo M, Bogyo C, et al. Accuracy and reliability of coronal and sagittal spinal curvature data based on patient-specific three-dimensional models created by the EOS 2D/3D imaging system. Spine J 12:1052-1059, 2012.

16. Ames CP, Smith JS, Scheer JK, et al. Impact of spinopelvic alignment on decision making in deformity surgery in adults: a review. J Neurosurg Spine 16:547-564, 2012.

17. Glassman SD, Berven S, Bridwell K, et al. Correlation of radiographic parameters and clinical symptoms in adult scoliosis. Spine 30:682-688, 2005.

18. Klineberg E, Schwab F, Smith JS, et al. Sagittal spinal pelvic alignment. Neurosurg Clin N Am 24:157-162, 2013.

19. El Fegoun AB, Schwab F, Gamez L, et al. Center of gravity and radiographic posture analysis: a preliminary review of adult volunteers and adult patients affected by scoliosis. Spine 30:1535-1540, 2005.

20. Gangnet N, Pomero V, Dumas R, et al. Variability of the spine and pelvis location with respect to the gravity line: a three-dimensional stereoradiographic study using a force platform. Surg Radiol Anat 25:424-433, 2003.

21. Lafage V, Schwab F, Skalli W, et al. Standing balance and sagittal plane spinal deformity: analysis of spinopelvic and gravity line parameters. Spine 33:1572-1578, 2008.

22. Legaye J, Duval-Beaupere G. Gravitational forces and sagittal shape of the spine. Clinical estimation of their relations. Int Orthop 32:809-816, 2008.

23. Mac-Thiong JM, Transfeldt EE, Mehbod AA, et al. Can C7 plumbline and gravity line predict health related quality of life in adult scoliosis? Spine 34:E519-E527, 2009.

24. Schwab F, Lafage V, Boyce R, et al. Gravity line analysis in adult volunteers: age-related correlation with spinal parameters, pelvic parameters, and foot position. Spine 31:E959-E967, 2006.

25. Wang J, Zhou Y, Zhang ZF, et al. Comparison of one-level minimally invasive and open transforaminal lumbar interbody fusion in degenerative and isthmic spondylolisthesis grades 1 and 2. Eur Spine J 19:1780-1784, 2010.

26. Beier G, Schuck M, Schuller E, et al. Determination of Physical Data of the Head I. Center of Gravity and Moments of Inertia of Human Heads. Arlington, VA: Office of Naval Research, 1979.

27. Lafage V, Schwab F, Patel A, et al. Pelvic tilt and truncal inclination: two key radiographic parameters in the setting of adults with spinal deformity. Spine 34:E599-E606, 2009.

28. Schwab F, Patel A, Ungar B, et al. Adult spinal deformity-postoperative standing imbalance: how much can you tolerate? An overview of key parameters in assessing alignment and planning corrective surgery. Spine 35:2224-2231, 2010.

29. Protopsaltis TS, Bronsard N, Smith JS, et al. The T1 pelvic angle (TPA), a novel radiographic measure of global sagittal deformity, accounts for both spinal inclination and pelvic tilt and correlates with HRQOL. J Bone Joint Surg (in press).

30. Harrison DE, Harrison DD, Cailliet R, et al. Cobb method or Harrison posterior tangent method: which to choose for lateral cervical radiographic analysis. Spine 25:2072-2078, 2000.

31. Polly DW Jr, Kilkelly FX, McHale KA, et al. Measurement of lumbar lordosis. Evaluation of intraobserver, interobserver, and technique variability. Spine 21:1530-1535; discussion 1535-1536, 1996.

32. Singer KP, Jones TJ, Breidahl PD. A comparison of radiographic and computer-assisted measurements of thoracic and thoracolumbar sagittal curvature. Skeletal Radiol 19:21-26, 1990.

33. Hardacker JW, Shuford RF, Capicotto PN, et al. Radiographic standing cervical segmental alignment in adult volunteers without neck symptoms. Spine 22:1472-1480; discussion 1480, 1997.

34. Chi JH, Tay B, Stahl D, et al. Complex deformities of the cervical spine. Neurosurg Clin N Am 18:295-304, 2007.

35. Mummaneni PV, Deutsch H, Mummaneni VP. Cervicothoracic kyphosis. Neurosurg Clin N Am 17:277-287, vi, 2006.

36. Steinmetz MP, Stewart TJ, Kager CD, et al. Cervical deformity correction. Neurosurgery 60:S90-S97, 2007.

37. Smith JS, Shaffrey CI, Lafage V, et al. Spontaneous improvement of cervical alignment after correction of global sagittal balance following pedicle subtraction osteotomy. J Neurosurg Spine 17:300-307, 2012.

38. Boachie-Adjei O. Role and technique of eggshell osteotomies and vertebral column resections in the treatment of fixed sagittal imbalance. Instr Course Lect 55:583-589, 2006.

39. Booth KC, Bridwell KH, Lenke LG, et al. Complications and predictive factors for the successful treatment of flatback deformity (fixed sagittal imbalance). Spine 24:1712-1720, 1999.

40. Kim YJ, Bridwell KH, Lenke LG, et al. Results of lumbar pedicle subtraction osteotomies for fixed sagittal imbalance: a minimum 5-year follow-up study. Spine 32:2189-2197, 2007.

41. Lu DC, Chou D. Flatback syndrome. Neurosurg Clin N Am 18:289-294, 2007.

42. Smith JS, Shaffrey CI, Lafage V, et al. Spontaneous improvement of cervical alignment after correction of global sagittal balance following pedicle subtraction osteotomy. J Neurosurg Spine 17:300-307, 2012.

43. Lee SH, Kim KT, Seo EM, et al. The influence of thoracic inlet alignment on the craniocervical sagittal balance in asymptomatic adults. J Spinal Disord Tech 25:E41-E47, 2012.

44. Scheer JK, Tang JA, Smith JS, et al. Cervical spine alignment, sagittal deformity, and clinical implications: a review. J Neurosurg Spine 19:141-159, 2013.

45. Legaye J, Duval-Beaupere G, Hecquet J, et al. Pelvic incidence: a fundamental pelvic parameter for three-dimensional regulation of spinal sagittal curves. Eur Spine J 7:99-103, 1998.

46. Boulay C, Tardieu C, Hecquet J, et al. Sagittal alignment of spine and pelvis regulated by pelvic incidence: standard values and prediction of lordosis. Eur Spine J 15:415-422, 2006.

47. Schwab F, Lafage V, Patel A, et al. Sagittal plane considerations and the pelvis in the adult patient. Spine 34:1828-1833, 2009.

48. Barrey C, Jund J, Noseda O, et al. Sagittal balance of the pelvis-spine complex and lumbar degenerative diseases. A comparative study about 85 cases. Eur Spine J 16:1459-1467, 2007.

49. Schwab FJ, Blondel B, Bess S, et al. Radiographical spinopelvic parameters and disability in the setting of adult spinal deformity: a prospective multicenter analysis. Spine 38:E803-E812, 2013.

50. Smith JS, Singh M, Klineberg E, et al. Surgical treatment of pathological loss of lumbar lordosis (flatback) in the setting of normal sagittal vertical axis (SVA) achieves similar clinical improvement as surgical treatment of elevated SVA. J Neurosurg Spine 21:160-170, 2014.

4

Relationship Between Spinopelvic Alignment, Imaging Studies, and Clinical Symptoms

Jeffrey L. Gum ▪ *Leah Yacat Carreon* ▪ *Virginie Lafage*
Steven D. Glassman

During the past two decades, awareness regarding the sagittal profile of the spine has increased. This emphasis has occurred in parallel with a shift in how treatment effectiveness is assessed or measured. A gradual transition has occurred from provider-perspective outcomes to patient-centered, health-related quality of life (HRQOL) outcomes. With these two developments, it has become more apparent that abnormal spinal processes, such as malalignment or imbalance, drive poor clinical outcomes and result in greater disability. As a result, health care providers have been able to more appropriately treat specific areas of spine pathology that are the primary drivers of clinical improvement, with research highlighting the importance of sagittal balance and alignment of the spine in HRQOL measures. In addition, the interaction of the sagittal alignment of specific regions of the spine to the overall global sagittal alignment is being extensively studied.

ORIGIN OF PELVIC PARAMETERS

Human bipedalism and an upright posture resulted in widening and verticalization of the pelvis, with reciprocal regional curves of the spine.[1,2] This has produced a neutral, upright posture that is ergonomically efficient for ambulation. Dubousset[3] helped to explain this in his description of a *cone of economy* or *cone of balance,* referring to the narrow range of posture that ensures energy-efficient standing and ambulation. Deviation from this range increases the work required to maintain an upright posture and presents a physiologic challenge to balance mechanisms. Dubousset et al[4] coined the term *pelvic vertebra,* emphasizing the importance of the pelvis as a link between the spine and lower extremities.

In 1985 During et al[5] introduced the term *pelvisacral angle,* which is defined as the angle between the line through the center of the hip joints to the middle of the sacral plate and a line tangent to the sacral plate. They described the pelvisacral angle as "of constructional origin; the suspension of the sacrum between the iliac wings cannot be influenced at will." Duval-Beaupère et al[6] subsequently introduced the complement to this pelvisacral angle, the *pelvic incidence.* Jackson et al[7] used lumbopelvic lordosis to assess pelvic morphology. These reports have led to the current use of the following radiographic measures of the pelvis: pelvic tilt (PT), sacral slope (SS), and pelvic incidence (PI).[8] The geometrical relationship of these parameters is as follows: Pelvic incidence = Pelvic tilt + Sacral slope.

AGE-DEPENDENT CHANGES IN PELVIC PARAMETERS

Studies have shown that pelvic incidence is a fixed parameter that does not change with position and remains relatively constant during adulthood.[9,10] After comparing the PI in different age groups, Marty et al[10] and Descamps et al[11] suggested that PI is relatively stable before 10 years of age and increases to its adult value during adolescent growth. In another study, Mangione and Sénégas[9] showed that PI increased linearly during childhood after the start of ambulation. More recently, Mac-Thiong et al[12] carried out a prospective evaluation of 180 children and reported a significant correlation between age and PI and hypothesized that the change in PI during childhood was a mechanism to maintain sagittal balance during growth. They concluded that PI tends to increase from 4 to 18 years of age, with a corresponding increase in PT and lumbar lordosis (LL), whereas SS is not significantly influenced by age after the start of ambulation. Berthonnaud et al[13,14] confirmed that the known interdependence between spinopelvic parameters is maintained for both adult and pediatric populations.

SPINAL ALIGNMENT AND SPINOPELVIC RELATIONSHIP

Overall, the spine and pelvis work to center the head over the pelvis. Although numerous ways to measure this have been reported, the current, most accepted method involves the sagittal vertical axis (SVA). This is the distance between a plumb line from the middle of the vertebral body of C7 and the posterosuperior endplate of S1. Jackson and McManus[15] reported that the mean SVA value in asymptomatic adults is 0.5 ± 2.5 cm. As we age, gravity slowly wins the conflict, with a vertical, erect spine and an increase in the SVA, that is, the SVA moves anteriorly. To offset imbalance, regional sagittal curves in the cervical, thoracic, and lumbar spines and the lumbopelvic junction work in concert. Pathologic changes in one region lead to reciprocal changes in another in an effort to compensate and maintain optimal balance. However, these compensatory mechanisms are limited by several factors, including the pathology itself, age, and location of the primary change in sagittal contour. For instance, the more caudal the pathology along the spinal axis, the more profound the overall effect on the SVA; this is a flagpole effect derived from the length of the lever arm.

Because PI is the only spinopelvic parameter that is static, its relationship with the other pelvic and sagittal spinal parameters has been extensively studied. Most notably, LL has been shown to be directly correlated with PI. A high PI necessitates a high LL to maintain ideal sagittal alignment. Using a cohort of asymptomatic adults, Boulay et al[16] proposed a complex formula to help predict the amount of LL. Schwab et al[17] simplified it as follows: LL = PI + 9 degrees ($\pm$9 degrees). This relationship is valuable when planning deformity surgical correction in the sagittal plane. It helps a surgeon to estimate the required amount of LL to match PI and achieve alignment in a patient's sagittal profile. Lafage et al[18] studied multilinear models based on a group of 219 adults with spine deformity and showed that thoracic kyphosis (TK), which is modifiable during deformity reconstruction, along with LL (modifiable) and PI (fixed), sagittal balance can be predicted in greater than 80% of cases. Additionally, Rose et al[19] examined the relationship between PI and LL in the setting of adult deformity and included TK. They reported the relationship of PI + LL + TK $\leq$45 degrees to be 91% sensitive for predicting ideal sagittal alignment.[20]

Recently, interest in the role of PT has increased, especially in the setting of spinal deformity.[8] PT is a dynamic parameter that changes through rotation about the hip axis. In the setting of sagittal malalignment or imbalance, retroversion of the pelvis is a compensatory mechanism that is reflected by an increased PT.[8,21] This compensatory retroversion requires hip extension and becomes more difficult as a person ages, secondary to osteoarthritis and decreased muscle forces about the pelvis. This increased awareness in PT is necessary to help explain the dynamic changes that occur in the pelvis and unfused spinal segments after sagittal realignment reconstructive procedures such as pedicle subtraction osteotomies. Lafage et al[18,22] incorporated PT to help predict SVA after a single-level pedicle subtraction osteotomy. In a comparison of five predictive formulas, the two Lafage formulas were found to predict postoperative SVA with the greatest accuracy[20]:

$$SVA = -52.87 + 5.90 \times PI - 5.13 \times (\text{maximal lumbar lordosis}) - 4.45 \times PT - 2.09 \times (\text{maximal thoracic kyphosis}) + 0.566 \times (\text{age})$$

$$PT = 1.14 + 0.71 \times (PI) - 0.52 \times (\text{maximal lumbar lordosis}) - 0.19 \times (\text{maximal thoracic kyphosis})$$

RELATIONSHIP BETWEEN SPINOPELVIC PARAMETERS AND SPECIFIC SPINAL DISEASES

The influence of spinopelvic parameters on isthmic spondylolisthesis has been studied in detail.[23-28] The role of PI and slip progression in patients with isthmic spondylolisthesis was first reported after studies showed that slip progression correlated poorly with the grade of spondylolisthesis.[28,29] A plausible biomechanical explanation is that a high PI tends toward a high LL, which places a high shear stress at the L5-S1 pars interarticularis, resulting in the defect. SS is increased in grade I to III slips but then decreases in grade IV and V slips as a compensatory mechanism; the pelvis retroverts in an attempt to balance the spine (Fig. 4-1). Hresko et al[30] classified high-grade patients with isthmic spondylolisthesis into two distinct groups based on SS and PT: a balanced group and an unbalanced group. The balanced group had near-normal pelvic parameters (low PT, high SS) and may tolerate less of a reduction, whereas the unbalanced group (high PT, low SS) comprised the patients who tried to compensate by retroverting the pelvis, resulting in increased lumbosacral kyphosis. The latter cohort required normalization of their pelvic parameters to achieve an optimal surgical outcome.[30,31] Overall, evidence suggested that an abnormally elevated PI contributes to the development, progression, and severity of isthmic spondylolisthesis.

Abnormal spinopelvic parameters have been implicated in several degenerative conditions such as chronic low back pain, lumbar degenerative disc disease, degenerative spondylolisthesis, and hip osteoarthritis.[15,32,33] Jackson and McManus[15] compared patients with chronic low back pain to asymptomatic, age-matched controls. They found that low back patients had less lumbar lordosis (56.3 versus 60.9 degrees), less sacral slope (47.2 versus 50.4 degrees), and more hip extension, but overall SVA and TK were comparable. This

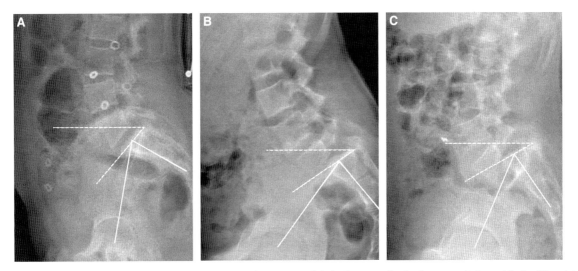

Fig. 4-1   **A** and **B**, Lateral radiographs showing isthmic spondylolisthesis and a higher sacral slope *(dashed lines)* in a Meyerding grade I patient and a Meyerding grade II patient, respectively. **C,** Sacral slope decreases as lumbar lordosis increases in a Meyerding grade IV patient as the pelvis retroverts in an attempt to balance the spine. The angle represented by the *solid lines* is the pelvic incidence.

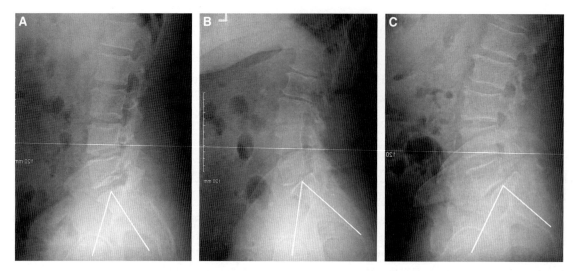

Fig. 4-2   Lateral radiographs of **A,** a patient with disc herniation, **B,** a patient with degenerative disc disease with mechanical disc collapse, and **C,** a patient with degenerative spondylolisthesis, respectively. The patient with degenerative spondylolisthesis has the highest pelvic incidence.

study helps to explain age-related versus pathologic changes and shows that compensation for the decreased lumbar lordosis comes by retroverting the pelvis (low SS) and extending the hips. In an age-matched comparison of three degenerative process (disc herniation, degenerative disc disease, and degenerative spondylolisthesis), Barrey et al[32] evaluated the relationship of PI and spinopelvic alignment. SS and LL were decreased in all three groups, consistent with the findings in the low back pain cohort discussed previously. PI was elevated in the degenerative spondylolisthesis group (60.0 degrees) but normal in both the disc herniation group (49.8 degrees) and degenerative disc disease (51.6 degrees) group, suggesting that a higher PI may predispose to development of degenerative spondylolisthesis (Fig. 4-2). In a long-term prospective observational study, Aono et al[34] followed 142 healthy, perimenopausal women without spine disease for over 8 years. The incidence of newly developed degenerative spondylolisthesis was 12.7%. These patients had an abnormally high baseline LL and PI. The multivariate analysis confirmed that PI was an independent risk factor. Yoshimoto et al[33] evaluated spinopelvic parameters in patients with low back pain and hip osteoarthritis and found that PI was greater in the latter cohort. They concluded that an abnormally high PI at a young age may contribute to osteoarthritis later in life because of anterior acetabulum uncovering.

Several studies investigating fixed sagittal imbalance or sagittal decompensation after lumbar spinal fusion enhanced our understanding of the relationship between pelvic parameters and adult deformity. Cho et al[35] noted a difference in PI between patients who maintained sagittal alignment versus patients who decompensated. The latter cohort had less LL, a greater incidence of pseudarthrosis, implant failure, and adjacent-segment disease. Similarly, Gottfried et al[36] described a characteristic spinopelvic profile in patients who developed fixed sagittal imbalance after lumbar spinal fusion. These patients had a high PI and reduced LL, attempting to compensate with reduced TK and increased pelvic retroversion (high PT). Fixed sagittal imbalance becomes more evident after fusion, because these patients have an iatrogenically induced inability to compensate by increasing LL[28] (Fig. 4-3). These two studies highlighted the importance of recognizing the presence of a PI-LL mismatch and planning appropriately for lumbar arthrodesis. Other causes of fixed sagittal imbalance have been shown to correlate with abnormal PI, including posttraumatic kyphosis, junctional kyphosis in Scheuermann's kyphosis, and kyphosis in ankylosing spondylitis.[37-39] A patient with a kyphotic deformity after a burst fracture can compensate by increasing LL, but only within the limits of the PI.[38] Sagittal decompensation will develop if more LL is required than that allowed by the PI. Debarge et al[37] found that patients with ankylosing spondylitis and symptomatic kyphotic deformities

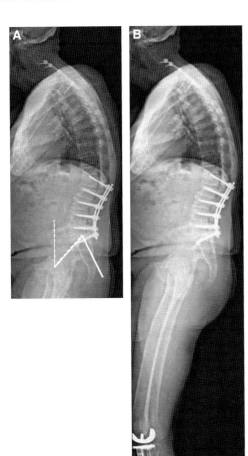

Fig. 4-3 **A,** Lateral radiograph of a patient with fixed sagittal imbalance with a large lumbar lordosis–pelvic incidence mismatch. **B,** The patient is attempting to compensate by retroverting the pelvis. This results in a large pelvic tilt, knee flexion, and hyperextension of the cervical spine.

had a higher PI compared with controls (61 versus 51 degrees).[28] Similar to patients with iatrogenic lumbar fusions, patients with autofusion can no longer compensate by increasing lumbar lordosis, and they subsequently decompensate. Lonner et al[39] showed that a third of patients who had surgery for Scheuermann's kyphosis developed junctional kyphosis, and the extent directly correlated with the magnitude of elevated PI.

Hong et al[40] reported a correlation between coronal deformity (Cobb angle) and spinopelvic parameters. They studied 108 elderly patients with adult degenerative scoliosis and grouped them according to coronal curve severity as follows: normal (Cobb angle less than 10 degrees), low grade (Cobb angle of 10 to 19 degrees), and high grade (Cobb angle of at least 20 degrees). They observed a significant difference for PI between the three groups and concluded that PI, PT, and S1 overhang are correlated with the magnitude of curvature in the coronal plane. (S1 overhang is the distance between the bicoxofemoral axis and the midpoint of the sacral endplate. Trigonometrically, it is in the PI.) They did not discuss the tighter correlation between PI and SVA in their results, which is better explained by the magnitude of the three-dimensional deformity reflected by the degree of coronal deformity measured.

Patients with adolescent idiopathic scoliosis, regardless of curve type, have a higher PI.[28,41-43] This is more extensively reported in adult scoliosis patients. Mac-Thiong et al[42] and Charlebois et al[44] both reported that PI determined LL but had less of an impact on other curve parameters. Overall, it is unclear whether PI plays a critical role in the development and/or progression of adolescent idiopathic scoliosis.

CORRELATION BETWEEN SPINOPELVIC PARAMETERS AND HEALTH-RELATED QUALITY OF LIFE

It has become increasingly evident that preoperative and postoperative outcomes or patient-reported HRQOL outcomes are affected by spinopelvic parameters. In 2000 Lazennec et al[45] performed one of the first studies to highlight this concept. They observed poor outcomes in patients with iatrogenic flat-back after lumbar fusion procedures. Eighty-one patients were evaluated before and after lumbosacral arthrodesis and were grouped as those with and those without pain. The patients with persistent back pain had a more vertical sacrum-pelvis with a decreased SS and an increased PT. The PT in the postfusion pain cohort was nearly double the normal value and significantly correlated with pain ($p = 0.0003$). The authors concluded that failing to correct or inducing excessive pelvic retroversion produces a sagittal alignment that replicates the sitting position and is accompanied by loss of LL, which is associated with chronic pain. After using more sophisticated HRQOL measures, Glassman et al[46,47] published their two landmark studies showing that sagittal balance (SVA) was the single most important driver of good outcomes in adult spinal deformity patients in the preoperative and postoperative settings. Subsequent studies have confirmed the importance of a proper sagittal profile not only in spinal deformity but in other spinal pathologies.[15,17,32,33] The studies discussed previously are responsible for encouraging the modern era of spinal alignment analysis to focus on spinopelvic parameters. As discussed earlier in the chapter, understanding the pelvis as the foundation of the spine is critical in determining overall spinal balance and alignment. Similar to performing osteotomies more caudally along the spinal axis, the pelvis provides a very powerful point for overall balance and alignment optimization. Clinically optimal sagittal alignment centers the head over the pelvis, restores level gaze, and creates ergonomically efficient standing and walking mechanics.

Ames et al[48] have popularized the previously mentioned formula based on the work of Duval-Beaupère et al[6] and Boulay et al[16] $LL = PI + 9 (\pm 9)$, and they have shown that it correlates not only with HRQOL outcomes but also with the success of realignment osteotomies. Similarly, the *Rose-Kim sagittal ideal* of PI + LL + TK ≤45 showed a 91% sensitivity for predicting ideal sagittal alignment at 2 years in a consecutive series of 40 pedicle subtraction osteotomies.[19] With a slightly more complicated model, Neal et al[49] used an age-matched adjustment derived from the work of Kuntz et al[50] on normative values to evaluate the ability to predict ideal spinopelvic alignment in a series of 41 spinal deformity patients. They devised the formula $r = PI/(LL + TK)$ to calculate a constant (r) for adult (18 to 60 years) and geriatric (older than 60 years) patients. Patients in both sagittal and spinopelvic balance had significantly better HRQOL outcomes. Overall, these relationships are becoming increasingly understood, and the equations are useful for surgical guidance, not as rules, and should be applied in context to the overall balance and alignment pathology.

Major realignment procedures have potential complications. Kim et al[51] recently showed that excessive lordosis and large SVA corrections led to proximal junctional kyphosis with subsequently worse HRQOL outcomes. They pointed out that although age has consistently been reported as a risk factor for proximal junctional kyphosis, normative data for age are lacking. For instance, the correction goal in LL and SVA in a 70-year-old versus that in a 50-year-old should not be the same.

More recently, an interest in the correlation of PT and HRQOL outcomes has emerged. In a series of 125 adult deformity patients, Lafage et al[21] reported a high correlation between PT (pelvic retroversion) (0.28 <r <0.42) and SVA (r = 0.64, p <0.001) with HRQOL outcome scores. Accordingly, Schwab et al[17] proposed threshold values of spinopelvic parameters using retrospectively collected HRQOL and radiographic data to be used in surgical planning to optimize satisfactory HRQOL outcomes. Schwab et al[52] performed a larger, prospective, multicenter study with 492 consecutive patients that compared nonoperative versus operative treatment in adult spinal deformity. They found that SVA, PT, and PI-LL were the parameters most strongly correlated with disability. A relative risk analysis revealed that patients with PI-LL mismatch had a 4.2-fold greater risk of pelvic retroversion (PT), a 10.9-fold greater risk of positive sagittal malalignment (SVA), and a 3.9-fold greater risk of severe disability. Linear regression models were employed to establish thresholds of radiographic spinopelvic parameters predictive of poor HRQOL outcomes, specifically using an Oswestry Disability Index (ODI) greater than 40. They suggested that a PT of at least 22 degrees, an SVA of at least 47 mm, and PI-LL of at least 11 degrees were predictive of disability and should help to guide patient assessment.

CONCLUSION

Arguably the largest advancements in the setting of spinal surgery over the last two decades have been the introduction of patient-centered HRQOL outcome measures and attention to the sagittal spinal profile, specifically spinopelvic parameters. Evolution of the understanding of the sagittal spinopelvic parameters has no doubt been motivated by optimization of HRQOL outcomes. Although there is more work to be done, we have made great strides in our comprehension of the vital role occupied by the *pelvic vertebra* and its relationship with the spine. Future direction will include *taking another step back* and looking at total body balance and the role played by the spine in our endless pursuit of an everlasting antigravity erect posture.

REFERENCES

1. Berge C. Heterochronic processes in human evolution: an ontogenetic analysis of the hominid pelvis. Am J Phys Anthropol 105:441-459, 1998.
2. Le Huec JC, Aunoble S, Philippe L, et al. Pelvic parameters: origin and significance. Eur Spine J 20(Suppl 5):S564-S571, 2011.
3. Dubousset J. Three-dimensional analysis of the scoliotic deformity. In Weinstein SL, ed. The Pediatric Spine Principles and Practice. New York: Raven Press, 1994.
4. Dubousset J, Charpak G, Dorion I, et al. Le système EOS. Nouvel imagerie ostéo-articulaire basse dose en position debout. e-mémoires de l'Académie Nationale de Chirurgie 4:22-27, 2005.
5. During J, Goudfrooij H, Keessen W, et al. Toward standards for posture. Postural characteristics of the lower back system in normal and pathologic conditions. Spine 10:83-87, 1985.
6. Duval-Beaupère G, Schmidt C, Cosson P. A Barycentremetric study of the sagittal shape of spine and pelvis: the conditions required for an economic standing position. Ann Biomed Eng 20:451-462, 1992.
7. Jackson RP, Kanemura T, Kawakami N, et al. Lumbopelvic lordosis and pelvic balance on repeated standing lateral radiographs of adult volunteers and untreated patients with constant low back pain. Spine 25:575-586, 2000.
8. Schwab F, Lafage V, Patel A, et al. Sagittal plane considerations and the pelvis in the adult patient. Spine 34:1828-1833, 2009.
9. Mangione P, Sénégas J. [Sagittal balance of the spine] Rev Chir Orthop Reparatrice Appar Mot 83:22-32, 1997.
10. Marty C, Boisaubert B, Descamps H, et al. The sagittal anatomy of the sacrum among young adults, infants, and spondylolisthesis patients. Eur Spine J 11:119-125, 2002.
11. Descamps H, Commare-Nordmann MC, Marty C, et al. Modifications des angles pelviens, dont l'incidence, au cours de la croissance humaine. Biom Hum Anthropol 17:59-63, 1999.
12. Mac-Thiong JM, Berthonnaud E, Dimar JR II, et al. Sagittal alignment of the spine and pelvis during growth. Spine 29:1642-1647, 2004.
13. Berthonnaud E, Labelle H, Roussouly P, et al. A variability study of computerized sagittal spinopelvic radiologic measurements of trunk balance. J Spinal Disord Tech 18:66-71, 2005.
14. Berthonnaud E, Dimnet J, Roussouly P, et al. Analysis of the sagittal balance of the spine and pelvis using shape and orientation parameters. J Spinal Disord Tech 18:40-47, 2005.
15. Jackson RP, McManus AC. Radiographic analysis of sagittal plane alignment and balance in standing volunteers and patients with low back pain matched for age, sex, and size. A prospective controlled clinical study. Spine 19:1611-1618, 1994.
16. Boulay C, Tardieu C, Hecquet J, et al. Sagittal alignment of spine and pelvis regulated by pelvic incidence: standard values and prediction of lordosis. Eur Spine J 15:415-422, 2006.
17. Schwab F, Patel A, Ungar B, et al. Adult spinal deformity-postoperative standing imbalance: how much can you tolerate? An overview of key parameters in assessing alignment and planning corrective surgery. Spine 35:2224-2231, 2010.

18. Lafage V, Schwab F, Vira S, et al. Spino-pelvic parameters after surgery can be predicted: a preliminary formula and validation of standing alignment. Spine 36:1037-1045, 2011.

19. Rose PS, Bridwell KH, Lenke LG, et al. Role of pelvic incidence, thoracic kyphosis, and patient factors on sagittal plane correction following pedicle subtraction osteotomy. Spine 34:785-791, 2009.

20. Smith JS, Bess S, Shaffrey CI, et al; International Spine Study Group. Dynamic changes of the pelvis and spine are key to predicting postoperative sagittal alignment after pedicle subtraction osteotomy: a critical analysis of preoperative planning techniques. Spine 37:845-853, 2012.

21. Lafage V, Schwab F, Patel A, et al. Pelvic tilt and truncal inclination: two key radiographic parameters in the setting of adults with spinal deformity. Spine 34:E599-E606, 2009.

22. Lafage V, Bharucha NJ, Schwab F, et al. Multicenter validation of a formula predicting postoperative spinopelvic alignment. J Neurosurg Spine 16:15-21, 2012.

23. Hanson DS, Bridwell KH, Rhee JM, et al. Correlation of pelvic incidence with low- and high-grade isthmic spondylolisthesis. Spine 27:2026-2029, 2002.

24. Huang RP, Bohlman HH, Thompson GH, et al. Predictive value of pelvic incidence in progression of spondylolisthesis. Spine 8:2381-2385, 2003.

25. Jackson RP, Phipps T, Hales C, et al. Pelvic lordosis and alignment in spondylolisthesis. Spine 28:151-160, 2003.

26. Vialle R, Ilharreborde B, Dauzac C, et al. Is there a sagittal imbalance of the spine in isthmic spondylolisthesis? A correlation study. Eur Spine J 16:1641-1649, 2007.

27. Mac-Thiong JM, Wang Z, de Guise JA, et al. Postural model of sagittal spino-pelvic alignment and its relevance for lumbosacral developmental spondylolisthesis. Spine 33:2316-2325, 2008.

28. Mehta VA, Amin A, Omeis I, et al. Implications of spinopelvic alignment for the spine surgeon. Neurosurgery 70:707-721, 2012.

29. Curylo LJ, Edwards C, DeWald RW. Radiographic markers in spondyloptosis: implications for spondylolisthesis progression. Spine 27:2021-2025, 2002.

30. Hresko MT, Hirschfeld R, Buerk AA, et al. The effect of reduction and instrumentation of spondylolisthesis on spinopelvic sagittal alignment. J Pediatr Orthop 29:157-162, 2009.

31. Labelle H, Roussouly P, Chopin D, et al. Spino-pelvic alignment after surgical correction for developmental spondylolisthesis. Eur Spine J 17:1170-1176, 2008.

32. Barrey C, Jund J, Noseda O, et al. Sagittal balance of the pelvis-spine complex and lumbar degenerative diseases. A comparative study about 85 cases. Eur Spine J 16:1459-1467, 2007.

33. Yoshimoto H, Sato S, Masuda T, et al. Spinopelvic alignment in patients with osteoarthrosis of the hip: a radiographic comparison to patients with low back pain. Spine 30:1650-1657, 2005.

34. Aono K, Kobayashi T, Jimbo S, et al. Radiographic analysis of newly developed degenerative spondylolisthesis in a mean twelve-year prospective study. Spine 35:887-891, 2010.

35. Cho KJ, Suk SI, Park SR, et al. Risk factors of sagittal decompensation after long posterior instrumentation and fusion for degenerative lumbar scoliosis. Spine 35:1595-1601, 2010.

36. Gottfried ON, Daubs MD, Patel AA, et al. Spinopelvic parameters in postfusion flatback deformity patients. Spine J 9:639-647, 2009.

37. Debarge R, Demey G, Roussouly P. Radiological analysis of ankylosing spondylitis patients with severe kyphosis before and after pedicle subtraction osteotomy. Eur Spine J 19:65-70, 2010.

38. Koller H, Acosta F, Hempfing A, et al. Long-term investigation of nonsurgical treatment for thoracolumbar and lumbar burst fractures: an outcome analysis in sight of spinopelvic balance. Eur Spine J 17:1073-1095, 2008.

39. Lonner BS, Newton P, Betz R, et al. Operative management of Scheuermann's kyphosis in 78 patients: radiographic outcomes, complications, and technique. Spine 32:2644-2652, 2007.

40. Hong JY, Suh SW, Modi HN, et al. Correlation of pelvic orientation with adult scoliosis. J Spinal Disord Tech 23:461-466, 2010.

41. Lonner BS, Auerbach JD, Sponseller P, et al. Variations in pelvic and other sagittal spinal parameters as a function of race in adolescent idiopathic scoliosis. Spine 35:E374-E377, 2010.

42. Mac-Thiong JM, Labelle H, Charlebois M, et al. Sagittal plane analysis of the spine and pelvis in adolescent idiopathic scoliosis according to the coronal curve type. Spine 28:1404-1409, 2003.

43. Upasani VV, Tis J, Bastrom T, et al. Analysis of sagittal alignment in thoracic and thoracolumbar curves in adolescent idiopathic scoliosis: how do these two curve types differ? Spine 32:1355-1359, 2007.

44. Charlebois M, Mac-Thiong JM, Huot MP, et al. Relation between the pelvis and the sagittal profile in adolescent idiopathic scoliosis: the influence of curve type. Stud Health Technol Inform 91:140-143, 2002.

45. Lazennec JY, Ramaré S, Arafati N, et al. Sagittal alignment in lumbosacral fusion: relations between radiological parameters and pain. Eur Spine J 9:47-55, 2000.

46. Glassman SD, Bridwell K, Dimar JR, et al. The impact of positive sagittal balance in adult spinal deformity. Spine 30:2024-2029, 2005.

47. Glassman SD, Berven S, Bridwell K, et al. Correlation of radiographic parameters and clinical symptoms in adult scoliosis. Spine 30:682-688, 2005.

48. Ames CP, Smith JS, Scheer JK, et al. Impact of spinopelvic alignment on decision making in deformity surgery in adults: a review. J Neurosurg Spine 16:547-564, 2012.

49. Neal CJ, McClendon J, Halpin R, et al. Predicting ideal spinopelvic balance in adult spinal deformity. J Neurosurg Spine 15:82-91, 2011.

50. Kuntz C IV, Shaffrey CI, Ondra SL, et al. Spinal deformity: a new classification derived from neutral upright spinal alignment measurements in asymptomatic juvenile, adolescent, adult, and geriatric individuals. Neurosurgery 63(3 Suppl):S25-S39, 2008.

51. Kim HJ, Bridwell KH, Lenke LG, et al. Patients with proximal junctional kyphosis requiring revision surgery have higher postoperative lumbar lordosis and larger sagittal balance corrections. Spine 39:E576-E580, 2014.

52. Schwab FJ, Blondel B, Bess S, et al; International Spine Study Group (ISSG). Radiographical spinopelvic parameters and disability in the setting of adult spinal deformity: a prospective multicenter analysis. Spine 38:E803-E812, 2013.

5

Neurodegenerative Spinal Deformity in Adults

Themistocles S. Protopsaltis ▪ *Anthony J. Boniello*
Emmanuelle Ferrero ▪ *Frank J. Schwab*

Neurodegeneration is an umbrella term that encompasses a range of pathologies caused by the progressive loss of structure or function of neurons, including the death of neurons. Patients with neurodegeneration present with variable symptoms related to cognitive impairment and postural and motor dysfunction. Neurodegenerative diseases that present with postural deformities and concurrent motor dysfunction include Parkinson's disease, multiple sclerosis, multiple system atrophy, myopathy, myositis, dystonia, and amyotrophic lateral sclerosis. Examples of disabling postural deformities frequently observed in this population include camptocormia, anterocollis, Pisa syndrome, and scoliosis. Given the prevalence of Parkinson's disease and the limited reports in the literature regarding spine surgery for other neurodegenerative disorders, we will highlight the surgical treatment of Parkinson's patients who have spinal deformities to explain how the approach and treatment differ from those of routine adult scoliosis patients. Patients with neurodegenerative disease and spinal deformity present unique challenges and have increased rates of complications and reoperations.

EPIDEMIOLOGY

Parkinson's disease is the second most common neurodegenerative disorder after Alzheimer's disease.[1] The prevalence of Parkinson's disease is about 0.3% in industrialized countries, rising from 1% in those over 60 years of age to 4% in those over 80 years of age.[1] From 2001 to 2010, thoracolumbar spinal fusion was performed in 1,347,359 patients (ICD9 8104-8108, 8134-8138) in the U.S. National Inpatient Sample (NIS) database, representing 20% of weighted U.S. hospitalizations. Of these patients, 146,268 (10.9%) were diagnosed with Parkinson's disease.

SPINAL DEFORMITY IN THE SETTING OF PARKINSON'S DISEASE

Postural deformities are frequent and disabling complications of Parkinson's disease. An accurate differentiation of these conditions during a diagnostic workup is critical, because treatment options vary considerably. This section describes the most frequently seen postural deformities, including anterocollis, Pisa syndrome, scoliosis, and camptocormia.[2] Clear diagnostic criteria are provided to aid in diagnosis.

Patients with anterocollis, or dropped-head syndrome, have a significant anteriorly leaning neck position in the sagittal plane, while in a neutral posture (Fig. 5-1). This anterior translation occurs as a minimum of 45 degrees of cervical flexion, which can be partially overcome by voluntary or passive movement, that is, patients are unable to fully extend the neck against gravity but are able to exert force against the resistance

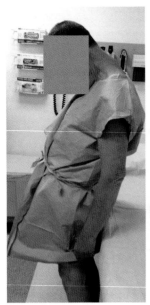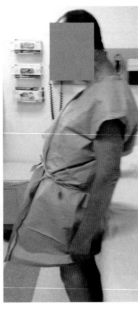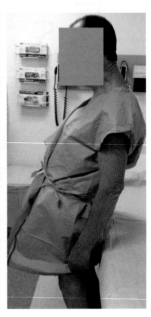

Fig. 5-1   This Parkinson's patient has anterocollis, as shown in a sagittal profile in flexion, neutral, and extension (from left to right). He has marked flexion in a neutral position, which can be partially overcome with voluntary extension.

of the examiner's hand.[2-4] The mechanism of dropped head in Parkinson's disease is considered to result from either dystonia of flexor neck muscles or weakness of extensor neck muscles.[5] Anterocollis develops in 5% to 6% of Parkinson's patients.[5-7]

Pisa syndrome is similar to anterocollis; however, the deformity involves the thoracolumbar region and occurs mostly in the coronal plane. The syndrome derives its name from the lateral lean (similar to that of the Tower of Pisa in Italy) that patients assume while in a neutral posture (Fig. 5-2). A minimum of 10 degrees of lateral thoracic flexion can be almost completely alleviated by passive mobilization or supine positioning.[2,8,9] Pisa syndrome is often idiopathic; however, its development in the absence of neurodegenerative disorders is associated commonly with neuroleptic treatment.[9] It has been proposed that Pisa syndrome might be a precursor to the development of scoliosis in Parkinson's.[2] Two percent of Parkinson's patients develop Pisa syndrome.[8]

Scoliosis is defined in the general population as curvature of the spine of at least 10 degrees, as measured by the Cobb method, and radiographic evidence of axial vertebral rotation[2,10] (Fig. 5-3). The pathophysiology of scoliosis in Parkinson's patients remains a great mystery. The risk of developing scoliosis is not related to L-dopa (or levodopa) treatment, the clinical manifestations of Parkinson's disease, or the severity of parkinsonian symptoms.[11] Furthermore, the direction of scoliosis convexity is not related to the laterality of initial parkinsonian symptoms.[11] Scoliosis is more common in Parkinson's patients (range 43% to 90%)[11-14] than in the general elderly population (range 6% to 30%).[11,15,16]

Camptocormia, derived from the Greek words *camptos* (bent) and *kormos* (trunk), is also known as *bent spine syndrome*.[17] Patients present with a significant anterior truncal flexion. Camptocormia is defined as a minimum of 45 degrees of thoracolumbar flexion in the sagittal plane that resolves almost completely when the patient is in a supine position[2,17-19] (Fig. 5-4). Originally described as a psychogenic disorder that was prevalent in World War I veterans of trench warfare,[20] camptocormia is now considered to be idiopathic or secondary to neuromuscular disease. Camptocormia secondary to a neuromuscular disorder is caused by axial dystonia.[21] It can be diagnosed by the use of EMG, demonstrating denervation of the paravertebral muscles; elevated creatinine kinase levels; a muscle biopsy, indicating extensive endomysial fibrosis and fat tissue with irregular degenerated fibers; and/or MRI that shows fatty infiltration of paravertebral muscles.[21] Camptocormia occurs in 3% to 17.6% of Parkinson's patients.[22-25]

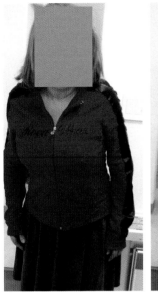
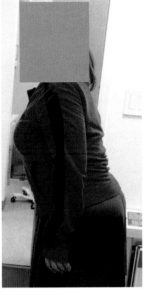

Fig. 5-2 This Parkinson's patient has Pisa syndrome. She has significant coronal thoraco-lumbar deformity with lateral flexion.

Fig. 5-3 AP and lateral radiographs of this 64-year-old woman with Parkinson's disease reveal coronal and sagittal deformities. Deep brain stimulation wires and batteries are evident.

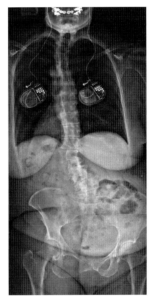
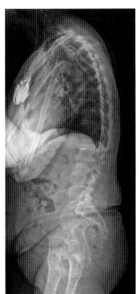

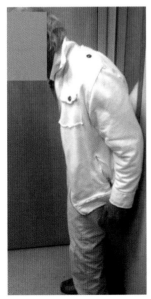
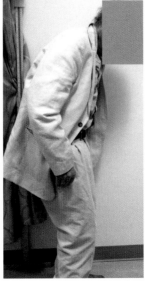

Fig. 5-4 This Parkinson's patient has camptocormia. His sagittal deformity corrects when he assumes a supine position.

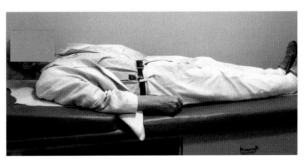

TREATMENT

CONSERVATIVE TREATMENT

Conservative management of spinal deformity in the setting of neuromuscular disease generally involves identification and maximization of the treatment of all potential underlying causes. Levodopa is effective for the treatment of parkinsonism symptoms such as rigidity and akinesia. However, levodopa has been found to worsen camptocormia and Pisa syndrome in some Parkinson's patients.[26,27] Conservative treatment modalities directed toward spinal disorders include bracing, injections, and physical therapy. Although deep brain stimulation is a surgical procedure, it is less invasive than spinal deformity correction and has been proposed as a precursor to all spine surgery procedures.[26,28-35] In this procedure, electrodes are implanted into the subthalamic nucleus or the globus pallidus internus.[35] In a review of deep brain stimulation performed to treat patients with camptocormia (in which data from nine reports were assessed), 16 of 24 patients (66.7%) with subthalamic nucleus stimulation showed categorical improvement of camptocormia (improved thoracolumbar angle), whereas two patients with globus pallidus internus stimulation showed improvement.[26]

Bracing with thoracopelvic anterior distraction (TPAD) involves an orthosis comprising two belts that encircle the pelvis and thorax and are linked by an anterior support.[36] A prospective case series reviewed 15 patients with camptocormia secondary to Parkinson's disease, Steinert's myopathy, and/or vertebral settling, who were treated with a TPAD orthosis.[36] At 90 days, patients benefited from a decrease in mean C7-S1 sagittal vertical alignment (SVA) from 18.3 to 7 cm ($p < 0.01$), a reduction on the VAS pain scale of 70% ($p < 0.01$), and an increase on the VAS quality of life scale of 92% ($p < 0.01$). Despite reported benefits, compliance was a challenge.

Botulinum toxin (BTX) A injections into the iliopsoas muscle guided by ultrasound (500 to 1500 mouse units [MU] per side) in 4- to 6-month intervals did not have favorable results.[37] In a small case series of three Parkinson's patients with camptocormia, the authors reported a clinical benefit in one patient based on improvement in posture, as measured by height.[37]

Lidocaine injection into the external oblique muscle has shown transient improvement in posture.[38] Eight of 12 patients (66.7%) with camptocormia showed improvement 90 days after the beginning of treatment (a single injection), and 9 of 12 patients (75%) showed improvement after repeated lidocaine injections.[38] The mean flexion angle decreased with repeated injections from 62.1 ± 13.4 to 49.0 ± 18.5 degrees ($p = 0.005$) at 90 days.[38]

OPERATIVE TREATMENT

Operative management can be categorized into short- and long-fusion constructs. Surgical treatment of Parkinson's patients requires consideration of many factors. For example, these patients have an inherent festinating gait, making postoperative rehabilitation difficult. Patients and physicians report a lack of motivation to ambulate in this population.[39] Parkinson's patients have shorter life expectancies and considerable disability with dramatic spinal deformities. Bone anchorage is an issue of great concern because of the high rate of osteoporosis. One study reported that 34% of Parkinson's patients were osteoporotic.[15] These challenges need to be considered when a spine surgery is contemplated.

Parkinson's patients often have major deformities that are localized to the thoracolumbar region. Alignment goals are frequently difficult to define, because patients have limited compensatory reserve. They generally are less able to compensate with pelvic retroversion or thoracic hypokyphosis, resulting in large sagittal deformities without increased pelvic tilt. Therefore the surgical goals should aim for optimal correction of the spinopelvic alignment parameters as follows: a pelvic tilt of less than 25 degrees,[40] C7-S1 sagittal vertical alignment of less than 50 mm,[40,41] a pelvic incidence minus lumbar lordosis of less than 10 degrees,[42-44] and a T1 pelvic angle of less than 20 degrees.[45] A T1 pelvic angle is defined as an angle formed by a line from the center of T1 to the femoral heads and a line from the femoral heads to the center of the S1 endplate.[46]

In a review of the challenges of spine surgery in Parkinson's patients, Upadhyaya et al[26] recommended that patients with camptocormia be evaluated for deep brain stimulation before spine surgery. The authors contended that spine surgery is not recommended for Parkinson's patients without radiculopathy or myelopathy because of the high rate of complications in this population. They recommended decompressions and fusions for patients with myelopathy or radiculopathy without motor fluctuations in whom nonoperative treatment was unsuccessful. The authors defined motor fluctuations as transient abnormal truncal postures associated with fluctuating expression of dystonia. Short-fusion constructs and decompressions were recommended for patients less motivated to walk, whereas long-fusion constructs and major deformity correction were suggested in patients who are highly motivated to walk and have minimal major comorbidities.

POTENTIAL COMPLICATIONS AND MANAGEMENT

Parkinson's patients are medically fragile and susceptible to commonly reported risks of spine surgery. They have higher rates of medical complications such as postoperative delirium, epidural hematomas, pulmonary emboli, cardiac events, and transfusion-related events. They also have high rates of surgical complications such as instrumentation failure, proximal junctional kyphosis (PJK), and adjacent-segment disease.

POSTOPERATIVE DELIRIUM

Postoperative delirium is a common and potentially dangerous condition for this patient population. One study in patients who had orthopedic procedures reported that in the general population postoperative delirium can increase other postoperative complications ($p = 0.01$), increasing the length of stay by about 1½ days.[46] Katus and Shtilbans[47] compared preoperative baseline scores on a Stamford Health Assessment Questionnaire with those obtained at 6 months and found that delirious patients were less likely to improve in function by 6 months postoperatively ($t = 6.43$, $p < 0.001$). Parkinson's patients have an increased risk of postoperative delirium and the attendant increase in other complications. The rate of postoperative delirium in the general population was 8.4 per 1000 patients having lumbar spine surgery versus 66.7% in a study of Parkinson's patients undergoing major spine surgery.[39,48]

INSTRUMENTATION FAILURE

The rate of instrumentation failures is reported to be as high as 29% to 33.3%.[39,49] Parkinson's patients are at increased risk of this complication, because the higher rate of osteoporosis and the nature of the neuromuscular disease itself create a relentless drive to forward sagittal tilting and place stress on the instrumentation construct.[39]

PROXIMAL JUNCTIONAL KYPHOSIS

According to the limited series in the literature, rates are high for revision surgery to treat PJK in Parkinson's patients after spine surgery.[39,50] The studies that report revisions because of PJK are relatively small case series, and most do not report the total rate of PJK. Babat et al[49] reported that 79% of patients who had any type of spine surgery required a reoperation to correct kyphosis or segmental instability at the operated or adjacent level. The higher rate of revision for PJK was probably a result of the higher rate of osteoporosis and the neuromuscular disease itself, which is more likely to result in major global deformity after PJK. Koller et al[50] reported a revision rate of 34.7%, with a revision rate for PJK of 16%. A postoperative sagittal vertical axis of more than 10 cm was found to be a risk factor for revision surgery. In 60% of the patients in the study who had an SVA of more than 10 cm, the authors attributed the loss of alignment to PJK or proximal junctional failure (PJF). The higher rate of PJK in the elderly population after long spine fusions may partly result from subclinical myopathies that can cause deformities in elderly patients to mimic those of patients with neurodegenerative disorders.[51]

REVISION SURGERY

Reported rates of revision surgery in Parkinson's patients vary from 50% to 86%.[39,49,50] Common diagnoses leading to revision surgery include instrumentation failure or pullout, proximal junctional kyphosis, adjacent-level instability, epidural hematomas, and infection.[39,49,50] The largest series of Parkinson's patients having spine surgery is a heterogenous group without consistent inclusion criteria. Some studies report a variety of cases, including simple decompressions and limited fusions in the cervical thoracic and lumbar spine, whereas others focus on patients with long fusions for deformity correction.[39,49,50] The common thread in these studies is the high rate of revision surgery regardless of the length of the fusion or the limited extent of the surgery.

REVIEW OF THE LITERATURE: SPINE SURGERY IN PARKINSON'S PATIENTS

Bourghli et al[39] reported a retrospective review of 12 consecutive Parkinson's patients with major spinal deformities who had long-segment posterior spinal fusion. The authors stated that no consensus existed regarding the management of Parkinson's patients with major spinal deformity. However, they argued for long arthrodesis because of the prevalence of osteoporosis and motor dysfunction of the spinal extensor muscles inherent in the disease. All patients were fused from T2 to the sacrum, with iliac screws and autologous graft. In revision cases, bone morphogenic protein was used. Six of 12 patients underwent pedicle subtraction osteotomy as part of the deformity correction, and a transforaminal lumbar interbody fusion was performed above and below the osteotomy level. The mean postoperative SRS-30 score was 114/150. Radiographic outcomes were excellent, with a decrease in sagittal vertical axis from 15.2 to 0.5 cm ($p < 0.0001$), an improvement in the pelvic tilt from 31 to 19 degrees, and improvement in the pelvic incidence minus lumbar lordosis from 34 to −3 degrees. Complications included eight cases (66.7%) of postoperative delirium and one pulmonary embolus. Six patients required revision (50%): three for instrumentation failure (33.3%) at the level of the pedicle subtraction osteotomy, two to correct PJK (16.7%), and one to treat an epidural hematoma.

Babat et al[49] published a retrospective review of 14 Parkinson's patients who underwent lumbar/ lumbosacral (8 patients), thoracolumbar (2 patients), and cervical (4 patients) spinal surgery. They reported a very high reoperation rate of 86%. Thirty-one revisions were performed in 12 patients. In 79% of the patients, additional procedures were needed for kyphosis or spinal instability at the operated or adjacent levels. The rate of hardware failure or pullout necessitating reoperations was 29%, and 4 patients had hardware pullout a total of 10 times. Six of 14 patients in the study had decompressions alone or uninstrumented fusions; all of these patients required revision fusions.

Koller et al[50] conducted a retrospective review of 23 Parkinson's patients treated surgically for spinal disorders. The rate of medical complications was 30.4%. These included appendicitis (1 patient), postoperative delirium (3 patients), liver decompensation with temporary hepatic encephalopathy (1 patient), pneumothorax (1 patient), akinetic crisis indicating intensive neurologic care (1 patient), and renal insufficiency (1 patient). The rate of postoperative complications was 52.2%, which included adjacent-segment collapse or fractures (17.6%), proximal junctional kyphosis (17.6%), and reoperation (58.8%).

GUIDELINES

IMMEDIATE POSTOPERATIVE GUIDELINES

Parkinson's patients are more susceptible to immobility, postoperative dysphagia, respiratory dysfunction, urinary retention, and postoperative delirium.[47] These susceptibilities lead to higher rates of pneumonia, urinary tract infections, deconditioning, and falls, compared with non-Parkinson's patients, as well as prolonged hospital stays and a greater need for rehabilitation after hospitalization.[47] Katus and Shtilbans[47] recommended limited duration of the NPO status, alternative routes of drug administration during the NPO status duration, avoidance of medications and drug interactions that can worsen parkinsonism, frequent assessment of swallowing ability, encouragement of incentive spirometry, frequent bladder scans, limited use of Foley catheters, and aggressive physical therapy. Bourghli et al[39] recommended surveillance of postoperative patients for at least 48 hours in the ICU to minimize the risk of postoperative pulmonary or cardiac complications.

LONG-TERM GUIDELINES

Because of the increased risk of postoperative complications in Parkinson's patients who have spinal fusion surgery, long-term rehabilitation is beneficial in this population. Bourghli et al[39] recommended that these patients wear a thoracolumbosacral orthosis for 3 months to prevent screw pullout, given the prevalence of osteoporosis. Aggressive physical therapy and ambulation in the postoperative period allow acclimation to new spinal alignment. Exercise has the potential to benefit both motor (gait, balance, and strength) and nonmotor (depression, apathy, fatigue, and constipation) aspects of Parkinson's disease and secondary complications of immobility (cardiovascular and osteoporosis).[52] Close follow-up with a neurology consult in the postoperative period is advisable to monitor parkinsonian symptoms and medication regimens.

PATIENT EXAMPLES

This 72-year-old man with Parkinson's disease had a past medical history significant for anxiety, depression, hyperlipidemia, and low back pain that was refractory to conservative management. At presentation the patient complained of severe lateral left leg pain that extended into his dorsal left foot, which had a partial response to targeted steroid injections. Preoperative radiographs were significant for an anteriorly displaced sagittal vertical axis, a pelvic incidence–lumbar lordosis mismatch, L2-3 retrolisthesis with degenerative disc disease, and facet arthropathy at L3-4, L4-5, and L5-S1, and foraminal stenosis (Fig. 5-5, *A* through *C*). The benefits of surgery were discussed, and the patient underwent an uneventful minimally invasive posterior spinal fusion with instrumentation and pedicle screws from L3-S1 and a left-sided laminoforaminotomy with a discectomy at L5-S1.

Two weeks postoperatively the patient had transient right thigh pain related to the surgical approach. His preoperative left leg pain had resolved. Radiographs showed excellent correction of the coronal balance and restoration of the lumbar lordosis, with hardware in good position without lucencies around the screws (Fig. 5-5, *D* through *F*). Eleven months postoperatively the patient complained of progressive back pain. He was stooping forward more and not walking regularly or participating in physical therapy. A brace had been prescribed, but compliance was difficult. Radiographs demonstrated PJK at the level above the surgery, with loss of sagittal alignment (Fig. 5-5, *G* and *H*). Twelve months postoperatively, a revision surgery was performed to extend the fusion more cephalad with posterior spinal fusion and instrumentation from T10-S1 with iliac fixation (Fig. 5-5, *I*). The surgery was completed without complications, and the patient was transferred to a subacute rehabilitation facility. Approximately 10 days after being transferred to this facility, the patient fell onto his back while attempting to get out of bed by himself. During the next 2 days, he developed progressive weakness in both legs, an inability to walk, and bowel and bladder incontinence. He was transferred to a local emergency department. An urgent MRI showed a T10 burst fracture with bony retropulsion and thoracic spinal cord compression (Fig. 5-5, *J*). Results of a neurologic examination were significant for some antigravity movement in both legs, although most was triple flexion, with an unclear amount of volitional movement. The patient was diagnosed with acute bilateral calf deep venous thrombosis.

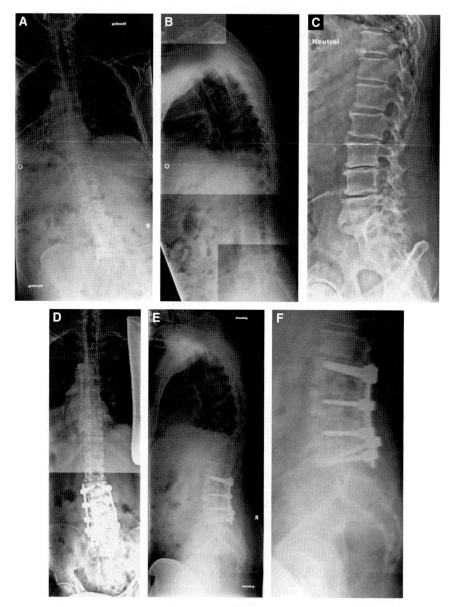

Fig. 5-5   **A** and **B,** AP and lateral radiographs of a 72-year-old man with Parkinson's disease. He had a mild degenerative scoliosis with coronal and sagittal truncal tilting. **C,** The lumbar lateral view demonstrated sacralization of the lowest lumbar vertebra. MIS fusion was performed from L3 to S1 with placement of lateral interbody cages and percutaneous screws. **D-F,** Two-week postoperative radiographs: AP and lateral scoliosis radiographs and a lateral lumbar radiograph, respectively. The patient had good correction of the sagittal and coronal plane deformities.

Thirteen days after the first revision surgery, he had a secondary revision surgery. Fusion was extended to T6, and T9-11 laminectomies were performed (Fig. 5-5, *K* and *L*). The surgery was completed without complications, and the patient was transferred to a subacute rehabilitation facility. Two months later he was discharged home, with home care established. Seven months after the second revision surgery, the patient is mostly wheelchair dependent, with full control of bowel and bladder. He has strength of 4/5 or better in his lower extremities, but he has not regained the ability to walk independently because of balance difficulty and his underlying neurodegenerative disorder.

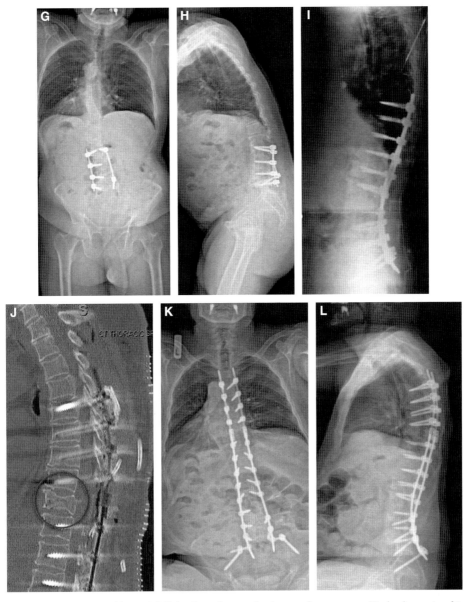

Fig. 5-5, cont'd   **G** and **H,** AP and lateral full-body radiographs 1 year after surgery. He had proximal junctional kyphosis at the L2-3 level with loss of sagittal alignment. **I,** A lateral intraoperative radiograph was obtained after revision fusion and instrumentation from T10 to S1 with iliac fixation. **J,** CT revealed a T10 burst fracture *(red circle)* sustained in a fall at a subacute nursing facility. The fracture resulted in spinal cord injury with paraplegia. The fusion was extended to T6, and T9-T11 laminectomies were performed. **K** and **L,** AP and lateral radiographs 4 months after the last revision surgery. The patient has regained strength to a score of 4/5 or better in the muscles of his lower extremities, but he is unable to walk independently because of balance difficulty and his underlying neurologic condition.

This 72-year-old woman presented with Parkinson's disease, adult scoliosis, and spinal stenosis (Fig. 5-6, *A* and *B*). The patient had an uncomplicated decompression and fusion from T2 to the sacrum, with iliac crest fixation, L4-5 and L5-S1 laminoforaminotomies, and grade II osteotomies at T10-11, T11-12, and T12-L1. At her 2-month follow-up, radiographs showed hardware in good position without lucencies around the screws (Fig. 5-6, *C* and *D*). At the 12-month follow-up, radiographs revealed PJK at T3-4 with loss of sagittal alignment (Fig. 5-6, *E* and *F*).

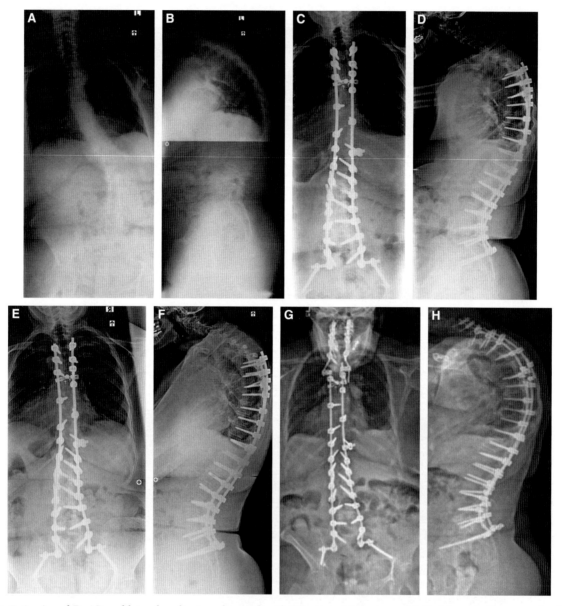

Fig. 5-6 **A** and **B,** AP and lateral scoliosis radiographs of a 72-year-old woman with Parkinson's disease and a degenerative thoracolumbar scoliosis. **C** and **D,** AP and lateral scoliosis radiographs 2 months after scoliosis correction and T4 to S1 fusion and instrumentation with iliac fixation. She had proximal junctional kyphosis, with loss of sagittal alignment at the cervicothoracic junction. **E** and **F,** AP and lateral scoliosis radiographs 1 year after scoliosis correction. Sagittal malalignment at the cervicothoracic junction had progressed. She was unable to compensate for the proximal junctional kyphosis with cervical hyperlordosis because of her underlying neurodegenerative disorder. **G** and **H,** AP and lateral scoliosis radiographs 1 year after revision surgery show extension of the fusion to C6. The cervical sagittal deformity has worsened because of the patient's underlying neurodegenerative disorder. An upper thoracic three-column osteotomy is recommended, but the patient refuses further surgical correction.

One year after her scoliosis correction surgery, an uncomplicated revision surgery was performed, involving kyphosis correction and extension of the fusion to C5, with a grade II posterior osteotomy at T3-4. Fig. 5-6, *G* and *H*, show the patient 1 year after her revision procedure. Fifteen months postoperatively the patient has worsening neck pain and further deterioration of her overall cervicothoracic alignment, with her head falling forward. She denied numbness, weakness, loss of hand dexterity, or balance difficulty. We have recommended a pedicle subtraction osteotomy at the cervicothoracic junction with extension of the fusion up to C2. However, the patient declines further surgery and chooses to continue physical therapy.

CONCLUSION

Patients with neurodegenerative disorders and spinal deformities present unique challenges to spine surgeons. Spinal deformities such as camptocormia, anterocollis, Pisa syndrome, and structural scoliosis are commonly associated with neurologic disorders, including Parkinson's disease, multiple sclerosis, multiple system atrophy, myopathy, myositis, and dystonia. A multidisciplinary approach is necessary in the care of these patients because of the high rates of medical complications. These include postoperative delirium and the need for extended care in an ICU setting. Close follow-up with a neurologic consult is recommended to optimize the medical management of neurologic disorders and to minimize postoperative metabolic encephalopathy. Compared with an average spinal deformity patient, the postoperative outcomes for these patients are fraught with higher rates of surgical complications such as instrumentation failure, PJK, and loss of correction. The high rates of PJK in our elderly population in particular may reflect subclinical, undiagnosed myopathy. Limited decompressions with or without fusions are as likely as long-fusion constructs to require revision surgery, emphasizing both the importance of tailoring surgical plans to the patients and the magnitude of the spinal deformity comorbidities. Because neurodegenerative patients have poor functional reserve and a limited ability to compensate for their spinal deformities with pelvic retroversion and thoracic hypokyphosis, the aim of major deformity corrections—when indicated—should be to optimize spinal alignment by established targets of correction.

REFERENCES

1. de Lau LM, Breteler MM. Epidemiology of Parkinson's disease. Lancet Neurol 5:525-535, 2006.
2. Doherty KM, van de Warrenburg BP, Peralta MC, et al. Postural deformities in Parkinson's disease. Lancet Neurol 10:538-549, 2011.
3. Quinn N. Disproportionate antecollis in multiple system atrophy. Lancet 1:844, 1989.
4. van de Warrenburg BP, Cordivari C, Ryan AM, et al. The phenomenon of disproportionate antecollis in Parkinson's disease and multiple system atrophy. Mov Disord 22:2325-2331, 2007.
5. Fujimoto K. Dropped head in Parkinson's disease. J Neurol 253(Suppl 7):VII21-VII26, 2006.
6. Ashour R, Jankovic J. Joint and skeletal deformities in Parkinson's disease, multiple system atrophy, and progressive supranuclear palsy. Mov Disord 21:1856-1863, 2006.
7. Kashihara K, Ohno M, Tomita S. Dropped head syndrome in Parkinson's disease. Mov Disord 21:1213-1216, 2006.
8. Bonanni L, Thomas A, Varanese S, et al. Botulinum toxin treatment of lateral axial dystonia in Parkinsonism. Mov Disord 22:2097-2103, 2006.
9. Villarejo A, Camacho A, García-Ramos R, et al. Cholinergic-dopaminergic imbalance in Pisa syndrome. Clin Neuropharmacol 26:119-121, 2003.
10. Schwab FJ, Smith VA, Biserni M, et al. Adult scoliosis: a quantitative radiographic and clinical analysis. Spine 27:387-392, 2002.
11. Baik JS, Kim JY, Park JH, et al. Scoliosis in patients with Parkinson's disease. J Clin Neurol 5:91-94, 2009.
12. Duvoisin RC, Marsden CD. Note on the scoliosis of Parkinsonism. J Neurol Neurosurg Psychiatry 38:787-793, 1975.
13. Grimes JD, Hassan MN, Trent G, et al. Clinical and radiographic features of scoliosis in Parkinson's disease. Adv Neurol 45:353-355, 1987.
14. Indo T, Ando K. [Studies on the scoliosis of Parkinsonism (author's transl)] Rinsho Shinkeigaku 20:40-46, 1980.

15. Robin GC, Span Y, Steinberg R, et al. Scoliosis in the elderly: a follow-up study. Spine 7:355-359, 1982.

16. Vanderpool DW, James JI, Wynne-Davies R. Scoliosis in the elderly. J Bone Joint Surg Am 51:446-455, 1969.

17. Orekhova OA, Fedorova NV, Gamaleia AA. [Camptocormia in patients with Parkinson's disease] Zh Nevrol Psikhiatr Im S S Korsakova 113(7 Pt 2):13-17, 2013.

18. Marinelli P, Colosimo C, Ferrazza AM, et al. Effect of camptocormia on lung volumes in Parkinson's disease. Respir Physiol Neurobiol 187:164-166, 2013.

19. Sato M, Sainoh T, Orita S, et al. Posterior and anterior spinal fusion for the management of deformities in patients with Parkinson's disease. Case Rep Orthop. 2013 Sep 2. [Epub ahead of print]

20. Souques A, Rosanoff-Saloff M. La camptocormie; incurvation du tronc, consecutive aux traumatismes du dos et des lombes; considerations morphologiques. Rev Neurol 28:937-939, 1914.

21. Lenoir T, Guedj N, Boulu P, et al. Camptocormia: the bent spine syndrome, an update. Eur Spine J 19:1229-1237, 2010.

22. Seki M, Takahashi K, Koto A, et al. Camptocormia in Japanese patients with Parkinson's disease: a multicenter study. Mov Disord 26:2567-2571, 2011.

23. Tiple D, Fabbrini G, Colosimo C, et al. Camptocormia in Parkinson disease: an epidemiological and clinical study. J Neurol Neurosurg Psychiatry 80:145-148, 2009.

24. Abe K, Uchida Y, Notani M. Camptocormia in Parkinson's disease. Parkinsons Dis, 2010.

25. Lepoutre AC, Devos D, Blanchard-Dauphin A, et al. A specific clinical pattern of camptocormia in Parkinson's disease. J Neurol Neurosurg Psychiatry 77:1229-1234, 2006.

26. Upadhyaya CD, Starr PA, Mummaneni PV. Spinal deformity and Parkinson disease: a treatment algorithm. Neurosurg Focus 28:E5, 2010.

27. Bloch F, Houeto JL, Tezenas du Montcel S, et al. Parkinson's disease with camptocormia. J Neurol Neurosurg Psychiatry 77:1223-1238, 2006.

28. Sako W, Nishio M, Maruo T, et al. Subthalamic nucleus deep brain stimulation for camptocormia associated with Parkinson's disease. Mov Disord 24:1076-1079, 2009.

29. Azher SN, Jankovic J. Camptocormia: pathogenesis, classification, and response to therapy. Neurology 65:355-359, 2005.

30. Schäbitz WR, Glatz K, Schuhan C, et al. Severe forward flexion of the trunk in Parkinson's disease: focal myopathy of the paraspinal muscles mimicking camptocormia. Mov Disord 18:408-414, 2003.

31. Micheli F, Cersósimo MG, Piedimonte F. Camptocormia in a patient with Parkinson disease: beneficial effects of pallidal deep brain stimulation. Case report. J Neurosurg 103:1081-1083, 2005.

32. Yamada K, Goto S, Matsuzaki K, et al. Alleviation of camptocormia by bilateral subthalamic nucleus stimulation in a patient with Parkinson's disease. Parkinsonism Relat Disord 12:372-375, 2006.

33. Hellmann MA, Djaldetti R, Israel Z, et al. Effect of deep brain subthalamic stimulation on camptocormia and postural abnormalities in idiopathic Parkinson's disease. Mov Disord 21:2008-2010, 2006.

34. Umemura A, Oka Y, Ohkita K, et al. Effect of subthalamic deep brain stimulation on postural abnormality in Parkinson disease. J Neurosurg 112:1283-1288, 2010.

35. Asahi T, Taguchi Y, Hayashi N, et al. Bilateral subthalamic deep brain stimulation for camptocormia associated with Parkinson's disease. Stereotact Funct Neurosurg 89:173-177, 2011.

36. De Sèze M-P, Creuzé A, de Sèze M, et al. An orthosis and physiotherapy programme for camptocormia: a prospective case study. J Rehabil Med 40:761-765, 2008.

37. von Coelln R, Raible A, Gasser T, et al. Ultrasound-guided injection of the iliopsoas muscle with botulinum toxin in camptocormia. Mov Disord 23:889-892, 2008.

38. Furusawa Y, Mukai Y, Kawazoe T, et al. Long-term effect of repeated lidocaine injections into the external oblique for upper camptocormia in Parkinson's disease. Parkinsonism Relat Disord 19:350-354, 2013.

39. Bourghli A, Guérin P, Vital JM, et al. Posterior spinal fusion from T2 to the sacrum for the management of major deformities in patients with Parkinson disease: a retrospective review with analysis of complications. J Spinal Disord Tech 25:E53-E60, 2012.

40. Lafage V, Schwab F, Patel A, et al. Pelvic tilt and truncal inclination: two key radiographic parameters in the setting of adults with spinal deformity. Spine 34:E599-E606, 2009.

41. Glassman SD, Bridwell K, Dimar JR, et al. The impact of positive sagittal balance in adult spinal deformity. Spine 30:2024-2029, 2005.

42. Smith JS, Klineberg E, Schwab F, et al; International Spine Study Group. Change in classification grade by the SRS–Schwab Adult Spinal Deformity Classification predicts impact on health-related quality of life measures: prospective analysis of operative and non-operative treatment. Spine 38:1663-1671, 2013.

43. Schwab F, Ungar B, Blondel B, et al. Scoliosis Research Society–Schwab adult spinal deformity classification: a validation study. Spine 37:1077-1082, 2012.

44. Bess S, Schwab F, Lafage V, et al. Classifications for adult spinal deformity and use of the Scoliosis Research Society–Schwab Adult Spinal Deformity Classification. Neurosurg Clin N Am 24:185-193, 2013.

45. Protopsaltis TS, Schwab FJ, Bronsard N, et al. The T1 pelvic angle (TPA), a novel radiographic measure of global sagittal deformity, accounts for both pelvic retroversion and truncal inclination and correlates strongly with HRQOL. Presented at the Forty-eighth Annual Meeting of the Scoliosis Research Society, Lyons, France, Sep 2013.

46. Rogers MP, Liang MH, Daltroy LH, et al. Delirium after elective orthopedic surgery: risk factors and natural history. Int J Psychiatry Med 19:109-121, 1989.

47. Katus L, Shtilbans A. Perioperative management of patients with Parkinson's disease. Am J Med 127:275-280, 2013.

48. Fineberg SJ, Nandyala SV, Marquez-Lara A, et al. Incidence and risk factors for postoperative delirium after lumbar spine surgery. Spine 38:1790-1796, 2013.

49. Babat LB, McLain RF, Bingaman W, et al. Spinal surgery in patients with Parkinsons disease: construct failure and progressive deformity. Spine 29:2006-2012, 2004.

50. Koller H, Acosta F, Zenner J, et al. Spinal surgery in patients with Parkinson's disease: experiences with the challenges posed by sagittal imbalance and the Parkinson's spine. Eur Spine J 19:1785-1794, 2010.

51. Kim YJ, Bridwell KH, Lenke LG, et al. Proximal junctional kyphosis in adult spinal deformity after segmental posterior spinal instrumentation and fusion: minimum five-year follow-up. Spine 33:2179-2184, 2008.

52. van der Kolk NM, King LA. Effects of exercise on mobility in people with Parkinson's disease. Mov Disord 28:1587-1596, 2013.

Comprehensive Classification of Spinal Deformity

Shian Liu ▪ *Bassel Diebo* ▪ *Frank J. Schwab* ▪ *Virginie Lafage*

Radiographs remain the basis for diagnostic approaches for most orthopedic pathologies, yet substantial variations in interpretation exist, creating challenges in physician communication and collaborative research. A classification of adult spinal deformity (ASD) should be based on established, clinically relevant parameters to ensure reliability and simplicity.

Although a radiographic categorization scheme for adolescent idiopathic scoliosis (AIS) exists, pain and disability are rarely noted in the pediatric population. Conversely, ASD treatment is driven by patient expectations to regain function and reduce pain; thus a classification of adults should also consider these aspects of the disease.

CLASSIFICATION EFFORTS TO DATE

Significant advances in the classification of scoliotic deformity are attributed to Lenke et al.[1] In a 2001 publication, their classification offered an updated approach to AIS, which was more comprehensive than the King classification[2] and considered the sagittal plane. Furthermore, the new AIS classification offered guidelines on surgical fusion levels using segmental fixation.

The classification of adult scoliosis[3] is more complex than that of AIS. Adult deformity has a wide variability of segmental, regional, and global malalignment, and symptoms range from minimal to severe.[4] Treatment is driven by disability and pain, the most common chief complaint in the initial presentation of ASD,[5-7] and not simply by the magnitude of radiographic deformity. Because ASD is a multifaceted disease, a clinically relevant radiographic classification has been difficult to design, and many attempts have been made.

One of the first studies aimed at isolating the pain generator in adult scoliosis was published in 2002.[8] This work by Schwab and colleagues was the first to correlate a lack of lumbar lordosis with results of the VAS, which is a patient-reported outcome. The results launched an ongoing effort at reconciling health-related quality of life (HRQOL) measures and the radiographic presentation of adult deformity. In 2005 a preliminary classification of adult scoliosis emphasized the importance of lumbar parameters, which correlated significantly with pain scores.[9] Lumbar endplate obliquity, intervertebral olisthesis, and lordosis reflect the level of regional instability and pathologic loading of spinal elements.

Another attempt at a clinically influential classification was made in 2006.[10] This system defined five coronal curve types and included a lumbar lordosis and subluxation modifier, proving that a classification with descriptive value and bearing on surgical strategy in adults with scoliosis is feasible. This classification further demonstrated higher surgical rates with higher modifiers, both increased lumbar hypolordosis and intervertebral subluxation. An increase in these modifiers was also associated with more disability on the SRS-22 questionnaire and ODI.[11]

Also in 2006 Lowe et al[3] published the initial SRS effort on classification and were the first to introduce a primary sagittal deformity category. Although interobserver and intraobserver reliability were excellent, this attempt was based on the translation of a pediatric classification to adults, and the clinical application of this system was not clear. In pediatric patients the driver is fear of coronal progression and cosmesis, whereas in adults the driver is disability.

These approaches led to the Spinal Deformity Study Group (SDSG) classification[4] (Table 6-1). This classification was based on outcome measures, and it refined prior complexities in classification. The classification hinged on the following elements:
- Basic coronal curve locations
- A sagittal plane deformity category
- Regional and global modifiers graded by HRQOL severity

Table 6-1   Spinal Deformity Study Group Adult Spinal Deformity Classification

Type: Location of the Deformity (apical level of the major curve OR sagittal plane only)	
Type I	Thoracic-only scoliosis (no thoracolumbar or lumbar component)
Type II	Upper thoracic major, apex T4-8 (with thoracolumbar or lumbar curve)
Type III	Lower thoracic major, apex T9-10 (with thoracolumbar/lumbar curve)
Type IV	Thoracolumbar major curve, apex T11-L1 (with any other minor curve)
Type V	Lumbar major curve, apex L2-4 (with any other minor curve)
Type K	Deformity in the sagittal plane only

Lordosis Modifier: Sagittal Cobb Angle From T12-S1	
A	Marked lordosis >40 degrees
B	Moderate lordosis 0-40 degrees
C	No lordosis present, Cobb <0 degrees

Subluxation Modifier: Frontal or Sagittal Plane (Anterior or Posterior), Maximum Value	
0	No subluxation
+	Subluxation 1-6 mm
++	Subluxation >7 mm

Global Balance Modifier: Sagittal Plane C7 Offset From Posterosuperior Corner S1	
N	Normal: 0-4 cm
P	Positive: 4-9.5 cm
VP	Very positive: >9.5 cm

From Schwab F, Lafage V, Farcy JP, et al. Surgical rates and operative outcome analysis in thoracolumbar and lumbar major adult scoliosis: application of the new adult deformity classification. Spine 32:2723-2730, 2007.

All aspects of this classification were based on HRQOL analysis. The thresholds between groups within each modifier were determined by the HRQOL measures, splitting the population into discrete groups based on the clinical impact of each parameter.

Although classification schemes evolved and began to successfully achieve the goal of offering a common language through which clinical results and treatment approaches could be evaluated, past efforts did not include the pelvis, a factor that had significant clinical implications.

THE SCOLIOSIS RESEARCH SOCIETY–SCHWAB CLASSIFICATION

The Scoliosis Research Society–Schwab adult spinal deformity classification is a recently updated system that was developed based on the latest research on alignment and correlations between radiographic parameters and clinical outcomes.[12] This improved version of the 2006 SDSG adult deformity classification was created in conjunction with the SRS and included parameters that were selected on the basis of clinical relevance, most notably the pelvic parameters.

Because treatment of patients with ASD centers on improvement of pain and disability, the parameters are strongly associated with HRQOL outcome scores. The cutoff values for the modifier grades were established using the outcome scores to achieve a strong clinical impact. Recent studies showed the impact of these modifiers on the health-related quality of life measures and the decision of pursuing operative or nonoperative treatment.[13,14]

Frontal and sagittal full-length radiographs were employed in the design to provide a standard basis for classification that is easy to use. Similar to the Lenke classification of AIS, the coronal curve type describes the relevant coronal aspects of the deformity and is the overriding classifier. To account for the sagittal plane and pelvic parameters, the lateral components of the deformity are characterized through the following three modifiers: pelvic incidence minus lumbar lordosis (PI-LL), pelvic tilt (PT), and sagittal vertical axis (SVA). The classification is shown in Fig. 6-1.[12]

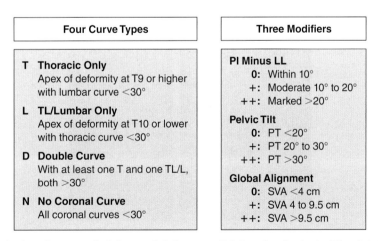

Fig. 6-1 SRS–Schwab classification of adult spinal deformity. (*LL,* Lumbar lordosis; *PI,* pelvic incidence; *PT,* pelvic tilt; *SVA,* sagittal vertical axis; *TL/L,* thoracolumbar/lumbar.) (Adapted from Schwab F, Ungar B, Blondel B, et al. Scoliosis Research Society–Schwab adult spinal deformity classification: a validation study. Spine 37:1077-1082, 2012.)

The curve type is the maximal coronal angle measured by the Cobb technique on a standard AP free-standing radiograph of the spine. The major curve has the largest Cobb angle. An apex of deformity at T9 or higher is classified as a thoracic curve. Curves whose apex of deformity is at T10 or lower are considered thoracolumbar or lumbar curves. The first sagittal modifier, PI-LL, indicates the importance of the harmonious relationship between the spine and pelvis. The PT modifier is an assessment the degree of pelvic retroversion, with higher values indicating increased retroversion and compensation; this parameter is highly correlated with pain and disability. The global alignment modifier groups patients based on thresholds of SVA, which increases with pain and disability. Radiographic examples are shown in Figs. 6-2 through 6-4.

This classification scheme has excellent intraobserver and interobserver reliability and clinical correlations to HRQOL instruments such as the ODI, SF-36, and SRS-22.[12,13] These patient-reported outcomes cover the gamut of region-specific, disease-specific, and general health status problems that patients with ASD can experience.

Recent studies have shown the clinical utility of the SRS–Schwab classification. Changes in classification category through surgery can affect a patient's HRQOL. In 2013 Smith et al[14] compared patients who improved in the SRS–Schwab sagittal modifiers (PT, SVA, or PI-LL) with those who deteriorated in sagittal modifiers. Patients who improved in PT grade also had significant improvement in ODI scores and SRS appearance. Furthermore, the clinical relevance of the improvement was notable, with an increased likelihood of achieving a minimal clinically important difference (MCID), which is the smallest change that is important to patients.[15] Patients with improvement in the PT modifier, SVA modifier, or PI-LL modifier were more likely to reach an MCID in ODI results, SRS activity, and SRS appearance than those who deteriorated or maintained the same classification. Furthermore, those who improved in the SVA modifier

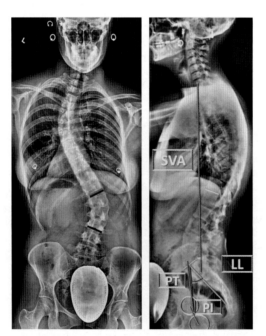

Fig. 6-2 This patient has an SRS–Schwab curve type of *D, PI − LL = ++*. Radiographic values are the following: thoracic Cobb angle = 50 degrees, thoracolumbar Cobb angle = 43 degrees, pelvic incidence *(PI)* = 62 degrees, lumbar lordosis *(LL)* = 36 degrees, pelvic incidence minus lumbar lordosis *(PI − LL)* = 26 degrees, pelvic tilt *(PT)* = 0 degrees, and sagittal vertical axis *(SVA)* = −0.1 cm.

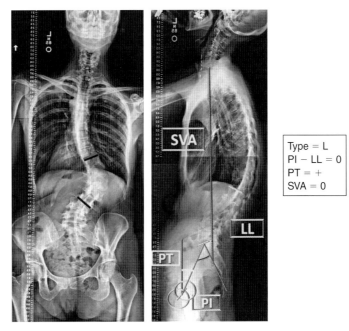

Fig. 6-3 This patient has an SRS–Schwab curve type of *L, PT* = +. Radiographic values are the following: thoracic Cobb angle = 29 degrees, thoracolumbar Cobb angle = 56 degrees, pelvic incidence *(PI)* = 42 degrees, lumbar lordosis *(LL)* = 41 degrees, pelvic incidence minus lumbar lordosis *(PI − LL)* = 1 degree, pelvic tilt *(PT)* = 25 degrees, and sagittal vertical axis *(SVA)* = −0.1 cm.

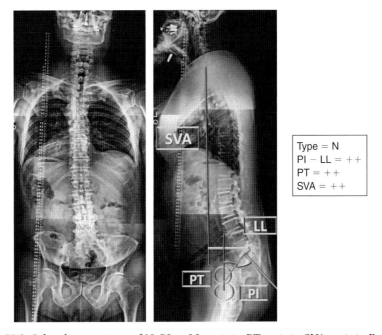

Fig. 6-4 This patient has an SRS–Schwab curve type of *N, PI − LL* = ++, *PT* = ++, *SVA* = ++. Radiographic values are as follows: thoracic Cobb angle = 0 degrees, thoracolumbar Cobb angle = 0 degrees, pelvic incidence *(PI)* = 65 degrees, lumbar lordosis *(LL)* = 18 degrees, pelvic incidence minus lumbar lordosis *(PI − LL)* = 47 degrees, pelvic tilt *(PT)* = 36 degrees, and sagittal vertical axis *(SVA)* = 14.0 cm.

were also more likely to reach an MCID threshold in SRS pain, and those who improved in the PI-LL modifier were more likely to reach an MCID threshold in SF-36 results and all SRS subdomains. This study clearly demonstrated that the patients with improved spinopelvic modifiers after surgical correction were more likely to have a clinically noticeable difference in HRQOL, as measured with ODI or SF-36 results or SRS activity and pain than those who deteriorated or remained the same in classification. Patterns of deformity, when classified carefully by clinical relevance, are more than just visually appealing and simple to understand; they are surgically applicable.

Research into surgical techniques by classification is already under way. Terran et al[13] showed that SRS–Schwab modifiers not only reflect severity of a disease state, but they also correlate with the important decision of whether to pursue operative or nonoperative treatment, with operative patients having significantly worse sagittal spinopelvic modifiers. Furthermore, of the patients who underwent surgery, operative approach and techniques significantly differed based on classification parameters. Patients with D-type and L-type deformities were more likely to have combined anterior/posterior procedures, whereas patients with T-type deformities were more likely to have posterior-only fusion. Patients with an N-type deformity were more likely to be treated with a major three-column osteotomy than those with overriding coronal deformities. Interbody fusion was more frequently performed in patients with type T or N deformities than in those with type D or T deformities. Patients with worse spinopelvic modifiers were significantly more likely to require a major osteotomy, iliac fixation, and decompression. This study provided evidence that surgical strategies vary based on the SRS–Schwab classification. It also offered an objective language to share results and set the stage for further study on treatment effectiveness in relation to classification.

CONCLUSION

ASD is an emerging health care issue of the twenty-first century. This is the result, in part, of increased awareness of its clinical impact and the aging population in Western societies.[16-18] A comprehensive classification of spinal deformity that is based on clinically relevant radiographic parameters is necessary to standardize a common language for patient care and to continue research in the adult population. Caring for patients with ASD involves skill not only in the clinical and surgical setting; like so much of what is accomplished in the advancement of medicine, it requires a willingness to partake in multidisciplinary and international teamwork and an evidence-based approach to patient care.

REFERENCES

1. Lenke LG, Betz R, Harms J, et al. Adolescent idiopathic scoliosis: a new classification to determine extent of spinal arthrodesis. J Bone Joint Surg Am 8:1169-1181, 2001.
2. King HA, Moe JH, Bradford DS, et al. The selection of fusion levels in thoracic idiopathic scoliosis. J Bone Joint Surg Am 65:1302-1313, 1983.
3. Lowe T, Berven S, Schwab F, et al. The SRS classification for adult spinal deformity: building on the King/Moe and Lenke classification systems. Spine 31(Suppl):S119-S125, 2006.
4. Schwab F, Lafage V, Farcy JP, et al. Surgical rates and operative outcome analysis in thoracolumbar and lumbar major adult scoliosis: application of the new adult deformity classification. Spine 32:2723-2730, 2007.
5. Kotwal S, Pumberger M, Hughes A, et al. Degenerative scoliosis: a review. HSS J 7:257-264, 2011.
6. Glassman SD, Bridwell K, Dimar JR, et al. The impact of positive sagittal balance in adult spinal deformity. Spine 30:2024-2029, 2005.
7. Bridwell KH, Cats-Baril W, Harrast J, et al. The validity of the SRS-22 instrument in an adult spinal deformity population compared with the Oswestry and SF-12: a study of response distribution, concurrent validity, internal consistency, and reliability. Spine 30:455-461, 2005.
8. Schwab FJ, Smith VA, Biserni M, et al. Adult scoliosis: a quantitative radiographic and clinical analysis. Spine 27:387-392, 2002.

9. Schwab F, el-Fegoun AB, Gamez L, et al. A lumbar classification of scoliosis in the adult patient: preliminary approach. Spine 30:1670-1673, 2005.

10. Schwab F, Farcy J, Bridwell K, et al. A clinical impact classification of scoliosis in the adult. Spine 31:2109-2114, 2006.

11. Schwab FJ, Lafage V, Farcy J, et al. Predicting outcome and complications in the surgical treatment of adult scoliosis. Spine 33:2243-2247, 2008.

12. Schwab F, Blondel B, Bess S, et al. Radiographical spinopelvic parameters and disability in the setting of adult spinal deformity: a prospective multicenter analysis. Spine 38:E803-E812, 2013.

13. Terran J, Schwab F, Shaffrey CI, et al. The SRS–Schwab adult spinal deformity classification: assessment and clinical correlations based on a prospective operative and nonoperative cohort. Neurosurgery 73:559-568, 2013.

14. Smith JS, Klineberg E, Schwab F, et al. Change in classification grade by the SRS–Schwab adult spinal deformity classification predicts impact on health-related quality of life measures: prospective analysis of operative and nonoperative treatment. Spine 38:1663-1671, 2013.

15. Copay AG, Subach BR, Glassman SD, et al. Understanding the minimum clinically important difference: a review of concepts and methods. Spine J 7:541-546, 2007.

16. Francis RS. Scoliosis screening of 3,000 college-aged women. The Utah Study—phase 2. Phys Ther 68:1513-1516, 1988.

17. Robin GC, Span Y, Steinberg R, et al. Scoliosis in the elderly: a follow-up study. Spine 7:355-359, 1982.

18. Grevitt M, Khazim R, Webb J, et al. The short form-36 health survey questionnaire in spine surgery. J Bone Joint Surg Br 79:48-52, 1997.

7

Measuring Clinical Outcomes in the Treatment of Spinal Deformity

Sigurd Berven

Clinical outcome is the end result of health care delivered to patients or populations. Measuring clinical outcomes may include metrics for quality of care, patient-centered assessment of health status, and costs and risks of providing care. Measuring outcomes is complex, and no single measure summarizes the patient's experience, the hospital perspective, the payer perspective, and the treating physician's perspective. Therefore outcomes need to be considered broadly and encompass a spectrum of perspectives and measures. The purpose of this chapter is to introduce and review methods for measuring clinical outcomes and to demonstrate the importance of these measures in considering new reimbursement models for care, in protecting access to care for our patients, and in guiding an evidence-based approach to care in the management of spinal deformity.

Accountability for the outcome of care is a priority for all health care providers and has specific relevance to the management of complex disorders of the spine. Patient safety, quality of care, and clinical outcomes in the care of patients with spinal deformity are important goals of care. Demonstration of comparative effectiveness and the value of care are important in defining the place of spinal interventions in a value-based health care economy. Outcome measurement is an important aspect of surgeon accountability and is vital in determining the value of health care interventions. Clinical outcomes include process measures, objective measures of function or performance, patient-reported assessment of health status, and complications and long-term consequences of care. *Value* is a broader measure that incorporates an analysis of clinical outcomes, costs, and risks of care. This chapter presents an overview of common clinical outcome measures used for spinal deformity surgery, along with data from the literature on outcomes in adult spinal deformity surgery.

PROCESS MEASURES

Process measures assess adherence to clinical pathways and performance of care with a focus on how care is delivered. It is not a patient-centered evaluation. Process measures are useful, because they can be easy to record and report, and they are an important proxy for quality of care if a clear correlation exists between the care pathway and the outcome of care. Examples of process measures in clinical outcomes include compliance with antibiotic or thromboembolic prophylaxis guidelines, adherence to surgical time-outs before surgery, preoperative risk assessments of patients, and implementation of postoperative care protocols for the prevention of common postoperative complications. The utility of process measures depends on how reliably they are linked to clinical outcomes. For example, measuring compliance with preoperative antibiotic guidelines is useful in that compliance should be associated with a reduction in the incidence of surgical site infections. Although process measures are an indirect measure of quality, the implementation and measurement of such processes are important in standardizing care and improving quality. Process measures are not a direct reflection of a patient's health care experience, and adherence to the most rigorous evidence-based processes of care may not improve patient-centered measures of outcome. Focus on patient-centered outcome remains the priority endpoint of accountability for surgeons and other health care providers.

FUNCTIONAL AND PERFORMANCE-BASED OUTCOME MEASURES

Functional and performance-based outcome measures are clinical health metrics that are centered on objective assessment of patient activity. Functional measures can comprise gait analysis, time to get up and go, time to walk a fixed distance, oxygen consumption during gait, and measures of patient activity, including time that a patient spends walking and out of bed. Functional measures may provide useful insight into the impairment and burden that spinal deformity imposes on patient activity and insight into the effect of management of deformity on improving activity tolerance and abilities. However, patient activity measures at baseline vary significantly. Many objective measures of function can be influenced dramatically by factors independent of spinal deformity, including comorbidities, concurrent musculoskeletal pathology, and patient motivation and vitality.

RADIOGRAPHIC OUTCOME MEASURES

Radiographic assessment of spinal deformity is important in classifying deformity and in quantifying the magnitude and location of spinal deformity. Radiographic measures include Cobb angle, regional measures of lordosis and kyphosis, sagittal vertical axis, spinopelvic parameters (pelvic incidence, pelvic tilt, and sacral slope), and the presence of solid arthrodesis. Radiographic measurements are important in the preoperative and postoperative assessment of spinal deformity. The correlation between radiographic measures and patient-centered assessment of health status is highest for measures of sagittal deformity, but radiographic measures are only one component of predictors of clinical outcome.

QUALITY MEASURES

Measurements of quality include outcomes such as operative time, length of hospital stay, and rates of complications, reoperations, and readmissions. Such measures provide important information that can be used to compare performance of individual providers and hospitals and to establish metrics for performance and goals for quality improvement. Quality metrics are valuable in identifying outliers and in improving care processes and pathways. However, overall quality measures are distinct from patient-centered clinical outcome measures. One important concern regarding reliance on quality measures is the possibility that measuring quality alone may lead to a focus on outcomes that are not patient-centered. If the target for outcome is length of stay or avoidance of readmission alone, then that goal might incentivize significant undertreatment of complex spinal disorders. Fig. 7-1 provides an example of a case in which a patient underwent a limited decompression and fusion for a complex spinal deformity. If measured by length of stay or complications of care alone, the procedure is rated as having a high-quality outcome. However, the patient had no improvement in her health status or in her deformity measures. She had a revision surgery 1 year after the index procedure and was treated with an asymmetrical transpedicular wedge resection osteotomy. The revision surgery resulted in a longer length of stay, higher cost, and more risk and potential for complication than the index surgery. However, the patient reported a dramatic improvement in health status that was not captured by the quality metrics alone. It is inappropriate to focus myopically on quality metrics without giving priority to patient-centered measures in measuring clinical outcomes in spinal deformity.

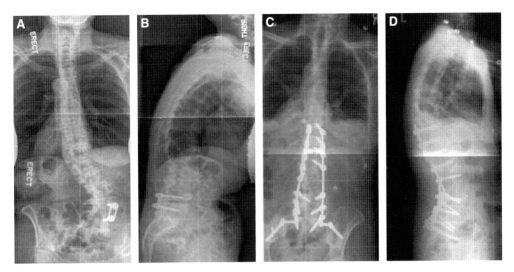

Fig. 7-1 **A** and **B,** This 68-year-old woman presented with sagittal and coronal plane deformity, back pain, and neurogenic claudication. She was treated with a limited decompression and fusion. Although the length of stay was 2 days, no complications occurred, and she was not readmitted within 90 days, no improvement in radiographic or patient-centered clinical outcomes was observed, and the patient was unable to resume her work as a nursing supervisor. **C** and **D,** Postoperative radiographs 1 year after revision surgery. The patient has significant improvement in coronal and sagittal global balance. Function is improved to the degree that she is able to return to work.

PATIENT-REPORTED OUTCOMES

Process measures, physiologic outcomes, and traditional quality metrics are important tools for assessing health care quality; however, they do not reflect a patient's health care experience or the impact of care on health-related quality of life (HRQOL). Patient-centered outcomes are the top priority for physician accountability in managing patients with spinal deformity. Patient-reported outcome measures may include a spectrum of domains to assess HRQOL. Frequently used domains include disability, function status, pain, appearance, emotional/psychological well-being, social function, general health status, and satisfaction with health care experience.

Measurement tools for patient-reported outcomes include both disease-specific and general health status measures. Disease-specific measures focus on domains associated with a particular condition or patient population. They have the advantage of increased responsiveness to change, compared with general health status measures. Examples of disease-specific outcome tools include the Scoliosis Research Society (SRS-22) questionnaire, the Oswestry Disability Index (ODI), and the Neck Disability Index (NDI).

General health status outcomes tools are useful, because they measure a patient's self-assessment of health status more broadly, and they allow comparisons across a spectrum of medical and surgical conditions. General health status measures provide an indirect measure of patient preference of a specific health state or the utility of a health state. The utility of a health state over time is the measure of a quality-adjusted life-year (QALY), which is the fundamental currency of health care economics. Examples of generic profiles include the Short-Form 36 (SF-36), Short-Form 6 Domains (SF-6D), EuroQOL five dimensions questionnaire (EQ-5D), and the Health Utilities Index (HUI).

General health status measures and specific disease-specific outcome tools can be useful as indirect measures to calculate utility scores. A utility score reflects societal preferences for a health state. Different health states are rated on a scale from 0 (death) to 1 (perfect health). Utility scores derived from patient-reported outcome questionnaires using validated instruments provide information on a patient's health status and the value that society places on that health state. Consideration of a utility score over time yields a QALY, calculated as the utility score multiplied by the number of years that health state is maintained. Thus the durability of an outcome results in increased QALYs over time. A QALY is an outcome measure that represents a standardized unit for comparison across fields and can be assigned a value.

The following instruments are commonly used patient-reported outcome measurements in adult spinal deformity that have validated conversions to utility scores/QALYs:

- The *SF-36* is a widely used generic health survey consisting of 36 questions with four physical health scales (physical functioning, physical role limitation, bodily pain, and general health) and four mental health scales (vitality, social functioning, emotional role limitation, and mental health). The SF-6D is an abbreviated version of the SF-36 that has been established as a preference-based health state classification and can be converted to a utility score.[1]
- The *EQ-5D* is another validated and widely used general health questionnaire that is used to establish a utility score. It includes five health dimensions: mobility, self-care, usual activities, pain/discomfort, and anxiety/depression.
- The *SRS questionnaire* measures how spinal deformity affects a patient's HRQOL based on five domains: pain, function, self-image, mental health, and satisfaction. The 22-item questionnaire (SRS-22) is the most widely used and validated version, although several other versions exist (SRS-24, SRS-29, and SRS-30). SRS-22 has been validated as a reliable instrument with high internal consistency, responsiveness, reproducibility, and discriminatory capacity for patients with adult deformity.[2,3] A model has been established for translating SRS-22 scores to SF-6D scores to determine utility scores.[4,5]
- The *ODI* measures HRQOL in patients with low back pain. It rates a patient's disability score based on 10 measures: pain, personal care, sitting, standing, walking, lifting, sleeping, sex life, social life, and traveling. Higher scores correspond to a greater degree of disability. ODI is a validated and widely used measure that can be reliably translated to a utility score.[6]

Patient-centered measures of health status are the most direct method for assessment of the effect of health care on HRQOL. The burden of spinal disorders and the impact of care on health status can be measured from a patient's perspective using these clinical outcome tools. If the goal of treatment is to improve HRQOL, including domains of pain, function, appearance, and mental health, then patient-centered measures are the metric for which providers are most accountable. However, for many conditions the impact of the disorder may be limited at present, and the goal of care is to prevent the adverse consequences of disease progression. Adolescent idiopathic scoliosis is an important example in which a patient can present with limited symptoms measurable by pain, disability, or health status compromise, but the goal of surgery is to prevent the consequences of deformity progression. Fig. 7-2 shows a 14-year-old female with a double-thoracic curve who presented with progressive deformity without significant compromise in self-assessment of health status. Surgery with deformity correction and fusion of the thoracic spine was performed to prevent deformity progression and the adult sequelae of adolescent deformity.

COST AND VALUE

In every health care economy with limited resources, cost is an important consideration in the assessment of health care interventions. Economic analyses of health care interventions include cost-minimization studies, cost-effectiveness analyses, and cost-utility analyses. An assessment of costs may include direct costs, charges, or reimbursements. Indirect costs such as loss of productivity because of time off of work, transportation to health care facilities, and the cost of caretakers can be included in cost analyses and incorporate a wider view of total costs from a societal perspective.

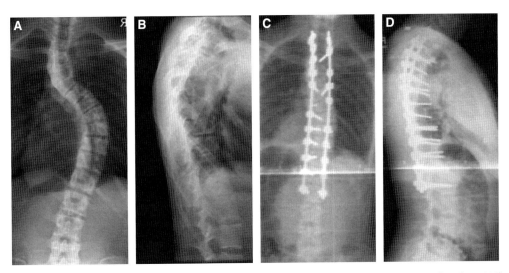

Fig. 7-2 **A** and **B,** Preoperative radiographs of a 14-year-old girl with a double-thoracic curve (Lenke 2AN) and progressive deformity. She had limited pain and disability related to her deformity. **C** and **D,** Postoperative radiographs demonstrate realignment of the spine in all planes. The patient's self-assessment of her health status is normal for her age and not significantly improved as a result of surgery.

Although cost in itself is an important consideration, the value of care provides the most meaningful assessment of a health care intervention. *Value of care* encompasses both outcome and cost and is defined as the net benefit of care relative to the net cost of care, in other words, what we get for what we spend. The measurement of benefits and costs in spine surgery is not uniform and varies depending on the perspective of the stakeholder in the health care economy. Hospitals and other health care facilities may emphasize outcomes and costs that affect a single admission or episode of care such as length of hospital stay, implant placement, and complications. Third-party payers often focus on outcomes and costs in a medium-term time frame, including readmissions within 90 days or the cost of outpatient care. The value of a health care intervention to a physician and patient is established over a longer time frame than a single admission—its impact is measured based on HRQOL over a lifetime.

Cost-utility studies provide the most useful information about the value of a health care intervention, because a utility score captures a patient's preference for different health states over time. An outcome measure that directly reflects HRQOL and is translatable across disease states, such as QOLY, is an important prerequisite for estimating the value of spinal care. The length of follow-up is an important consideration when measuring value, because the cost of a single episode of care will be significantly discounted by the duration of the benefit.

OUTCOMES OF ADULT SPINAL DEFORMITY SURGERY

Clinical outcomes studies in adult spinal deformity surgery provide valuable insight into the impact of deformity on health status and the impact of care on changing health status. Patient populations, outcome measures, and duration and completeness of follow-up over time vary significantly. The heterogeneity of the adult deformity population and the outcome measures recorded limit our ability to make firm conclusions regarding comparative effectiveness of specific surgical strategies or approaches to care. Estimates of the prevalence of adult spinal deformity in the United States range from 2.5% to more than 50%.[7] Population-based studies on adult deformity are limited, and many patients with spinal deformity may not seek or access medical care for their condition. Nonoperative care of adult spinal deformity is highly variable and includes physical therapy, conditioning, pain medications, injections, and alternative modalities such as behavioral therapies, acupuncture, and chiropractic care. In the absence of neural compromise, instability, or progressive deformity, nonoperative care is the initial approach to management of symptomatic deformity. However, there is limited evidence to demonstrate a significant or reliable effect of nonoperative care in symptomatic deformity. Surgery is most appropriate for patients with progressive deformity, neural compromise, pain, and disability that are unresponsive to nonoperative treatment. Studies of operative and nonoperative management of adult spinal deformity have demonstrated improved patient-reported outcomes with surgical management, compared with nonoperative approaches.[8-12]

In a review article on adult spinal deformity, Youssef et al[13] summarized findings of 49 studies reporting outcomes for various surgical strategies. These included decompression alone versus decompression with fusion; anterior, posterior, or combined surgical approaches; the use of vertebral osteotomies; and levels of instrumented vertebrae. A variety of outcome measurements were reported for each technique.

RADIOGRAPHIC OUTCOMES

Yadla et al[14] conducted a systematic review of adult scoliosis outcomes in a series of 49 articles published between 1950 and 2009, with a minimum follow-up of 2 years. They found a range in Cobb angle correction from 9.1 to 53.9 degrees (mean 26.6 degrees, representing an average 40.7% curve correction).

Radiographic outcomes have been compared between different surgical approaches. Crandall and Revella[15] found no significant difference in coronal curve correction between patients having posterior instrumented fusion in addition to either anterior lumbar interbody fusion (average correction of 69.5%) or transforaminal lumbar interbody fusion (average correction of 68.7%). Based on a literature review, Mundis et al[16] reported improved coronal and sagittal correction with a lateral transpsoas approach, compared with open anterior procedures. Pateder et al[17] retrospectively compared patients who underwent posterior-only surgery (n = 45) with patients who had combined anterior-posterior surgery (n = 35). They reported no significant difference in coronal or sagittal curve correction between the two groups.

Youssef et al[13] reviewed radiographic outcomes for different types of posterior osteotomies, including Smith-Petersen osteotomy (SPO), pedicle subtraction osteotomy (PSO), and vertebral column resection (VCR). These techniques are performed to achieve varying degrees of lordosis correction and restoration of sagittal balance. SPO achieves the smallest degree of curve correction (up to 10 degrees of lordosis per vertebral level); however, multilevel osteotomies may achieve a large overall correction. Reports of PSO have demonstrated an average of 30 degrees of lordotic correction per level. In a comparison of SPO with PSO, Cho et al[18] found an average total correction of 33 degrees for patients who had three or more SPOs and 31.7 degrees for patients who had PSO. However, improvement in sagittal balance was significantly lower in the SPO group than the PSO group. VCR achieves the highest degree of curve correction. Suk et al[19] reported a mean deformity correction of 59% (from 109.0 to 45.6 degrees) in 16 patients who underwent posterior VCR. Papadopoulos et al[20] reported outcomes of 45 patients who had posterior VCR. Deformity correction was 44.5%.

Radiographic measurements are most important in helping surgeons to predict clinical impact. Sagittal balance, measured in millimeters of deviation from the C7 plumb line, is one such parameter that has been shown to correlate with clinical health outcomes. Glassman et al[21] performed a retrospective review of 752 patients, 352 of whom had a positive sagittal balance that ranged from 1 to 271 mm (mean 57.7 ± 51.2). Positive sagittal balance was highly correlated with a deterioration of patient-reported health outcomes, including SRS-29, SF-12, and ODI. As the magnitude of positive sagittal balance increased, health status measures demonstrated significantly increased pain and decreased function. This study emphasized that sagittal balance is an important radiographic parameter to evaluate for the treatment of adult spinal deformity. The C7 sagittal vertical axis alone may underestimate sagittal imbalance in patients who use compensatory mechanisms, including extension of the hips, bending the knees, and thoracic hyperextension. Inclusion of lumbopelvic parameters such as pelvic tilt and pelvic incidence is important to accurately quantify global sagittal alignment. Schwab et al[22] demonstrated that radiographic measures of sagittal alignment, including pelvic tilt, matching of lumbar lordosis with pelvic incidence, and sagittal vertical axis are the most significant predictors of health status in adults with spinal deformity. Smith and members of the International Spine Study Group[23] showed the utility of the Schwab–SRS Radiographic Classification System in measuring outcomes of adult spinal deformity. In a multicenter prospective study, the authors reported that classification modifiers were associated with preoperative health status, and patient-centered changes in health status were responsive to changes in radiographic classification modifiers.

COMPLICATIONS

The incidence of complications is an important quality measure in adult spinal deformity. Reported complication rates for spinal deformity surgery are high; however, a standardized definition or classification for reporting complications has not been established in the literature. Complication rates have been classified in various ways, including major versus minor complications, early versus late complications, and surgical versus medical complications. Reported complications in deformity surgery include pseudarthrosis, adjacent-segment disease, dural tears, superficial or deep wound infections, implant complications, neurologic deficits, epidural hematoma, wound hematoma, pulmonary embolism, deep venous thrombosis, systemic complications, and death. The incidence of complications can be influenced by patient factors (for example, age, comorbidities, and severity of deformity) or surgical factors (for example, approach type, need for osteotomy, and number of levels fused).

Yadla et al[14] reviewed 49 articles and reported complication rates ranging from 0% to 53%, with a combined total of 897 complications among 2175 patients (41.2%). Charosky et al[24] reported an overall 39% complication rate among 306 patients 50 years of age or older, who had adult deformity surgery with either an anterior only, posterior only, or combined approach. Sansur et al[25] reviewed a total 4980 cases of adult scoliosis from the SRS morbidity and mortality database and found an overall complication rate of 13.4% and a mortality rate of 0.3%. Significantly higher complication rates resulted from revision surgeries, osteotomies, and combined anterior-posterior surgery.

Youssef et al[13] summarized a number of studies reporting complication rates of various procedures. Transfeldt et al[26] reported a 10% complication rate among adult deformity patients who underwent decompression alone, compared with 56% in patients who had decompression and fusion. Burneikiene et al[27] reported a 31% incidence of systemic complications and a 49% incidence of hardware or surgical technique complications in 29 patients who had transforaminal lumbar interbody fusion. Complications of anterior lumbar interbody fusion can include vascular injuries, ilioinguinal and iliohypogastric nerve injuries, damage to the bladder or ureters, pseudarthrosis and subsidence, ileus, lymphocele, and retrograde ejaculation.[13,28] Most of these complications are uncommon, although rates of major and minor complications vary in the literature. In a study of 447 patients, McDonnell et al[29] noted a complication rate of 11% for major complications and 24% for minor complications. Complications of the lateral transpsoas approach are often related to manipulation of the lumber plexus. In a prospective multicenter evaluation of 107 adult degenerative scoliosis patients undergoing extreme lateral interbody fusion, Isaacs et al[30] reported a 12.1% major complication rate.

Reoperations

Scheer et al[31] analyzed data from a prospective, multicenter adult spinal deformity database to examine the rates, indications, timing, and risk factors for reoperation and the effect of reoperation on HRQOL measures. In a cohort of 352 patients (268 with at least 1 year of follow-up), they found a total reoperation rate of 17%, most of which occurred within 1 year of the index operation. The most common indications for reoperation included instrumentation complications and radiographic failure. The reoperation rate was a 19% for patients undergoing a three-column osteotomy, and the reoperation rate was 16% for patients not requiring three-column osteotomy. However, a three-column osteotomy was not significantly predictive of reoperation at 1 year. The uppermost instrumented vertebra was not predictive of reoperation. No significant differences were reported between patients who did not undergo reoperation and those who did require reoperation for American Society of Anesthesiologists or ASA grade, Charlson comorbidity index, preoperative BMI, or smoking history. Patients who needed reoperation within 1 year had worse ODI and SRS-22 scores at the 1-year follow-up than patients not needing reoperation. However, no significant difference was noted in HRQOL scores at 2 years between patients who required reoperation at 1 year and those who did not.

Other studies have demonstrated similar reoperation rates, ranging from 10% to 21%.[24,32-34] Reasons for revision surgery in adult spinal deformity include pseudarthrosis, curve progression, infection, painful/prominent implants, adjacent-segment disease, implant failure, and neurologic deficits.[32,33]

Health-Related Quality of Life Outcomes

Despite high complication and reoperation rates in adult spinal deformity surgery, patient satisfaction with these procedures is high. Both condition-specific and general HRQOL outcomes that can be converted to utility scores and compared across the literature are important prerequisites for determining the value of spinal deformity surgery.

Multiple prospective multicenter studies have demonstrated the benefits of operative treatment of adult spinal deformity, compared with nonoperative care, with regard to patient-reported health measures including ODI, SRS-22, EQ-5D, and numeric rating scale (NRS) scores for leg and back pain.[8-12] Bridwell et al[12] performed a prospective observational cohort study of adult patients with symptomatic lumbar scoliosis who had operative or nonoperative treatment. At a minimum 2-year follow-up, the operative cohort showed statistically significant improvements over both the matched and unmatched nonoperative groups in all quality of life measures, including SRS, ODI, and NRS back and leg pain scores. Patients treated operatively had significantly improved in all quality of life measures at the 2-year follow up, whereas the nonoperative cohort showed no significant change in these measures. This study was limited by poor follow-up of nonoperatively treated patients (45%), compared with a 95% follow-up rate of operatively treated patients. However, patients with a 2-year follow-up were identical to those who did not follow up with regard to age, gender, curve size, SRS, ODI, and NRS back and leg pain scores. This study provided important evidence for the benefit of operative compared with nonoperative management of adult symptomatic lumbar scoliosis.

Based on the 49 studies included in their systematic review, Yadla et al[14] reported ODI and SRS as the most commonly used patient-based outcome instruments. Eleven studies reported preoperative and postoperative ODI scores, and 10 studies reported preoperative and postoperative SRS scores. The ODI score decreased by an average of 15.7 points (range 3.1 to 32.3) in 911 patients. This improvement in disability outcome correlated with previous reports of significant clinical improvement of ODI scores ranging from 4 to 15 points.[35] In the study by Yadla et al, of the 999 patients with preoperative and postoperative SRS scores, the mean increase in SRS scores was 23.1 points, well above the minimal important difference for SRS scores of 13 points reported by Bagó et al.[36]

Youssef et al[13] summarized results of studies reporting HRQOL outcomes for patients undergoing various surgical approaches. The authors reviewed literature indicating a high rate of complications in adult deformity surgery but overall high patient satisfaction and improvement in health status. Crandall and Revella[15] found nonsignificant differences in VAS and ODI outcomes between patients having posterior fusion with either anterior lumbar interbody fusion or transforaminal lumbar interbody fusion. Mundis et al[16] reported significantly improved VAS and ODI scores in a literature review of the lateral approach for adult spinal deformity. Various studies have noted improved patient-reported outcomes after posterior lumbar interbody fusion, including improved ODI, SF-36, and VAS scores.[37-39] Good et al[40] reported similar SRS and ODI scores for both posterior-only and combined fusions, and both had improvements at the 2-year follow-up.

COST AND VALUE

Several recent articles have reported on the costs of adult spinal deformity surgery. McCarthy et al[41] studied the total costs of 484 patients who had operative treatment of adult spinal deformity. The average follow-up was 4.8 years, and the average total hospital cost was $120,394. Total cost for primary surgery averaged $103,143, which increased to $111,807 at the 1-year follow-up and $126,323 at 4-year follow-up. Hospital readmission was required for 130 patients (27%), with an average readmission cost of $67,262. In another cost analysis, McCarthy et al[42] observed higher direct costs with increasing age, length of hospital stay, length of fusion, and fusions to the pelvis.

Cost-utility studies of adult spinal deformity are lacking in the literature. Although several recently published systematic reviews reported on cost-utility analyses in spine care,[43,44] none of the reviewed articles included value assessments in adult deformity. Glassman et al[45] examined the costs and benefits of nonoperative care for adult scoliosis. They found a $10,815 mean treatment cost over a 2-year period with no significant change in HRQOL. This led them to question the value of nonoperative treatment. McCarthy et al[42] reported on a health economic analysis of adult deformity surgery in which they identified age, length of fusion, and primary diagnosis as important predictors of the direct costs of surgery. In a subsequent study on the incremental cost-effectiveness of surgery compared with nonoperative care for adult spinal deformity, the authors demonstrated that durability of the surgical intervention and deterioration of health status with nonoperative care were important determinants of cost-effectiveness of operative care.[46] Durability of surgical intervention and limited need for revision surgery are important challenges for improvement in approaches to adult scoliosis.

IMPROVING OUTCOMES IN DEFORMITY SURGERY

Measurement of clinical outcomes and value is an important goal in spine surgery and is critical in establishing accountability for the end result of care. Ernest A. Codman was a surgeon in the early twentieth century and a pioneer in advocating for outcome measurement and reporting. He advocated for an "end results system" in which patients' symptoms, diagnosis, treatment, and outcomes could be tracked over time in an effort to reduce complications and improve quality of care. At the time, Codman's ideas were seen as radical and met with strong resistance, leading to his dismissal from his faculty position at Massachusetts General Hospital. Although great strides have been made since Codman's time in recognizing the importance of outcome measurement, there is much room for improvement in the effort to establish regular and reliable systems for outcome measurement and reporting.

Surgical rates, surgical strategies, and costs of spine surgery vary significantly.[47-49] High variability indicates a lack of consensus on the optimal treatment strategy and a need for further comparative effectiveness research. Reducing variability in spine surgery requires an evidence-based approach to care. The establishment of large multicenter procedural- and diagnosis-based registries for spine surgery has been an important step to improving outcome measurement and reporting. These registries provide a reliable system for the reporting of complications, clinical outcomes, and HRQOL outcomes and facilitate the evaluation of alternative *interventions* in comparative effectiveness research. With the accurate measurement of complications, quality can be improved through the establishment of clinical protocols based on standards of care in an effort to reduce complications. The widespread use of patient-reported outcome tools that can be translated to a utility score is necessary to address the lack of cost-utility analyses and value-based assessments in adult spinal deformity. An increased emphasis on measuring and improving value in spine care will result in improved outcomes and reduced costs over time. Although we advocate for an effort to reduce variability in spine surgery through an evidence-based approach to care, we also recognize that care is not monolithic, and patient and physician preference must be considered to obtain optimal outcomes.

REFERENCES

1. Brazier JE, Roberts J, Deverill M. The estimation of a preference-based measure of health from the SF-36. J Health Econ 21:271-292, 2002.
2. Berven S, Deviren V, Demir-Deviren S, et al. Studies in the modified Scoliosis Research Society Outcomes Instrument in adults: validation, reliability, and discriminatory capacity. Spine 28:2164-2169; discussion 2169, 2003.
3. Bridwell KH, Berven S, Glassman S, et al. Is the SRS-22 instrument responsive to change in adult scoliosis patients having primary spinal deformity surgery? Spine 32:2220-2225, 2007.
4. Bridwell KH, Cats-Baril W, Harrast J, Berven S, et al. The validity of the SRS-22 instrument in an adult spinal deformity population compared with the Oswestry and SF-12: a study of response distribution, concurrent validity, internal consistency, and reliability. Spine 30:455-461, 2005.
5. Brazier JE, Roberts J. The estimation of a preference-based measure of health from the SF-12. Med Care 42:851-859, 2004.
6. Carreon LY, Glassman SD, McDonough CM, Berven S, et al. Predicting SF-6D utility scores from the Oswestry disability index and numeric rating scales for back and leg pain. Spine 34:2085-2089, 2009.
7. United States Bone and Joint Initiative. The Burden of Musculoskeletal Diseases in the United States: Prevalence, Societal, and Economic Cost, ed 2. Rosemont, IL: American Academy of Orthopaedic Surgeons, 2011.
8. Everett CR, Patel RK. A systematic literature review of nonsurgical treatment in adult scoliosis. Spine 32(19 Suppl):S130-S134, 2007.
9. Smith JS, Shaffrey CI, Berven S, et al; Spinal Deformity Study Group. Improvement of back pain with operative and nonoperative treatment in adults with scoliosis. Neurosurgery 65:86-94, 2009.
10. Li G, Passias P, Kozanek M, et al. Adult scoliosis in patients over sixty-five years of age: outcomes of operative versus nonoperative treatment at a minimum two-year follow-up. Spine. 34:2165-2170, 2009.
11. Smith JS, Shaffrey CI, Berven S, et al; Spinal Deformity Study Group. Operative versus nonoperative treatment of leg pain in adults with scoliosis: a retrospective review of a prospective multicenter database with two-year follow-up. Spine 34:1693-1698, 2009.
12. Bridwell KH, Glassman S, Horton W, et al. Does treatment (nonoperative and operative) improve the two-year quality of life in patients with adult symptomatic lumbar scoliosis: a prospective multicenter evidence-based medicine study. Spine 34:2171-2178, 2009.
13. Youssef J, Orndorff D, Patty C, et al. Current status of adult spinal deformity. Global Spine J 3:51-62, 2012.
14. Yadla S, Maltenfort MG, Ratliff JK, et al. Adult scoliosis surgery outcomes: a systematic review. Neurosurg Focus 28:E3, 2010.
15. Crandall DG, Revella J. Transforaminal lumbar interbody fusion versus anterior lumbar interbody fusion as an adjunct to posterior instrumented correction of degenerative lumbar scoliosis: three year clinical and radiographic outcomes. Spine 34:2126-2133, 2009.
16. Mundis GM, Akbarnia BA, Phillips FM. Adult deformity correction through minimally invasive lateral approach techniques. Spine 35(26 Suppl):S312-S321, 2010.
17. Pateder DB, Kebaish KM, Cascio BM, et al. Posterior only versus combined anterior and posterior approaches to lumbar scoliosis in adults: a radiographic analysis. Spine 32:1551-1554, 2007.
18. Cho KJ, Bridwell KH, Lenke LG, et al. Comparison of Smith-Petersen versus pedicle subtraction osteotomy for the correction of fixed sagittal imbalance. Spine 30:2030-2037; discussion 2038, 2005.

19. Suk SI, Chung ER, Kim JH, et al. Posterior vertebral column resection for severe rigid scoliosis. Spine 30:1682-1687, 2005.

20. Papadopoulos EC, Boachie-Adjei O, Hess WF, et al; Foundation of Complex Spine and Orthopedics, New York, NY. Early outcomes and complications of posterior vertebral column resection. Spine J. 2013 Apr 25. [Epub ahead of print]

21. Glassman SD, Bridwell K, Dimar JR, Berven S, et al. The impact of positive sagittal balance in adult spinal deformity. Spine 30:2024-2029, 2005.

22. Schwab F, Farcy JP, Bridwell K, Berven S, et al. A clinical impact classification of scoliosis in the adult. Spine 31:2109-2114, 2006.

23. Smith JS, Klineberg E, Schwab F, et al; International Spine Study Group. Change in classification grade by the SRS–Schwab Adult Spinal Deformity Classification predicts impact on health-related quality of life measures: prospective analysis of operative and nonoperative treatment. Spine 38:1663-1671, 2013.

24. Charosky S, Guigui P, Blamoutier A, et al; Study Group on Scoliosis. Complications and risk factors of primary adult scoliosis surgery: a multicenter study of 306 patients. Spine 37:693-700, 2012.

25. Sansur CA, Smith JS, Coe JD, Berven SH, et al. Scoliosis Research Society morbidity and mortality of adult scoliosis surgery. Spine 36:E593-E597, 2011.

26. Transfeldt EE, Topp R, Mehbod AA, et al. Surgical outcomes of decompression, decompression with limited fusion, and decompression with full curve fusion for degenerative scoliosis with radiculopathy. Spine 35:1872-1875, 2010.

27. Burneikiene S, Nelson EL, Mason A, et al. Complications in patients undergoing combined transforaminal lumbar interbody fusion and posterior instrumentation with deformity correction for degenerative scoliosis and spinal stenosis. Surg Neurol Int 3:25, 2012.

28. Than KD, Wang AC, Rahman SU, et al. Complication avoidance and management in anterior lumbar interbody fusion. Neurosurg Focus 31:E6, 2011.

29. McDonnell MF, Glassman SD, Dimar JR II, et al. Perioperative complications of anterior procedures on the spine. J Bone Joint Surg Am 78:839-847, 1996.

30. Isaacs RE, Hyde J, Goodrich JA, et al. A prospective, nonrandomized, multicenter evaluation of extreme lateral interbody fusion for the treatment of adult degenerative scoliosis: perioperative outcomes and complications. Spine 35(26 Suppl):S322-S330, 2010.

31. Scheer JK, Tang JA, Smith JS, et al; International Spine Study Group. Reoperation rates and impact on outcome in a large, prospective, multicenter, adult spinal deformity database: clinical article. J Neurosurg Spine 19:464-470, 2013.

32. Pichelmann MA, Lenke LG, Bridwell KH, et al. Revision rates following primary adult spinal deformity surgery: six hundred forty-three consecutive patients followed-up to twenty-two years postoperative. Spine 35:219-226, 2010.

33. Kelly MP, Lenke LG, Bridwell KH, et al. The fate of the adult revision spinal deformity patient: a single institution experience. Spine 38:E1196-E1200, 2013.

34. Acosta FL, McClendon J, O'Shaughnessy BA, et al. Morbidity and mortality after spinal deformity surgery in patients 75 years and older: complications and predictive factors. J Neurosurg Spine 15:667-674, 2011.

35. Fairbank JC, Pynsent PB. The Oswestry Disability Index. Spine 25:2940-2952; discussion 2952, 2000.

36. Bagó J, Pérez-Grueso FJ, Les E, et al. Minimal important differences of the SRS-22 Patient Questionnaire following surgical treatment of idiopathic scoliosis. Eur Spine J 18:1898-1904, 2000.

37. Wu CH, Wong CB, Chen LH, et al. Instrumented posterior lumbar interbody fusion for patients with degenerative lumbar scoliosis. J Spinal Disord Tech 21:310-315, 2008.

38. Zimmerman RM, Mohamed AS, Skolasky RL, et al. Functional outcomes and complications after primary spinal surgery for scoliosis in adults aged forty years or older: a prospective study with minimum two-year follow-up. Spine 35:1861-1866, 2010.

39. Tsai TH, Huang TY, Lieu AS, et al. Functional outcome analysis: instrumented posterior lumbar interbody fusion for degenerative lumbar scoliosis. Acta Neurochir (Wien) 153:547-555, 2010.

40. Good CR, Lenke LG, Bridwell KH, et al. Can posterior-only surgery provide similar radiographic and clinical results as combined anterior (thoracotomy/thoracoabdominal)/posterior approaches for adult scoliosis? Spine 35:210-218, 2010.

41. McCarthy I, Hostin R, Ames C, et al. Total hospital costs of surgical treatment for adult spinal deformity: an extended follow-up study. Spine J. 2014 Jan 24. [Epub ahead of print]

42. McCarthy IM, Hostin RA, O'Brien MF, Berven SH, et al; International Spine Study Group. Analysis of the direct cost of surgery for four diagnostic categories of adult spinal deformity. Spine J 13:1843-1848, 2013.

43. Indrakanti SS, Weber MH, Takemoto SK, Berven SH, et al. Value-based care in the management of spinal disorders: a systematic review of cost-utility analysis. Clin Orthop Relat Res 470:1106-1123, 2012.

44. Kepler CK, Wilkinson SM, Radcliff KE, et al. Cost-utility analysis in spine care: a systematic review. Spine J 12:676-690, 2012.

45. Glassman SD, Carreon LY, Shaffrey CI, et al. The costs and benefits of nonoperative management for adult scoliosis. Spine 35:578-582, 2012.

46. McCarthy I, O'Brien M, Ames C, et al; International Spine Study Group. Incremental cost-effectiveness of adult spinal deformity surgery: observed quality-adjusted life years with surgery compared with predicted quality-adjusted life years without surgery. Neurosurg Focus 36:E3, 2014.

47. Irwin ZN, Hilibrand A, Gustavel M, et al. Variation in surgical decision making for degenerative spinal disorders. I. Lumbar spine. Spine 30:2208-2213, 2005.

48. Sanders JO, Haynes R, Lighter D, et al. Variation in care among spinal deformity surgeons: results of a survey of the Shriners hospitals for children. Spine 32:1444-1449, 2007.

49. Deyo RA, Mirza SK. Trends and variations in the use of spine surgery. Clin Orthop Relat Res 443:139-146, 2006.

PART II

Anatomic, Radiographic, and Surgical Considerations of Global Alignment

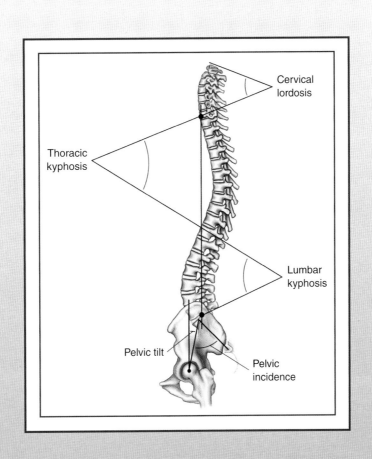

8

Clinical and Radiographic Considerations of Global Spinopelvic Alignment

Justin S. Smith ▪ *Christopher P. Ames* ▪ *John Paul Kelleher*
Regis W. Haid, Jr. ▪ *Christopher I. Shaffrey*

An unprecedented demographic shift toward an older population in the United States and many other developed countries is leading to an increased prevalence of adult spinal deformity (ASD), with recent studies suggesting rates as high as 70% among the elderly.[1] For many with ASD, this deformity may be asymptomatic or produce only limited symptoms, whereas others have significant symptoms.[2-10] The most common presentations of symptomatic ASD include back pain, radicular pain, and disability.[11] These symptoms can result from a combination of disc degeneration, facet arthropathy, nerve root compression, deconditioning, or as a direct consequence of the deformed spine.[12] Treatment of these pathologies requires recognition and assessment of spinopelvic alignment parameters, which have been shown to correlate significantly with standardized measures of health-related quality of life (HRQOL)[13-18] and are critical during surgical treatment planning.[19]

The spine, defined by the vertebrae, discs, and surrounding soft tissues, performs multiple important functions in the human body, including maintenance of upright posture. There has been a growing appreciation of the role of the pelvis as the foundation for the spine and a key determinant of spinal alignment.[15,17-19,20-24] Although pelvic morphology varies in the population, it remains essentially static once the skeleton is matured, and this morphology determines a chain of sagittal alignment correlations that extends to the lumbar, thoracic, and cervical spine.[25,26] Dubousset has coined the term *pelvic vertebra* in recognition of the fundamental role the pelvis serves as a link between the spine and lower extremities and to emphasize the necessity to include the pelvis when considering spinal alignment.[28]

Although the coronal component of spinal deformity may be the most apparent and has traditionally been the target of correction, multiple studies have shown that sagittal alignment demonstrates stronger correlations with symptomatology and HRQOL in ASD both before and after surgery.[13,17,27] Dubousset[28] introduced the concept of a *cone of economy* to describe the fundamentals of optimal standing balance and posture. The cone is centered at the feet of a standing individual and projects upward and outward, defining the range of standing postures for which the body can remain balanced with minimal effort and free from external support. As the body moves toward the periphery of this cone, which often occurs in patients with spinal deformities, additional effort and energy expenditure are necessary to maintain balance. Beyond the periphery, external support, such as a cane, crutch, or walker, may be necessary to prevent a person from falling. The substantially greater energy required to maintain an unsupported standing posture that approaches the periphery of the cone of economy or goes beyond can produce fatigue, pain, and disability.

Multiple radiographic measures have been defined for the assessment of spinopelvic alignment.[3] This chapter provides a brief overview of these measures and a discussion of the relationships between changes in spinopelvic alignment and changes in HRQOL.

SPINOPELVIC ALIGNMENT PARAMETERS

THORACIC KYPHOSIS AND LUMBAR LORDOSIS

Regional sagittal alignment of the thoracolumbar spine is commonly assessed based on thoracic kyphosis (TK) and lumbar lordosis (LL). Overall TK is typically measured from the superior endplate of T2 to the inferior endplate of T12; proximal TK can be measured from the superior endplate of T2 to the inferior endplate of T5, and mid-lower TK can be measured from the superior endplate of T5 to the inferior endplate of T12 (Fig. 8-1).[29] Although the normal range of mid-lower TK has been suggested to be 10 to 40 degrees (with positive [+] and negative [−] measurements reflecting kyphosis and lordosis, respectively),[29] the amount of TK that is normal for an individual has not been well defined. Compensatory measures can affect TK, including reduction of TK to compensate for global positive sagittal malalignment, and reciprocal changes in TK can occur after spinal fusions with an uppermost instrumented vertebra (UIV) in the upper lumbar or lower thoracic region.[30] In addition, TK tends to increase with age.[25]

LL is typically measured from the superior endplate of L1 to the superior endplate of S1 (see Fig. 8-1). Normal values for LL have been suggested to be 40 to 60 degrees[29]; however, more recently it has become clear that the morphology of the pelvis in each person is a better determinant of the amount of LL necessary rather than averages and ranges based on normative populations. Many authors have shown that pelvic morphology, as assessed by the pelvic incidence (PI), determines the amount of LL needed to optimize spinopelvic alignment.[19,21,31] Individuals with greater PI require more LL, whereas those with lower PI need less LL. Schwab and colleagues[15,17] have suggested that the LL should be within approximately 11 degrees of the PI (that is, LL = PI ± 11 degrees).

SAGITTAL VERTICAL AXIS

The sagittal vertical axis (SVA) is measured based on the horizontal distance between a vertical plumb line dropped from the center of the C7 vertebral body and the posterosuperior corner of the sacrum (Fig. 8-2). Based on convention, with full-length, standing radiographs displayed with the patient facing toward the right, C7 plumb lines that fall in front of the posterosuperior corner of the sacrum are designated with positive (+) values, and those that fall behind this corner are designated with negative (−) values. Although the normal value for SVA likely depends in part on patient age and other factors, a threshold of +5 cm or less has been suggested to be normal.[17]

T1 PELVIC ANGLE

Established measures of sagittal spinopelvic alignment, including SVA, T1 spinopelvic inclination (see Fig. 8-2), and PT, can be affected by means of postural compensation, such as pelvic retroversion, knee flexion, and the use of assistive devices for standing upright. Protopsaltis et al[32] and Ryan et al[33] recently introduced a novel radiographic measure of sagittal alignment that is less dependent on postural factors. This measurement, the T1 pelvic angle (TPA), simultaneously accounts for both truncal inclination and pelvic retroversion. The TPA is defined as the angle between a line from the femoral head axis to the centroid of T1 and a line from the femoral head axis to the middle of the S1 endplate (Fig. 8-3). In contrast to the SVA,

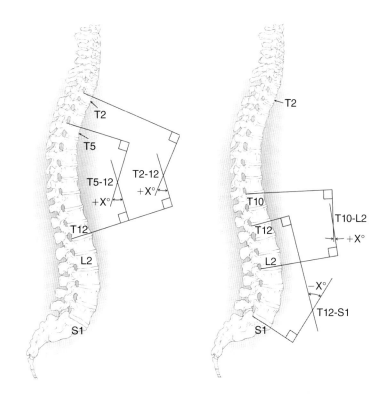

Fig. 8-1   Methods to assess regional sagittal spinal alignment, including T2-12 thoracic kyphosis, T5-12 thoracic kyphosis, T10-L2 thoracolumbar junction alignment, and lumbar lordosis (T12-S1). (+X°, Kyphosis, −X°, lordosis.) (Courtesy of K.X. Probst/Xavier Studio, 2012, with permission.)

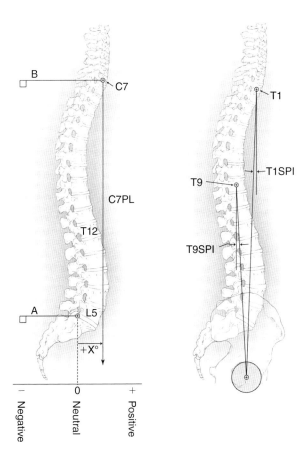

Fig. 8-2   Sagittal view of the spine demonstrating techniques to measure sagittal alignment based on the sagittal vertical axis, which is the horizontal distance *(+X°)* between the posterosuperior corner of the sacrum and the C7 plumb line *(C7PL) (left)*. The image on the *right* shows techniques to measure T1 and T9 spinopelvic inclination *(SPI)*, which are alternative measures of global sagittal alignment that do not rely on imaging scaling. (Courtesy of K.X. Probst/Xavier Studio, 2012, with permission.)

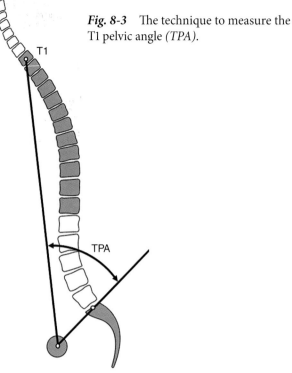

Fig. 8-3   The technique to measure the T1 pelvic angle *(TPA)*.

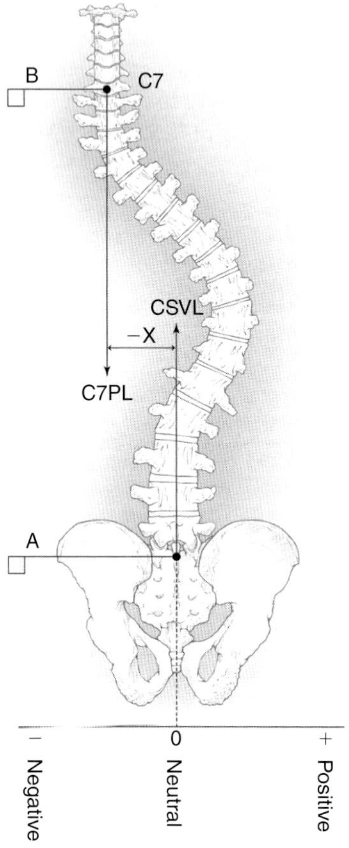

Fig. 8-4   This coronal view of the spine shows a technique to measure coronal alignment, which is the horizontal distance *(−X)* between the C7 plumb line *(C7PL)* and the central sacral vertical line *(CSVL)*. (Courtesy of K.X. Probst/Xavier Studio, 2012, with permission.)

TPA is an angular measure and does not require calibration of the radiograph. Based on 559 consecutive ASD patients, Protopsaltis et al[32] demonstrated that TPA correlated with SVA (r = 0.837), PI-LL mismatch (r = 0.889), and pelvic tilt (PT) (r = 0.933), and increasing TPA correlated significantly with progressive worsening of multiple measures of HRQOL. In addition, based on linear regression analysis, a threshold TPA of 20 degrees was found to correspond to an ODI of higher than 40, and the meaningful change that corresponded to one minimal clinically important difference (MCID) was 4.1 degrees.[32]

GLOBAL CORONAL ALIGNMENT

Global coronal alignment is assessed based on the horizontal distance between a vertical plumb line dropped from the center of the C7 vertebral body and the central sacral vertical line (CSVL) (Fig. 8-4). C7 plumb lines that fall to the left or right of the CSVL are designated with negative (−) or positive (+) values, respectively. Although normal global coronal alignment is 0 cm, a range in values from −2 cm to +2 cm is generally tolerated. Offset of the C7 plumb line, either to the left or the right of the CSVL, is referred to as coronal decompensation (see Fig. 8-4).

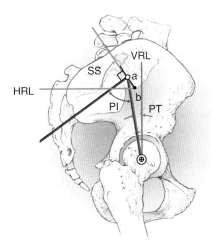

Fig. 8-5 Measurement of sagittal pelvic alignment, including pelvic incidence *(PI)*, pelvic tilt *(PT)*, and sacral slope *(SS)*. (*a,* Center of the sacral endplate; *b,* sacral promontory; *HRL,* horizontal reference line; *VRL,* vertical reference line.) (Courtesy of K.X. Probst/Xavier Studio, 2012, with permission.)

PELVIC INCIDENCE

PI is defined as the angle subtended by a line drawn from the center of the femoral head to the sacral endplate and a line drawn perpendicular to the center of the sacral endplate (Fig. 8-5). The PI is a morphologic parameter that reflects the relationship of the sacrum to the pelvis and remains relatively unchanged once the skeleton is mature. Recently, Schwab et al[15,17] and Boulay et al[31] reported on the role of PI in determining the degree of LL. Based on the work of Legaye et al,[34] they supported a formula in which LL should be within approximately 10 degrees of the PI.

PELVIC TILT

PT is defined as the angle subtended by a line drawn from the midpoint of the sacral endplate to the center of the bicoxofemoral axis and a vertical plumb line extended from the bicoxofemoral axis (see Fig. 8-4). In contrast to PI, which is a morphologic parameter, PT is a compensatory parameter. With progressive positive sagittal malalignment, the pelvis can be retroverted (increased PT) in an effort to maintain an upright posture. Increased PT has been shown to correlate with impairment in walking tolerance and disability measures and should be accounted for in surgical planning.[14,17,19] A high PT can mask the true magnitude of positive sagittal malalignment if only the SVA is considered; this can lead to an underestimation of the amount of sagittal alignment correction necessary when planning surgery.[18,19]

SACRAL SLOPE

Sacral slope (SS) is defined as the angle subtended by a line drawn along the endplate of the sacrum and a horizontal reference line extended from the posterior superior corner of S1 (see Fig. 8-4). The mathematical relationship of PI, PT, and SS are shown in the following equation: PI = PT + SS. As PT increases, the SS decreases, because the sacrum assumes a more vertical position about the femoral head axis (pelvic retroversion).

PELVIC OBLIQUITY

Pelvic obliquity is a coronal plane parameter that often plays a crucial role in surgical planning.[19] It is estimated by measuring the angle formed between a horizontal reference line and a line drawn between the

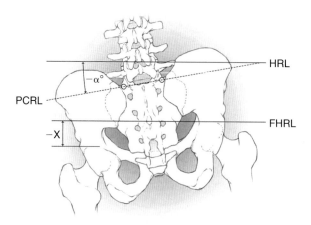

Fig. 8-6   The technique to measure pelvic obliquity ($-\alpha°$) or leg-length discrepancy ($-X$). (*FHRL,* Femoral horizontal reference line; *HRL,* horizontal reference line; *PCRL,* pelvic coronal reference line.) (Courtesy of K.X. Probst/ Xavier Studio, 2012, with permission.)

two inferior points of the sacral alae on an AP radiograph (Fig. 8-6). Pelvic obliquity can be a result of leg-length discrepancy from congenital or acquired conditions or from sacropelvic deformity, either of which can produce a compensatory lumbar curve to balance the spine. Correction of this lumbar curve without correction of the underlying pelvic obliquity can lead to coronal decompensation. Similarly, pelvic obliquity can be a secondary problem (for example, resulting from attempts to compensate for a spinal scoliotic curve). In these cases, the curve correction should be of sufficient magnitude to allow the pelvis to relax in the coronal plane after surgery. All patients should be evaluated clinically and radiographically for a leg-length discrepancy. If one is identified, the patient should be fitted for a shoe lift and then reevaluated both clinically and radiographically to assess how the spine and pelvis respond to correction of the discrepancy. Patients with a flexible curve from pelvic obliquity as a result of a leg-length discrepancy may respond well to the addition of a shoe lift only or surgical treatment of the leg-length discrepancy. If the spinal curve is rigid, it will not correct after the addition of a shoe lift, and this should be considered during surgical planning.

RELATIONSHIPS BETWEEN CHANGES IN SPINOPELVIC ALIGNMENT AND CHANGES IN HEALTH-RELATED QUALITY OF LIFE

Adults with spinal deformity characteristically present with pain and disability, a key drive of which is sagittal spinal malalignment.[3,8,9,14-19,35] Glassman and colleagues[13,27] were among the first to show a significant correlation between global SVA and HRQOL based on a large population of operatively and nonoperatively treated adults with spinal deformity. Specifically, with increasingly positive SVA measurements, standardized measures of pain and disability reflected significantly poorer HRQOL. Several subsequent studies, including that of Lafage et al,[14] have confirmed this significant correlation.

Although the importance of SVA has been clearly established, more recently it has become evident that assessment of SVA alone does not fully account for global alignment. Improved understanding of the role of the pelvis as a key determinant of spinal alignment and as a source of compensation has led to an expanded appreciation of spinopelvic alignment.[8,14-19,22,35-37] To better understand the correlations between spinopelvic alignment and HRQOL scores, Schwab et al[17] recently assessed correlations between radiographic parameters, both coronal and sagittal, and HRQOL scores in 492 adults with spinal deformity. Of the broad array of radiographic parameters reviewed, the three with the strongest correlations to HRQOL scores were the mismatch between the PI and LL (PI-LL), SVA, and PT. In addition, linear regression mod-

Four Coronal Curve Types	Three Sagittal Modifiers

T Thoracic Only
Apex of deformity at T9 or higher with lumbar curve <30°
 	
L TL/Lumbar Only
Apex of deformity at T10 or lower with thoracic curve <30°
 	
D Double Curve
With at least one T and one TL/L, both >30°
 	
N No Coronal Curve
All coronal curves <30°
	PI Minus LL
	  0: Within 10°
	  +: Moderate 10° to 20°
	  ++: Marked >20°
	
	Pelvic Tilt
	  0: PT <20°
	  +: PT 20° to 30°
	  ++: PT >30°
	
	Global Alignment
	  0: SVA <4 cm
	  +: SVA 4 to 9.5 cm
	  ++: SVA >9.5 cm

Fig. 8-7 SRS–Schwab classification of adult spinal deformity. (*LL,* Lumbar lordosis; *PI,* pelvic incidence; *PT,* pelvic tilt; *SVA,* sagittal vertical axis; *TL/L,* thoracolumbar/lumbar.) (Adapted from Schwab F, Ungar B, Blondel B, et al. Scoliosis Research Society–Schwab adult spinal deformity classification: a validation study. Spine 37:1077-1082, 2012.)

els demonstrated threshold radiographic spinopelvic parameters for an ODI of more than 40 (moderate to severe disability) to be the following: PT of at least 22 degrees (r = 0.38), SVA of at least 47 mm (r = 0.47), PI-LL mismatch of at least 11 degrees.[17] Collectively, this study not only further demonstrated the significant clinical impact of sagittal spinopelvic malalignment on HRQOL scores, but it also established thresholds of disability for these radiographic parameters that may prove useful in surgical planning.

Multiple attempts have been made to establish a clinically useful classification system for ASD, including the Scoliosis Research Society (SRS) system and the Schwab system.[38-40] Recently, an updated and improved version of the Schwab adult deformity classification, created in conjunction with the SRS, has been reported (Fig. 8-7).[41] The parameters for the SRS–Schwab classification were selected based on clinical relevance. The system includes four coronal curve type descriptors (T: thoracic curve, L: thoracolumbar/lumbar curve, D: double curve, and N: all coronal curves of less than 30 degrees) and three sagittal spinopelvic modifiers (see Fig. 8-7). The spinopelvic descriptors are PI-LL mismatch, global alignment (SVA), and PT. These were selected based on the previous work of Schwab et al,[17] which demonstrated these parameters to have the strongest correlations with HRQOL scores. For each sagittal modifier, a score of 0, +, or ++ is assigned, indicating normal, moderately abnormal, or markedly abnormal, respectively. The SRS–Schwab classification has been shown to have excellent intraobserver and interobserver agreement, suggesting that its application is sufficiently easy and reliable.[41]

Terran et al[42] prospectively assessed the clinical relevance of the SRS–Schwab classification based on correlations with HRQOL measures and the decision to pursue operative versus nonoperative treatment in 527 adults with spinal deformity. They noted significant differences in HRQOL scores based on the SRS–Schwab curve type, with poorer health status and greater disability associated with thoracolumbar primary sagittal deformities. Operative patients had significantly poorer grades for all three sagittal spinopelvic modifiers. For all of the parameters, progressively higher grades were associated with significantly poorer HRQOL scores. They also reported that patients with worse sagittal spinopelvic modifier grades were significantly more likely to require major osteotomies, iliac fixation, and decompression.

Smith et al[43] prospectively assessed the responsiveness of the SRS–Schwab ASD classification to changes in HRQOL measures 1 year after operative or nonoperative treatment. Based on results in 341 patients (177 operative and 164 nonoperative), they found that changes in modifier grades were significantly associated with changes in standardized measures of HRQOL. Patients with improvement of PI-LL mismatch, SVA, or PT classification modifier grades were significantly more likely to achieve MCID for ODI, the SF-36 physical component score (SVA and PI-LL only), the SRS activity subscore, and the SRS pain subscore

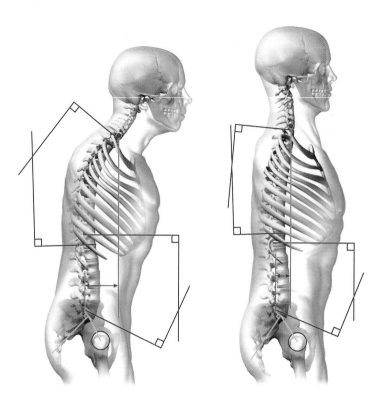

Fig. 8-8   Decompensated _(left)_ and compensated _(right)_ sagittal spinopelvic malalignment (SSM). In decompensated SSM, the global sagittal alignment (sagittal vertical axis [SVA]) is abnormally high (greater than 5 cm). In contrast, in compensated SSM, the SVA is not abnormal, but the magnitude of the pelvic incidence to lumbar lordosis mismatch (PI-LL) is abnormally high (greater than 10 degrees). (Courtesy of K.X. Probst/Xavier Studio, 2012, with permission.)

(PI-LL only). They concluded that the SRS–Schwab classification modifiers are responsive to changes in disease state and reflect significant changes in patient-reported outcomes.

It has been well established that abnormally elevated SVA correlates with pain and disability in adults with spinal deformity, and many of these patients also have a flat-back deformity (PI-LL mismatch of more than 10 degrees). Numerous reports have documented the potential for surgical correction of this positive sagittal malalignment to result in improved HRQOL, and this condition is considered a primary indication for surgery.[13,27,35,44] However, a subset of patients with flat-back deformity retain sagittal compensation with normal SVA (Fig. 8-8). Smith et al[35] recently reported on a comparison between decompensated (SVA of greater than 5 cm) and compensated (SVA of less than 5 cm and PI-LL mismatch larger than 10 degrees) adult deformity patients. In 125 patients (98 decompensated and 27 compensated), they found that the decompensated group was older and had less scoliosis, greater SVA, greater PI-LL mismatch, and poorer HRQOL (ODI, SF-36 physical component score, and SRS-22 total score). Notably, although baseline HRQOL differences between these groups reached statistical significance, only the mean difference in SF-36 physical component score reached a threshold for MCID. One year after surgery, the decompensated and compensated groups demonstrated significant improvement in key radiographic measures of alignment (coronal Cobb angle, TK, SVA, PT, and PI-LL mismatch) and in all measures of HRQOL assessed (ODI, SF-36 physical and mental component scores, SRS-22 total score, and all SRS-22 subscores). In addition, no significant differences were noted between the compensated and decompensated groups in the magnitude of HRQOL improvement or the percentages of patients achieving MCID for each of the clinical outcomes measures assessed. Collectively, these data clearly demonstrated the importance of evaluating pelvic parameters and the potential improvement in clinical outcome that can be achieved through correction of abnormal sagittal spinopelvic alignment.

CONCLUSION

Adults with spinal deformity characteristically present with pain and disability. Many reports have clearly shown that sagittal spinopelvic malalignment is a key cause of pain and disability in this population, and correction of spinopelvic malalignment correlates with improvement of HRQOL. Surgical correction goals have been suggested to include a PT of at least 22 degrees, SVA of at least 47 mm, and PI-LL mismatch of 11 degrees or more. Failure to recognize and integrate spinopelvic parameters into surgical planning can lead to suboptimal clinical outcomes.

REFERENCES

1. Schwab F, Dubey A, Pagala M, et al. Adult scoliosis: a health assessment analysis by SF-36. Spine 28:602-606, 2003.
2. Aebi M. The adult scoliosis. Eur Spine J 14:925-948, 2005.
3. Bess S, Boachie-Adjei O, Burton D, et al. Pain and disability determine treatment modality for older patients with adult scoliosis, while deformity guides treatment for younger patients. Spine 34:2186-2190, 2009.
4. Bridwell KH, Baldus C, Berven S, et al Changes in radiographic and clinical outcomes with primary treatment adult spinal deformity surgeries from two years to three- to five-years follow-up. Spine 35:1849-1854, 2010.
5. Smith JS, Kasliwal MK, Crawford A, et al. Outcomes, expectations, and complications overview for the surgical treatment of adult and pediatric spinal deformity. Spine Deform (Preview Issue):4-14, 2012.
6. Smith JS, Shaffrey CI, Berven S, et al. Improvement of back pain with operative and nonoperative treatment in adults with scoliosis. Neurosurgery 65:86-93; discussion 93-84, 2009.
7. Smith JS, Shaffrey CI, Berven S, et al. Operative versus nonoperative treatment of leg pain in adults with scoliosis: a retrospective review of a prospective multicenter database with two-year follow-up. Spine 34:1693-1698, 2009.
8. Smith JS, Shaffrey CI, Fu KM, et al. Clinical and radiographic evaluation of the adult spinal deformity patient. Neurosurg Clin N Am 24:143-156, 2013.
9. Smith JS, Shaffrey CI, Glassman SD, et al. Risk-benefit assessment of surgery for adult scoliosis: an analysis based on patient age. Spine 36:817-824, 2011.
10. Smith JS, Shaffrey CI, Glassman SD, et al. Clinical and radiographic parameters that distinguish between the best and worst outcomes of scoliosis surgery for adults. Eur Spine J 22:402-410, 2013.
11. Smith JS, Fu KM, Urban P, et al. Neurological symptoms and deficits in adults with scoliosis who present to a surgical clinic: incidence and association with the choice of operative versus nonoperative management. J Neurosurg Spine 9:326-331, 2008.
12. Fu KM, Rhagavan P, Shaffrey CI, et al. Prevalence, severity, and impact of foraminal and canal stenosis among adults with degenerative scoliosis. Neurosurgery 69:1181-1187, 2011.
13. Glassman SD, Berven S, Bridwell K, et al. Correlation of radiographic parameters and clinical symptoms in adult scoliosis. Spine 30:682-688, 2005.
14. Lafage V, Schwab F, Patel A, et al. Pelvic tilt and truncal inclination: two key radiographic parameters in the setting of adults with spinal deformity. Spine 34:E599-E606, 2009.
15. Schwab F, Lafage V, Patel A, et al. Sagittal plane considerations and the pelvis in the adult patient. Spine 34:1828-1833, 2009.
16. Schwab F, Patel A, Ungar B, et al. Adult spinal deformity-postoperative standing imbalance: how much can you tolerate? An overview of key parameters in assessing alignment and planning corrective surgery. Spine 35:2224-2231, 2010.
17. Schwab FJ, Blondel B, Bess S, et al. Radiographical spinopelvic parameters and disability in the setting of adult spinal deformity: a prospective multicenter analysis. Spine 38:E803-E812, 2013.
18. Smith JS, Bess S, Shaffrey CI, et al. Dynamic changes of the pelvis and spine are key to predicting postoperative sagittal alignment after pedicle subtraction osteotomy: a critical analysis of preoperative planning techniques. Spine 37:845-853, 2012.
19. Ames CP, Smith JS, Scheer JK, et al. Impact of spinopelvic alignment on decision making in deformity surgery in adults: a review. J Neurosurg Spine 16:547-564, 2012.
20. Labelle H, Roussouly P, Berthonnaud E, et al. The importance of spino-pelvic balance in L5-s1 developmental spondylolisthesis: a review of pertinent radiologic measurements. Spine 30:S27-S34, 2005.

21. Legaye J, Duval-Beaupère G. Sagittal plane alignment of the spine and gravity: a radiological and clinical evaluation. Acta Orthop Belg 71:213-220, 2005.
22. Roussouly P, Gollogly S, Berthonnaud E, et al. Classification of the normal variation in the sagittal alignment of the human lumbar spine and pelvis in the standing position. Spine 30:346-353, 2005.
23. Schwab F, Lafage V, Boyce R, et al. Gravity line analysis in adult volunteers: age-related correlation with spinal parameters, pelvic parameters, and foot position. Spine 31:E959-E967, 2006.
24. Vaz G, Roussouly P, Berthonnaud E, et al. Sagittal morphology and equilibrium of pelvis and spine. Eur Spine J 11:80-87, 2002.
25. Ames CP, Blondel B, Scheer JK, et al. Cervical radiographical alignment: comprehensive assessment techniques and potential importance in cervical myelopathy. Spine 38:S149-S160, 2013.
26. Skalli W, Zeller RD, Miladi L, et al. Importance of pelvic compensation in posture and motion after posterior spinal fusion using CD instrumentation for idiopathic scoliosis. Spine 31:E359-E366, 2006.
27. Glassman SD, Bridwell K, Dimar JR, et al. The impact of positive sagittal balance in adult spinal deformity. Spine 30:2024-2029, 2005.
28. Dubousset J. Three-dimensional analysis of the scoliotic deformity. In Weinstein SL, ed. The Pediatric Spine: Principles and Practice. New York: Raven Press 1994.
29. O'Brien MF, Kuklo TR, Blanke KM, eds. Spinal Deformity Study Group Radiographic Measurement Manual. Memphis, TN: Medtronic Sofamor Danek, 2005.
30. Klineberg E, Schwab F, Ames C, et al. Acute reciprocal changes distant from the site of spinal osteotomies affect global postoperative alignment. Adv Orthop 2011:415946, 2011.
31. Boulay C, Tardieu C, Hecquet J, et al. Sagittal alignment of spine and pelvis regulated by pelvic incidence: standard values and prediction of lordosis. Eur Spine J 15:415-422, 2006.
32. Protopsaltis T, Schwab F, Bronsard N, et al. The T1 pelvic angle (TPA), a novel radiographic measure of global sagittal deformity, accounts for both spinal inclination and pelvic tilt and correlates with HRQOL. J Bone Joint Surg Am (in press).
33. Ryan DJ, Protopsaltis T, Ames C, Hostin R, Klineberg E, Mundis G, et al. T1 pelvic angle (TPA) effectively evaluates sagittal deformity and assesses radiographic surgical outcomes longitudinally. Spine (in press).
34. Legaye J, Duval-Beaupère G, Hecquet J, et al. Pelvic incidence: a fundamental pelvic parameter for three-dimensional regulation of spinal sagittal curves. Eur Spine J 7:99-103, 1998.
35. Smith JS, Singh M, Klineberg E, et al. Surgical treatment of pathological loss of lumbar lordosis (flatback) in the setting of normal sagittal vertical axis (SVA) achieves similar clinical improvement as surgical treatment of elevated SVA. J Neurosurg Spine (in press).
36. Lafage V, Bharucha NJ, Schwab F, et al. Multicenter validation of a formula predicting postoperative spinopelvic alignment. J Neurosurg Spine 16:15-21, 2012.
37. Schwab FJ, Blondel B, Bess S, Hostin R, Shaffrey CI, Smith JS, Boachie-Adjei O, Burton DC, Akbarnia BA, Mundis GM, Ames CP, et al. Radiographic spinopelvic parameters and disability in the setting of adult spinal deformity: a prospective multicenter analysis. Spine 38:E803-E812, 2013.
38. Lowe T, Berven SH, Schwab FJ, et al. The SRS classification for adult spinal deformity: building on the King/Moe and Lenke classification systems. Spine 31:S119-S125, 2006.
39. Schwab F, Farcy JP, Bridwell K, et al. A clinical impact classification of scoliosis in the adult. Spine 31:2109-2114, 2006.
40. Smith JS, Shaffrey CI, Kuntz Ct, et al. Classification systems for adolescent and adult scoliosis. Neurosurgery 63:16-24, 2008.
41. Schwab F, Ungar B, Blondel B, et al. Scoliosis Research Society–Schwab adult spinal deformity classification: a validation study. Spine 37:1077-1082, 2012.
42. Terran J, Schwab F, Shaffrey CI, et al. The SRS–Schwab adult spinal deformity classification: assessment and clinical correlations based on a prospective operative and nonoperative cohort. Neurosurgery 73:559-568, 2013.
43. Smith JS, Klineberg E, Schwab F, et al. Change in classification grade by the SRS–Schwab Adult Spinal Deformity Classification predicts impact on health-related quality of life measures: prospective analysis of operative and nonoperative treatment. Spine 38:1663-1671, 2013.
44. Smith JS, Sansur CA, Donaldson WF III, et al. Short-term morbidity and mortality associated with correction of thoracolumbar fixed sagittal plane deformity: a report from the Scoliosis Research Society Morbidity and Mortality Committee. Spine 36:958-964, 2011.

9

Craniocervical Region

Yakov Gologorsky ▪ *Michael W. Groff*

During the past decade interest in the vital importance of sagittal balance and its importance in clinical outcome has increased tremendously. A growing emphasis is being placed on the preservation or restoration of neutral upright sagittal spinal alignment, partly because the ability to comfortably stand upright and maintain horizontal gaze is inherent to the human condition.[1,2] Many recent articles have demonstrated that the regional and global alignment of the spine after fusion is a major factor in postoperative clinical outcomes.[3,4]

Kuntz et al[1,2] reviewed the English-language literature to identify studies that evaluated neutral upright sagittal spinal (occiput-pelvis) alignment in asymptomatic adult volunteers with no spinal disease. They reported 23 angles and displacements that represented neutral upright sagittal occiput-pelvis alignment. They found wide variations in the undulating lordotic and kyphotic regional curves from the occiput to the pelvis. Despite these wide regional variations, global sagittal spinal balance was maintained in a much narrower range for preservation of horizontal gaze and balance of the spine and pelvis over the femoral heads. The chin-brow vertical angle, a common measurement representing horizontal gaze, was maintained within very few degrees, highlighting the significance of this particular parameter (Fig. 9-1).

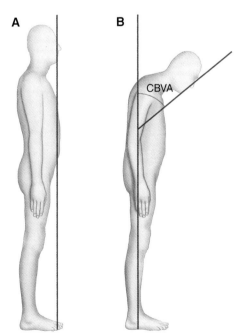

Fig. 9-1 The chin-brow vertical angle is defined as the angle subtended by a vertical reference line and a line drawn parallel to the chin and brow, with the neck in a neutral or fixed position and the knees and hips extended. It is a clinical measurement of the total flexion deformity of the spine and the effect on horizontal gaze. **A,** Demonstrates a normal angle. **B,** Demonstrates an abnormally kyphotic angle.

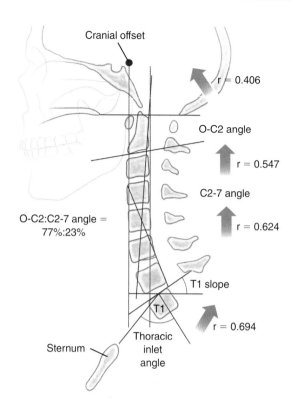

Fig. 9-2   The sequential linkage of significant correlations from the thoracic inlet angle to the cranial offset and craniocervical alignment. The r values within the arrows between the segments represent Pearson's correlation coefficient between the two segments. The sequential correlations between adjacent segments link the correlation between the thoracic inlet angle and the cranial offset. (*O-C2,* Occipitocervical angle.)

Regional curves do not function independently of one another but are rather closely interrelated.[3-6] The sagittal alignment of the cranium and cervical spine can be influenced by the shape and orientation of the thoracic inlet to maintain a balanced, upright posture and horizontal gaze, similar to the relationship between the pelvic incidence and lumbar lordosis. Lee et al[5] found significant correlations between the thoracic inlet angle and both the cranial offset and craniocervical alignment[4] (Fig. 9-2).

Hardacker et al[7] reported that the relative contributions of the occiput-C2 and the C2-7 angles to overall cervical lordosis in asymptomatic individuals are 77% and 23%, respectively. Consequently, a fusion operation that fixates the occiput to the cervical spine in poor alignment will place undue stresses on the remaining cervical spine and can result in adjacent-level/regional compensatory deformity to maintain neutral horizontal gaze. Cervical kyphotic deformity, in turn, is associated with neck pain, poorer outcomes in health-related quality of life indices, and less postoperative neurologic improvement.[3]

ANATOMIC AND BIOMECHANICAL CONSIDERATIONS

The craniovertebral junction is a complex region that incorporates the occiput–C1-2 portions of the spine. The occiput–C1-2 complex functions as a single unit, with the atlas acting as a washer between the occiput and the rest of the cervical spine. It is the most mobile portion of the cervical spine and acts as a transition between the cranium and the subaxial cervical spine.[8-10] The anatomy and motions afforded by the occiput-C1 (O-C1) and C1-2 articulations are vastly different. The mechanical properties of O-C1 are largely determined by bony elements, whereas those of the C1-2 segment are largely controlled by ligamentous elements. The two motion segments, however, are intimately linked, and the motion is always coupled.[8-10]

The atlantooccipital joints (O-C1) are anteromedially oriented, concave spheroid articulations connected by very tight capsules. Their mechanical properties are chiefly determined by the shape of the bony elements. The primary movement at O-C1 is flexion and extension, with a total range of movement from 20 to

25 degrees.[8-10] Flexion is limited by impingement of the tip of the dens on the foramen magnum, whereas extension is limited by the tectorial membrane. Lateral bending ranges from 3 to 5 degrees per side. This movement is resisted by the O-C1 articulation and the alar ligaments. Axial rotation ranges from 1 to 7.2 degrees per side and is also limited by the O-C1 articulation and the alar ligaments. The instantaneous axis of rotation for axial movement is ventral to the foramen magnum.[8-10]

The atlantoaxial complex (C1-2) is composed of four joints: two atlantoaxial lateral joints, the atlantoaxial median joint (between the anterior arch of the atlas and the dens axis), and the joint between the posterior aspect of the dens and the transverse ligament. Stability of this highly complex structure is mainly determined by ligamentous structures.[8-10] The primary movement at C1-2 is axial rotation, with mean rotational movement of approximately 40 degrees to each side. Movement is limited by the C1-2 articulation, the ipsilateral transverse ligament, the contralateral alar ligament, and the capsular ligaments. Axial rotation at C1-2 is negatively coupled to rotation at O-C1, that is, axial rotation at C1-2 induces axial rotation of lesser magnitude and in the opposite direction at O-C1. The instantaneous axis of rotation is located in the central portion of the dens. Flexion-extension ranges from 10 to 30 degrees.[8-10] Flexion is limited by the transverse ligament, and extension is limited by the tectorial membrane and the C1-2 articulation. In flexion and extension, the instantaneous axis of rotation is located midway between the tip and base of the dens near its dorsal cortex. Lateral bending is checked by the alar ligaments and is inconsequential under normal conditions, but can reach 7 degrees in pathologic states. Ventral sagittal translation is primarily limited by the transverse ligament, and secondary stabilizers include the alar and capsular ligaments. Posterior sagittal translation is limited by abutment of the dens on the ventral arch and is usually less than 3 mm in adults.[8-10]

The center of mass of the head in the sagittal plane directly overlies the occipital condyle, approximately 1 cm above and anterior to the external auditory canal; any deviations from the normal alignment of the mass of the head result in an increase in cantilever loads, which subsequently induces an increase in muscular energy expenditure.[4] The weight of the head is borne through the condyle to the lateral masses of C1 and then to the two lateral C1-2 joints. This load is then divided via the C2 articular pillars to the anterior column (which includes the C2-3 disc) and the posterior column (which includes the C2-3 facets). Most of the load is transmitted to the C2-3 disc space and less to the facets[9] (Fig. 9-3). In the subaxial spine, however, the load distribution is primarily in the posterior columns, with 36% in the anterior column and 64% in the two posterior columns. The force transmission has critical areas in which overload results in fracture. The first area is in the *washer* ring of C1. When overloaded, the atlas bursts, resulting in Jefferson fractures. The next critical area is at the isthmus of the C2 pars interarticularis, where an axial force overload results in a hangman-type fracture.[9]

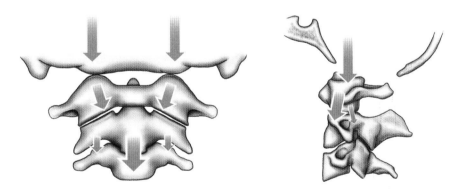

Fig. 9-3   The weight of the head is borne through the condyle to the lateral masses of C1 and then to the two lateral C1-2 joints. This load is then divided via the C2 articular pillars to the anterior column (which includes the C2-3 disc) and the posterior column (which includes the C2-3 facets). Most of the load is transmitted to the C2-3 disc space and less to the facets.

INDICATIONS FOR FUSION

Indications for occipitocervical fixation include myriad causes that result in occipitocervical instability. Essentially, instability is defined as a condition in which the spine is unable to resist physiologic loads without pain, deformity, and/or neurologic deficit. Causes include arthropathies such as rheumatoid arthritis, congenital deformity such as those seen with Down's syndrome or os odontoideum, basilar invagination, trauma, tumor, infection/osteomyelitis, degenerative spine disease, or iatrogenic instability after particular transcondylar or transoral approaches for skull-base surgery.[11-14] Many cases involve fusion or assimilation of the occiput and atlas; consequently, atlantoaxial fusion results effectively in occipitocervical fusion.

PREOPERATIVE EVALUATION AND PLANNING

PHYSICAL EXAMINATION

A complete history should be obtained and a thorough physical examination performed. The patient's medical history should be reviewed carefully, and a general review of systems helps to identify conditions such as renal, respiratory, and cardiac abnormalities that can be associated with spinal abnormality and may necessitate additional evaluation.[14] Cervical range of motion is evaluated, and the entire spine is inspected and palpated. Neurologic assessment includes cranial nerves, motor strength, sensation, muscle tone, reflexes (peripheral and pathologic), coordination, proprioception, and gait.

Preoperative nutritional status is evaluated.[14] Patients with brainstem or cranial nerve compromise may have impaired swallowing and impaired nutritional status that could negatively affect wound healing and osseous fusion. Patients with evidence of poor nutritional status may benefit from preoperative nutritional support. Pulmonary function can be affected in patients with significant brainstem or lower cranial nerve impairment, in particular cranial nerves IX, X, and XII. Preoperative tracheostomy is occasionally appropriate in these patients.[13,14]

RADIOGRAPHIC WORKUP AND PREOPERATIVE IMAGING

Multimodality radiographic imaging of the craniovertebral junction is integral to preoperative surgical planning. However, not all modalities are necessary for each patient. Many centers separate indications into broader degenerative, traumatic, and neoplastic categories.[15] For patients with degenerative causes (of which rheumatoid arthritis is by far the most common), standard, neutral, noncontrast MRI allows visualization of soft tissues, neural, and vascular structures. Dynamic MRI views in flexion and extension can be considered to identify the best position to obviate neural compression.[13,14] If bony relationships are obscured on plain radiographs, thin-slice CT imaging with coronal, sagittal, and three-dimensional reconstructions are obtained. These best define the often-complex osseous anatomy and are supplemented with flexion-extension lateral plain radiographs. The occipitocervical angle and other relevant parameters are best calculated on CT imaging.[15] In preparation for screw fixation, angiographic studies such as CT-angiography or MR-angiography may be useful. For patients with traumatic causes, thin-cut CT is crucial to identify fractures, and MRI imaging reveals neural compression and ligamentous injury. Finally, in patients with neoplastic disease of the craniovertebral junction, contrast-enhanced MRI is performed in addition to the modalities discussed previously. Occasionally, with invasive tumors, catheter-based angiography is indicated to further define the vascular anatomy, to rule out vascular invasion, or for preoperative embolization.[15]

IMPORTANT ANGLES AND MEASUREMENTS

The occipitocervical angle has been widely studied and described in both asymptomatic individuals and in patients with occipitocervical or atlantoaxial instability. Unfortunately, because many methods are available to measure this angle, the range of normal values is wide. This has introduced confusion into the literature. The three main ways to calculate this angle are described as follows:

- The O-C2 angle itself can be calculated by three different methods.[16] The first line is drawn parallel to the inferior endplate of C2. The second line is one of the following three: (1) Chamberlain's line[17] (from the posterosuperior aspect of the hard palate to the opisthion [Fig. 9-4]), (2) McRae's line[18] (from the basion and the opisthion [Fig. 9-5]), or (3) McGregor's line[19] (from the posterosuperior aspect of the hard palate to the most caudal point on the midline occipital curve [Fig. 9-6]). The subtended angle between these lines defines the O-C2 angle. Shoda et al[16] compared the reliability of these three methods and concluded that McGregor's line is the most reproducible and reliable method for measuring the occipitocervical angle. Using this technique, the mean neutral O-C2 angle is approximately 15 degrees, with normal ranging from approximately 5 to 25 degrees.[1,2,20-22]
- The O-C3 angle is formed by McRae's line (see above) and a line drawn parallel to the superior endplate of C3.[23] Using this definition, the mean occipitocervical angles are 24.2 degrees, 44.0 degrees, and 57.2 degrees in flexion, neutral, and extension views, respectively.[23]

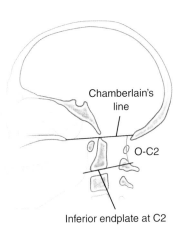

Fig. 9-4   Chamberlain's line is drawn from the posterosuperior aspect of the hard palate to the opisthion. The occipitocervical angle *(O-C2)* is formed by the intersection of this line with a line parallel to the inferior endplate of C2.

Fig. 9-5   McRae's line is drawn from the basion to the opisthion. The occipitocervical angle *(O-C2)* is formed by the intersection of this line with a line parallel to the inferior endplate of C2.

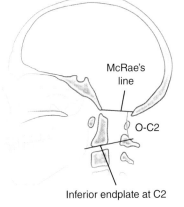

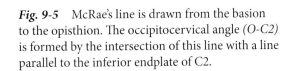

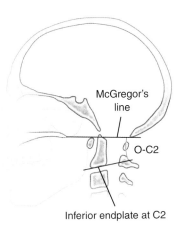

Fig. 9-6   McGregor's line is drawn from the posterosuperior aspect of the hard palate to the most caudal point on the midline occipital curve. The occipitocervical angle *(O-C2)* is formed by the intersection of this line with a line parallel to the inferior endplate of C2.

- The posterior occipital cervical angle[24] is the angle formed by a line drawn tangential to the posterior aspect of the occipital protuberance and a line determined by the posterior aspect of the facets of the third and fourth cervical vertebrae. Using this method, the posterior occipital cervical angle measures 109.7 degrees, with 80% of normal from 101 to 119 degrees.[24]

Atlantoaxial fusion is often performed for C1-2 instability. In instances of assimilation of the atlas to the occiput, fusion of the C1-2 joint effectively results in occipitocervical fusion. In these circumstances, measurement of other angles such as the C1-2 angle is critically important. This angle is formed by a line passing through the centers of the anterior and posterior arches of C1 and its intersection with a line parallel to the inferior endplate of C2.[25] A similar angle is formed by a line passing through the bottoms of the anterior and posterior arches of C1 and its intersection with a line parallel to the inferior endplate of C2.[26]

Generally, atlantoaxial fusion is performed for patients with basilar invagination. Basilar invagination can often be difficult to diagnose with plain radiography in patients with rheumatoid arthritis. Numerous radiographic criteria have been described, and the most frequently used are the following:

- *McRae's line:* Protrusion of the tip of the odontoid process above this line indicates basilar invagination.[18,27]
- *Chamberlain's line:* Protrusion of the odontoid tip more than 3 mm above this line indicates basilar invagination.[17,27]
- *McGregor's line:* Basilar invagination is diagnosed when the apex of the odontoid process rises more than 4.5 mm above this line.[19,27]
- *Fischgold-Metzger line:* A line is drawn between the tips of the mastoid processes on an anteroposterior open-mouth odontoid radiograph. Protrusion of the tip of the odontoid process above this line indicates basilar invagination.[27,28]
- *Wackenheim clivus baseline* (also referred to as the *basilar line*): A line is drawn along the clivus and projected inferiorly into the upper cervical spinal canal. This line should lie tangent to the posterior aspect of the tip of the odontoid process. Protrusion of the odontoid tip posterior to the projection of this line indicates basilar invagination.[27,29]
- *Clark's station:* The station of the atlas is determined by dividing the odontoid process into three equal parts in the sagittal plane. If the anterior ring of the atlas is level with either the middle (station II) or the caudal third (station III) of the odontoid process, a diagnosis of basilar invagination is made[27,30] (Fig. 9-7).

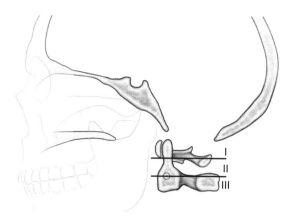

Fig. 9-7   Clark's station for diagnosing basilar invagination. The station of the atlas is determined by dividing the odontoid process into three equal parts in the sagittal plane. If the anterior ring of the atlas is level with either the middle (station II) or the caudal third (station III) of the odontoid process, a basilar invagination is diagnosed.

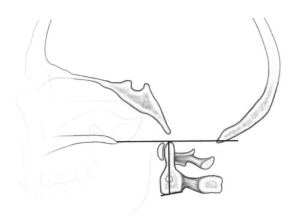

Fig. 9-8   Redlund-Johnell criterion for diagnosing basilar invagination. The distance between McGregor's line and the midpoint of the caudal margin of the second cervical vertebral body is measured. A measurement of less than 34 mm in males and less than 29 mm in females indicates basilar invagination.

Fig. 9-9   Ranawat criterion for diagnosing basilar invagination. The distance between the center of the second cervical pedicle and the transverse axis of the atlas is measured along the axis of the odontoid process. A measurement of less than 15 mm in males and less than 13 mm in females indicates basilar invagination.

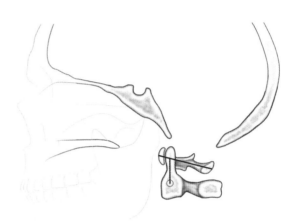

- *Redlund-Johnell criterion:* The distance between McGregor's line and the midpoint of the caudal margin of the second cervical vertebral body is measured. A measurement of less than 34 mm in males and less than 29 mm in females indicates basilar invagination[27,31] (Fig. 9-8).
- *Ranawat criterion:* The distance between the center of the second cervical pedicle and the transverse axis of the atlas is measured along the axis of the odontoid process. A measurement of less than 15 mm in males and less than 13 mm in females indicates basilar invagination[27,32] (Fig. 9-9).

Riew et al[27] compared these eight radiographic criteria for basilar invagination in 131 rheumatoid patients. They found that no single test had a sensitivity of higher than 90%, which is the desired sensitivity for any plain radiographic criterion used to screen for basilar invagination. However, this objective was reached when the Clark station, the Redlund-Johnell criterion, and the Ranawat criterion were measured. When at least one of these tests was positive for basilar invagination, the sensitivity increased to 94%, with a negative predictive value of 91%.

PREOPERATIVE TRACTION AND HALO PLACEMENT

Before surgical treatment, patients with basilar invagination occasionally undergo a trial of axial cervical traction to assess the degree to which the odontoid can be reduced.[14] Traction should be used cautiously, starting with low weights and with close assessment of neurologic status and reducibility. Lateral plain films are obtained after the addition of any weights to monitor reduction and to note inadvertent joint subluxation or overdistraction. With any change in neurologic examination results, traction should be decreased or possibly removed. The direction of traction is optimized to relieve the neural compression. Prior reports suggest that adequate reduction of basilar invagination or atlantoaxial subluxation is possible in most patients.[13,14]

Bagley et al[33] advocated the use of preoperative halo immobilization in patients having occipitocervical fusion. This allows patients to determine if they are able to tolerate the proposed new head position, and it allows the surgeon to adjust the head position before permanent fixation. The authors reported that in their experience, this method ensured physiologic craniocervical neutrality and prevented permanent postoperative dysphagia or patient dissatisfaction with postoperative head position.

SURGICAL CONSIDERATIONS

Patients are intubated in a carefully controlled manner, maintaining neutral alignment of the occipito-cervical junction and subaxial spine at all times.[11,34] In patients with severe instability and/or significant spinal cord compression, the use of awake fiberoptic intubation should be considered. A brief neurologic examination can be performed after intubation but before patient sedation.

Although no compelling scientific evidence supports the use of intraoperative monitoring in occipitocervi-cal or atlantoaxial fusions, it has become the routine practice in many centers.[11] Somatosensory evoked potentials (SSEPs) and motor evoked potentials (MEPs) can be assessed during surgery to monitor neurologic function. In cases of high foramen magnum compression, basilar invagination, and/or lower cranial nerve dysfunction, brainstem auditory evoked potentials can also be used. In patients with severe myelopathy, a baseline SSEP and MEP signal is obtained immediately after intubation while the patient is still supine and before manipulation of the cervical spine.[11] The choice of anesthetic agents is critical when evoked potentials are monitored. Long-acting paralytic agents cannot be used in these cases, because they blunt the MEPs. Likewise, nitrous oxide cannot be used, because it blunts evoked potentials. One minimum alveolar concentration of vapor can also blunt evoked potentials. Consequently, anesthesia is induced with propo-fol and a short- or intermediate-acting paralytic agent such as rocuronium. After induction, total intrave-nous anesthesia is maintained with a combination of propofol and sufentanil infusions, with or without additional use of dexmedetomidine. This combination is least likely to affect evoked potentials. In adults, a mean arterial pressure of greater than 85 to 90 mm Hg is maintained to prevent spinal cord ischemia.[11]

Once adequate anesthesia has been established and baseline monitoring signals obtained, the patient is placed in a Mayfield head clamp, Gardner-Wells tongs, or a modified Mayfield fixation device if a halo brace was placed preoperatively.[34] The patient is then carefully turned to a prone position, and the head is secured. All pressure points are checked. C-arm fluoroscopy is performed to confirm satisfactory alignment of the craniovertebral junction. Specifically, adequate reduction of C1-2 or basilar invagination should be confirmed.[25,34] If manipulation of the head clamp or repositioning of the head is required for further internal reduction, repeat C-arm fluoroscopy is required to confirm proper alignment before fixation and fusion.[34]

All efforts to achieve a neutral anatomic position should be made, because this is critical in maintaining sagittal balance.[20,25,26,33,35-38] Immediate complications of fixation of a patient's neck in exaggerated extension can include difficulty seeing low objects, and difficulty walking, eating, and self-cleaning of the perineum.[11] Fixation in exaggerated flexion can cause a patient to bend the torso backward to see the surrounding environment or the person he or she is speaking with.[11] Overall, the occipitocervical angle must be checked to confirm that it is unchanged from the preoperative, neutral value, or has up to 15 degrees of lordosis.[20,37,39]

POSTOPERATIVE CARE

Before extubation, the endotracheal cuff is deflated to ensure that the patient can breathe around the tube. A tube-exchange technique can be used before complete extubation. In this technique, a smaller-diameter tube is inserted through the existing endotracheal tube, which is then removed over the exchanger.[13,40] If the patient breathes well with the exchanger in place, then it is removed. The exchanger can serve as a stylette for reintubation if needed, which will prevent difficulty with reintubation if necessary. In patients with preoperative lower cranial nerve dysfunction or those in whom prolonged prone positioning resulted in airway edema, delayed extubation should be considered. Before this maneuver is performed, a routine cervical spine radiograph is obtained to check for soft tissue swelling.[13] In routine surgeries, a postoperative cervical collar is not necessary. However, in patients with poor bone quality, or when instrumentation is tenuous, a cervical collar or halo vest can be worn until fusion is evident clinically and radiographically.

OUTCOMES AND COMPLICATIONS

SAGITTAL BALANCE

Preoperative assessment of upright sagittal spinal alignment is increasingly recognized as an important determinant of clinical outcome.[1-4] Matsunaga et al[20] performed a retrospective study of 38 patients with rheumatoid arthritis, who underwent occipitocervical fusion with a 5-year follow-up. They demonstrated that patients who were fused in an abnormal lordotic occipitocervical angle tended to develop subaxial kyphosis or swan-neck deformity in the subaxial spine. In contrast, patients fused in an abnormal kyphotic occipitocervical angle developed subaxial subluxation (most often at C4-5 and occasionally at C5-6 and C7-T1) within 3 years[20] (Fig. 9-10). Of the patients in whom the occipitocervical angle was fixed within the normal range, none developed kyphosis or swan-neck deformity, and only one developed subaxial subluxation.

In a similar patient population with rheumatoid arthritis, Kraus et al[41] reported that the incidence of subaxial subluxation after occipitocervical fusion was 36% at an average of 2.6 years after surgery. In contrast, only 5.5% of rheumatoid arthritis patients undergoing atlantoaxial (C1-2) fusion for isolated atlantoaxial instability had subaxial subluxation at an average of 9 years after fusion.

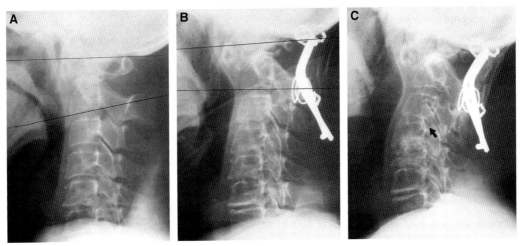

Fig. 9-10 This 56-year-old woman had advanced rheumatoid arthritis. **A,** Her preoperative O-C2 angle was +15 degrees. **B,** Her postoperative angle was −5 degrees, indicating fixation in an abnormally kyphotic angle. **C,** Two years after surgery, C3-4 subaxial subluxation *(arrow)* developed. (From Matsunaga S, Onishi T, Sakou T. Significance of occipitoaxial angle in subaxial lesion after occipitocervical fusion. Spine 26:161-165, 2001.)

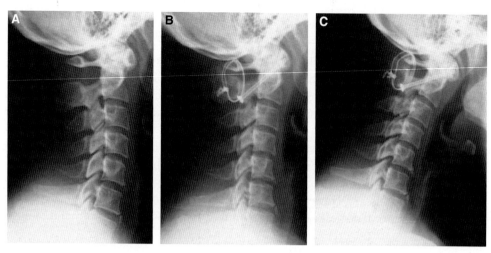

Fig. 9-11 This 43-year-old woman with myelopathy from os odontoideum underwent C1-2 fusion. **A,** Before surgery the C1-2 and C2-7 angles were 11 degrees and 18 degrees, respectively. **B,** Immediately after surgery the C1-2 and C2-7 angles were changed to 24 degrees and 10 degrees. **C,** Although the C1-2 angle was maintained until bony fusion, the C2-7 angle was −8 degrees at the final follow-up, suggesting development of subaxial cervical kyphotic deformity. This patient complained of pain and fatigue at the nuchal region. (From Yoshimoto H, Ito M, Abumi K, et al. A retrospective radiographic analysis of subaxial sagittal alignment after posterior C1-C2 fusion. Spine 29:175-181, 2004.)

Likewise, Yoshimoto et al[25] analyzed the subaxial sagittal alignment of 76 consecutive patients who had isolated C1-2 fusion for atlantoaxial instability secondary to multiple causes, including rheumatoid arthritis, trauma, os odontoideum, and idiopathic factors. They identified a linear correlation between postoperative C1-2 fixation angle and postoperative kyphosis of the C2-7 angle. The overall C1-7 angle changed little throughout the preoperative and postoperative periods. The authors inferred that hyperlordosis of the C1-2 angle resulted in progressive kyphotic deformity of the subaxial spine. They emphasized the vital importance of using intraoperative fluoroscopy to ensure appropriate fixation angles at C1-2[25] (Fig. 9-11).

Similarly, Mukai et al[42] investigated 28 patients with rheumatoid arthritis, who had C1-2 transarticular fixation. In all cases, the subaxial spine became less lordotic postoperatively, and a negative linear correlation was noted between the C1-2 fixation angle and subaxial alignment. Four of 28 patients (14%) went on to develop postoperative kyphotic subaxial deformity, and 4 other patients (14%) suffered neurologic deterioration because of postoperative subaxial subluxation.

Special consideration should be given to skeletally immature children who have occipitocervical fusion.[36,43] In this patient population, increasing lordosis occurs at the occipitocervical junction after fusion. The mechanism behind this phenomenon has been speculated to involve a crankshaft phenomenon in which asymmetrical growth of the anterior and posterior columns results in lordotic deformity.[36,43] Wills et al[36] found that as the fusion mass extended distally (that is, as more vertebral bodies were included in the fusion mass), lordotic deformity increased. In this particular patient population, they suggested fusion in a neutral to slightly flexed position, and at all costs, avoiding fusion in a hyperextended position.[36]

Postoperative Dyspnea and Dysphagia

Another severe and feared complication of occipitocervical fusion is the development of oropharyngeal stenosis leading to trismus,[35] severe dysphagia,[22,35,39,44,45] and life-threatening dyspnea.[22,38-40,44,46] The oropharynx is the area from the soft palate to the upper border of the epiglottis. It forms an upper aerodigestive tract with many functions, including deglutition, respiration, and phonation.[39,44] In the oropharynx, a complex and precisely coordinated succession of muscular contractions and relaxations occurs. The tongue root provides the primary force for the movement of food from the oropharynx, around the epiglottis, and into the laryngopharynx. The soft palate is elevated to seal the nasopharynx, and the suprahyoid muscles pull the larynx up and forward. The epiglottis moves downward to cover the airway, while striated pharyngeal muscles contract to move the food bolus.[39]

Anatomically, the oropharyngeal space is bounded by bony structures: the mandible anteriorly and laterally and the cervical spine posteriorly. The mechanism of postoperative dysphagia and dyspnea after occipitocervical fusion has been postulated to involve reduction in the cross-sectional area of the oropharynx.[39,44,46] Reduction in the occipitocervical angle results in a shift of the mandible posteriorly, decreasing the cross-sectional area of the oropharynx. This leads to dysphagia in mild cases and to dyspnea in more severe reductions. Misawa et al[35] reported on a patient who developed trismus after atlantoaxial fusion in a relatively flexed position, superimposed on contact of the C1 screw heads with the occiput, effectively resulting in occipitocervical fusion. Ota et al[22] showed that a 10-degree decrease in the O-C2 angle caused a reduction of the narrowest oropharyngeal airway space in the neutral position of approximately 37% in normal subjects. Conversely, Ataka et al[47] have demonstrated that rheumatoid patients with obstructive sleep apnea have significant improvements after occipitocervical fusion in a slightly extended (lordotic) position, presumably from enlargement of the oropharyngeal space.

Miyata et al[39] demonstrated that even in patients undergoing short occipitocervical fusion (O-C2 or O-C3), impaired deglutition occurs in excessively flexed (kyphotic) positions as a consequence of combined mechanical bony stenosis of the oropharynx and changes in the soft tissue around the epiglottis. In a flexed position, the tongue root is displaced downward, resulting in narrowing of the oropharynx and impairment of adequate motion of the epiglottis. Because this happened in the context of short occipitocervical fusion, the authors inferred that these complications were much more closely related to the alignment of the upper cervical spine, rather than to that of the middle or lower cervical spine[39] (Fig. 9-12) In their series, all patients undergoing occipitocervical fusion with a postoperative O-C2 angle of more than 10 degrees of kyphosis, compared with a neutral preoperative baseline, showed more than a 40% increase in oropharyngeal stenosis with resultant dyspnea and/or dysphagia after surgery. Conversely, no patients who were fused in extension, compared with a preoperative neutral baseline, developed these complications. They concluded that the O-C2 angle is a key factor in preventing dyspnea and dysphagia after posterior occipitocervical fusion and suggested that patients be fused in the neutral or slightly extended position.[39]

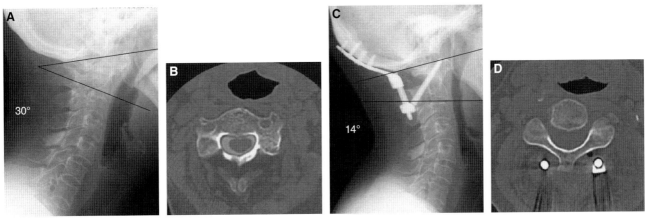

Fig. 9-12 This patient developed postoperative dysphagia after fusion in a kyphotic position, as shown in lateral radiographs and axial CT images just proximal to the epiglottis. **A and B,** Before surgery the O-C2 angle was 30 degrees, and the cross-sectional area of the oropharynx was 282 mm². **C and D,** After surgery the O-C2 angle is 14 degrees, and the cross-sectional area of the oropharynx is 145 mm². (From Miyata M, Neo M, Fujibayashi S, et al. O-C2 angle as a predictor of dyspnea and/or dysphagia after occipitocervical fusion. Spine 34:184-188, 2009.)

Fusion in a hyperextended position can similarly impede normal deglutition. Morishima et al[48] demonstrated a delay in the pharyngeal phase of swallowing when normal volunteers were placed in a halo vest in slight extension, compared with the neutral position. They provided three hypotheses to explain the differences in swallowing function. First, head position influences tonic neck reflexes, which alter genioglossal muscle activity. Second, head position alters tongue position and the relationship of structures of the posterior oropharyngeal cavity. Third, the length of the suprahyoid muscles may be longer in the extended position; therefore biomechanical efficiency is compromised.[33,48] In a cineradiographic study of 53 patients with dysphagia, Ekberg[49] showed that swallowing with the head extended increased defective closure of the laryngeal vestibule and decreased efficient movement of the epiglottis, contributing to aspiration in this group of patients. Finally, patients who have been in a fixed kyphotic position for a prolonged period of time can have contractures of the suprahyoid musculature, causing biomechanical compromise in a relatively neutral position that is similar to that described from hyperextension under normal conditions.[33]

Ota et al[22] demonstrated that the occipital–upper cervical alignment (O-C2 angle) has a great impact on the oropharyngeal space, but that the middle–lower cervical alignment (C2-6 angle) does not. Independent of the O-C2 angle, reduction of the anterior atlantoaxial subluxation can decrease the oropharyngeal cross-sectional area, although the precise relationship between the anterior atlantodental interval and the cross-sectional area is less clear.[46] Thus they encouraged surgeons to pay special attention to both the O-C2 angle and to changes to the oropharyngeal space when positioning patients in the operating room.

Patients with rheumatoid arthritis are particularly prone to postoperative dysphagia and dyspnea.[38,39] Keenan et al[50] reported that the relative shortening of the neck secondary to the vertical migration of the dens causes the soft tissue of the pharynx to become redundant, compromising the airway. Redlund-Johnell[51] suggested that a reduction in the size of the upper airway can occur in patients with rheumatoid arthritis in association with temporomandibular joint destruction. Acquired laryngeal deviation, laryngeal mucosal abnormalities, and the frequent existence of cricoarytenoid and cricothyroid arthritis also distort the anatomy of the airway in patients with rheumatoid arthritis.[38,39] Finally, compression of the brainstem associated with the vertical subluxation of the odontoid process can cause central dyspnea or dysphagia.[39] Intubation of many rheumatoid arthritis patients is difficult, resulting in airway trauma and edema. Rheumatoid arthritis is a major risk factor for postoperative oropharyngeal space obstruction.

PATIENT EXAMPLES

This 37-year-old woman had a past medical history notable for Saethre-Chotzen syndrome, left-sided hearing loss, and hypothyroidism. She was referred by a neurologist for evaluation of a Chiari I malformation, which was diagnosed after a workup for progressive neck pain, headaches, swallowing difficulties, loss of balance and dexterity, and Lhermitte's phenomenon.

A sagittal T2-weighted MRI image of her cervical spine showed 16 mm tonsillar ectopia down to the level of the C2 dentocentral synchondrosis, without evidence of a syrinx (Fig. 9-13, A). Plain radiographs of her cervical spine in flexion and extension demonstrated widening of the atlantodental interval (Fig. 9-13, B and C). CT of the cervical spine showed assimilation of C1 to the occiput (Fig. 9-13, D). Her preoperative O-C2 angle, measured by subtending the angle of McGregor's line and a line parallel to the inferior endplate of C2, measured approximately 24 degrees (Fig. 9-13, E). She underwent a suboccipital craniectomy, expansile duraplasty, and fusion of C1-3. Great care was taken intraoperatively to maintain her neutral preoperative O-C2 angle, and this was confirmed immediately before fixation (Fig. 9-13, F). Her postoperative course was routine, and she went home on postoperative day 2. Her balance and dexterity improved tremendously, and Lhermitte's phenomenon was no longer present. Postoperative CT confirmed maintenance of the O-C2 angle, and 3-month follow-up flexion and extension films show maintenance of normal subaxial cervical spine alignment (Fig. 9-13, G through I).

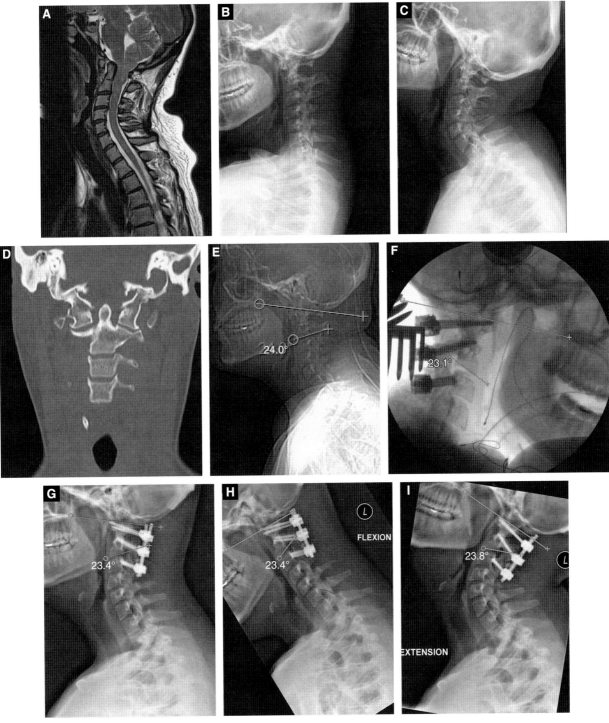

Fig. 9-13   **A,** This preoperative sagittal T2-weighted MRI image of the cervical spine demonstrated 16 mm tonsillar ectopia down to the level of the C2 dentocentral synchondrosis, without evidence of a syrinx. The atlantodental interval was widened, and the cervicomedullary junction was compressed. **B** and **C,** Plain radiographs of the cervical spine in flexion and extension revealed widening of the atlantodental interval. **D,** Coronal CT reconstruction of the cervical spine showed fusion of the occipital condyles to the lateral masses of C1 bilaterally. **E,** On a lateral CT scout film, the preoperative O-C2 angle, measured by subtending the angle of McGregor's line and a line parallel to the inferior endplate of C2, was approximately 24 degrees. **F,** Intraoperative fluoroscope obtained before fixation confirmed maintenance of the neutral preoperative O-C2 angle. **G-I,** Three months postoperatively, normal subaxial cervical spinal alignment is maintained, and the neutral preoperative O-C2 angle is preserved in neutral, flexion, and extension films.

This 65-year-old man with long-standing history of rheumatoid arthritis presented for neurosurgical evaluation of basilar invagination, which was diagnosed after a workup for clumsiness of his hands, difficulty buttoning buttons, difficulty with his handwriting and opening jars, and imbalance. Sagittal T1-weighted MRI of the cervical spine showed obvious basilar invagination (Fig. 9-14, *A*). CT confirmed the diagnosis using all of the previously mentioned criteria, and demonstrated fusion of the occiput to C1 (Fig. 9-14, *B*). The O-C2 angle was approximately 14 degrees, measured by subtending the angle of McRae's line and a line parallel to the inferior endplate of C2 (Fig. 9-14, *C*). The patient underwent a C1-2 fusion and reduction of basilar invagination. Preoperative MEPs and SSEPs were obtained, and Gardner-Wells tongs were placed. The patient was then positioned prone in a horseshoe head holder, with 15 pounds of in-line traction placed. Fluoroscopy was used to confirm appropriate occipitocervical alignment (Fig. 9-14, *D*). Every 5 minutes, an additional 5 pounds of traction was added, followed by repeated fluoroscopy and confirmation of unchanged MEPs until a total of 35 pounds of traction was placed. A C1 laminectomy was performed. Because of the cranial translocation of the odontoid, the C2 nerve roots prohibited access to the C1-2 space and were subsequently dissected and ligated. The C1-2 joints were then visualized and gradually distracted with a lumbar interbody intradiscal distractor to achieve 1 cm of distraction bilaterally. Carbon fiber Concord cages (Depuy-Synthes Spine, Raynham, MA) 10 mm high, 9 mm wide, and 23 mm long were placed bilaterally and filled with local autograft and demineralized bone matrix. A final intraoperative fluoroscope confirmed maintenance of the patient's preoperative O-C2 angle (Fig. 9-14, *E*). His postoperative course was routine, and he went home on postoperative day 4. A CT scan shows excellent decompression of the foramen magnum and preservation of his preoperative O-C2 angle (Fig. 9-14, *F* through *I*).

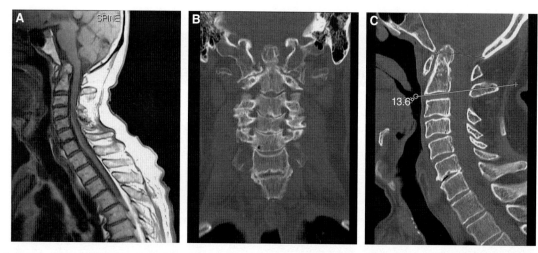

Fig. 9-14 **A,** Preoperative sagittal T1-weighted MRI of the cervical spine showed basilar invagination and compression of the cervicomedullary junction. **B,** Coronal CT reconstruction of the cervical spine revealed fusion of the occipital condyles to the lateral masses of C1 bilaterally. The tip of the odontoid process protruded significantly above a line drawn between the tips of the mastoid processes (Fischgold-Metzger line), suggesting basilar invagination. **C,** Sagittal CT reconstruction of the cervical spine demonstrated the anterior tubercle of C1 at station II. This indicated that the patient had basilar invagination by Clark's criteria. The tip of the odontoid process protruded above McRae's line. The O-C2 angle was approximately 14 degrees, measured by subtending the angle of McRae's line and a line parallel to the inferior endplate of C2.

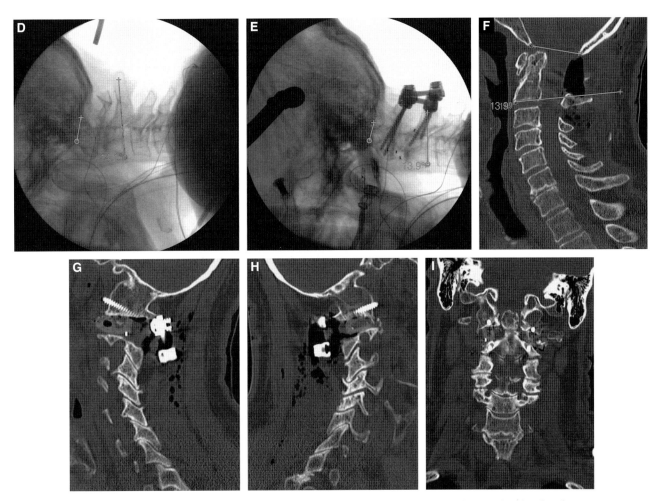

Fig. 9-14, cont'd   **D** and **E,** Intraoperative fluoroscopy obtained at positioning and immediately after fixation confirmed maintenance of the patient's preoperative O-C2 angle. **F,** Postoperative sagittal CT reconstruction of the cervical spine demonstrates much improved basilar invagination with resolution of ventral cervicomedullary compression. The anterior tubercle of C1 is at station I. The neutral preoperative O-C2 angle is preserved. **G-I,** Postoperative sagittal (right and left side) and coronal CT reconstructions, respectively, of the cervical spine show distraction of the C1-2 joints with placement of bilateral carbon fiber Concord cages. High-riding vertebral arteries are evident bilaterally, along with bilateral C2 pedicle screws and bicortically placed C1 lateral mass screws.

CONCLUSION

Sagittal balance and maintenance of neutral upright horizontal gaze are vitally important to good outcomes in occipitocervical and atlantoaxial fusion surgeries. It is increasingly recognized that regional spinal curves are not independent but are rather closely interrelated. Changes in any curve are compensated by adjacent curves in the body's attempt to maintain neutral gaze. Patients fused in abnormal lordotic occipitocervical or atlantoaxial angles develop subaxial kyphosis or swan-neck deformity in the subaxial spine. In contrast, patients fused in abnormally kyphotic angles tend to develop subaxial subluxation. In addition, fusion in abnormally kyphotic angles results in critical stenosis of the oropharyngeal space with resultant postoperative dyspnea, dysphagia, and trismus. Therefore preoperative measurement of a patient's occipitocervical or atlantoaxial angles is critical. It is equally important to maintain this angle or an additional 15 degrees of lordosis to minimize postoperative complications. This can be accomplished by meticulous attention to fluoroscopic images and intraoperative measurement of the angle before fixation or by preoperative halo immobilization with maintenance of this position in the operating room.

REFERENCES

1. Kuntz C IV, Levin LS, Ondra SL, et al. Neutral upright sagittal spinal alignment from the occiput to the pelvis in asymptomatic adults: a review and resynthesis of the literature. J Neurosurg Spine 6:104-112, 2007.

2. Kuntz C IV, Shaffrey CI, Ondra SL, et al. Spinal deformity: a new classification derived from neutral upright spinal alignment measurements in asymptomatic juvenile, adolescent, adult, and geriatric individuals. Neurosurgery 63:25-39, 2008.

3. Ames CP, Blondel B, Scheer JK, et al. Cervical radiographical alignment: comprehensive assessment techniques and potential importance in cervical myelopathy. Spine 38:S149-S160, 2013.

4. Scheer JK, Tang JA, Smith JS, et al. Cervical spine alignment, sagittal deformity, and clinical implications: a review. J Neurosurg Spine 19:141-159, 2013.

5. Lee SH, Kim KT, Seo EM, et al. The influence of thoracic inlet alignment on the craniocervical sagittal balance in asymptomatic adults. J Spinal Disord Tech 25:E41-E47, 2012.

6. Tang JA, Scheer JK, Smith JS, et al. The impact of standing regional cervical sagittal alignment on outcomes in posterior cervical fusion surgery. Neurosurgery 71:662-669; discussion 669, 2012.

7. Hardacker JW, Shuford RF, Capicotto PN, et al. Radiographic standing cervical segmental alignment in adult volunteers without neck symptoms. Spine 22:1472-1480; discussion 1480, 1997.

8. Steinmetz MP, Mroz TE, Benzel EC. Craniovertebral junction: biomechanical considerations. Neurosurgery 66:7-12, 2010.

9. Suchomel P, Buchvald P. Biomechanical remarks. In Suchomel P, Choutka O, eds. Reconstruction of Upper Cervical Spine and Craniovertebral Junction. Berlin: Springer-Verlag, 2011.

10. Suchomel P, Choutka O, Barsa P. Surgical anatomy In Suchomel P, Choutka O, eds. Reconstruction of Upper Cervical Spine and Craniovertebral Junction. Berlin: Springer-Verlag, 2011.

11. Lu DC, Roeser AC, Mummaneni VP, et al. Nuances of occipitocervical fixation. Neurosurgery 66:141-146, 2010.

12. Martin MD, Bruner HJ, Maiman DJ. Anatomic and biomechanical considerations of the craniovertebral junction. Neurosurgery 66:2-6, 2010.

13. Menezes AH. Craniocervical fusions in children. J Neurosurg Pediatr 9:573-585, 2012.

14. Smith JS, Shaffrey CI, Abel MF, et al. Basilar invagination. Neurosurgery 66:39-47, 2010.

15. Choutka O, Suchomel P. Special radiology. In Suchomel P, Choutka O, eds. Reconstruction of Upper Cervical Spine and Craniovertebral Junction. Berlin: Springer-Verlag, 2011.

16. Shoda N, Takeshita K, Seichi A, et al. Measurement of occipitocervical angle. Spine 29:E204-E208, 2004.

17. Chamberlain WE. Basilar impression (platybasia): a bizarre developmental anomaly of the occipital bone and upper cervical spine with striking and misleading neurologic manifestations. Yale J Biol Med 11:487-496, 1939.

18. McRae DL, Barnum AS. Occipitalization of the atlas. Am J Roentgenol Radium Ther Nucl Med 70:23-46, 1953.

19. McGregor M. The significance of certain measurements of the skull in the diagnosis of basilar impression. Br J Radiol 21:171-181, 1948.

20. Matsunaga S, Onishi T, Sakou T. Significance of occipitoaxial angle in subaxial lesion after occipitocervical fusion. Spine 26:161-165, 2001.

21. Nojiri K, Matsumoto M, Chiba K, et al. Relationship between alignment of upper and lower cervical spine in asymptomatic individuals. J Neurosurg 99:80-83, 2003.

22. Ota M, Neo M, Aoyama T, et al. Impact of the O-C2 angle on the oropharyngeal space in normal patients. Spine 36:E720-E726, 2011.

23. Phillips FM, Phillips CS, Wetzel FT, et al. Occipitocervical neutral position. Possible surgical implications. Spine 24:775-778, 1999.

24. Riel RU, Lee MC, Kirkpatrick JS. Measurement of a posterior occipitocervical fusion angle. J Spinal Disord Tech 23:27-29, 2010.

25. Yoshimoto H, Ito M, Abumi K, et al. A retrospective radiographic analysis of subaxial sagittal alignment after posterior C1-C2 fusion. Spine 29:175-181, 2004.

26. Yoshida G, Kamiya M, Yoshihara H, et al. Subaxial sagittal alignment and adjacent-segment degeneration after atlantoaxial fixation performed using C-1 lateral mass and C-2 pedicle screws or transarticular screws. J Neurosurg Spine 13:443-450, 2010.

27. Riew KD, Hilibrand AS, Palumbo MA, et al. Diagnosing basilar invagination in the rheumatoid patient. The reliability of radiographic criteria. J Bone Joint Surg Am 83:194-200, 2001.

28. Fischgold H, Metzger J. [Radio-tomography of the impression fractures of the cranial basis] Rev Rhum Mal Osteoartic 19:261-264, 1952.
29. Thiebaut F, Wackenheim A, Vrousos C. [Definition of antero-posterior displacement of the odontoid process of the axis with the aid of the basilar line] Acta Radiol Diagn 1:811-813, 1963.
30. Clark CR, Goetz DD, Menezes AH. Arthrodesis of the cervical spine in rheumatoid arthritis. J Bone Joint Surg Am 71:381-392, 1989.
31. Redlund-Johnell I, Pettersson H. Radiographic measurements of the cranio-vertebral region. Designed for evaluation of abnormalities in rheumatoid arthritis. Acta Radiol Diagn 25:23-28, 1984.
32. Ranawat CS, O'Leary P, Pellicci P, et al. Cervical spine fusion in rheumatoid arthritis. J Bone Joint Surg Am 61:1003-1010, 1979.
33. Bagley CA, Witham TF, Pindrik JA, et al. Assuring optimal physiologic craniocervical alignment and avoidance of swallowing-related complications after occipitocervical fusion by preoperative halo vest placement. J Spinal Disord Tech 22:170-176, 2009.
34. Papadopoulos SM, ed. Manual of Cervical Spine Internal Fixation. Philadelphia: Lippincott Williams & Wilkins, 2004.
35. Misawa H, Tanaka M, Sugimoto Y, et al. Development of dysphagia and trismus developed after c1-2 posterior fusion in extended position. Acta Med Okayama 67:185-190, 2013.
36. Wills BP, Auerbach JD, Glotzbecker MP, et al. Change in lordosis at the occipitocervical junction following posterior occipitocervical fusion in skeletally immature children. Spine 31:2304-2309, 2006.
37. Wolfla CE. Anatomical, biomechanical, and practical considerations in posterior occipitocervical instrumentation. Spine J 6(6 Suppl):225S-232S, 2006.
38. Yoshida M, Neo M, Fujibayashi S, et al. Upper-airway obstruction after short posterior occipitocervical fusion in a flexed position. Spine 32:E267-E270, 2007.
39. Miyata M, Neo M, Fujibayashi S, et al. O-C2 angle as a predictor of dyspnea and/or dysphagia after occipitocervical fusion. Spine 34:184-188, 2009.
40. Tagawa T, Akeda K, Asanuma Y, et al. Upper airway obstruction associated with flexed cervical position after posterior occipitocervical fusion. J Anesth 25:120-122, 2011.
41. Kraus DR, Peppelman WC, Agarwal AK, et al. Incidence of subaxial subluxation in patients with generalized rheumatoid arthritis who have had previous occipital cervical fusions. Spine 16(10 Suppl):S486-S489, 1991.
42. Mukai Y, Hosono N, Sakaura H, et al. Sagittal alignment of the subaxial cervical spine after C1-C2 transarticular screw fixation in rheumatoid arthritis. J Spinal Disord Tech 20:436-441, 2007.
43. Rodgers WB, Coran DL, Kharrazi FD, et al. Increasing lordosis of the occipitocervical junction after arthrodesis in young children: the occipitocervical crankshaft phenomenon. J Pediatr Orthop 17:762-765, 1997.
44. Izeki M, Neo M, Takemoto M, et al. The O-C2 angle established at occipito-cervical fusion dictates the patient's destiny in terms of postoperative dyspnea and/or dysphagia. Eur Spine J 23:328-336, 2014.
45. Takami T, Ichinose T, Ishibashi K, et al. Importance of fixation angle in posterior instrumented occipitocervical fusion. Neurol Med Chir (Tokyo) 48:279-282; discussion 282, 2008.
46. Izeki M, Neo M, Ito H, et al. Reduction of atlantoaxial subluxation causes airway stenosis. Spine 38:E513-E520, 2013.
47. Ataka H, Tanno T, Miyashita T, et al. Occipitocervical fusion has potential to improve sleep apnea in patients with rheumatoid arthritis and upper cervical lesions. Spine 35:E971-E975, 2010.
48. Morishima N, Ohota K, Miura Y. The influences of Halo-vest fixation and cervical hyperextension on swallowing in healthy volunteers. Spine 30:E179-E182, 2005.
49. Ekberg O. Posture of the head and pharyngeal swallowing. Acta Radiol Diagn 27:691-696, 1986.
50. Keenan MA, Stiles CM, Kaufman RL. Acquired laryngeal deviation associated with cervical spine disease in erosive polyarticular arthritis. Use of the fiberoptic bronchoscope in rheumatoid disease. Anesthesiology 58:441-449, 1983.
51. Redlund-Johnell I. Upper airway obstruction in patients with rheumatoid arthritis and temporomandibular joint destruction. Scand J Rheumatol 17:273-279, 1988.

10

Cervical Region

Ricardo B. V. Fontes ▪ *Vincent C. Traynelis*

Cervical deformity is directly related to several quality of life metrics and is now recognized as a significant clinical challenge for spine surgeons.[1,2] Although deformities in the coronal plane occur, sagittal plane deformities, particularly kyphosis, are far more frequent and clinically relevant.[3] Tumors, trauma, neuromuscular diseases, rheumatologic conditions, and infection can lead to cervical deformity, but the cause of sagittal plane imbalance for most patients is either iatrogenic or degenerative. Kyphosis has long been recognized as a long-term complication of posterior decompressive interventions.[4] Most of the normal cervical lordosis is localized at C1-2; in the subaxial spine, it is conferred by the wedge-shaped cervical discs, with different anterior and posterior heights. In healthy, young individuals, cervical lordosis averages 15 degrees and it usually increases slightly with age, reaching 23 degrees in the seventh decade.[1,5] As opposed to the lumbar spine, load is shared equally between the vertebral body and the articular processes in the cervical spine in the setting of normal alignment.[6] The biomechanical properties of the cervical subaxial segment have been shown to be altered with as minimal a surgical intervention as resection of 50% of the facet capsule, and segmental hypermobility can result after bilateral resection of as little as 50% of the facet joints.[7,8] Disruption of the posterior tension band places the extensor musculature at a mechanical disadvantage. Fatigue eventually occurs, leading to axial pain and failure to maintain further alignment. A commonly cited tenet of cervical alignment is that kyphosis begets kyphosis.[3] Once the cervical spine assumes a kyphotic posture, the cord becomes draped over the posterior aspect of the vertebral bodies, leading to microvascular compromise of the spinal cord without compression necessarily being present.[9,10] Myelopathy may be apparent clinically at this stage, and if microvascular compromise persists, neuronal death and myelomalacia occur, with few possibilities of recovery.

TECHNIQUES FOR EVALUATION OF CERVICAL ALIGNMENT

One of the first clinically useful measurements designed to assess global deformity is the chin-brow angle. This was developed to evaluate horizontal gaze in patients with fixed kyphotic deformity, of which the prototype is ankylosing spondylitis. Unlike most patients with focal deformities, those with ankylosing spondylitis cannot maintain horizontal gaze by compensating with other spinal segments. The chin-brow angle provides meaningful functional information and is helpful for evaluating global alignment. It is assessed clinically or radiographically by measuring the angle between a line touching the chin and brow of the patient and a line perpendicular to the ground[11] (Fig. 10-1).

Cervical lordosis can be assessed using Cobb angles, the Ishihara Index, and the Harrison posterior tangent method. The Cobb angle method involves drawing lines parallel to the superior and inferior vertebrae of the region of interest. Secondary lines that are perpendicular to the initial lines are determined, and the angle at the intersection of these perpendicular lines is recorded as the Cobb angle. In the cervical spine, Cobb angles are usually reported as encompassing C1 to C7 or more frequently C2 to C7. The Cobb angle from C1 to C7 can overestimate lordosis, which is understandable given the tremendous sagittal influ-

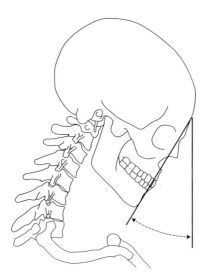

Fig. 10-1   Chin-brow angle.

Fig. 10-2   A, C2-7 flexion measured using the Cobb angle method. **B,** C2-7 extension measured using the Drexler method.

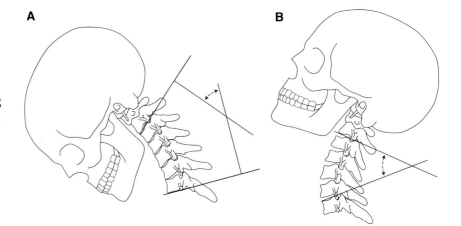

A

B

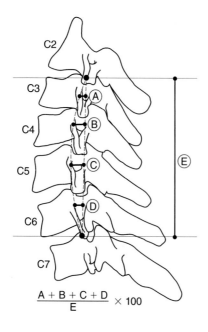

Fig. 10-3   Ishihara Index.

$$\frac{A + B + C + D}{E} \times 100$$

ence exerted by the C1-2 segment. Conversely, the Cobb angle from C2 to C7 may underestimate overall lordosis. However, because this is the region usually treated with corrective surgery, it is a very important parameter.[12] Cobb angles were useful in the era of plain radiographs. Now with more sophisticated digital imaging, most surgeons employ the technique described by Drexler, which involves drawing lines tangent to the endplates of the vertebrae of interest and measuring the angle between them.[13] Theoretically this angle should equal the Cobb angle (Fig. 10-2).

Other manners of assessing cervical lordosis have a more historical value. The Ishihara Index is calculated on a standing, neutral, lateral cervical radiograph and was once very popular in Japanese literature.[14] A line between the posterior edges of the inferior endplates of C2 and C7 is traced (line E); distances from this line to the inferior endplates of C3, C4, C5, and C6 are then measured. The Ishihara Index is then calculated according to the following formula: $(A + B + C + D)/E \times 100$ (Fig. 10-3). The Ishihara Index in a normal population is estimated to be approximately 10.[15,16]

The Harrison posterior tangent method defines an angle that is determined from the summation of segmental angles derived from a series of lines drawn parallel to the posterior surfaces of each of the cervical vertebra from C2 to C7.[12]

Translation in the sagittal plane is evaluated by measuring the distance from a plumb line originating from a cervical vertebra (usually the anterior tubercle of C1, the centroid of C2, or the posterosuperior aspect of C7) to the posterosuperior corner of the first sacral vertebra. The resulting distance is the C1 (or C2 or C7) sagittal vertical axis (SVA). The distance between the C1 (or C2) and C7 SVA can be applied regionally to assess cervical translation; the C2-7 SVA was recently associated with worse outcomes after posterior arthrodesis[2] (Fig. 10-4).

Cervical alignment parameters have been increasingly studied in conjunction with more caudal segments of the vertebral column. It is evident today that not only do cervical alignment parameters reflect imbalances in the thoracic and lumbar spines, but they may spontaneously correct after thoracolumbar deformity corrections.[17] Cervical lordosis has long been known to positively correlate with thoracic kyphosis and positive spinopelvic malalignment to maintain horizontal gaze.[17-19] In 2012 Lee et al[20] described the thoracic inlet angle (TIA), T1 slope, and neck tilt (NT) based on an analogy between the thoracic inlet and

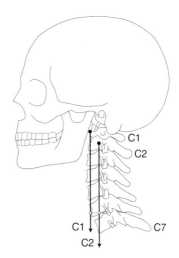

Fig. 10-4   C1 and C2 sagittal vertical axis.

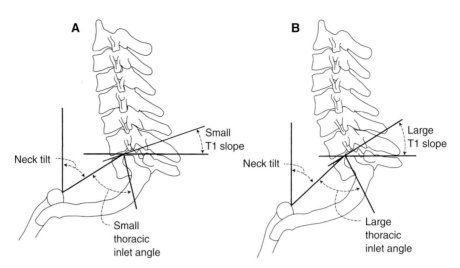

Fig. 10-5   A, Thoracic inlet angle, neck tilt, and T1 slope. The T1 slope is relatively small in this example, and a normal C2 SVA can be achieved with relatively little cervical lordosis. **B,** Thoracic inlet angle, neck tilt, and T1 slope. The T1 slope is relatively large in this example; therefore more cervical lordosis is required to achieve a normal C2 SVA than is required in **A.**

the pelvis, comparing them to fixed bases where a mobile segment lies. As in the case of spinopelvic parameters, the central point for measuring these parameters is the center of the superior T1 endplate. TIA is the angle defined by a line perpendicular to this point and another line between this point and the manubrium (Fig. 10-5). NT is defined by the line between the center point of the T1 superior endpoint and the manubrium and a line perpendicular to the ground. T1 slope is the angle between the superior T1 endplate and a line parallel to the ground. In a manner analogous to spinopelvic parameters, where pelvic incidence (PI) = pelvic tilt (PT) + sacral slope (SS), TIA = T1 slope + NT. T1 slope can be an important factor in determining the degree of cervical lordosis necessary to maintain horizontal gaze and optimize C1 or C2 SVA, but its exact significance in preoperative planning of deformity correction has not been fully defined.[21]

CLINICAL CORRELATIONS

In cases of lumbosacral deformity, considerable evidence suggests that PI may be used as a rough guide to estimate the amount of lumbar lordosis to be restored based on the anatomy of the pelvis. However, a formula to individually calculate the ideal amount of cervical lordosis based on the TIA or any other parameter has not been identified yet. A general rule is to restore cervical lordosis to at least a neutral value.[3] Most outcome studies focus on regional (frequently C2-7) lordosis. Cervical kyphosis has been identified as an indicator of worse recovery for myelopathy.[22-24] Literature results regarding improvement for neck pain based solely on the measurement of cervical lordosis have been somewhat conflicting but point in a direction of worse NDI in situations of global cervical kyphosis.[25-27] Increased T1 slope has been found to correlate with development of postoperative kyphosis after laminoplasty and offers an opportunity for future research in cervical alignment parameters.[28]

The identification of positive sagittal malalignment as a poor prognostic factor for thoracolumbar deformity was one of the most important advances in recent years. For these patients, positive sagittal malalignment defined as a C7 SVA greater than 40 mm has been correlated with worse quality of life.[29,30] In the cervical spine, such correlations have only recently begun to be identified. Smith et al[31] demonstrated that severity of myelopathy, exemplified by worse modified Japanese Orthopaedic Association (mJOA) scale, correlates negatively with C2-7 SVA but not with C2-7 Cobb angle. Tang et al[2] have further analyzed SVA measure-

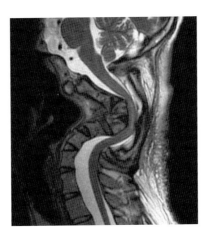

Fig. 10-6 Hyperlordosis below a kyphotic region allows a patient to maintain horizontal gaze.

ments and quality of life metrics (neck disability index and SF-36 physical component score) in patients undergoing posterior instrumented cervical fusions. In their retrospective analysis, positive sagittal malalignment was correlated with worse functional outcomes and suggested a threshold value of 40 mm for C2-7 SVA, beyond which correlations were most significant.

PREOPERATIVE PLANNING AND POSTOPERATIVE CARE

Preoperative planning involves a full physical examination, with particular attention to the patient's posture. In adult global deformity, the ability to compensate with other spinal segments is decreased as discussed previously. Therefore patients will often compensate by flexing their knees, which is an extremely energy-consuming technique that quickly leads to fatigue. Cervical hyperlodosis can be present and is an attempt to maintain horizontal gaze (Fig. 10-6). Cervical kyphosis may be apparent clinically; an extreme of this pathology can result in so-called chin-on-chest deformity. Assessment of the rigidity of cervical kyphosis is important, because it can dictate a different surgical strategy with an initial posterior release. These patients should therefore be examined in the standing and supine positions. A complete neurologic examination is critical, and signs of myelopathy are of special importance to localize the site of cord pathology and ensure that thoracic myelopathy is not a concern.

Every patient with cervical myelopathy is assessed with MRI and cervical flexion and extension radiographs. In the event of a contraindication to MRI, a CT-myelogram is performed to delineate cord anatomy. If deformity is clinically or radiographically suspected, standing long-cassette (3 feet) scoliosis radiographs are obtained, with special care to ensure that the femoral heads are visible.[22] In the case of prior or spontaneous arthrodesis, osseous anatomy can be specifically studied with a cervical spine CT. The presence of solid facet fusion or competent posterior instrumentation may dictate the need for initial posterior release in a multistage procedure (posterior-anterior-posterior approach).

Correction of cervical deformities requires meticulous preoperative planning. The workup for patients undergoing a repeat anterior cervical spine intervention includes examination of vocal cord motion through fiberoptic inspection and/or specific planning to approach the spine from the same side of prior interventions to prevent bilateral recurrent laryngeal nerve injury. A left-sided approach is preferred for the same reason.[32] Adequate cardiac and general medical preoperative clearance is of paramount importance given the extent of surgery for correction of adult deformity and reported rates of medical complications.[33] At our institution, postoperative care is given in the intensive care unit if multistage correction is performed or medical comorbidities dictate this need. Airway management is the most important part of postoperative management of such patients. Lack of a specific extubation protocol in this setting can be catastrophic, with mortality rates reported in the literature of up to 33%.[34-36] In our extubation protocol, both intensive care and spine surgery teams need to confer and agree on extubation before a time cutoff to allow monitoring and reintubation during working hours when all the hospital resources can be marshaled in timely fashion. Assurance of viable air flow around the endotracheal tube is ensured through the presence of an audible leak measuring at least 150 ml with standardized ventilatory parameters. Our personal experience with this protocol has resulted in zero reintubations. If a patient fails to achieve such parameters, a trial extubation may be attempted with immediate access for an infraglottic airway, or the patient is offered a tracheostomy on day 10. Approximately 10% of patients required temporary placement of a gastric tube for enteral nutrition when having complete subaxial reconstruction. Most patients treated with multilevel 360-degree surgery resume eating several days after extubation. In rare instances a tracheostomy and/or a G-tube is necessary, but we have not treated any patients in whom the tracheostomy or the gastric tube was removed within 3 months postoperatively.[37]

PATIENT EXAMPLE

Cervical deformities can be corrected with a posterior-only approach in selected cases, particularly if the deformity is mobile or a pedicle subtraction osteotomy is performed. Anterior approaches allow solid column reconstruction, indirect foraminal enlargement, and additional internal fixation. Our surgical strategy frequently involves 360- or 540-degree operations for the management of cervical deformities, as depicted in the following case.

This middle-aged patient developed significant neck and lower back pain and myelopathy after a posterior cervical surgery. She did not improve with physical therapy or medications. Radiographs demonstrated an instrumented fusion from C3 to C7 and a laminectomy from C3 to C6 with significant kyphosis particularly at the C4-5 level (Fig. 10-7, *A*). Her preoperative C2-7 SVA was 68 mm, and she had 38 degrees of kyphosis. Her C7 plumb line was −84 mm (Fig. 10-7, *C*). Surgical correction was accomplished by first removing the instrumentation and performing complete bilateral facetectomies at C3-4, C4-5, and C6-7. Anterior discectomies were performed at C2-3, C3-4, C4-5, C5-6, C6-7, and C7-T1. Lordotic grafts were placed at each level, and a 110 mm anterior plate was placed. The procedure was completed with placement of posterior instrumentation from C2 to T1. Postoperatively her myelopathy improved, and her pain scores were markedly decreased. She was corrected to 28 degrees of C2-7 lordosis, and her C2-7 SVA reduced to 45 mm. Her C7 plumb line was +17 mm (Fig. 10-7, *B* and *D*).

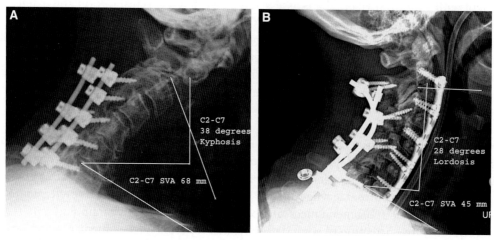

Fig. 10-7   **A** and **B,** Preoperative and postoperative neutral standing lateral cervical radiographs. (*SVA,* Sagittal vertical axis.)

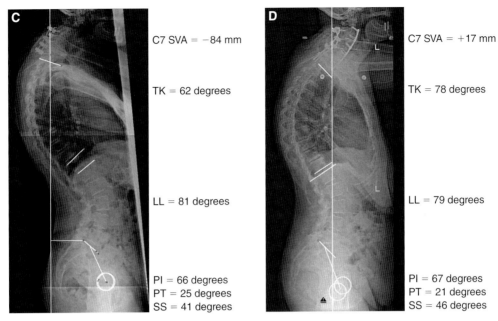

Fig. 10-7, cont'd C and D, Preoperative and postoperative spinal alignment. (*LL,* Lumbar lordosis; *PI,* pelvic incidence; *PT,* pelvic tilt; *SS,* sacral slope; *SVA,* sagittal vertical axis; *TK,* thoracic kyphosis.)

CONCLUSION

Global and regional cervical alignment should be considered in every patient undergoing evaluation for any cervical intervention involving arthrodesis. Even patients who are candidates for purely decompressive procedures such as foraminotomy can be at risk for developing delayed instability.[1,7] With increasing life expectancy, adjacent-level degeneration is a significant concern, and a straightforward, single-level anterior cervical discectomy and fusion in a young person may be only the beginning of a long series of interventions over a life span.

REFERENCES

1. Scheer JK, Tang JA, Smith JS, et al. Cervical spine alignment, sagittal deformity, and clinical implications: a review. J Neurosurg Spine 19:141-159, 2013.
2. Tang JA, Scheer JK, Smith JS, et al. The impact of standing regional cervical sagittal alignment on outcomes in posterior cervical fusion surgery. Neurosurgery 71:662-669; discussion 669, 2012.
3. Steinmetz MP, Stewart TJ, Kager CD, et al. Cervical deformity correction. Neurosurgery 60(1 Suppl 1):S90-S97, 2007.
4. Albert TJ, Vacarro A. Postlaminectomy kyphosis. Spine 23:2738-2745, 1998.
5. Gore DR, Sepic SB, Gardner GM. Roentgenographic findings of the cervical spine in asymptomatic people. Spine 11:521-524, 1986.
6. Pal GP, Sherk HH. The vertical stability of the cervical spine. Spine 13:447-449, 1988.
7. Zdeblick TA, Zou D, Warden KE, et al. Cervical stability after foraminotomy. A biomechanical in vitro analysis. J Bone Joint Surg Am 74:22-27, 1992.
8. Zdeblick TA, Abitbol JJ, Kunz DN, et al. Cervical stability after sequential capsule resection. Spine 18:2005-2008, 1993.
9. Breig A, el-Nadi AF. Biomechanics of the cervical spinal cord. Relief of contact pressure on and overstretching of the spinal cord. Acta Radiol Diagn (Stockh) 4:602-624, 1966.
10. Masini M, Maranhão V. Experimental determination of the effect of progressive sharp-angle spinal deformity on the spinal cord. Eur Spine J 6:89-92, 1997.

11. Suk KS, Kim KT, Lee SH, et al. Significance of chin-brow vertical angle in correction of kyphotic deformity of ankylosing spondylitis patients. Spine 28:2001-2005, 2003.

12. Harrison DE, Harrison DD, Cailliet R, et al. Cobb method or Harrison posterior tangent method: which to choose for lateral cervical radiographic analysis. Spine 25:2072-2078, 2000.

13. Drexler L. Röntgenanatomische Untersuchringen uber Krumming der Halswirbelsaule in der verschiedenen Lebensaltern. Stuttgart: Hippokrates, 1962.

14. Motosuneya T, Maruyama T, Yamada H, et al. Long-term results of tension-band laminoplasty for cervical stenotic myelopathy: a ten-year follow-up. J Bone Jt Surg Br 93:68-72, 2010.

15. Ishihara A. [Roentgenographic studies on the normal pattern of the cervical curvature] Nihon Seikeigeka Gakkai Zasshi 42:1033-1044, 1968.

16. Takeshita K, Murakami M, Kobayashi A, et al. Relationship between cervical curvature index (Ishihara) and cervical spine angle (C2-7). J Orthop Sci 6:223-226, 2001.

17. Smith JS, Shaffrey CI, Lafage V, et al; International Spine Study Group. Spontaneous improvement of cervical alignment after correction of global sagittal balance following pedicle subtraction osteotomy. J Neurosurg Spine 17:300-307, 2010.

18. Berthonnaud E, Dimnet J, Roussouly P, et al. Analysis of the sagittal balance of the spine and pelvis using shape and orientation parameters. J Spinal Disord Tech 18:40-47, 2005.

19. Vialle R, Levassor N, Rillardon L, et al. Radiographic analysis of the sagittal alignment and balance of the spine in asymptomatic subjects. J Bone Joint Surg Am 87:260-267, 2005.

20. Lee SH, Kim KT, Seo EM, et al. The influence of thoracic inlet alignment on the craniocervical sagittal balance in asymptomatic adults. J Spinal Disord Tech 25:E41-E47, 2012.

21. Lee SH, Son ES, Seo EM, et al. Factors determining cervical spine sagittal balance in asymptomatic adults: correlation with spinopelvic balance and thoracic inlet alignment. Spine J 2013 Sep 7. [Epub ahead of print]

22. Ames CP, Blondel B, Scheer JK, et al. Cervical radiographical alignment: comprehensive assessment techniques and potential importance in cervical myelopathy. Spine 38:S149-S160, 2013.

23. Kawakami M, Tamaki T, Yoshida M, et al. Axial symptoms and cervical alignments after cervical anterior spinal fusion for patients with cervical myelopathy. J Spinal Disord 12:50-56, 1999.

24. Naderi S, Ozgen S, Pamir MN, et al. Cervical spondylotic myelopathy: surgical results and factors affecting prognosis. Neurosurgery 43:43-49; discussion 49-50, 1998.

25. Guérin P, Obeid I, Gille O, et al. Sagittal alignment after single cervical disc arthroplasty. J Spinal Disord Tech 25:10-16, 2012.

26. Jagannathan J, Shaffrey CI, Oskouian RJ, et al. Radiographic and clinical outcomes following single-level anterior cervical discectomy and allograft fusion without plate placement or cervical collar. J Neurosurg Spine 8:420-428, 2008.

27. Kwon B, Kim DH, Marvin A, et al. Outcomes following anterior cervical discectomy and fusion: the role of interbody disc height, angulation, and spinous process distance. J Spinal Disord Tech 18:304-308, 2005.

28. Kim TH, Lee SY, Kim YC, et al. T1 slope as a predictor of kyphotic alignment change after laminoplasty in patients with cervical myelopathy. Spine 38:E992-E997, 2013.

29. Glassman SD, Berven S, Bridwell K, et al. Correlation of radiographic parameters and clinical symptoms in adult scoliosis. Spine 30:682-688, 2013.

30. Mac-Thiong JM, Transfeldt EE, Mehbod AA, et al. Can c7 plumbline and gravity line predict health related quality of life in adult scoliosis? Spine 34:E51-E527, 2009.

31. Smith JS, Lafage V, Ryan DJ, et al. Association of myelopathy scores with cervical sagittal balance and normalized spinal cord volume: analysis of 56 preoperative cases from the AOSpine North America Myelopathy study. Spine 38(22 Suppl 1):S161-S170, 2013.

32. Jung A, Schramm J. How to reduce recurrent laryngeal nerve palsy in anterior cervical spine surgery: a prospective observational study. Neurosurgery 67:10-15; discussion 15, 2015.

33. Schwab FJ, Hawkinson N, Lafage V, et al. Risk factors for major peri-operative complications in adult spinal deformity surgery: a multi-center review of 953 consecutive patients. Eur Spine J 21:2603-2610, 2012.

34. Emery SE, Smith MD, Bohlman HH. Upper-airway obstruction after multilevel cervical corpectomy for myelopathy. J Bone Joint Surg Am 73:544-551, 1991.

35. Epstein NE, Hollingsworth R, Nardi D, et al. Can airway complications following multilevel anterior cervical surgery be avoided? J Neurosurg 94(2 Suppl):185-188, 2001.

36. Kwon B, Yoo JU, Furey CG, et al. Risk factors for delayed extubation after single-stage, multi-level anterior cervical decompression and posterior fusion. J Spinal Disord Tech 19:389-393, 2006.

37. Traynelis VC. Total subaxial reconstruction. J Neurosurg Spine 13:424-434, 2010.

11

Cervicothoracic Region

Anthony C.W. Lau ▪ *Nabeel S. Alshafai* ▪ *Michael G. Fehlings*

The cervical region of the human spine is the most mobile. It normally adopts a lordotic configuration, with the center of gravity (COG) of the head over the femoral heads at rest to remain mechanically efficient. Minor changes in the steady state conformation can often be accommodated because of the flexibility of the cervical spine. However, a marked deviation in cervical alignment associated with degeneration, disease, or trauma can cause the cranial COG to move outside of the conceptual *cone of balance* described by Dubousset[1] (Fig. 11-1), leading to increasing energy demands to maintain adequate posture. Sustained imbalances in alignment precipitate progressive spinal deformity, leading to spinal cord pathology.

Cervical spondylotic myelopathy (CSM) is the leading cause of spinal cord dysfunction in the elderly worldwide[2] and is the result of a complex interplay of mechanical dynamic and static factors.[3] Static factors include hypertrophy of the ligamentum flavum, osteophyte formation, and malalignment of the cervical spine. When sufficiently severe, CSM can cause symptoms ranging from radiculopathy to quadriplegia. Surgical intervention is the mainstay of treatment for CSM and has been shown to improve clinical outcomes significantly.[4] However, one of the lingering problems in the study of CSM has been the contribution of abnormal sagittal alignment to the pathophysiology and surgical outcomes of CSM.[5] This chapter reviews the methodology for quantifying alignment in the cervical spine and the contribution of sagittal malalignment to the pathophysiology and surgical outcomes in CSM. Case examples are presented to reinforce these concepts.

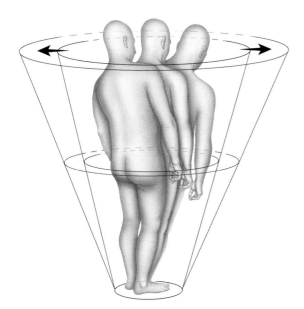

Fig. 11-1 The cone of balance described by Dubousset. Any deviation outside of this conceptual cone leads to increased energy expenditure to maintain balance and posture (Adapted from Dubousset J. Three-dimensional analysis of the scoliotic deformity. In Weinstein SL, ed. The Pediatric Spine: Principles and Practice. New York: Raven Press, 1994.)

RADIOGRAPHIC MEASURES OF CERVICAL ALIGNMENT

Several methods of estimating alignment of the cervical spine have been published. Ames et al[6] provide an excellent review of these methods. Traditional measures of cervical spine alignment estimate the degree of cervical curvature or sagittal translation. However, increasing evidence supports the notion that alterations in parameters of adjacent[7] or remote[6] regions of the spine can influence cervical alignment.

CERVICAL CURVATURE

The Cobb Angle

The Cobb angle can be measured from either the C1 or C2 level using C7 as a point of reference. Both a C1-7 Cobb angle and a C2-7 Cobb angle have been described. A C1-7 angle is formed by drawing a line from the anterior tubercle and extending it posteriorly through the C1 spinous process (Fig. 11-2, *A*). To measure a C2-7 Cobb angle, a line is drawn parallel to the inferior endplate of C2 (Fig. 11-2, *B*). In both cases, a second line is drawn parallel to the inferior endplate of C7 and extended posteriorly. Lines perpendicular to the C1 (or C2) line and the C7 line are then drawn to form an angle (see Fig. 11-2, *A* and *B*). According to convention, a negative Cobb angle represents lordosis, whereas a positive angle represents kyphosis.

The concept of *segmental* or *regional kyphosis* has been investigated on plain radiographs. In these studies, a regional or segmental angle is reported. However, the methodology for measuring the degree of segmental disease can vary. For example, Ferch et al[8] defined their regional angle as the Cobb angle produced from the superior endplate of the first diseased segment to the inferior endplate of C7 (Fig. 11-2, *C*), whereas other studies have used the superior endplate of the level above and the inferior endplate of the level below the pathology as points of reference for measurements[9] (Fig. 11-2, *D*). In either case, a perpendicular line is drawn from both endplates, and the intersecting angle is reported.

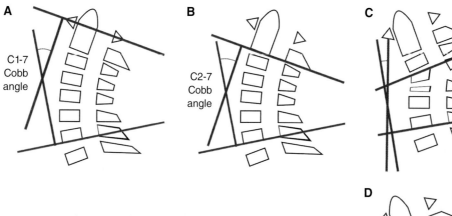

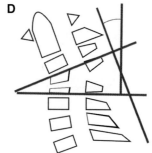

Fig. 11-2   Applications of the Cobb angle. **A,** C1-7 Cobb angle. **B,** C2-7 Cobb angle. **C,** Segmental Cobb angle in which C7 is used as a reference and compared with the first superior endplate above the pathologic level. **D,** Segmental Cobb angle in which the superior endplate above the pathologic level is used as a reference and compared with the inferior endplate below the pathologic level.

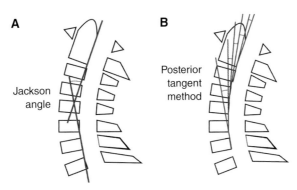

Fig. 11-3 The posterior tangent method. **A,** The Jackson angle is the angle at the intersection of two lines that extend from the posterior aspect of C2 and C7. **B,** The Harrison posterior tangent method measures the angle between these lines at each adjacent level.

The Cobb angle was originally designed to describe the severity of scoliotic deformity in the coronal plane,[10] but it has since been adapted to estimate the degree of lordosis/kyphosis in the cervical spine. Because of its simplicity and high interrater and intrarater reliability, the Cobb angle is believed to be the most widely used method of estimating cervical curvature.[11]

The Harrison and Jackson Posterior Tangent Angles

The Jackson angle was originally published in 1957 and is determined by measuring the angle between two intersecting lines derived from parallel lines drawn along the posterior aspect of the C2 and C7 vertebral bodies[12] (Fig. 11-3, *A*). The Harrison angle is an extension of the Jackson angle and is measured by drawing lines along the posterior aspect of each vertebral body from C2 through C7 inclusive (Fig. 11-3, *B*). The angle between each level can be added to yield the C2-7 Harrison angle or Jackson angle.

Harrison et al[13] popularized the Harrison angle as a more descriptive method of measuring curvature in the lumbar spine. Since its application in the cervical spine, it has been suggested that it is the most accurate method of measuring cervical curvature.[14]

Sagittal Translation
Global Sagittal Vertical Axis

The best measure of global sagittal translation requires standing lateral views encompassing the head to the sacrum. A plumb line (a vertical line along gravitational forces) is drawn starting from the middle of the C2 vertebral body or the C7 vertebral body. Alternatively, a plumb line from the anterior margin of the external auditory canal or meatus (EAM) can be used as an estimate of the cranial COG.[15] These lines are extended down to the level of the sacrum, and a second horizontal line is drawn from the most posterosuperior aspect of the S1 body to these plumb lines. The distance from the sacrum to the plumb line of C2, C7, and the EAM provides the C2, C7, and COG sagittal vertical axis (SVA), respectively (Fig. 11-4, *A*). The C2 and EAM (COG) SVA are estimates of the global sagittal balance, whereas the C7 plumb line is an estimate of thoracolumbar sagittal alignment.

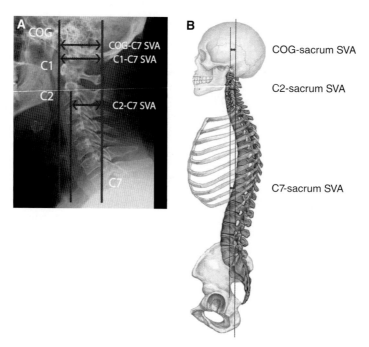

Fig. 11-4   Local and global sagittal vertical axis *(SVA)*. **A,** The cervical SVA can be measured by comparing a plumb line from the cranial center of gravity *(COG)*, the anterior tubercle of *C1*, or the centroid of *C2 (short red line)* with a plumb line from the centroid of *C7 (blue line)*. In this example, the COG and C1 plumb line *(long red line)* are identical. **B,** Global SVA can be estimated by drawing a plumb line from the COG or C2 centroid and comparing it with a plumb line generated at the most posterosuperior aspect of the S1 body. The C7-sacrum SVA is derived by comparing a plumb line from the centroid of C7 with an S1 plumb line. The C7-sacrum SVA is more appropriate for estimating thoracolumbar kyphosis.

Cervical Sagittal Vertical Axis

To measure the regional sagittal balance, the distance from a plumb line drawn from the anterior tubercle of C1, the center of C2, or the anterior margin of the EAM to the plumb line of the centroid of C7 (Fig. 11-4, *B*) provides the C1-7, C2-7, or COG-C7 SVA, respectively. These measures are better suited to estimate the contribution of the cervical region of the spine alone to overall sagittal translation.

Other Related Radiographic Measures

The complexity of the cervical spine is compounded at its ends by the cranium at the rostral end and the thoracic cage at its caudal end. Each of these regions is associated with a separate set of radiographic measurements and can exert influence over the overall alignment of the cervical region.

C0-2 Slope and Chin-Brow Vertical Angle

The cranial-C2 slope is the angle created by two lines: one is perpendicular to a line drawn from the basion to the clivus and one is perpendicular to a line parallel to the inferior endplate of C2 (Fig. 11-5, *A*). This angle estimates the amount of flexion attributable to the occipital cervical junction. The chin-brow vertical angle is derived from the angle formed between a vertical line and a line drawn from the brow to the chin on a lateral radiograph or photograph (Fig. 11-5, *B*). This angle is believed to be the most clinically relevant, because large angles require an individual to compensate dramatically to achieve and maintain horizontal gaze.[16]

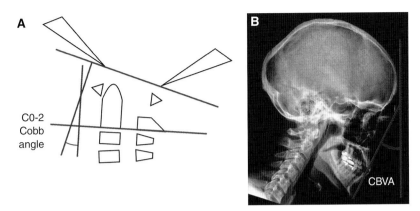

Fig. 11-5 Craniocervical parameters. **A,** The C0-2 angle is used for estimating the craniocervical kyphosis or lordosis attributable mostly to the C1-2 articulation. It is the angle created at the intersection of two perpendicular lines: one is perpendicular to the endplate of C2 and the other is perpendicular to a line that connects the inferiormost aspect of the basion to the clivus. **B,** The chin-brow vertical angle *(CBVA)* is usually measured with photographs (not lateral skull radiographs) of an upright patient. It is the angle created by a line from the chin to the brow and a vertical line.

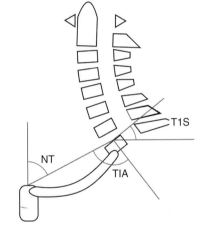

Fig. 11-6 Cervicothoracic parameters. Neck tilt *(NT)* is the angle created by a line drawn from the middle of the superior endplate of T1 to the superiormost aspect of the manubrium and a vertical line. The thoracic inlet angle *(TIA)* is the angle formed between a line perpendicular to the superior endplate of T1 and a line that extends from the superior endplate of T1 to the superiormost aspect of the manubrium. The T1 slope *(T1S)* is the angle formed by a line parallel to the superior endplate of T1 and a horizontal line.

Thoracic Inlet Angle, T1 Slope, and Neck Tilt

The thoracic inlet angle is a novel radiographic estimate thought to be analogous to the pelvic incidence in the lumbar spine.[7] In this respect, it is a static measurement regardless of posture. The thoracic inlet angle defined as the angle between a perpendicular line to the superior endplate of T1 and a line drawn from the midpoint of the superior endplate of T1 to the uppermost aspect of the manubrium (Fig. 11-6). The T1 slope is defined as the angle created by a line parallel to the T1 vertebral body and an arbitrary horizontal line. Neck tilt is the angle created by a vertical line and a line drawn from the center of the T1 superior endplate to the top of the manubrium.

DISCUSSION OF CERVICAL PARAMETERS
Cervical Measurement Values in Asymptomatic Individuals

The average cervical lordosis in asymptomatic individuals is approximately −40 degrees, as measured using a C1-7 Cobb angle[17] and −14 degrees using the C2-7 Cobb angle.[18] Values for each segment are provided in Table 11-1. These were derived using Cobb angle and Harrison methods. Approximately 75% to 80% of the normal cervical lordosis is localized to the C1-2 level, emphasizing the degree of mobility that is pos-

Table 11-1   Normal Segmental Values Based on Cobb Angle and Posterior Tangent Methods

	Cobb Angle Method[17]		Posterior Tangent Method[14]	
	Mean (degrees)	SD	Mean (degrees)	SD
0-C1	2.1	5	NA	NA
C1-2	−32.2	7	NA	NA
C2-3	−1.9	5.2	−6.4	5.4
C3-4	−1.5	5	−6.9	5.1
C4-5	−0.6	4.4	−6.8	5
C5-6	−1.1	5.1	−6.6	5.3
C6-7	−4.5	4.3	−7.8	6

NA, Not applicable; *SD*, standard deviation.

Table 11-2   Normal Age Values for Cervical Lordosis

	Cobb Angle Method[18]					Posterior Tangent Method[19]			
	Male		Female			Male		Female	
Age (years)	Mean (degrees)	SD	Mean (degrees)	SD	Age (years)	Mean (degrees)	SD	Mean (degrees)	SD
20	10.8	17.5	5.2	11.4	20-25	16	16	15	10
30	10.7	14.7	7.0	11.2	30-35	21	14	16	16
40	14.1	14.4	9.9	11.2	40-45	27	14	23	17
50	18.4	12.8	15.7	12.2	50-55	22	15	25	11
60	18.4	10.9	16.9	10.8	60-65	22	13	25	16
70	20.7	14.0	18.7	10.6					

SD, Standard deviation.

sible at the C1-2 junction. With the Jackson angle method, the average C2-7 lordosis is −23 degrees.[19] The average C2-7 SVA is 15.6 ± 11.2 mm, and the average C2-sacrum SVA is 13.2 ± 29.5 mm.[17]

With increasing age, the predisposition toward cervical lordosis increases, as measured by the posterior tangent method[19] and the Cobb angle method[18] (Table 11-2). Park et al[20] similarly reported increasing cervical lordosis with age, as indicated by the C2-7 Cobb angle (−8.98 versus −13.70 degrees). Their study included an analysis of the C2-7 plumb line with aging that included two study populations defined as *young* (20 to 29 years of age) and *older* (older than 60 years of age). The authors reported a statistically significant difference between the young and older groups in T1 slope (23.76 versus 19.96 degrees, respectively) and the C7-sacrum SVA (1.27 mm versus 20.54 mm, respectively), but not in the C2-7 plumb line (13.21 mm versus 13.68 mm, respectively). These studies favor a model of *normal* spinal aging that results in increasing cervical lordosis to accommodate decreasing lumbar lordosis to maintain sagittal balance.

Relationships of Cervical Parameters

The spine is an extremely adaptable complex of joints. Under normal circumstances, the conformation of the spine remains within the cone of balance described by Dubousset. However, during aging, degenerative and pathologic processes can alter the conformation so that it lies outside of this theoretical cone, leading to further degeneration, pathology, and disability. To minimize disability, regions remote to the level of deformity can adopt new conformations to maintain balance or revert to normal conformations as remote deformity is corrected.[21] The new equilibrium achieved to accommodate pathologic processes can be far from an ideal state and can lead to progressive deformity as seen in ankylosing spondylitis, rheumatoid arthritis, and other degenerative diseases.

Because of the increasing awareness of the holistic nature of the spine, recent interest had developed in quantifying the relationships between cervical spine parameters and other remote regions of the spine. Lee et al[7] published a study exploring the relationship of the thoracic inlet angle with several cervical spine parameters. In a study population of 77 asymptomatic individuals, the authors reported a statistically significant correlation between the thoracic inlet angle and T1 slope (r = 0.694), the T1 slope and the C2-7 Cobb angle (r = 0.624), the C2-7 Cobb angle, the C0-2 Cobb angle (r = 0.547), and the C0-2 angle and cranial offset, measured by the COG-C7 SVA (r = 0.406) (Fig. 11-7, A). Moreover, because the thoracic cage is a fixed reference point, the authors further suggested that the T1 slope and thoracic inlet angle can be used to predict the optimal cervical lordosis necessary during correction of deformity. The ideas introduced in this paper were recently extended to include the entire spine.[6] The authors retrospectively analyzed radiographs of 55 asymptomatic patients and determined a statistically significant correlation between pelvic incidence and lumbar lordosis (r = −0.52), lumbar lordosis and thoracic kyphosis (r = −0.34), and thoracic kyphosis and cervical lordosis (r = −0.51) (Fig. 11-7, B). These results reinforced the notion that the regions of the spine cannot be studied in isolation, and care must be taken to establish the primary cause of the deformity especially in cases of multilevel/multiregional disease.

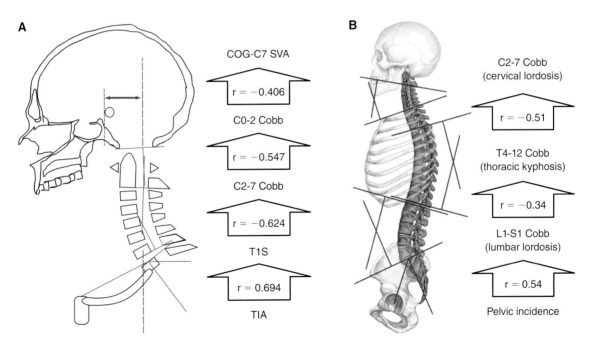

Fig. 11-7 Relationships between spinal parameters. All correlations are reported in Pearson correlation coefficients *(r)*. **A,** Relationships between various parameters from the cranium to the thoracic spine, as reported by Lee et al.[7] **B,** The associations in spinal parameters globally, as reported by Ames et al.[6] (*COG,* Center of gravity; *SVA,* sagittal vertical axis; *T1S,* T1 slope; *TIA,* thoracic inlet angle.)

Clinical Outcome Measures and Cervical Spine Alignment

The degree of kyphosis in the cervical spine affects clinical outcomes after surgery. In the trauma population, Jenkins et al[22] reported a significantly higher degree of neck pain complaints with kyphotic fusions of equal to or more than 20 degrees. Kawakami et al[23] reported that patients with axial symptoms had significantly less lordosis, compared with those without axial symptoms. However, several studies of the possible correlation between the degree of cervical curvature and clinical outcomes have been negative. Ferch et al[8] showed no relationship between C2-7 Cobb angles or segmental angles and baseline preoperative myelopathy scores with the modified Japanese Orthopaedic Association (mJOA) scale. Similarly, Uchida et al[24] found no significant correlation with the degree of cervical curvature, as measured with the Jackson angle and preoperative JOA scale in a Japanese population.

The lack of linear correlation between the angle of cervical lordosis and clinical outcome measures suggests that the contribution of cervical lordosis to clinical outcomes is much more complex. Minor changes in cervical lordosis can be tolerated to some extent by accommodation; thus it may not correlate linearly with clinical outcome measures. However, poor clinical outcomes will be associated with kyphosis beyond a particular degree, as reported by Jenkins et al.[22] In contrast, preliminary evidence suggests that a correlation exists between sagittal translation and clinical outcomes. Tang et al[25] reported a Pearson correlation coefficient of 0.20 in a comparison of the C2-7 SVA and the neck disability index (NDI) in 108 patients after posterior cervical laminectomy and fusion. These results raised the possibility that the overall sagittal translation rather than curvature is more important to clinical outcomes.

Pathophysiology of Cervical Spondylotic Myelopathy

The pathobiology of CSM is complex and involves both static and dynamic factors.[3] The static factors involved in the progression of CSM largely encompass the structural changes in the cervical spine that often accompany aging. These changes include disc degeneration; facet joint osteoarthritis and laxity; and posterior longitudinal ligament hypertrophy, laxity, and ossification. With time, the resultant biomechanical changes can lead to pathologic kyphosis and exacerbation of the dynamic factors contributing to CSM. The dynamic factors contributing to CSM include the repetitive motion of the cervical spine, which leads to mechanical stress and ischemia of the spinal cord.

Microvasculature changes leading to ischemia of the spinal cord in the context of mechanical stretch and increasing compression[26] have long been implicated in the pathogenesis of CSM. Animal models of CSM have shown evidence of ischemia[3] and reduced blood flow to the cord,[27] whereas postmortem histologic analysis of CSM spinal cords demonstrated cord necrosis and gray matter cavitations consistent with ischemic injury.[28] As mentioned previously, compression of the spinal cord can lead to microvasculature-mediated ischemic changes in the spinal cord, and a narrow spinal canal is a risk factor in the development of symptomatic CSM.[29] However, recent evidence suggests that chronic compression can also cause significant endothelial cell dysfunction, leading to increasing pathologic permeability and inflammation in animal models, with progressive gait deficits. Persistent elevation in matrix metallopeptidase–9 (MMP-9) has been implicated in maintenance of the blood-spinal cord barrier disruption in animal and human tissue.[30] Ensuing inflammation and accumulation of macrophages and microglia appear to be mediated by the release of a chemokine CX3CL1 from injured neurons,[31] further exacerbating neuronal injury. In addition to endothelial cells, compressive forces can exert a direct effect on cultured neurons, and sublethal mechanical stretching of neurons has been shown to cause apoptotic cell death and an increased susceptibility to glutamatergic insults and secondary injury.[32] In an animal model of CSM, apoptosis was seen in the late stages of cervical cord compression.[33] This can be reduced with the application of riluzole, a glutamate-sodium channel blocker.[34] A clinical trial is currently under way to examine the efficacy of riluzole, an antiglutamatergic drug used in the treatment of amyotrophic lateral sclerosis in CSM patients.[35] A very basic summary of these mechanisms is shown in Fig. 11-8.

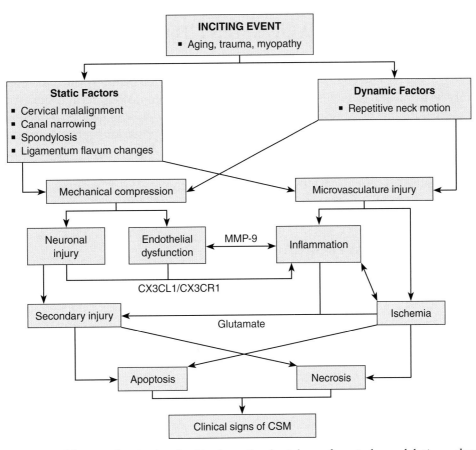

Fig. 11-8 Overview of the complexities involved in the pathophysiology of cervical spondylotic myelopathy. (*CSM,* Cervical spondylotic myelopathy; *MMP-9,* matrix metallopeptidase–9.)

Pathologic Consequences of Cervical Malalignment

The reversal of cervical lordosis to kyphosis has many physiologic and structural consequences, including draping of the spinal cord onto the back of the vertebral bodies of the apex of the cervical spine. In experimental models, it has been shown that mechanical stress on the cord increases with worsening kyphosis,[36] leading to deformation of the spinal cord, neuronal loss, and demyelination in animal models.[37] Similarly, Chavanne et al[38] demonstrated increasing cord pressures in a cadaveric model, with worsening kyphosis beginning at +7 degrees; this became exponentially higher with kyphosis larger than +21 degrees. The degree of kyphosis was assessed using the posterior tangent method.

Dynamic factors can further exacerbate the already-compromised cord in malaligned patients. With the use of MRI in asymptomatic patients, Muhle et al[39] demonstrated a 43% decrease in ventral subarachnoid space with flexion of the cervical spine and a reduction of dorsal subarachnoid space by 17% with extension. Moreover, this was associated with a 14% decrease in sagittal diameter of the cord. In patients with CSM, extension increased spinal stenosis by 48%, compared with flexion, which worsened cervical stenosis by 24%.[40] Recently, Zhang et al[41] showed that flexion of the cervical spine in CSM patients can lead to stretching of the spinal cord, which has been demonstrated to cause loss of spinal cord evoked potentials in an animal model.[42] Evidence supports the notion that cervical spine malalignment can act synergistically with dynamic insults, leading to progressive neurologic disability and myelopathy.

CONTRIBUTION OF MALALIGNMENT TO SURGICAL MANAGEMENT

Cervical malalignment is caused by a variety of pathologies. The overall guiding principles in spine surgery are to decompress the neural elements, stabilize the spine, and promote long-term fusion. An additional goal in kyphotic deformities is the restoration of cervical lordosis as close to neutral as possible.[43] In most cases, these surgical goals can be achieved by either an anterior or posterior approach. In addition, all of these techniques have been shown to improve clinical outcomes. A direct comparison of these techniques is not the purpose of this review. Rather, the advantages and disadvantages of these techniques with respect to sagittal alignment will be discussed. Other nontraditional techniques such as cervical disc replacement, skip laminectomies, and oblique corpectomies are presented elsewhere.[44]

ANTERIOR SURGICAL APPROACHES

Anterior cervical discectomy and fusion (ACDF) is described in detail elsewhere.[45] It is a prevalent technique in the treatment of anterior pathology in the cervical spine. The procedure has many variations, including the choice of graft and the application of an anterior plate. However, the overall principles are the same. The cervical spine is approached from an anterior neck incision, respecting the natural surgical planes. A discectomy is then performed, and an interbody fusion device with or without an anterior plate is implanted (Fig. 11-9). It has been shown that placement of some type of interbody device is preferable to discectomy alone to prevent increasing rates of segmental kyphosis.[46]

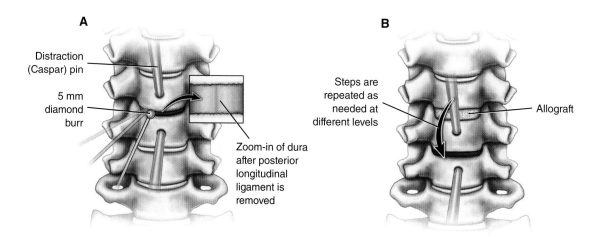

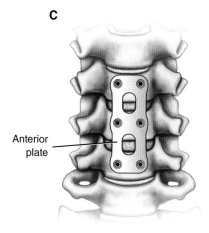

Fig. 11-9   For anterior cervical discectomy and fusion at multiple levels, we make a linear incision along the medial border of the sternocleidomastoid muscle. A traditional anterior cervical exposure is performed, and adequate visualization of all levels to be decompressed and fused is confirmed. The anterior longitudinal ligament and superficial disc material are removed before distraction pins are placed. **A,** A 5 mm diamond burr is used to drill the endplates and disc down to the posterior longitudinal ligament, which is removed along with posterior osteophytes with a Cloward punch to visualize the dura. **B,** An appropriately sized allograft is placed into the disc space, the anterior longitudinal ligament and superficial disc material of the next level are removed, and the distraction pins are moved to the next level. This step is repeated as needed. **C,** An anterior plate is placed over the segments to be fused.

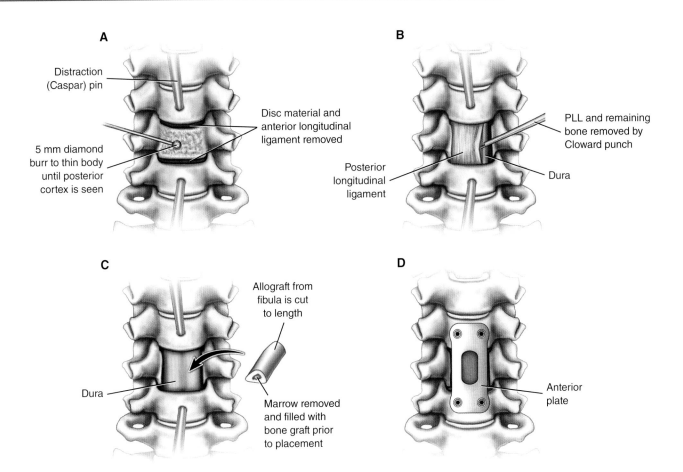

A

Distraction
(Caspar) pin

5 mm diamond
burr to thin body
until posterior
cortex is seen

Disc material and
anterior longitudinal
ligament removed

B

PLL and remaining
bone removed by
Cloward punch

Posterior
longitudinal
ligament

Dura

C

Allograft from
fibula is cut
to length

Dura

Marrow removed
and filled with
bone graft prior
to placement

D

Anterior
plate

Fig. 11-10   Anterior cervical corpectomy and fusion. A traditional anterior cervical exposure is performed, ensuring visualization of the entire vertebral bodies of the level above and below the corpectomy. **A,** The anterior longitudinal ligament and superficial disc material are removed from the disc space above and below the proposed corpectomy level before the insertion of distraction pins. The bulk of the corpectomy is achieved by drilling away the vertebral body using a coarse 5 mm diamond burr. **B,** A posterior longitudinal ligament defect is created with a blunt hook, and the rest of the ligament is removed with any remaining bone using a Cloward punch to visualise the dura. **C,** An allograft is crafted with a slight angle to promote physiologic lordosis and to prevent it from slipping posteriorly. **D,** The distraction pins are removed and an anterior plate is placed.

In cases of vertebral body pathology or retrovertebral disease, a corpectomy or hybrid procedure may be indicated (Fig. 11-10). A systemic review comparing multilevel discectomies, corpectomies, and hybrid procedures was recently published.[47] It was postulated that a disc-based approach allows better sagittal correction and potentially less blood loss, whereas a corpectomy-based approach may achieve better decompression and possibly fusion. Overall, the evidence suggested that multilevel discectomies result in better clinical outcomes and sagittal correction than corpectomies and hybrids alone; however, the strength of the evidence is low. In addition, the analysis revealed that C5 nerve palsies are rarer with multiple discectomies alone.

POSTERIOR SURGICAL APPROACHES

Many posterior approaches are available to achieve the surgical principles of neural decompression, acute spinal stabilization, and promotion of long-term fusion. However, one pitfall of the posterior approaches is an inability to achieve significant sagittal correction, which occurs with anterior approaches (discussed later).

Laminectomy With or Without Fusion

A laminectomy alone can be useful to remove the lamina of spinal column and underlying ligamentum flavum to reduce compression on the spinal cord. This approach has traditionally been employed in cases with multilevel degeneration and minimal kyphosis. However, multilevel posterior laminectomies alone can lead to an iatrogenic progressive kyphosis,[48] with an estimated incidence of 21% after laminectomies in lordotic spines and even higher rates in cervical spines with minimal lordosis (that is, straight spines) or kyphosis.[49] Currently, most cases of posterior decompression are followed by stabilization with lateral mass screws and rods or plates (Fig. 11-11). Roy-Camille and Saillant[50] and Jeanneret et al[51] have described two popular methods of lateral mass screw placement. These have been reviewed in detail.[52]

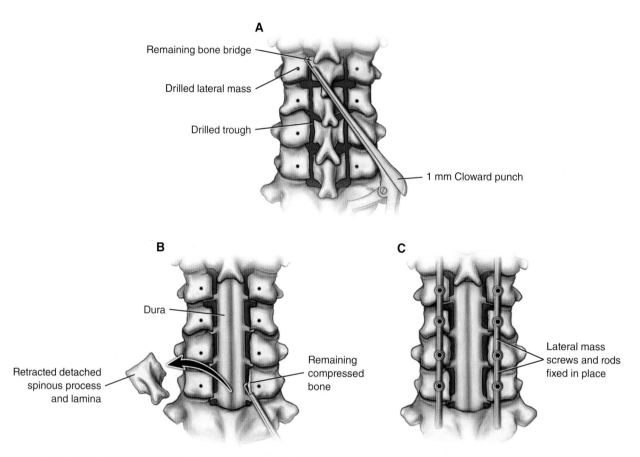

Fig. 11-11   Posterior cervical decompression and fusion. A classic posterior exposure is performed with monopolar cautery. Care is taken to expose the lateral border of all the lateral masses to be fused without disruption of facet joints. **A,** According to the technique described by Jeanneret et al,[51] starting points for lateral mass screws are drilled and tapped before the decompression. Bone wax can be used for hemostasis. Troughs are drilled along the lateral borders of the lamina to be removed down to the ligamentum flavum. Along the troughs, remaining bone bridges are removed with a 1 mm Cloward punch. **B,** The detached spinous processes and lamina are retracted and removed away from the dura. Remaining soft tissue and ligamentum attachments are freed with sharp or blunt dissection. All remaining compressive bone or soft tissue is removed with a Cloward punch. **C,** Lateral mass screws and rods are then fixed into position.

Laminoplasty

Laminoplasty is a procedure in which the lamina of one or more spinal levels in the cervical spine is detached from the bony attachment to the lateral masses and expanded in a bilateral (French door) or unilateral (barn door) fashion.[53] A detailed technical review of the laminoplasty has been published.[54] This method was developed to reduce the need for fusion of the cervical spine but also to reduce the possibility of progressive iatrogenic kyphosis after laminectomy alone. This method largely accomplishes a posterior decompression of the spinal cord, but it can do little to restore sagittal malalignment. Recent studies have estimated that the maximum kyphotic angle possible for a successful laminoplasty is 13 degrees.[55] However, Uchida et al[24] published a case series comparing anterior and posterior approaches to cervical myelopathy. They reported no difference in JOA scores between ACDF and laminoplasty approaches even though the laminoplasty group had a mean kyphotic angle of 16 degrees.

Pedicle Subtraction Osteotomy

A pedicle subtraction osteotomy (PSO) is not a traditional technique for treating CSM. However, it can be very effective in treating kyphotic deformities of the cervical spine. A pedicle osteotomy in the cervical spine involves removal of the posterior and middle column elements of a cervical level and removal of a wedge of the cervical vertebral body of the same level. Deviren et al[56] have published a detailed technical discussion of the cervical PSO procedure. A PSO alone can restore a large degree of lordosis to the spine but can do little to decompress the spine in multilevel disease. An additional procedure is required for this purpose.

SURGICAL MANAGEMENT DISCUSSION

Anterior Versus Posterior Techniques: A General Overview

Anterior approaches can cause a number of general problems, including pseudarthrosis, adjacent-level stress, swallowing difficulty, and construct failure. Komotar et al[57] reported increasing failure rates with three or more levels of fusion. However, a multicenter prospective study led by Fehlings et al[58] demonstrated no major differences in complication rates between the anterior and posterior surgical approaches, except for a slightly higher infection rate with the posterior approach. Major complications were associated with several factors, including age and combined approaches. Combined anterior-posterior approaches resulted in significantly increased rates of dysphagia.

In a recent systematic review, Lawrence et al[59] attempted to address the long-standing debate as to whether an anterior or posterior approach to spinal surgery was favored for multilevel CSM. Eight comparative studies were included in their analysis, which encompassed a variety of anterior and posterior approaches. Overall, the authors concluded that evidence was insufficient in the literature to support either an anterior or posterior surgical approach. However, they stressed that the important factors to consider included: ventral versus dorsal compression, sagittal alignment, focal versus diffuse disease, the presence or absence of axial pain or radiculopathy, age, comorbidities, and the surgeon's preference/familiarity with procedures.[60] The authors further reinforced the earlier notion that an individualized approach is absolutely critical for the successful treatment of patients with cervical pathology.[61]

Surgical Approach: Sagittal Alignment

An anterior approach is believed to achieve better correction than a posterior (nonosteotomy) approach alone in fixed deformities. Ferch et al[8] presented a case series of 28 patients who had an ACDF for cervical kyphotic deformity. ACDF resulted in a mean angular correction of −14 degrees locally and −11 degrees regionally. Twenty-six percent of these patients had a correction of more than −20 degrees locally. By comparison, the posterior laminectomy and fusion technique had a modest effect on cervical curvature.[62]

This retrospective study of 56 patients showed a change of lordosis from -6.8 to -9.0 with lateral mass screws and rod fixation. This study was not designed to examine the extent of kyphotic deformity correction possible with a posterior approach, although the authors reported a mean change of 6.5 degrees in patients with preoperative kyphosis.

To our knowledge no studies have been designed specifically to assess the maximum degree of sagittal correction achievable with a posterior (nonosteotomy) approach. However, a number of retrospective studies comparing anterior and posterior approaches in patients with CSM have reported significant differences in cervical curvature with anterior and posterior approaches. A retrospective analysis comparing ADCF with laminoplasty for treatment of CSM showed a mean reduction of kyphosis from 17.0 to 7.1 degrees with the ACDF approach and from 15.6 to 12.6 degrees with laminoplasty.[24] A similar retrospective study comparing anterior corpectomy and posterior multilevel laminectomies showed improvement of lordosis from -5.3 to -14.1 degrees in the corpectomy group, compared with a worsened lordotic angle from -12.4 to -5.9 in the posterior laminectomy group.[63] A laminoplasty alone was estimated to increase cervical lordosis by 1.8 degrees on average.[64] In contrast, a PSO in the cervical spine can achieve an average correction of -49.9 degrees, as estimated by a Cobb angle method from C2-T1, and a C2-7 SVA correction of 4.5 cm.[56] These values were achieved in patients with fixed deformity. Surgical correction of cervical malalignment in patients with flexible deformities are limited largely by the degree of flexion/extension achievable by the patient, as seen in the case discussion later in the chapter.

Surgical Approach: Adjacent-Level Disease

Any surgical intervention requiring fusion in the cervical spine results in increasing physical forces on adjacent levels.[65] In addition, some types of surgical intervention can lead to different disc stresses and posterior facet loads. With the use of a finite element model, Hussain et al[66] demonstrated that disc stresses and posterior facet loads at adjacent segments were greatest after combined instrumentation followed by posterior instrumentation, and they were lowest with anterior instrumentation. The clinical significance of this difference in forces is unclear with respect to approach; but regardless of the individual contributions of surgical interventions in the cervical spine, adjacent-level disease is a known complication with all of them, with an estimated incidence of symptomatic adjacent-level disease of 1.6% to 4.2% per year and 0.8% requiring reoperation.[67] Unfortunately, the definition of adjacent-level disease varies from study to study, further complicating interpretation.[68]

Malalignment of the spine in cadaveric models increases forces to adjacent-level discs, particularly with flexion or kyphosis.[69] Thus a reasonable conclusion is that malalignment of the cervical spine can predispose patients to adjacent-level disease. Ishihara et al[70] performed a retrospective study of adjacent-level disease in ACDF patients. They reported no difference in sagittal alignment between patients who developed adjacent-segment disease versus those who did not. In contrast, Katsuura et al[71] categorized postoperative cervical spine conformations into lordotic, kyphotic, straight, or sigmoidal and determined that lordotic alignment had significantly lower rates of adjacent-level disease, compared with other alignments. A systematic review published in 2012 was performed to determine the evidence for or against malalignment as a contributing factor to adjacent-level disease.[72] The authors recommended that sagittal lordosis be maintained after cervical spine surgery, though the overall evidence was low.

Surgical Correction, Alignment, and Clinical Outcomes

Given the complex nature of the cervical spine and related radiologic measures, it is reasonable to think that a correlation between surgical outcomes, sagittal alignment, and clinical outcomes will be difficult to delineate. Jagannathan et al[73] reported no relationship between the clinical outcome and segmental sagittal alignment after ACDF. Similarly, Gum et al[9] showed no correlation between the NDI and C2-7 Cobb angle or segmental angles after ACDF. However, the surgical correction in sagittal alignment in this study was minimal.

Naderi et al[74] conducted a retrospective study of 27 patients who had cervical laminectomies for CSM. They reported initial evidence that sagittal alignment influenced postoperative outcomes. The improvement in mJOA scores in patients with a lordotic spine were significantly increased, whereas the change in preoperative and postoperative mJOA scores in kyphotic patients was not significantly different. In a more recent study, Villavicencio et al[75] attempted to determine whether a clinical difference existed with the use of parallel versus lordotic allografts in anterior cervical decompression and fusions. Although no significant difference was seen in the parallel or lordotic allograft groups, the authors noted that patients who maintained or had improved segmental sagittal alignment, as measured by the segmental angle at the level of fusion, had significantly improved clinical outcomes, as measured by the NDI. However, cervical sagittal alignment, as measured by the Jackson method, did not correlate with the same clinical improvement. The authors further postulated that the degree of the postoperative angle achieved (the average postsurgical change in segmental angle was 1 degree) was not as important as the maintenance or improvement of the sagittal alignment. As mentioned previously, Tang et al[25] reported a Pearson correlation coefficient of 0.20 in a comparison of the C2-7 SVA and the NDI in 108 patients after posterior cervical laminectomy and fusion, suggesting that sagittal translation rather than curvature is important to clinical outcomes.

In summary, no one surgical technique is optimal for every case. Of the techniques described here, the anterior approach (either discectomy or corpectomy) has the advantage of moderate deformity correction and decompression, whereas the PSO can result in large, fixed deformity correction without decompression. A laminectomy and fusion (or laminoplasty) technique provides the least degree of sagittal correction, but can achieve the widest decompression.[76] The angles obtained by the posterior approach appear more stable than those of the anterior approach overall, but the clinical and statistical significance of this is unclear. The wide range of achievable goals with various techniques further reinforces the importance of individualized clinical decision-making as a goal of patient care for cervical deformity and myelopathy.

PATIENT EXAMPLE

DROPPED-HEAD SYNDROME

Clinical Presentation

This 39-year-old woman presented with a 12-year history of worsening chronic neck pain, progressive neck deformity, and gait abnormalities. Her gait and ambulation problems were largely secondary to difficulty elevating her head. Although the patient's symptoms had been long-standing, she reported that her neck deformity had worsened during the 3 to 4 months before her clinic visit. Martin et al[77] presented this case in greater detail.

Physical Examination

On examination, the patient had pronounced cervical kyphosis with hypertrophic neck extensors. The deformity was reducible manually by the examiner, but active cervical flexion and extension was reduced by 50%, compared with normal range of motion. Results of her cranial nerve examination were normal, and she had no ocular or facial muscle weakness. Her motor examination showed no abnormalities in muscle bulk or tone, and power was normal in all four limbs. The patient demonstrated global hyperreflexia with a positive Hoffman's sign bilaterally. Results of a sensory examination were normal in all modalities, including light touch, pinprick, vibration, and position sense. Her cerebellar examination results and gait were normal.

Initial Investigations

The patient's initial MRI showed cervical spondylosis with spinal canal stenosis that was worst across the C2-4 segments of the cervical spine (Fig. 11-12, *A*). Plain radiographs of the cervical spine with the patient upright showed marked kyphosis and sagittal translation (Fig. 11-13, *A* through *D*). A comparison of her cervical parameters with normal values is shown in Table 11-3. Findings of initial electrodiagnostic studies were nonspecific. A trapezius muscle biopsy was performed to rule out primary muscle disease. It showed no evidence of inflammatory myopathy and nonspecific atrophic changes with fibrosis.

Management

The patient was not offered operative treatment initially, because no overt neurologic findings were noted; thus we elected to follow her closely clinically. Over the next 2 years, she developed additional symptoms and signs, including worsening walking distance, increasing hyperreflexia, and T2 cord signal change on MRI (see Fig. 11-12, *B*). More important, subsequent repeat EMG studies demonstrated fibrillations and small-amplitude polyphasic potentials in paraspinal muscles, suggestive of idiopathic neck extensor myopathy (INEM) as the cause of this patient's dropped-head syndrome (DHS).

Table 11-3   Comparison of Preoperative, Postoperative, and Normal Values

	Preoperative Value	Postoperative Value	Normal Value
C2-7 Cobb angle (degrees)	57.7	−4.6	−9.6[17]
Jackson angle (degrees)	66	−9.9	−23[19]
COG-C7 SVA (cm)	11.7	3.8	NA
C2-7 SVA (cm)	7.6	3.3	1.6[17]
Neck tilt (degrees)	44.6	41	43.7[7]
Thoracic inlet angle (degrees)	64.3	70.2	69.5[7]
T1 slope (degrees)	19.3	29.6	25.7[7]

COG, Center of gravity; *NA,* not applicable; *SVA,* sagittal vertical axis.

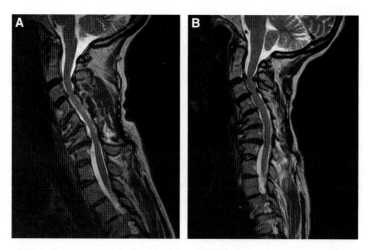

Fig. 11-12   Preoperative MRI of a patient with dropped-head syndrome. **A,** The initial T2-weighted MRI scan demonstrates kyphosis and canal narrowing, but without T2 signal change. **B,** After a period of conservative treatment, the patient returned with increasing myelopathy and T2 signal change on MRI.

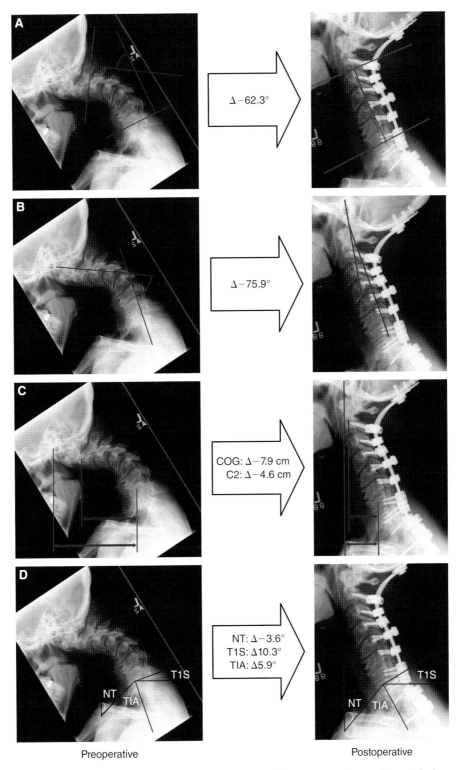

Preoperative   Postoperative

Fig. 11-13 Comparison of preoperative and postoperative cervical parameters in a patient with dropped-head syndrome. This is the same patient shown in Fig. 11-12. **A,** Upright lateral radiographs of the patient at presentation showed marked kyphosis, which was corrected postoperatively by −62.3 degrees. **B,** Cervical curvature measured by the Jackson angle showed a correction of −75.9 degrees. **C,** Sagittal translation, as measured by COG-C7 SVA and C2-C7 SVA, was corrected dramatically by −7.9 cm and −4.6 cm, respectively. **D,** Thoracic parameters of neck tilt *(NT),* T1 slope *(TIS),* and thoracic inlet angle *(TIA)* changed postoperatively by −3.6 degrees, 10.3 degrees, and 5.9 degrees, respectively.

Because of these new radiologic and clinical changes, the patient was offered an occiput-T6 posterior instrumented fusion and decompression from C2 to T1. Reduction of the cervical deformity with neutral head alignment was achieved intraoperatively via direct visualization and lateral radiographs. The surgical procedure was uncomplicated. Motor and sensory evoked potentials were maintained throughout the surgery. Intraoperative EMG recordings showed transient spiking activity, which resolved spontaneously. Postoperatively, the patient wore a cervicothoracic brace for 8 weeks.

Follow-Up

Postoperatively, fibrillations in the paraspinal muscles were resolved on a repeat EMG study. CT confirmed good positioning of all hardware and anatomic alignment with increased space in the spinal canal. Standing radiographs demonstrated a marked reduction in kyphosis and normalization of sagittal balance (see Fig. 11-13).The preoperative and postoperative corrected cervical parameter values are shown on Table 11-3. Cervical curvature and sagittal translation were dramatically corrected, though the thoracic parameters remained relatively stable. Eight months postoperatively, the patient has recovered full mobility and reports significant improvement in her activities of daily living.

Discussion

This case illustrates the uncommon spinal condition of patients with DHS, which is a subtype of camptocormia specific to the neck.[78] This condition is characterized by severe kyphotic deformity of the cervicothoracic spine, which results from a variety of pathologies (Table 11-4) and leads to significant disability.

The clinical management of this group of patients is complicated and requires thorough investigations. A comprehensive multidisciplinary workup is critical to determine whether a medically treatable primary cause is present before a decision can be made to proceed with surgical intervention. Oftentimes, conservative management, including physiotherapy, massage, and acupuncture, can maximize function and slow progression of symptoms. Nonsurgical options for mechanical stabilization and correction of DHS include removable soft or hard collars, a sternal occipital mandibular immobilizer (SOMI) brace, or a halo vest. These external orthotic devices can provide temporary stabilization and partially correct the deformity; however, they can be cumbersome and lead to further deconditioning and deterioration of neck extensor musculature. Therefore they are considered only temporary solutions except in elderly patients or those deemed too high risk for surgery. In time, kyphosis of the cervical spine leads to accelerated degenerative changes. In this case, we observed vertebral body height loss in the subaxial spine (most noticeable at C6) and paraspinal muscle atrophy and fat infiltration appreciable on T2-weighted MRI (see Fig. 11-12, *B*).

When medical and physical treatment options have been exhausted, surgical correction of DHS may be needed to maintain a reasonable quality of life for the patient. Unfortunately, because of the rarity of the disease and referral patterns favoring medical neurologists, most are treated conservatively.[79] Simmons et al[80] described a case series of six patients who were treated surgically. They advocated either anterior (anterior muscle release and a halo vest for a long-standing condition) or posterior resection (of the inferior facets to achieve restoration of normal extension). In the largest case report series, Gerling et al[81] reported on nine patients with DHS and cervical myopathy who were managed either through posterior instrumented fusion from C2 to thoracic levels (T1-5) or anterior cervical releases. Only one of nine patients presented without myelopathy, and this patient was not decompressed during surgery. The main presenting symptoms were loss of horizontal gaze and axial neck pain. Overall, the authors reported good outcomes at the 2-year follow-up in seven patients and fair outcomes in two. Petheram et al[79] described a series of seven patients with DHS, six of whom were treated nonoperatively. The only patient who was

Table 11-4 Conditions Associated With Dropped-Head Syndrome

Type of Condition	Specific Diagnosis
Neurologic	Amyotrophic lateral sclerosis Parkinson's disease* Multiple-system atrophy Cervical dystonia Cervical myelopathy Chronic inflammatory polyneuropathy Tardive dyskinesia
Neuromuscular	Myasthenia gravis Lambert-Eaton myasthenic syndrome
Muscular Primary inflammatory	Polymyositis, scleromyositis Isolated inflammatory axial myopathy*
Primary noninflammatory	Nemaline myopathy, mitochondrial myopathy, fascioscapulo- humeral dystrophy, isolated neck extensor myopathy
Secondary	Postradiation myopathy† Postbotulinum toxin injection Cushing's syndrome,* hypothyroidism,* hyperparathyroidism,* hypokalemia*
Other	Malignancy Postsurgical

*Patients with these conditions are likely to show improvement when treated medically.
†This causes focal structural changes that are poorly suited to medical treatment.

treated surgically was unhappy because of decreased neck mobility and difficulty walking after surgery. The six patients treated nonoperatively did not fare well. Amin et al[82] presented a single patient with a good outcome and independence after 3 months of rehabilitation. The patient, who was 79 years old and had DHS and severe osteoporosis, was fused from C2 to T11. Kawaguchi et al[83] reported a case of DHS caused solely by cervical myelopathy secondary to spondylosis. Posterior decompressive laminectomy alone was sufficient to lead to full recovery. Because of the rarity of this disease and its numerous causes, it is recommended that DHS be approached on a case-by-case basis.

Three main factors require consideration during surgical management of patients with this illness: the neurologic presentation (especially the presence of myelopathy), the stability of the spine, and the presence of a fixed versus flexible deformity. The patient presented previously had a flexible deformity. However, patients with fixed deformity often necessitate a combined anterior and posterior approach, as seen in the patient in Fig. 11-14, *A*. The changes in this patient's preoperative and postoperative cervical parameters are presented numerically in Table 11-5 and radiographically in Fig. 11-14, *B* through *D*. In summary, treatment of DHS requires a thorough medical workup and treatment of reversible causes before surgical intervention is contemplated. Once the decision is made to intervene surgically, successful clinical outcomes can be achieved by adhering to core principles of surgical spine treatment, specifically, decompression of neural elements (if necessary), stabilization and promotion of long-term fusion, and correction of deformity.

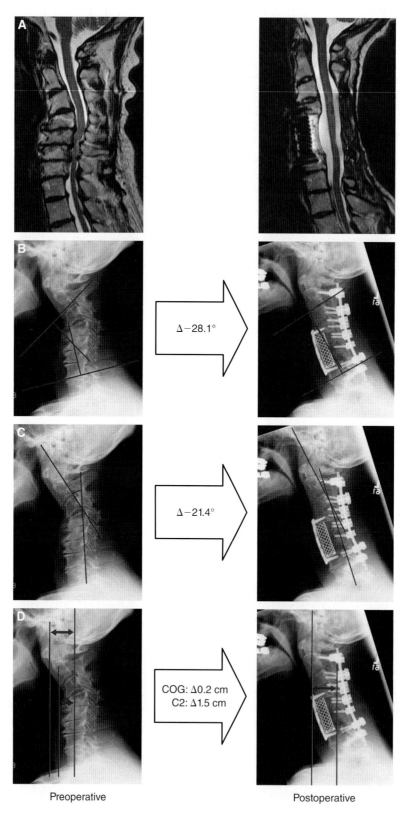

Preoperative   Postoperative

Fig. 11-14   Preoperative and postoperative images of a patient with a fixed kyphotic deformity. **A,** T2-weighted MRI showed severe cervical stenosis with kyphotic deformity preoperatively *(left)*. The patient is seen after a combined anterior-posterior correction *(right)*. **B,** Cervical kyphosis is corrected by –28.1 degrees, as measured by the C2-7 Cobb angle method. **C,** Cervical kyphosis is corrected by –21.4 degrees, as measured by the Jackson angle method. **D,** Postoperative changes in the COG-C7 and C2-7 SVA parameters are minimal.

Table 11-5 Fixed Deformity Case: Preoperative, Postoperative, and Normal Values

	Preoperative Value	Postoperative Value	Normal Value
C2-7 Cobb angle (degrees)	31.2	3.1	−9.6[17]
Jackson angle (degrees)	31.4	10.0	−23[19]
COG-C7 SVA (cm)	3.0	3.2	NA
C2-7 SVA (cm)	1.7	3.2	1.6[17]

COG, Center of gravity; *NA*, not applicable; *SVA*, sagittal vertical axis.

CONCLUSION

Postoperative cervical spine alignment has long been presumed to be a clinical indicator of surgical outcomes. Many cervical parameters are available to quantify the degree of cervical curvature; however, a correlation of these parameters with clinical outcomes is lacking. Recently, evidence has increased to support a possible correlation of sagittal translation with clinical outcomes after surgery. The correlation of cervical parameters with thoracic and lumbar parameters is also becoming an increasingly important concept in surgical planning. These correlations reflect the importance of determining the primary cause of spinal deformity pathology before committing a patient to a regional fusion.

Surgery remains the mainstay of treatment in patients who have failed conservative management. The many techniques available in the cervical spine have advantages and disadvantages with respect to sagittal correction and spinal decompression, but the overall surgical goals are the same. The case illustration in this chapter highlights the importance of a thorough understanding and investigation of the primary cause of spinal deformity before surgical intervention. In addition, it reinforces the necessity of individualized clinical decision-making for cervical deformity and myelopathy. Finally, continued research is necessary to further delineate the contribution of cervical malalignment to disease progression and surgical outcomes in cervical spine disease.

REFERENCES

1. Dubousset J. Three-dimensional analysis of the scoliotic deformity. In Weinstein SL, ed. The Pediatric Spine: Principles and Practice. New York: Raven Press, 1994.
2. Young WF. Cervical spondylotic myelopathy: a common cause of spinal cord dysfunction in older persons. Am Fam Physician 62:1064-1070, 2000.
3. Fehlings MG, Skaf G. A review of the pathophysiology of cervical spondylotic myelopathy with insights for potential novel mechanisms drawn from traumatic spinal cord injury. Spine 23:2730-2737, 1998.
4. Fehlings MG, Wilson JR, Kopjar B, et al. Efficacy and safety of surgical decompression in patients with cervical spondylotic myelopathy: results of the AOSpine North America prospective multi-center study. J Bone Joint Surg Am 95:1651-1658, 2013.
5. Shamji MF, Ames CP, Smith JS, et al. Myelopathy and spinal deformity: relevance of spinal alignment in planning surgical intervention for degenerative cervical myelopathy. Spine 38(22 Suppl 1):S147-S148, 2013.
6. Ames CP, Blondel B, Scheer JK, et al. Cervical radiographical alignment: comprehensive assessment techniques and potential importance in cervical myelopathy. Spine 38(22 Suppl 1):S149-S160, 2013.
7. Lee SH, Kim KT, Seo EM, et al. The influence of thoracic inlet alignment on the craniocervical sagittal balance in asymptomatic adults. J Spinal Disord Tech 25:E41-E47, 2012.
8. Ferch RD, Shad A, Cadoux-Hudson TA, et al. Anterior correction of cervical kyphotic deformity: effects on myelopathy, neck pain, and sagittal alignment. J Neurosurg 100(1 Suppl Spine):S13-S19, 2004.

9. Gum JL, Glassman SD, Douglas LR, et al. Correlation between cervical spine sagittal alignment and clinical outcome after anterior cervical discectomy and fusion. Am J Orthop 41:E81-E84, 2012.

10. Cobb JR. Outline for the study of scoliosis. In The American Academy of Orthopedic Surgeons Instructional Course Lectures, vol 5. Ann Arbor, MI: JW Edwards, 1948.

11. Polly DW Jr, Kilkelly FX, McHale KA, et al. Measurement of lumbar lordosis. Evaluation of intraobserver, interobserver, and technique variability. Spine 21:1530-1535; discussion 1535-1536, 1996.

12. Jackson R, ed. The Cervical Syndrome. Springfield, IL: Charles C. Thomas, 1957.

13. Harrison DD, Cailliet R, Janik TJ, et al. Elliptical modeling of the sagittal lumbar lordosis and segmental rotation angles as a method to discriminate between normal and low back pain subjects. J Spinal Disord 11:430-439, 1998.

14. Harrison DE, Harrison DD, Cailliet R, et al. Cobb method or Harrison posterior tangent method: which to choose for lateral cervical radiographic analysis. Spine 25:2072-2078, 2000.

15. Vital JM, Senegas J. Anatomical bases of the study of the constraints to which the cervical spine is subject in the sagittal plane. A study of the center of gravity of the head. Surg Radiol Anat 8:169-173, 1986.

16. Suk KS, Kim KT, Lee SH, et al. Significance of chin-brow vertical angle in correction of kyphotic deformity of ankylosing spondylitis patients. Spine 28:2001-2005, 2003.

17. Hardacker JW, Shuford RF, Capicotto PN, et al. Radiographic standing cervical segmental alignment in adult volunteers without neck symptoms. Spine 22:1472-1479, 1997.

18. Yukawa Y, Kato F, Suda K, et al. Age-related changes in osseous anatomy, alignment, and range of motion of the cervical spine. Part I: Radiographic data from over 1,200 asymptomatic subjects. Eur Spine J 21:1492-1498, 2012.

19. Gore D, Sepic SB, Gardner GM. Roentgenographic findings of the cervical spine in asymptomatic people. Spine 11:521-524, 1986.

20. Park MS, Moon SH, Lee HM, et al. The effect of age on cervical sagittal alignment: normative data on 100 asymptomatic subjects. Spine 38:E458-E463, 2013.

21. Smith JS, Shaffrey CI, Lafage V, et al; International Spine Study Group. Spontaneous improvement of cervical alignment after correction of global sagittal balance following pedicle subtraction osteotomy. J Neurosurg Spine 17:300-307, 2012

22. Jenkins LA, Capen DA, Zigler JE, et al. Cervical spine fusions for trauma. A long-term radiographic and clinical evaluation. Orthop Rev Suppl:13-19, 1994.

23. Kawakami M, Tamaki T, Yoshida M, et al. Axial symptoms and cervical alignments after cervical anterior spinal fusion for patients with cervical myelopathy. J Spinal Disord 12:50-56, 1999.

24. Uchida K, Nakajima H, Sato R, et al. Cervical spondylotic myelopathy associated with kyphosis or sagittal sigmoid alignment: outcome after anterior or posterior decompression. J Neurosurg Spine 11:521-528, 2009.

25. Tang JA, Scheer JK, Smith JS, et al; ISSG. The impact of standing regional cervical sagittal alignment on outcomes in posterior cervical fusion surgery. Neurosurgery 71:662-669, 2012.

26. Breig A, El-Nadi AF. Biomechanics of the cervical spinal cord: Relief of contact pressure on and overstretching of the spinal cord. Acta Radiol Diagn 4:602-624, 1966.

27. Kurokawa R, Murata H, Ogino M, et al. Altered blood flow distribution in the rat spinal cord under chronic compression. Spine 36:1006-1009, 2011.

28. Baron EM, Young WF. Cervical spondylotic myelopathy: a brief review of its pathophysiology, clinical course, and diagnosis. Neurosurgery 60(1 Suppl 1):S35-S41, 2007.

29. Morishita Y, Naito M, Hymanson H, et al. The relationship between the cervical spinal canal diameter and the pathological changes in the cervical spine. Eur Spine J 18:877-883, 2009.

30. Karadimas SK, Klironomos G, Papachristou DJ, et al. Immunohistochemical profile of NF-κB/p50, NF-κB/p65, MMP-9, MMP-2, and u-PA in experimental cervical spondylotic myelopathy. Spine 38:4-10, 2013.

31. Donnelly DJ, Longbrake EE, Shawler TM, et al. Deficient CX3CR1 signaling promotes recovery after mouse spinal cord injury by limiting the recruitment and activation of Ly6Clo/iNOS+ macrophages. J Neurosci 31:9910-9922, 2011.

32. Arundine M, Aarts M, Lau A, et al. Vulnerability of central neurons to secondary insults after in vitro mechanical stretch. J Neurosci 24:8106-8123, 2004.

33. Karadimas SK, Moon ES, Yu WR, et al. A novel experimental model of cervical spondylotic myelopathy (CSM) to facilitate translational research. Neurobiol Dis 54:43-45, 2013.

34. Wu Y, Satkunendrarajah K, Teng Y. Delayed post-injury administration of rilazole as neuroprotective in a preclinical rodent model of cervical spinal cord injury. J Neurotrauma 30:441-452, 2013.

35. Fehlings MG, Wilson JR, Karadimas SK, et al. Clinical evaluation of a neuroprotective drug in patients with cervical spondylotic myelopathy undergoing surgical treatment: design and rationale for the CSM-Protect trial. Spine 38(22 Suppl 1):S68-S75, 2013.

36. Masini M, Maranhão V. Experimental determination of the effect of progressive sharp-angle spinal deformity on the spinal cord. Eur Spine J 6:89-92, 1997.

37. Shimizu K, Nakamura M, Nishikawa Y, et al. Spinal kyphosis causes demyelination and neuronal loss in the spinal cord: a new model of kyphotic deformity using juvenile Japanese small game fowls. Spine 30:2388-2392, 2005.

38. Chavanne A, Pettigrew DB, Holtz JR, et al. Spinal cord intramedullary pressure in cervical kyphotic deformity: a cadaveric study. Spine 36:1619-1626, 2011.

39. Muhle C, Wiskirechen J, Weinert D, et al. Biomechanical aspects of the subarachnoid space and cervical cord in healthy individuals examined with kinematic resonance imaging. Spine 23:556-567, 1998.

40. Muhle C, Weinert D, Falliner A, et al. Dynamic changes of the spinal canal in patients with cervical spondylosis at flexion and extension using magnetic resonance imaging. Invest Radiol 33:444-449, 1998.

41. Zhang L, Zeitoun D, Rangel A, et al. Preoperative evaluation of the cervical spondylotic myelopathy with flexion-extension magnetic resonance imaging: about a prospective study of fifty patients. Spine 36:E1134-E1139, 2011.

42. Owen JH, Naito M, Bridwell KH. Relationship among level of distraction, evoked potentials, spinal cord ischemia and integrity, and clinical status in animals. Spine 15:852-857, 1990.

43. Steinmetz MP, Stewart TJ, Kager CD, et al. Cervical deformity correction. Neurosurgery 60(1 Suppl 1):S90-S97, 2007.

44. Traynelis VC, Arnold PM, Fourney DR, et al. Alternative procedures for the treatment of cervical spondylotic myelopathy: arthroplasty, oblique corpectomy, skip laminectomy: evaluation of comparative effectiveness and safety. Spine 38(22 Suppl 1):S210-S231, 2013.

45. Smith GW, Robinson RA. The treatment of certain cervical-spine disorders by anterior removal of the intervertebral disc and interbody fusion. J Bone Joint Surg Am 40:607-624, 1958.

46. Xie JC, Hurlbert RJ. Discectomy versus discectomy with fusion versus discectomy with fusion and instrumentation: a prospective randomized study. Neurosurgery 61:107-116, 2007.

47. Shamji MF, Massicotte EM, Traynelis VC, et al. Comparison of anterior surgical options for the treatment of multilevel cervical spondylotic myelopathy: a systematic review. Spine 38(22 Suppl 1):S195-S209, 2013.

48. Sim FH, Svien HJ, Bickel WH, et al. Swan-neck deformity following extensive cervical laminectomy. A review of twenty-one cases. J Bone Joint Surg Am 56:564-580, 1974.

49. Kaptain GJ, Simmons NE, Replogle RE, et al. Incidence and outcome of kyphotic deformity following laminectomy for cervical spondylotic myelopathy. J Neurosurg 93(2 Suppl):S199-S204, 2000.

50. Roy-Camille R, Saillant G. [Surgery of the cervical spine. 4. Osteosynthesis of the upper cervical spine] Nouv Presse Med 1:2847-2849, 1972.

51. Jeanneret B, Magerl F, Ward EH, et al. Posterior stabilization of the cervical spine with hook plates. Spine 16(3 Suppl):S56-S63, 1991.

52. Stemper BD, Marawar SV, Yoganandan N, et al. Quantitative anatomy of subaxial cervical lateral mass: an analysis of safe screw lengths for Roy-Camille and Magerl techniques. Spine 33:893-897, 2008.

53. Lee DG, Lee SH, Park SJ, et al. Comparison of surgical outcomes after cervical laminoplasty: open-door technique versus French-door technique. J Spinal Disord Tech 26:E198-E203, 2013.

54. Wang MY, Green BA. Open-door cervical expansile laminoplasty. Neurosurgery 54:119-123, 2004.

55. Suda K, Abumi K, Ito M, et al. Local kyphosis reduces surgical outcomes of expansive open-door laminoplasty for cervical spondylotic myelopathy. Spine 28:1258-1262, 2003.

56. Deviren V, Scheer JK, Ames CP. Technique of cervicothoracic junction pedicle subtraction osteotomy for cervical sagittal imbalance: report of 11 cases. J Neurosurg Spine 15:174-181, 2011.

57. Komotar RJ, Mocco J, Kaiser MG. Surgical management of cervical myelopathy: indications and techniques for laminectomy and fusion. Spine J 6(6 Suppl):252S-267S, 2006.

58. Fehlings MG, Smith JS, Kopjar B, et al. Perioperative and delayed complications associated with the surgical treatment of cervical spondylotic myelopathy based on 302 patients from the AOSpine North America Cervical Spondylotic Myelopathy Study. J Neurosurg Spine 16:425-432, 2012.

59. Lawrence BD, Jacobs WB, Norvell DC, et al. Anterior versus posterior approach for treatment of cervical spondylotic myelopathy: a systematic review. Spine 38(22 Suppl 1):S173-S182, 2013.

60. Lawrence BD, Shamji MF, Traynelis VC, et al. Surgical management of degenerative cervical myelopathy: a consensus statement. Spine 38(22 Suppl 1):S171-S172, 2013.

61. Fehlings MG, Kopjar B, Massicotte E, et al. Surgical treatment for cervical spondylotic myelopathy: one year outcomes of a prospective multicenter study of 316 patients. Spine J 8(Suppl):S33-S34, 2008.

62. Heary RF, Choudhry OJ, Jalan D, et al. Analysis of cervical sagittal alignment after screw-rod fixation. Neurosurgery 72:983-991, 2013.

63. Cabraja M, Abbushi A, Koeppen D, et al. Comparison between anterior and posterior decompression with instrumentation for cervical spondylotic myelopathy: sagittal alignment and clinical outcome. Neurosurg Focus 28:E15, 2010.

64. Machino M, Yukawa Y, Hida T, et al. Cervical alignment and range of motion after laminoplasty: radiographical data from more than 500 cases with cervical spondylotic myelopathy and a review of the literature. Spine 37:E1243-E1250, 2012.

65. Hilibrand AS, Yoo JU, Carlson GD, et al. The success of anterior cervical arthrodesis adjacent to a previous fusion. Spine 22:1574-1579, 1997.

66. Hussain M, Nassr A, Natarajan RN, et al. Biomechanics of adjacent segments after a multilevel cervical corpectomy using anterior, posterior, and combined anterior-posterior instrumentation techniques: a finite element model study. Spine J 13:689-696, 2013.

67. Lawrence BD, Hilibrand AS, Brodt ED, et al. Predicting the risk of adjacent segment pathology in the cervical spine: a systematic review. Spine 37(22 Suppl):S52-S64, 2012.

68. Kraemer P, Fehlings MG, Hashimoto R, et al. A systematic review of definitions and classification systems of adjacent segment pathology. Spine 37(22 Suppl):S31-S39, 2012.

69. Park DH, Ramakrishnan P, Cho TH, et al. Effect of lower two-level anterior cervical fusion on the superior adjacent level. J Neurosurg Spine 7:336-340, 2007.

70. Ishihara H, Kanamori M, Kawaguchi Y, et al. Adjacent segment disease after anterior cervical interbody fusion. Spine J 4:624-628, 2004.

71. Katsuura A, Hukuda S, Saruhashi Y, et al. Kyphotic malalignment after anterior cervical fusion is one of the factors promoting the degenerative process in adjacent intervertebral levels. Eur Spine J 10:320-324, 2001.

72. Hansen MA, Kim HJ, Van Alstyne EM, et al. Does postsurgical cervical deformity affect the risk of cervical adjacent segment pathology? A systematic review. Spine 37(22 Suppl):S75-S84, 2012.

73. Jagannathan J, Shaffrey CI, Oskouian RJ, et al. Radiographic and clinical outcomes following single-level anterior cervical discectomy and allograft fusion without plate placement or cervical collar. J Neurosurg Spine 8:420-428, 2008.

74. Naderi S, Ozgen S, Pamir MN, et al. Cervical spondylotic myelopathy: surgical results and factors affecting prognosis. Neurosurgery 43:43-49, 1998.

75. Villavicencio AT, Babuska JM, Ashton A, et al. Prospective, randomized, double-blind clinical study evaluating the correlation of clinical outcomes and cervical sagittal alignment. Neurosurgery 68:1309-1316, 2011.

76. Liu T, Yang HL, Xu YZ, et al. ACDF with the PCB cage-plate system versus laminoplasty for multilevel cervical spondylotic myelopathy. J Spinal Disord Tech 24:213-220, 2011.

77. Martin AR, Rajesh R, Fehlings MG. Dropped head syndrome: diagnosis and management. Evid Based Spine Care J 2:41-47, 2011.

78. Gourie-Devi M, Nalini A, Sandhya S. Early or late appearance of "dropped head syndrome" in amyotrophic lateral sclerosis. J Neurol Neurosurg Psychiatry 2:683-686, 2003.

79. Petheram TG, Hourigan PG, Emran IM, et al. Dropped head syndrome: a case series and literature review. Spine 33:47-51, 2008.

80. Simmons EH, Bradley DD. Neuro-myopathic flexion deformities of the cervical spine. Spine 2:756-762, 1988.

81. Gerling MC, Bohlman HH. Dropped head deformity due to cervical myopathy: surgical treatment outcomes and complications spanning twenty years. Spine 33:E739-E745, 2008.

82. Amin A, Casey AT, Etherington G. Is there a role for surgery in the management of dropped head syndrome? Br J Neurosurg 18:289-293, 2004.

83. Kawaguchi A, Miyamoto K, Sakaguchi Y, et al. Dropped head syndrome associated with cervical spondylotic myelopathy. J Spinal Disord Tech 17:531-534, 2004.

12

Thoracolumbar Region

Megan M. Jack ▪ *Kyle A. Smith* ▪ *Elizabeth A. Friis*
Erin M. Mannen ▪ *Paul M. Arnold*

Spinal deformity is a group of complex disorders relating to regional abnormalities of spinal imbalance and overall global alignment of the spine. The spectrum of disease includes spinal deformities with coronal, sagittal, and rotational imbalance.[1-3] The broad range of disorders that encompass spinal deformity includes adult and pediatric idiopathic scoliosis, degenerative scoliosis, posttraumatic injury, iatrogenic deformity, and postinfectious complications.[1,4,5] Despite the diversity of the disorders, each involves abnormal physiologic spinal misalignment that can cause cosmetic deformity, pain, neurologic deficits, and functional disability.[1] Traditionally, deformity correction has focused on prevention of curve progression.[6-8] Recently, our knowledge has expanded to understanding the role of global spinal alignment and sagittal plane deformity in spinal deformity correction. Proper spinal alignment is critical for successful surgical outcomes, patient satisfaction, and overall clinical and functional improvement of patients.[9-11]

The intricate nature of normal spinal curvatures produces even more complex pathology. Surgeons need to understand normal regional and global spinal alignment to grasp the complexity of spinal deformity. Each segment of the vertebral column contributes to the overall global alignment. It is important to understand not only the regional alignment of each spinal segment but also how each region contributes to and affects overall spinal stability and function.[12-13]

The thoracolumbar junction is a key transitional zone between the kyphotic thoracic spine and the lordotic, mobile lumbar spine.[3] This region has its own distinct alignment and biomechanical properties. Sagittal alignment in the thoracolumbar region is generally measured from the cranial endplate of T10 to the caudal endplate of L2.[14,15] This area is typically neutral to slightly lordotic.[3] The thoracic segment above the thoracolumbar region is kyphotic and fairly rigid because of the articulation with the rib cage. On the other hand, the lumbar segment is lordotic and highly flexible. Given the nature of the transition zone and resulting stress concentrations, this area is at high risk for injury and other pathology that often leads to deformity.[16]

EVOLUTION OF TECHNIQUE

Spinal deformity was one of the earliest conditions recognized and recorded to afflict humans. Bracing, casting, and early versions of spinal traction were the primary means for treating disorders of the spine.[7] The surgical treatment of thoracolumbar deformity was first developed shortly after the discovery of X-rays in the early 1900s. Russell Hibbs[7] performed the first fusion in 1911. This event revolutionized spinal deformity surgery by showing that the surgical procedure was safe, and fusion procedures could halt curve progression; however, postoperative management required lengthy periods of bracing and casting to achieve solid arthrodesis and successful outcomes.[7,8] The Harrington rod system, developed in 1953, was used to successfully stabilize pathologic scoliotic spinal curvature and other disorders, but was fraught with many complications, including hardware failure and postoperative sagittal imbalance.[7,17] In 1959 Cotrel and Dubousset[8] advanced the technique with the introduction of the transpedicular approach, which maximized fixation and correction of coronal and sagittal deformities. The universal pedicle screw system was introduced in 1991 and allowed surgical correction in the sagittal and coronal planes and shorter segment fusions than prior techniques.[8] Pedicle screw development has been carried even further to fixed and variable-axis screws for a broader repertoire of instrumentation. Over the last three decades, many new and improved approaches and techniques have been developed, including combined anteroposterior fusions, osteotomy procedures, and minimally invasive approaches for correction of thoracolumbar deformity.[18]

ADVANTAGES AND DISADVANTAGES

Sagittal imbalance, coronal deformity, and global alignment are now recognized as factors contributing to pain generation, neurologic deficits, and functional decline of patients. Thoracolumbar deformity can prevent proper spinal alignment. Abnormal alignment prevents proper posture for normal sitting, lying flat, or standing via flexion of hip and knee joints.[16] Hence surgical correction is performed in an attempt to modify these spinal parameters. The goals of spinal deformity surgery include correction of sagittal and coronal balance, spinal stabilization, improved cosmesis, relief of pain, and restoration of function. However, surgical correction is not without risks. Often, corrective surgery can have long operative times with the risk of significant perioperative morbidity and mortality. Therefore proper patient selection is crucial, including definitive indications and contraindications, operative technique, postoperative complication risks, and management of thoracolumbar correction with the overall goal of normalizing global spinal alignment.

INDICATIONS AND CONTRAINDICATIONS

The goals of surgical treatment differ depending on the population and pathology of the spinal deformity. Pain is a common complaint of patients with spinal curvature and is a common indication for corrective surgery.[7] Patients who fail conservative management and continue to have pain and/or neurologic deficits are appropriate candidates for surgical intervention. Cosmetic concerns about spinal curves may be an indication for surgery; however, the risks of surgery must be weighed carefully in these patients if this is the only indication. Patients need to understand the indications and goals of surgery before a procedure.[4] The ultimate goal of spinal deformity surgery is to provide successful arthrodesis with adequate regional imbalance repair and global spinal alignment correction in all three dimensions.[19] This requires evaluating and selecting patients who are appropriate for reconstructive surgical correction and determining patients who are not appropriate for surgical intervention.[20] Patients with multiple comorbidities who are not good surgical candidates or are at high risk for morbidity and mortality should not undergo surgical correction of thoracolumbar deformity. In particular, severe osteopenia or osteoporosis can impede proper fusion of spinal instrumentation and grafts, leading to complications and often the need for revision surgery; thus patients with underlying bone disorders may not be appropriate for reconstructive surgery requiring instrumentation. Similarly, patients who smoke are at high risk for pseudarthrosis and should be advised to refrain from smoking for at least 6 weeks before surgery. Obesity is another challenging consideration. Nutritional status is important particularly regarding postoperative complications, because poor nutrition can result in poor wound healing and pseudarthrosis.

PATIENT PROFILE

This 38-year-old woman had a past medical history of idiopathic scoliosis, irritable bowel syndrome, obesity with previous lap band surgery, and hypertension. She presented with long-standing back and right radicular pain that began 9 months ago. Past treatments included physical therapy, pain management,

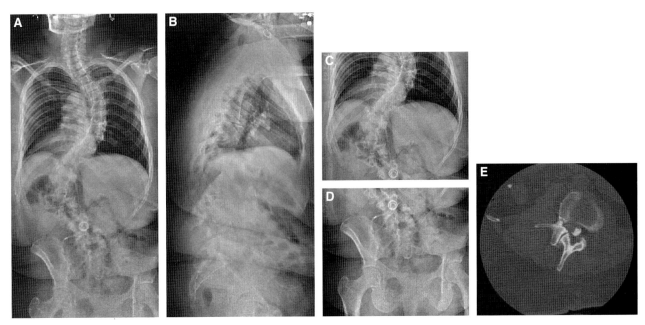

Fig. 12-1   **A** and **B,** Upright and lateral scoliosis radiographs. **C** and **D,** Thoracic and lumbar regional films. Preoperatively the patient had a 76-degree left-sided thoracolumbar curve and a 66-degree right-sided curvature of her thoracic spine with gibbus deformity at the thoracolumbar junction. **E,** A CT-myelogram of the lumbar spine showed spinal stenosis within the right L2-3 lateral recess.

epidural steroid injections, and unsuccessful placement of a spinal cord stimulator. None provided good relief. The patient was on Social Security disability because of her back pain. Physical examination revealed a forward-flexed posture with good strength in all extremities. Radiography demonstrated a 76-degree left convexity curvature of the lumbar spine and a 66-degree right convexity curvature of the thoracic spine with gibbus deformity at the thoracolumbar junction. The patient had positive sagittal balance of 61 mm. A CT-myelogram showed left lateral subluxation of L2 on L3 with right lateral recess stenosis at L2-3 (Fig. 12-1). Because she had significant disability related to clinically symptomatic deformity and had failed conservative treatments, surgical correction was an appropriate option.

PREOPERATIVE PLANNING AND EVALUATION OF SPINAL ALIGNMENT

A detailed clinical history is essential to establish the nature, severity, and clinical progression of deficits. Symptoms of bowel/bladder incontinence, discrete lower extremity weakness, gait disturbances, and altered sensation can affect patients with thoracolumbar spinal deformity. Adult patients with spinal deformity often present for surgical consultation with symptoms of pain, radiculopathy, and functional disability, whereas pediatric patients typically present because of cosmetic concerns.[14] For older patients the description of the pain, including intensity, quality, location, and aggravating and alleviating factors, will help to determine whether thoracolumbar curves are symptomatic and might require surgical treatment. It is also important to understand the course of curve progression. This can manifest as a change in height, or the patient may notice that clothes fit abnormally. Similarly, the previous course and success of nonoperative treatment are investigated. Beyond the focus of spinal curves, general medical health should be assessed to determine whether a patient is fit enough to undergo spinal deformity surgery.[19] Adequate workup with both cardiac and pulmonary clearance is necessary if clinically indicated. It is also important to document previous surgical history that may have contributed to or can complicate future deformity surgery.

PHYSICAL EXAMINATION

Physical examination should focus on neurologic function. A comprehensive neurologic examination should be conducted with key emphasis on motor and sensory modalities, reflexes, long tract signs, evidence of myelopathy, and gait. Patients should be asked their functional status at baseline and whether any changes have occurred recently that are attributable to spinal deformity. The necessity of using walking aids is discussed, because these can indicate progressive function loss. Key aspects of the spinal deformity, especially spinal alignment, should be assessed. Patients should be examined while standing, sitting, and lying down, with particular attention to overall spinal balance.[14] Flexibility of the curve is evaluated on flexion, extension, and lateral bending.[1] Similar to radiographic assessment, examination of standing posture is helpful for appreciating coronal and sagittal curves, though some smaller curves may not be appreciated on visual assessment. Although the thoracolumbar junction is relatively neutral on the sagittal plane, kyphotic deformity or positive sagittal malformation can cause a patient to pitch forward.[14] These patients may attempt to flex their knees and extend their hips to manually improve overall sagittal balance.[10] In the coronal plane, the iliac crests and unilateral rib cage prominence can indicate thoracolumbar malalignment.

RADIOGRAPHIC WORKUP AND PREOPERATIVE IMAGING

Initial radiographic assessment of thoracolumbar deformity begins with upright and recumbent frontal and lateral 36-inch radiographs (Fig. 12-2). Radiographs should include C7 proximally and bilateral femoral heads distally to allow accurate measurements of global and regional balance and alignment. Patient positioning should be standardized and facilitate clear visualization of all spinal levels within the thoracolumbar region and adjacent segments. Standing radiographs are essential to determine the degree of deformity.[1] Curves will be most severe on weight-bearing radiographs. The hips and knees need to be fully extended for accurate assessment of spinal alignment.[7] A comparison of weight-bearing to supine radiographs provides information about the flexibility of the spinal deformity. For instance, lateral bending radiographs or flexion-extension radiographs may be required to evaluate coronal and kyphotic deformities. Standard radiographs are of key importance, as they provide more detail to interpret regional alignment.

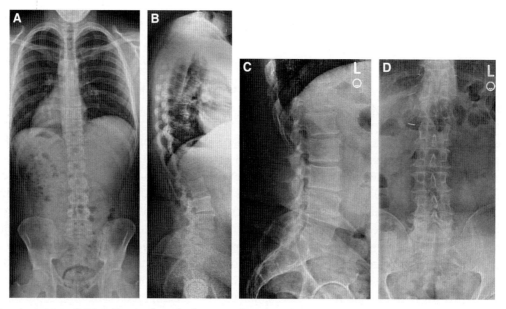

Fig. 12-2   **A,** A 36-inch PA radiograph with clear visualization of C7 to the pelvis is used to evaluate coronal alignment of the entire spine. **B,** Lateral spine radiographs demonstrate the normal spinal curvature and are used to assess sagittal balance. **C** and **D,** Dedicated lumbar plain radiographs are necessary to evaluate coronal and sagittal regional alignment of the thoracolumbar junction.

Standard radiographs are viewed under several conventions for normalization of findings across different examiners. Frontal radiographs are viewed from posterior to anterior so that the patient's left side is on the left of the radiograph; sagittal radiographs are obtained with the patient facing right (see Fig. 12-2). Displacements of curvature are defined in direction. Frontal radiographs define curves by the direction of the apex. Angular displacement is described by clockwise and counterclockwise or rightward and leftward displacement, respectively. Linear displacement such as sagittal imbalance is described in the directional terms of *positive* or *negative*. For example, positive or rightward displacement notes sagittal imbalance that shifts the C7 plumb line (C7PL) anterior to the sacrum on conventional rightward-facing radiographs. Vertebral rotation can be visualized on frontal radiographs, because the relationship of the pedicles to the lateral vertebral body can be assessed.[15]

Coronal Alignment

The regional location, alignment, and imbalance of the spinal curvature should be determined in the coronal plane using standing radiographs. The *apex* of the curve is defined as the maximally displaced and minimally angulated vertebra in the coronal plane. For thoracolumbar deformities, the apex of the curve is located between T10 and L2. The displacement of the apical vertebra or apical vertebral translation (AVT) in the thoracolumbar region is measured from the central sacral vertical line (CSVL), which is a vertical reference line drawn through the midpoint of the S1 endplate (Fig. 12-3). *AVT* is defined as the horizontal distance of the vertebral apex from the CSVL. Overall coronal balance is determined by the C7PL in reference to the CSVL. These lines are calculated from the left edge of the radiograph, and the difference is obtained for coronal alignment. Positive values define overall displacement to the right, whereas negative values correspond to leftward displacement.

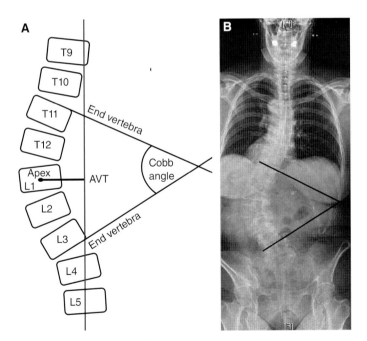

Fig. 12-3 **A,** The Cobb angle is used to measure the degree of coronal deformity. The end vertebrae are the last vertebral bodies to be tilted into the curve, whereas the apex is typically the most neutral body in the curve. Lines are drawn from the proximal endplate of the superior end vertebra and the distal endplate of the most inferior vertebral body to determine the angle. **B,** A PA scoliosis radiograph demonstrates a coronal thoracolumbar deformity with the Cobb angle denoted by *black lines*. (*AVT,* Apical vertebral translation.)

Coronal spinal balance is measured by determining the angular degree of the curve. The Cobb angle is used to measure the deformity angle in the coronal plane (see Fig. 12-3). The *end vertebrae* are defined as the maximally angled vertebrae in the curve and are often the most minimally rotated vertebrae in the coronal plane. In this technique, the proximal endplate of the cephalad vertebra and the distal endplate of the caudal vertebra are used to determine the angle of the curve (see Fig. 12-3). *Scoliosis* is defined as curvatures of the spine that are greater than 10 degrees in the coronal plane.

Sagittal Alignment

Kyphotic and lordotic curves are defined in the sagittal plane. Overall sagittal alignment is determined by the C7PL on lateral radiographs. The position of the C7PL in reference to the posterosuperior corner of the sacrum accounts for sagittal balance (Fig. 12-4). These points are calculated from the left edge of the radiograph, and the difference is obtained for sagittal alignment. Conventionally, positive sagittal balance is defined by positive values, and negative sagittal balance is defined by negative values. Sagittal alignment of the thoracolumbar region is either neutral or slightly lordotic[3] (see Fig. 12-4, *B* and *C*). Sagittal balance should be evaluated preoperatively. Furthermore, establishing the flexibility of the imbalance provides guidance on the possible degree of correction.[21] Flexible deformities can be corrected with instrumented fusions in proper position, and inflexible deformities can require ancillary maneuvers such as an osteotomy.[21]

First-line management is nonsurgical. Although the efficacy of nonsurgical management is not well established, it should be offered to all patients.[22,23] Options include physical therapy, aerobic exercise, core strengthening, and nonsteroidal antiinflammatory drugs. Bracing is controversial, because it is ineffective in preventing spinal curve progression in adults.[1] Injection therapy such as epidural steroids often provide symptomatic improvement. However, nonoperative management has less successful patient outcomes in Oswestry Disability Index (ODI) and Numeric Rating Scale scores compared with surgical treatment.[1,23]

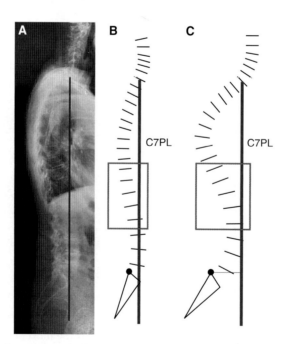

Fig. 12-4   **A,** A lateral plain radiograph with the red C7 plumb line *(C7PL)* shows appropriate sagittal alignment. **B,** Normal global sagittal alignment and neutral thoracolumbar alignment are denoted by the *box*. **C,** This spinal column shows overall positive sagittal balance, particularly in the thoracolumbar region. The *box* demonstrates the degree of imbalance.

OPERATIVE TECHNIQUE

PATIENT POSITIONING

Patient positioning is a crucial portion of spinal procedures and is determined by the surgical approach selected. Regardless of position, all bony prominences should be padded, and eyes should be protected. Sequential compression devices should be placed for adequate circulation and prevention of deep venous thrombosis. Antibiotics are given per normal routine within 1 hour of incision. Neuromonitoring is performed at the discretion of the operating surgeon. Monitoring is potentially of benefit when spinal implants are placed or the spinal column is lengthened.[24,25] No Class I evidence exists for the use of neurophysiologic monitoring in deformity surgery.[8] Neuromonitoring is, however, becoming commonplace in many operative facilities for these procedures. Care is needed to prevent limb compression injuries or nerve stretch injuries, as previously described. Posterior approaches generally involve prone positioning for access to the midline.[26] Hips should be relatively extended to ensure lumbar lordosis. Lumbar kyphosis can be predisposed in surgery by flexion at the hips.

INCISION PLACEMENT

Incision placement routinely involves a midline craniocaudal incision for dissection of bony anatomy and adequate lateral exposure to either side of the spine. Localization with intraoperative lateral radiograph or radiographs for confirmation of surgical level minimizes error and can result in less intraoperative blood loss, surgical incisional pain, and tissue healing burden. Anterior approaches generally involve positioning in the supine or lateral decubitus position. Flexion of the hips can improve access to the anterolateral lumbar spine via relaxation of the iliopsoas muscles.[27,28]

Operative management involves restoration of spinal alignment and balance. In cases of failed nonsurgical management or patients with clear indications for surgery, surgical options should be explored. Surgery should encompass curve correction for restoration of spinal alignment and balance.[29,30] Surgical techniques within the thoracolumbar spine are quite varied and are approached anteriorly, posteriorly, or both. Posterior-only approaches are generally sufficient for younger adult patients with flexible curves or in cases of balanced spinal curves.[27] Anterior approaches are rarely indicated alone. Anterior-only curves can lead to kyphosis or loss of sagittal balance or lordosis.[27,31] A combined anterior-posterior approach is useful in cases of rigid curves and is common in cases of adult spinal deformity. This combination provides the benefits of anterior procedures, which include anterior release of the spine with correction and fusion from a posterior procedure. In recent years, minimally invasive techniques have been used for deformity correction.[32-37]

Decompression is an option for claudication or radiculopathy in cases of small degenerative malalignment without instability. Complications have been reported to be lower with decompression alone versus decompression with fusion.[1] However, in one study, patient outcomes were higher in decompression with fusion rather than in decompression alone.[1]

An anterior approach is an option either alone or in combination with a posterior approach. The classic anterior approach in general is anterior lumbar interbody fusion (ALIF) with anterior instrumentation. In selected patients, an anterior approach with spine fusion provides good patient results and deformity correction.[1] An anterior approach allows direct visualization of the entire intervertebral disc space and insertion of disc spacers to induce fusion and correct spinal alignment. These structural grafts or cages maintain distraction between endplates, stimulate bony fusion, and help to restore lordosis.[7] Anterior approaches and these structural implants should be considered in lower thoracic and lumbar regions.[7] Benefits of anterior approaches include good deformity correction, patient satisfaction, and enhanced fusion.[7] Potential disadvantages include incisional dissatisfaction or pain, vascular damage, abdominal hernia, graft displacement, ureteral damage, and retrograde ejaculation.[1]

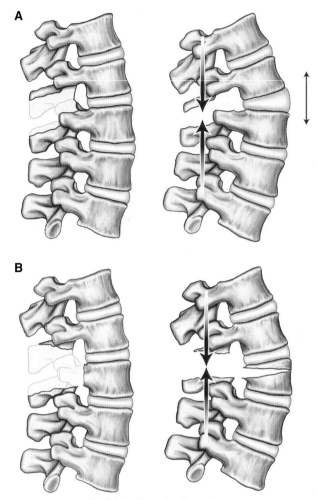

Pedicle-Subtraction Osteotomy

Fig. 12-5   Smith-Petersen and pedicle subtraction osteotomies. **A,** A Smith-Petersen osteotomy is used to correct kyphotic deformity by releasing posterior spinal articulations. **B,** A pedicle subtraction osteotomy involves removal of the posterior elements, pedicle, and a portion of the vertebral body to restore normal lumbar lordosis.

The workhorse of spinal deformity surgery has been the posterior approach. Posterior surgery generally involves posterior instrumentation with optional use of transforaminal or posterior lumbar interbody fusion (TLIF or PLIF), but it also offers the option of performing an osteotomy.[38] Several studies evaluating posterior approaches such as TLIF and PLIF have demonstrated improved patient outcomes and radiographic measurements, and ODI scores improve with posterior surgical correction of degenerative spinal disease.[1] A major benefit of posterior approaches is the ability to correct via bending of the rods and distribution of force over a larger area.[7] Additionally, pedicle screws used with rods allow control of all three columns of the spine in a single construct and shorter constructs; however, disadvantages include a learning curve for placement, potential toggle and loosening over time, damage with screw malplacement, and minimum pedicle diameter required to reduce the risk of fracture or breach during screw insertion.[7]

In major-degree spinal curvature, combined anterior-posterior approaches are an option. Combined approaches may provide the best option for correction of curvature with imbalance. Studies show better correction, fusion rates, and patient outcomes.[1,7] These improved results can come at a price, because dual approaches expose patients to the potential complications of either approach and longer operative times.[7]

Adjuncts to the standard approaches include osteotomies in which vertebral bone is resected to increase degrees of correction. Options include Smith-Petersen osteotomy (SPO), pedicle subtraction osteotomy (PSO), and vertebral column resection (VCR) (Fig. 12-5). SPO is technically the easiest osteotomy to perform and generally allows up to 10 degrees of lordosis correction per level. PSO is much more challenging, but a much greater degree of correction is possible. VCR has limited applications, because it is normally used in cases of deformity that cannot be corrected with PSO or SPO.[1,39]

POTENTIAL COMPLICATIONS AND MANAGEMENT

Complications after thoracolumbar surgery are generally reported to be higher in scoliosis surgery than in other elective spine surgeries, primarily because of the extent of the operations and the larger number of comorbid conditions that coexist with thoracolumbar deformity.[7,40,41] Complications in thoracolumbar operations are varied, and overall incidence is approximately 15%.[42,43] One recent review article estimated an overall complication rate in thoracolumbar surgery at 16.4%, twice as high as in cervical surgery.[42] Causes of complications can be both direct and indirect. Direct causes include compression, laceration, avulsion, and traction injury. Indirect causes primarily result from ischemia. Overall complications include pseudarthrosis, adjacent-level disease, infection, durotomy, implant failure, neurologic deficit, hardware failure, pulmonary embolism, vascular injury, bowel perforation, or systemic complication.[44-46]

Among the most common perioperative complications is compression injury from positioning.[42] Limb compression can affect individual nerves at compressible sites or plexuses at stretch-prone sites.[42] Compressive nerve injuries occur with the ulnar nerve at the elbow and peroneal nerve at the fibular neck. Prevention is critical, and these vulnerable sites should be evaluated before tissue is incised. Risk regions should be padded appropriately, and shoulders should be relaxed without excessive shoulder or cervical traction. Neutral positioning generally allows the least harm. Stretch injury is a risk, particularly at the brachial plexus. Risk for injury increases with either lateral decubitus positioning with dependent shoulder compression or supine positioning with excessive shoulder abduction.[42] The overall rate of iatrogenic nerve injury is 0.14%, 38% of which are brachial plexus injuries, and in general prognosis is fairly favorable, although recovery can take several months.[42]

In spinal instrumentation, complications can result from direct trauma. For instance, malpositioning of screws, hooks, or implants can occur. The rate of malpositioning was estimated to be 4.2%.[42] Exposure entails risk to neurovascular structures, which include medullary radicular arteries in the thoracolumbar region.[27] Vascular injury risk increases in anterior approaches; complication rates in prior studies range from 0% to 18%.[27] Relatively few of these injuries result in massive blood loss. Intimal dissection can occur after retraction of vessels. Sympathetic plexus nerves are within the dissection plane, particularly in the anterior approach, and should be protected. Careful blunt dissection and judicious use of bipolar cautery or sharp instrumentation is needed. Exposure and retraction should be used cautiously. Excessive retraction of the dural sac or nerve roots can induce direct or ischemic damage.

Accidental durotomy occurs at an estimated rate of 5.1%.[42] Most dural tears are without neurologic consequence. Approximately 7.7% of dural tears result in neurologic complications, and these tears are three times more likely to occur in revision surgery.[42] Durotomy repair is essential and can be completed primarily or secondarily. Primary repair includes suturing in interrupted or running fashion. Various autografts such as muscle or fat and allografts such as patches and glues are available for closure of the dura.

Infections in thoracolumbar surgery occur at an overall rate of 3.7%, including superficial and deep infections.[1] The rates tend to increase with repeat surgery and with fusions. Because these surgeries generally include instrumentation, foreign bodies add to the risk for infection. Judicious use of antibiotic irrigation and perioperative antibiotics are key practices to prevent postoperative infection.[47] Application of vancomycin powder into the wound before closing has shown good results in decreasing surgical site infections.[48,49]

Pseudarthrosis is one of the most common complications after surgery for scoliosis, with rates as high as 40%. This problem is even more exaggerated in revision surgery. Factors associated with pseudarthrosis include diabetes, smoking, use of allograft, poor technique, and use of immunosuppressant drugs. Techniques to overcome these obstacles include application of an autograft, meticulous surgical technique, and rh-BMP as a graft material.[50-55]

Ocular complications in spine surgery are primarily related to positioning. Corneal lesions are among the most common ocular complications, occurring 10 times more frequently with dependent positioning compared to lateral positioning.[42] Generally, maintaining the head in a slightly raised position and avoiding compression at the eyes prevents abrasions and ocular edema.

OUTCOMES

Outcomes are quite good for surgical intervention in patients with thoracolumbar deformity. When patients have failed conservative or nonoperative interventions, surgery is warranted for appropriate candidates. In general, the literature reports positive outcomes both clinically and radiographically for operative intervention compared with nonoperative management.[1,11,22,56,57] Adults who are older than 65 have shown improvement after surgical management based on self-assessment questionnaires.[11] Therefore the goal of treatment should be deformity correction with decompression and stabilization for pain and quality of life improvement.

In one study of 128 patients, outcomes were followed over 2 years after posterior fusion with osteotomy for thoracolumbar deformity correction.[58] Radiographic outcomes demonstrated near-complete scoliosis correction in 13% of patients and kyphosis correction in 49%, with mean kyphosis correction of 8.8 degrees per osteotomy level. Perhaps of more importance, ODI scores improved from 34.4 ± 17 to 23.6 ± 18, and normalized SRS-30 scores improved from 63.7 ± 13 to 76.4 ± 15, demonstrating improved quality of life for these patients. Another study of 784 adult scoliosis patients addressed the change on self-assessment questionnaires after operative intervention.[59] Patients were grouped by degree of sagittal imbalance, and all groups showed improvement in ODI, Scoliosis Research Society Outcomes Instrument-22 (SRS-22), and the 12-item Short Form Health Survey (SF-12) between baseline and one year. Additionally, 45 patients in the two-year follow-up group showed statistically significant improvement in ODI, SRS-22, and SF-12 measures compared with baseline ($p < 0.005$). However, no statistical improvement was noted between 1-year and 2-year follow-up marks for these 45 patients. Patients who had osteotomy showed a statistically significant correlation with SF-12 scores and improved health status at 1-year and 2-year follow-up assessments after surgery. Given these positive outcomes for radiographic and clinical follow-up, one study evaluated the association of quality of life with individual elements of spinal deformity assessment. Factors most significantly associated with and affecting quality of life were C7PL, degree of lumbar lordosis, thoracic kyphosis, and pelvic tilt and incidence; factors most associated with general health and well-being were degree of lumbar lordosis, thoracic kyphosis, and C7PL.[60] Therefore surgical management requires correction of these root elements of deformity for improved clinical outcomes.

PATIENT EXAMPLES

This 34-year-old man initially presented in 2009 after a motor vehicle accident, with a T11 burst fracture and complete paraplegia. Initial management included T10-12 posterior instrumented fusion (Fig. 12-6, *A*). He did well and presented again in 2011 with low back pain that worsened with movement and a grinding sensation below the fusion level. The patient was paraplegic and wheelchair bound with kyphosis. Flexion-extension radiographs demonstrated movement below T12 with marked kyphosis of the thoracolumbar curve involving T12-L1 (Fig. 12-6, *B*). Deformity surgery was completed and involved T11 laminotomy, T11 PSO, and T8-L3 posterior instrumented fusion for correction of kyphosis and decompression of the central canal. Postoperative imaging demonstrates good placement of hardware and solid fusion, with reversal of kyphosis from approximately 42 to 22 degrees (Fig. 12-6, *C* through *F*).

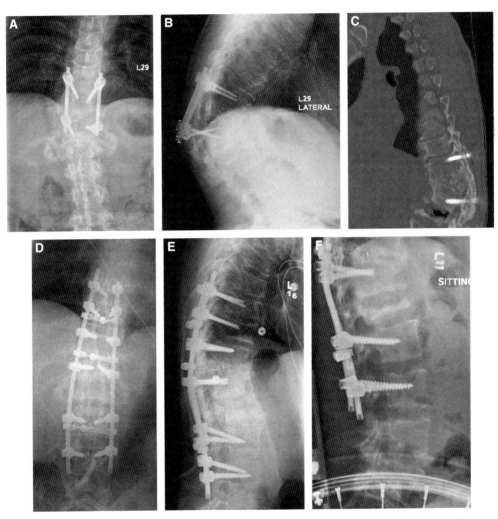

Fig. 12-6   **A,** A preoperative AP lumbar radiograph demonstrated T10-12 posterior instrumented fusion after a previous T11 burst fracture. **B,** A lateral radiograph showed significant kyphosis at T12-L1. **C,** Sagittal CT of the thoracic spine revealed breakdown below the previously placed construct. **D,** A postoperative AP lumbar radiograph shows T8-L3 posterior instrumented fusion and correction of kyphosis. **E,** A lateral lumbar radiograph demonstrates T11 laminectomy, T8-L3 posterior fusion, and T11 pedicle subtraction osteotomy. **F,** A magnified lateral lumbar radiograph details the procedure at the level of the burst fracture and the caudal extent of fusion.

This 62-year-old man had no significant past medical history except several prior joint surgeries and a fall from 20 feet, which resulted in an L1 compression fracture that was treated by a thoracolumbar spinal orthotic. The patient presented 6 months later with acute worsening of back pain. Examination was normal with the exception of back pain and tenderness to palpation at the thoracolumbar junction. MRI demonstrated T12-L1 discitis (Fig. 12-7, *A* and *B*). A peripherally inserted central line was placed, and the patient was treated with intravenous antibiotics. Three months later, pain symptoms persisted with intermittent thigh numbness. Follow-up MRI revealed osteomyelitis of T12-L1 and T12-L1 disc space edema and enhancement with severe central canal stenosis. Lateral views showed kyphotic deformity at the thoracolumbar junction (Fig. 12-7, *C* through *E*). Procedures included staged posterior-anterior operations of T12-L1, laminectomy with an SPO, L4-5 laminectomy, and T10-pelvis posterior instrumented fusion with T12-L1 corpectomy via an anterior approach (Fig. 12-7, *F* and *G*).

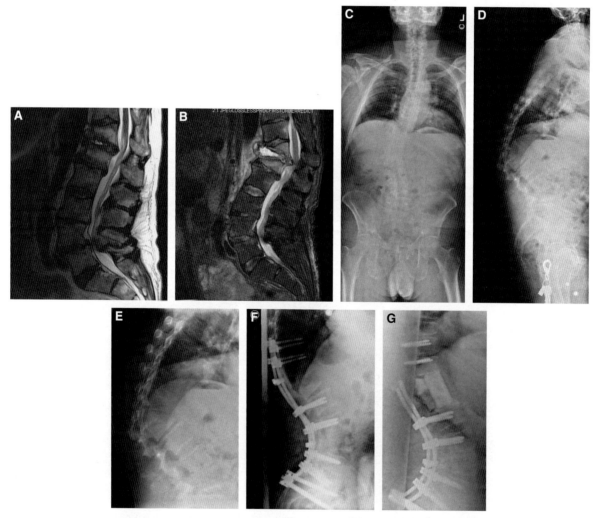

Fig. 12-7   **A,** Sagittal T2 MRI showed T12-L1 discitis with bony destruction. **B,** Repeat sagittal T2 MRI 3 months later revealed osteomyelitis of T12-L1 and T12-L1 disc space edema and enhancement with severe central canal stenosis. **C-E,** A PA radiograph, lateral scoliosis radiograph, and a thoracolumbar lateral plain radiograph showed thoracolumbar kyphotic deformity. **F,** A postoperative lateral lumbar radiograph shows a T12-L1 Smith-Petersen osteotomy with laminectomy and T10-sacrum posterior instrumentation. **G,** A postoperative thoracolumbar lateral radiograph after a staged approach with a T12-L1 corpectomy and previous instrumentation.

This 64-year-old woman had a history of idiopathic scoliosis since early adolescence. She had undergone noninstrumented fusion in 1961 by a previous surgeon; however, details of the operation were difficult to obtain. She presented for evaluation with low back pain radiating into the right lower extremity, which had progressively worsened over the past 3 years. Pain was described as worse with standing and walking. Conservative measures such as epidural steroid injections failed to provide relief. Examination demonstrated mild tenderness to palpation along spinal musculature. Standing balance was good with a 27-degree right thoracic angle of trunk inclination (ATI) as measured by a scoliometer. Her trunk was shifted rightward 6 cm and was unchanged from 3 years previously. Motor examination demonstrated full strength. Reflexes were normal. Scoliosis radiographs indicated good coronal and sagittal balance with lateral translation of L2-3 (Fig. 12-8, *A* through *D*). A CT-myelogram revealed stenosis at L4-5. Surgical procedures included posterior instrumentation from T7-S1 with T12-S1 arthrodesis, laminectomy at L3-5, and SPOs at L3-4 and L4-5 (Fig. 12-8, *E* and *F*).

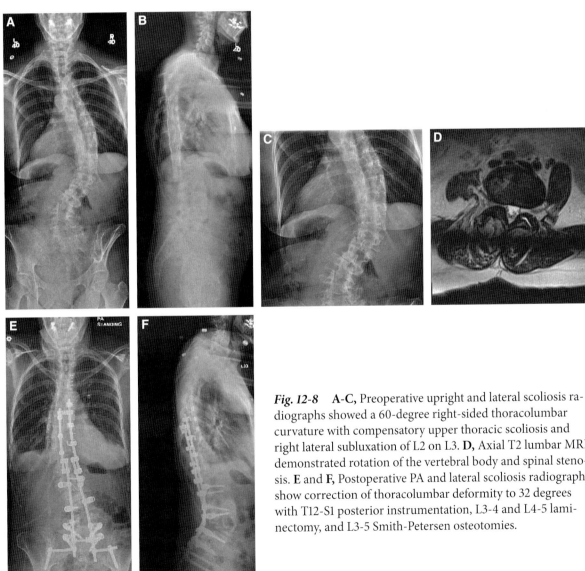

Fig. 12-8 **A-C,** Preoperative upright and lateral scoliosis radiographs showed a 60-degree right-sided thoracolumbar curvature with compensatory upper thoracic scoliosis and right lateral subluxation of L2 on L3. **D,** Axial T2 lumbar MRI demonstrated rotation of the vertebral body and spinal stenosis. **E and F,** Postoperative PA and lateral scoliosis radiographs show correction of thoracolumbar deformity to 32 degrees with T12-S1 posterior instrumentation, L3-4 and L4-5 laminectomy, and L3-5 Smith-Petersen osteotomies.

CONCLUSION

As the population ages, the incidence and prevalence of spinal deformity in adults will significantly increase. Recent studies have estimated the prevalence of this condition to be higher than 60%.[29,61] This highlights the clinical and economic impact that spinal deformity has and will continue to have on the health care system. Appropriate surgical correction is a key aspect of alleviating clinical deterioration. Correction of both sagittal and coronal spinal imbalance is clearly important for achievement of overall improved functional status.[62]

ACKNOWLEDGMENT

We would like to thank Karen K. Anderson, BS (Department of Neurosurgery, University of Kansas Medical Center), for her assistance with chapter preparation and editing.

REFERENCES

1. Youssef JA, Orndorff DO, Patty CA, et al. Current status of adult spinal deformity. Global Spine J 3:51-62, 2013.
2. Bess S, Schwab F, Lafage V, et al. Classifications for adult spinal deformity and use of the Scoliosis Research Society–Schwab Adult Spinal Deformity Classification. Neurosurg Clin N Am 24:185-193, 2013.
3. Herkowitz HN, Dvorák J, Bell GR, et al, eds. The Lumbar Spine: Official Publication of the International Society for the Study of the Lumbar Spine, ed 3. Philadelphia: Lippincott Williams & Wilkins, 2004.
4. Aebi M. The adult scoliosis. Eur Spine J 14:925-948, 2005.
5. Vaccaro AR, Silber JS. Post-traumatic spinal deformity. Spine 26(24 Suppl):S111-S118, 2001.
6. Ames CP, Smith JS, Scheer JK, et al. Impact of spinopelvic alignment on decision making in deformity surgery in adults: a review. J Neurosurg Spine 16:547-564, 2012.
7. Heary RF, Madhavan K. The history of spinal deformity. Neurosurgery 63(3 Suppl):5-15, 2008.
8. Kanter AS, Bradford DS, Okonkwo DO, et al. Thoracolumbar spinal deformity. I. A historical passage to 1990: historical vignette. J Neurosurg Spine 11:631-639, 2009.
9. Yadla S, Maltenfort MG, Ratliff JK, et al. Adult scoliosis surgery outcomes: a systematic review. Neurosurg Focus 28:E3, 2010.
10. Heary RF, Kumar S, Bono CM. Decision making in adult deformity. Neurosurgery 63(3 Suppl):69-77, 2008.
11. Li G, Passias P, Kozanek M, et al. Adult scoliosis in patients over sixty-five years of age: outcomes of operative versus nonoperative treatment at a minimum two-year follow-up. Spine 34:2165-2170, 2009.
12. Berven SH, Lowe T. The Scoliosis Research Society classification for adult spinal deformity. Neurosurg Clin N Am 18:207-213, 2007.
13. Panjabi MM. Clinical spinal instability and low back pain. J Electromyogr Kinesiol 13:371-379, 2003.
14. Smith JS, Shaffrey CI, Fu KM, et al. Clinical and radiographic evaluation of the adult spinal deformity patient. Neurosurg Clin N Am 24:143-156, 2013.
15. Angevine PD, Kaiser MG. Radiographic measurement techniques. Neurosurgery 63(3 Suppl):40-45, 2008.
16. Heary RF, Albert TJ, eds. Spinal Deformities: The Essentials. New York: Thieme Medical Publishers, 2007.
17. Mohan AL, Das K. History of surgery for the correction of spinal deformity. Neurosurg Focus 14:e1, 2003.
18. Lam FC, Kanter AS, Okonkwo DO, et al. Thoracolumbar spinal deformity. II. Developments from 1990 to today: historical vignette. J Neurosurg Spine 11:640-650, 2009.
19. Heary RF. Evaluation and treatment of adult spinal deformity. Invited submission from the Joint Section Meeting on Disorders of the Spine and Peripheral Nerves, March 2004. J Neurosurg Spine 1:9-18, 2004.
20. Mok JM, Hu SS. Surgical strategies and choosing levels for spinal deformity: how high, how low, front and back. Neurosurg Clin N Am 18:329-337, 2007.
21. Angevine PD, Bridwell KH. Sagittal imbalance. Neurosurg Clin N Am 1:353-363, 2006.
22. Smith JS, Shaffrey CI, Berven S, et al; Spinal Deformity Study Group. Operative versus nonoperative treatment of leg pain in adults with scoliosis: a retrospective review of a prospective multicenter database with two-year follow-up. Spine 34:1693-1698, 2009.
23. Smith JS, Shaffrey CI, Berven S, et al; Spinal Deformity Study Group. Improvement of back pain with operative and nonoperative treatment in adults with scoliosis. Neurosurgery 65:86-93, 2009.

24. Pastorelli F, Di Silvestre M, Plasmati R, et al. The prevention of neural complications in the surgical treatment of scoliosis: the role of the neurophysiological intraoperative monitoring. Eur Spine J 20 (Suppl 1):S105-S114, 2011.

25. Quraishi NA, Lewis SJ, Kelleher MO, et al. Intraoperative multimodality monitoring in adult spinal deformity: analysis of a prospective series of one hundred two cases with independent evaluation. Spine 34:1504-1512, 2009.

26. Harimaya K, Lenke LG, Mishiro T, et al. Increasing lumbar lordosis of adult spinal deformity patients via intra-operative prone positioning. Spine 34:2406-2412, 2009.

27. Marquez-Lara A, Nandyala SV, Hassanzadeh H, et al. Sentinel events in lumbar spine surgery. Spine. 2014 Jan 29. [Epub ahead of print]

28. Erickson MM, Currier BL. Surgical management of complex spinal deformity. Orthop Clin North Am 43:109-122, 2012.

29. Blondel B, Wickman AM, Apazidis A, et al. Selection of fusion levels in adults with spinal deformity: an update. Spine J 13:464-474, 2013.

30. Pekmezci M, Berven SH, Hu SS, et al. The factors that play a role in the decision-making process of adult deformity patients. Spine 34:813-817, 2009.

31. Kim YB, Lenke LG, Kim YJ, et al. The morbidity of an anterior thoracolumbar approach: adult spinal deformity patients with greater than five-year follow-up. Spine 34:822-826, 2009.

32. Wang MY. Improvement of sagittal balance and lumbar lordosis following less invasive adult spinal deformity surgery with expandable cages and percutaneous instrumentation. J Neurosurg Spine 18:4-12, 2013.

33. Deukmedjian AR, Dakwar E, Ahmadian A, et al. Early outcomes of minimally invasive anterior longitudinal ligament release for correction of sagittal imbalance in patients with adult spinal deformity. ScientificWorldJournal 2012:789698, 2012.

34. Anand N, Baron EM. Minimally invasive approaches for the correction of adult spinal deformity. Eur Spine J 22(Suppl 2):S232-S241, 2013.

35. Schwab FJ, Hawkinson N, Lafage V, et al; International Spine Study Group. Risk factors for major peri-operative complications in adult spinal deformity surgery: a multi-center review of 953 consecutive patients. Eur Spine J 21:2603-2610, 2012.

36. Mundis GM, Akbarnia BA, Phillips FM. Adult deformity correction through minimally invasive lateral approach techniques. Spine 35(26 Suppl):S312-S321, 2010.

37. Wang MY, Mummaneni PV. Minimally invasive surgery for thoracolumbar spinal deformity: initial clinical experience with clinical and radiographic outcomes. Neurosurg Focus 28:E9, 2010.

38. Hsieh PC, Ondra SL, Grande AW, et al. Posterior vertebral column subtraction osteotomy: a novel surgical approach for the treatment of multiple recurrences of tethered cord syndrome. J Neurosurg Spine 10:278-286, 2009.

39. Dorward IG, Lenke LG. Osteotomies in the posterior-only treatment of complex adult spinal deformity: a comparative review. Neurosurg Focus 28:E4, 2010.

40. Bhagat S, Vozar V, Lutchman L, et al. Morbidity and mortality in adult spinal deformity surgery: Norwich Spinal Unit experience. Eur Spine J 22(Suppl 1):S42-S46, 2013.

41. Glassman SD, Hamill CL, Bridwell KH, et al. The impact of perioperative complications on clinical outcome in adult deformity surgery. Spine 32:2764-2770, 2007.

42. Garreau de Loubresse C. Neurological risks in scheduled spinal surgery. Orthop Traumatol Surg Res 100(1 Suppl):S85-S90, 2014.

43. Cho SK, Bridwell KH, Lenke LG, et al. Major complications in revision adult deformity surgery: risk factors and clinical outcomes with 2- to 7-year follow-up. Spine 37:489-500, 2012.

44. Daubs MD, Lenke LG, Cheh G, et al. Adult spinal deformity surgery: complications and outcomes in patients over age 60. Spine 32:2238-2244, 2007.

45. DeWald CJ, Stanley T. Instrumentation-related complications of multilevel fusions for adult spinal deformity patients over age 65: surgical considerations and treatment options in patients with poor bone quality. Spine 31(19 Suppl):S144-S151, 2006.

46. Baron EM, Albert TJ. Medical complications of surgical treatment of adult spinal deformity and how to avoid them. Spine 31(19 Suppl):S106-S118, 2006.

47. Pull ter Gunne AF, van Laarhoven CJ, Cohen DB. Incidence of surgical site infection following adult spinal deformity surgery: an analysis of patient risk. Eur Spine J 19:982-988, 2010.

48. Sweet FA, Roh M, Sliva C. Intrawound application of vancomycin for prophylaxis in instrumented thoracolumbar fusions: efficacy, drug levels, and patient outcomes. Spine 36:2084-2088, 2011.

49. Heller A, McIff TE, Lai SM, et al. Intrawound vancomycin powder decreases staphylococcal surgical site infections following posterior instrumented spinal arthrodesis. J Spinal Disord Tech. 2013 Oct 30. [Epub ahead of print]

50. Kim HJ, Buchowski JM, Zebala LP, et al. RhBMP-2 is superior to iliac crest bone graft for long fusions to the sacrum in adult spinal deformity: 4- to 14-year follow-up. Spine 38:1209-1215, 2013.

51. Pichelmann MA, Lenke LG, Bridwell KH, et al. Revision rates following primary adult spinal deformity surgery: six hundred forty-three consecutive patients followed-up to twenty-two years postoperative. Spine 35:219-226, 2010.

52. Maeda T, Buchowski JM, Kim YJ, et al. Long adult spinal deformity fusion to the sacrum using rhBMP-2 versus autogenous iliac crest bone graft. Spine 34:2205-2212, 2010.

53. Mulconrey DS, Bridwell KH, Flynn J, et al. Bone morphogenetic protein (RhBMP-2) as a substitute for iliac crest bone graft in multilevel adult spinal deformity surgery: minimum two-year evaluation of fusion. Spine 33:2153-2159, 2008.

54. Kim YJ, Bridwell KH, Lenke LG, et al. Pseudarthrosis in adult spinal deformity following multisegmental instrumentation and arthrodesis. J Bone Joint Surg Am 88:721-728, 2006.

55. Kim YJ, Bridwell KH, Lenke LG, et al. Pseudarthrosis in long adult spinal deformity instrumentation and fusion to the sacrum: prevalence and risk factor analysis of 144 cases. Spine 31:2329-2336, 2006.

56. Everett CR, Patel RK. A systematic literature review of nonsurgical treatment in adult scoliosis. Spine 32(19 Suppl):S130-S134, 2007.

57. Bridwell KH, Glassman S, Horton W, et al. Does treatment (nonoperative and operative) improve the two-year quality of life in patients with adult symptomatic lumbar scoliosis: a prospective multicenter evidence-based medicine study. Spine 34:2171-2178, 2009.

58. Dorward IG, Lenke LG, Stoker GE, et al. Radiographic and clinical outcomes of posterior column osteotomies in spinal deformity correction. Spine. 2014 Feb 27. [Epub ahead of print]

59. Schwab F, Lafage V, Farcy JP, et al. Surgical rates and operative outcome analysis in thoracolumbar and lumbar major adult scoliosis: application of the new adult deformity classification. Spine 32:2723-2730, 2007.

60. Wang TP, Zheng ZM, Liu H, et al. Correlation of adult spinal sagittal imbalance and life quality. Zhonghua yi xue za zhi 92:1481-1485, 2012.

61. Schwab F, Farcy JP, Bridwell K, et al. A clinical impact classification of scoliosis in the adult. Spine 31:2109-2114, 2006.

62. Bridwell KH, Baldus C, Berven S, et al. Changes in radiographic and clinical outcomes with primary treatment adult spinal deformity surgeries from two years to three- to five-years follow-up. Spine 35:1849-1854, 2010.

13

Lumbar Region

Prokopis Annis ▪ *Darrel S. Brodke*

Adult spinal deformity is one of the most complex spinal pathologies, and its management is a challenge for every spine surgeon. The most common forms of adult spinal deformity in the lumbar spine are degenerative or de novo scoliosis, adult idiopathic scoliosis, isthmic and degenerative spondylolisthesis, and iatrogenic sagittal and/or coronal deformity. Very often coronal and sagittal deformities coexist. Recent data have confirmed the negative impact of sagittal plane malalignment on patients' self-reported disability and pain, whereas coronal deformity has been shown to contribute less than previously thought.[1-6]

Current emphasis is increasing on restoration and maintenance of physiologic sagittal alignment, given the strong correlation with better health-related quality of life (HRQOL) outcomes.[7,8] Focus was initially placed on the restoration of lumbar lordosis (LL), thoracic kyphosis (TK), and the C7 plumb line (C7PL). The critical role of pelvic shape in guiding and regulating spinal sagittal alignment is now well understood.[9-18]

Understanding the principles of sagittal balance requires knowledge of the normal spinopelvic relationships that provide insight into the normal ranges for regional and global alignment during standing posture. It also requires recognition of compensatory mechanisms that lead to apparent sagittal balance. Failure to recognize sagittal malalignment when planning surgical treatment for spinal disorders can lead to treatment failures, higher rate of revision surgeries, and increased health care cost.

This chapter focuses on the principles of spinopelvic alignment, normal values for lumbosacral alignment, and the presence of compensatory mechanisms in cases of sagittal malalignment. An algorithm is proposed for preoperative planning for lumbar deformity reconstruction using radiographic spinopelvic and global balance parameters.

ASSESSMENT OF SPINOPELVIC ALIGNMENT

Long 36-inch standing radiographs with the knees extended are indispensable for assessment of both coronal and sagittal plane balance. Poor arm positioning can lead to underestimation of sagittal alignment.[19] Positioning of the arms with 30 degrees of shoulder flexion has less impact on sagittal alignment.[20] Placement of the hands on the clavicles during both AP and lateral radiographs usually provides a good standing posture for assessment.

Coronal Balance

Global coronal alignment of the spine is assessed by the horizontal distance between the coronal C7PL and the center sacral vertical line (CSVL), which is a vertical line that passes through the center of the sacral endplate (Fig. 13-1). A C7PL-CSVL distance of 0 to 4 cm is considered to be normal. *Coronal malalignment* is defined as an offset of more than 5 cm and has been associated with increased disability.[21]

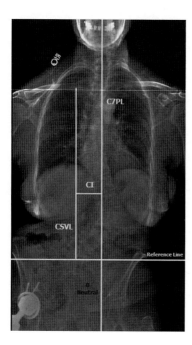

Fig. 13-1   Coronal alignment is assessed by measuring the distance between the C7 plumb line and center sacral vertical line.

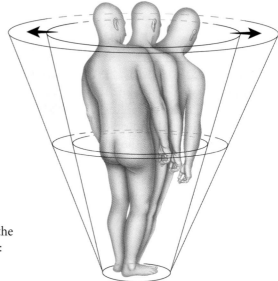

Fig. 13-2   The cone of economy, described by Dubousset. (Adapted from Dubousset J. Three-dimensional analysis of the scoliotic deformity. In Weinstein SL, ed. The Pediatric Spine: Principles and Practice. New York: Raven Press, 1994.)

Pelvic obliquity is defined as the angle formed between a horizontal reference line and a line connecting the two inferior points of the sacral alae. It represents either a compensatory mechanism of coronal imbalance caused by a scoliotic curve when the patient stands with one knee bent, or it is the result of a leg-length discrepancy. This must be carefully evaluated when coronal alignment is assessed.

Clavicle angle is defined as the angle between a line connecting the two clavicles and the horizontal line used to measure shoulder asymmetry.

Sagittal Balance

Assessment of sagittal alignment should include analysis of global and regional spinopelvic parameters.

Cone of Economy

Dubousset[22] introduced the concept of the *cone of economy* to describe the principles of ideal sagittal alignment and posture in the standing position. The ability to maintain erect position is fundamental for activities of daily living. The cone of economy defines a range of postures (within this cone) in which standing position is maintained with minimal effort and no requirement of external support, thus it is an economic position[22] (Fig. 13-2). Positions of the body outside the cone of economy require additional effort to maintain balance, which can produce muscle fatigue. In this case, an external support such as a cane or walker is often necessary to maintain standing or walking balance. Deviations of posture outside the cone in either the sagittal or coronal plane are commonly seen in significant spinal deformity.

Global Sagittal Alignment Parameters

One of the most important steps in the assessment of sagittal balance is evaluation of global balance. Multiple radiographic parameters have been described to assess global sagittal alignment. The most common is the *sagittal vertical axis* (SVA), defined as the horizontal distance between the posterior corner of the sacral endplate and the C7PL.[23-26] SVA is referred to as *positive* (+) or *negative* (−) if the C7PL falls, respectively, anterior or posterior to the ventral S1 vertebra. Normative values of SVA in young asymptomatic people have been established to be 0.5 cm (±2.5 cm).[25,27] The values of SVA tend to increase with age. It is the most commonly used measure to determine global balance, but the magnitude of the SVA is prone to magnification errors if the radiograph is not calibrated, and it does not take into consideration the position of the femoral heads or overall pelvic alignment.[19]

T1 and T9 spinopelvic inclination angles (T1 SPI and T9 SPI) were proposed as more reliable measures of assessing global sagittal alignment and provide an angular value of malalignment rather than only a horizontal distance.[28] These two angles are subtended from the C7PL and the line that connects T1 and T9, respectively, to the center of the femoral heads. Normative values of T1 SPI have been reported to be less than 0 degrees. Although these measures provide an angular value of global spinal balance, they do not take pelvic alignment into account.

The T1 pelvic angle (TPA) was very recently proposed to better assess global sagittal deformity, because it accounts for both pelvic retroversion and trunk forward inclination. It has been found to strongly correlate with HRQOL measures.[29] This angle is formed by a line connecting the center of the T1 vertebra to the center of the femoral heads and the line connecting the center of femoral heads with the center of the S1 endplate (Fig. 13-3). TPA is the sum of the T1 SPI angle and PT (TPA = T1 SPI + PT). Unlike the SVA, TPA measures sagittal deformity independent of the presence of postural compensatory mechanisms. TPA values greater than 19.8 degrees correlated strongly with disability (ODI greater than 40), whereas values of 14 degrees or less correlated with ODI less than 20. A meaningful ODI change (Δ ODI of more than 15)

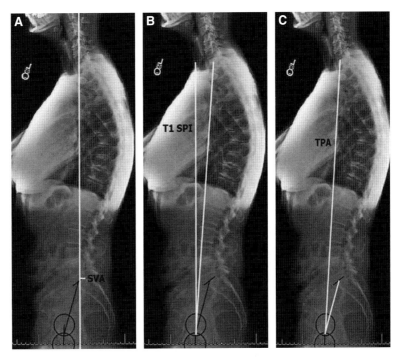

Fig. 13-3 Examples of three radiographic parameters used for the assessment of global sagittal alignment: the sagittal vertical access *(SVA)*, the T1 spinopelvic inclination *(T1 SPI)*, and the T1 pelvic angle *(TPA)*.

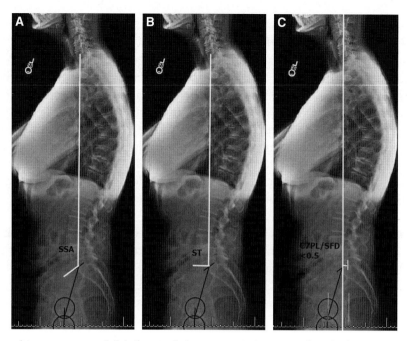

Fig. 13-4   Radiographic parameters of global sagittal alignment. **A,** Sacrospinal angle *(SSA).* **B,** Spinal tilt *(ST).* **C,** C7 plumb line/sacrofemoral distance *(C7PL/SFD)* ratio.

corresponded to a Δ TPA of 4.1. TPA can be used as a preoperative planning tool in adult deformity reconstruction surgery with the goal of a TPA of less than 15 degrees.

Another method to assess global sagittal alignment, described by French researchers, is through spinal tilt (ST) and sacrospinal angle (SSA).[30] ST is the angle formed by a line connecting the center of C7 to the center of the sacral endplate and the horizontal plane. Values less than 90 degrees suggest that C7 is anterior to the sacrum, whereas values greater than 90 degrees indicate that the center of C7 is behind the center of the sacral endplate. SSA corresponds to the angle formed by a line that connects the center of C7 with the center of the sacral endplate and a line parallel to the sacral endplate. ST reflects the global orientation of the spine, and SSA is a morphologic parameter that reflects global kyphosis of the spine. ST and SSA are related through the equation SSA = ST + SS. Normal values of ST and SSA have been reported to be 90.8 degrees ± 4 degrees and 130.4 degrees ± 8.1 degrees, respectively.[31]

The C7PL/sacrofemoral distance (C7PL/SFD) ratio has been proposed for the evaluation of global sagittal alignment and makes intuitive sense for the assessment of global alignment.[30] Based on the C7PL/SFD ratio, global sagittal alignment can be classified as in *balanced, balanced-compensated,* or *unbalanced* depending on the severity of the imbalance.[32] In a balanced spine the C7PL/SFD ratio is less than 0.5; in a balanced-compensated spine the C7PL/SFD ratio is less than 0.5 because of successful compensatory mechanisms. In an unbalanced spine the C7PL/SFD ratio is greater than 0.5, because the compensatory mechanisms are not efficient to maintain a balanced sagittal alignment (Fig. 13-4).

SPINOPELVIC PARAMETERS

One of the unique characteristics of human beings is the ability to maintain an erect position. LL is an exclusive characteristic of the human spine and is not found in other species. A normal human spine has successive opposing curves that allow a stable and ergonomic posture. The transformation of a quadruped to a biped gait has been associated with tremendous morphologic changes that within a short period contributed to the evolution of the human species.[33,34]

THE ROLE OF THE PELVIS IN THE EVOLUTION OF SAGITTAL BALANCE

The morphologic changes of the human pelvis that resulted in its broadening and more vertical position have played an extremely important role in the assumption of a vertical, bipedal position[33,35] (Fig. 13-5). The pelvis developed increased sacral slope as lumbar lordosis increased with upright posture, and pelvic tilt decreased. The pelvis, which acts as an intercalary unit between the spine and the lower extremities, directly influences the shape of the lumbar spine and constitutes the foundation of the spine that is critical for the maintenance of an upright posture.

PELVIS AND SPINOPELVIC RELATIONS

Legaye et al[17] and Duval-Beaupère et al[36] first underlined the importance of pelvic morphology in regulating standing balance. The description of three pelvic parameters—the pelvic incidence (PI), the pelvic tilt (PT), and the sacral slope (SS) angles—helped to characterize shape, geometry, and orientation of the pelvis and its relation with the sacral plateau (Fig. 13-6).

- PI is a morphologic parameter that is stable in adult life and reflects the shape of the pelvis and the relation of the sacrum to the acetabulae. PI is not affected by changes in the position of the lower extremities.[37] It is defined as the angle subtended by a line drawn between the center of the femoral heads and the center of the sacral plateau (or endplate) and a line drawn perpendicular to the center of the sacral plateau.

- PT is a positional parameter. It is defined as the angle subtended by a line drawn from the center of the sacral plateau to the center of the femoral heads and a vertical line extended from the center of the femoral heads.

- SS is a positional parameter and refers to the orientation of the sacral endplate in relation to a horizontal line. It is defined by an angle subtended by a line drawn parallel with the sacral plateau and a horizontal reference line.

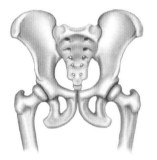
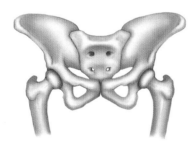

Fig. 13-5 Morphologic changes of the pelvis with acquisition of the biped gait. Broadening and more vertical position of the pelvis. (Adapted from Skoyles JR. Human balance, the evolution of bipedalism and dysequilibrium syndrome. Med Hypotheses 66:1060-1068, 2006.)

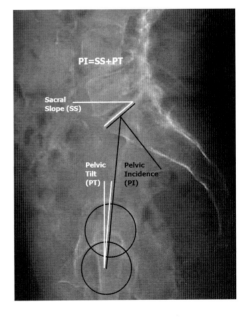

Fig. 13-6 Pelvic parameters. Pelvic incidence is the sum of sacral slope and pelvic tilt.

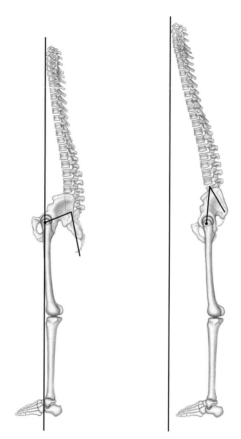

Fig. 13-7   Examples of two patients with low and higher pelvic incidence *(PI)* values. Individuals with higher values are better able to compensate for sagittal malalignment by retroversion of the pelvis.

These three angles are geometrically related in that PI is equal to the sum of the two positional variables, SS and PT (PI = SS + PT).[38] In standing position, the values of SS and PT vary in relation to each other, and normal values depend to some extent on the value of PI. Pelvic retroversion (or PT increase) is commonly reported as one of the most powerful mechanisms to compensate for forward tilt of the spine with aging, sagittal imbalance, loss of lordosis, or increased kyphosis and acts to maintain spinopelvic alignment in an economic position. This mechanism is limited by the amount of available hip extension. Individuals with a higher PI angle have greater ability for pelvic retroversion and therefore greater ability to compensate for sagittal malalignment (Fig. 13-7).

The shape of the pelvis changes from infancy to adulthood. The correlation between age and PI is linear until PI stabilizes.[1,39-41] PI is low at birth, but it increases during growth, with the acquisition of gait. The main identifiable factor for this change is the change in the inclination of the sacral plateau, which continues to increase until adulthood.[42] The mean value of PI is reported to be 30.6 degrees in newborns[41] and increases to 48 degrees in normal pediatric subjects.[1] In adulthood, the value of PI is believed to remain fixed. Legaye[43] recently reported an increased PI value in adults older than 60 years of age with chronic back pain and sagittal imbalance as a result of changes induced in the sacroiliac joint. The PI angle after skeletal maturity measures approximately 52 degrees (range 27 to 84 degrees), whereas the mean values of SS and PT are 40 degrees (range 20 to 65 degrees) and 13 degrees (range 5 to 30 degrees), respectively[44-51] (Table 13-1).

Several studies have presented the relationships between the shape of the pelvis (PI) and the regional sagittal parameters.[17,23,37,51-57] Roussouly et al[51] evaluated normal spinopelvic relationships in 160 asymptom-

Table 13-1 Normative Values of Radiographic Spinopelvic Parameters

	Mac-Thiong et al[31]	Roussouly et al[30]	Vialle et al[52]	Boulay et al[10]	Legaye et al[17]
No. of subjects	709	153	300	149	49
Mean age (years) (range)	37 ± 14.3 (18-81)	27 (18-48)	35 ± 12 (20-70)	31 ± 6 (19-50)	24 ± 6 (19-50)
Global					
Sagittal vertical axis (mm) (range)	—	35 ± 19 (–18-81)	—	—	—
T1 Spinopelvic inclination (degrees) (range)	—	—	(–)1.4 ± 2.7 (–9.2--7.12)	—	—
T9 Tilt (degrees) (range)	—	—	(–)10.35 ± 3 (–19.8--1.7)	—	—
Sacrospinal angle (degrees) (range)	130 ± 8.1 (114.2-146.5)	—	—	—	—
Spinal tilt (degrees) (range)	91 ± 3.4 (84.1-97.5)	—	—	—	—
C7 Plumb line/sacrofemoral distance (range)	1.1 ± 11.3 (–23.7-21.6)	—	—	—	—
Pelvic					
Pelvic incidence (degrees) (range)	—	51 ± 10 (28-83)	55 ± 10.6 (33-82)	53 ± 9 (34-78)	52 ± 10
Sacral slope (degrees) (range)	—	40 ± 8 (18-63)	41 ± 8.4 (17-63)	41 ± 7 (0.6-20)	11 ± 5.5
Pelvic tilt (degrees) (range)	—	11 ± 6 (–3-24)	13 ± 6 (–4.5-27)	12 ± 7 (–2-30)	40 ± 8.5
Regional					
Lumbar lordosis (degrees) (range)	—	61 ± 9 (40-84)	60 ± 10.3 (–89--30)	66 ± 10 (45-87)	60 ± 10
Thoracic kyphosis (degrees) (range)	—	46 ± 10 (23-66)	40.6 ± 10 (0-69)	54 ± 10 (32-84)	43 ± 13

—, Not measured or not reported.

atic individuals. Six classes of PI were reported from lower to higher values, along with the corresponding values of PT, SS, LL, and TK. The greater the values of PI, the greater the values of SS and LL. PT values were approximately a fourth of the values of PI. TK remained stable overall, between 44 and 45 degrees independent of the PI values. LL was approximately equal to PI ± 10 degrees, as previously proposed by Duval-Beaupère et al.[36] Because of the strong correlations between LL and SS and between PI and SS, it can be assumed that the shape of the pelvis guides the shape of LL and is a strong determinant of sagittal orientation of the pelvis in standing position.[37]

Regional and Segmental Parameters

The spine and pelvis in the sagittal plane can be considered as an open linear chain linking the head to the pelvis. A change in the orientation or shape of one spinal segment will induce a change in adjacent segments in an effort to restore or maintain normal alignment and minimize energy expenditure.[37]

Typically, sagittal curves are measured from C1 or C2 down to C7 for cervical alignment; from T1, T2, or T5 down to T12 for thoracic alignment; and from T12 or L1 down to S1 for lumbar alignment, respectively. Mean values of LL and TK have been reported by several studies to be 41 degrees (30 to 89 degrees) and 60 degrees (23 to 87 degrees), respectively* (see Table 13-1).

The traditional way to measure sagittal curves does not always reflect morphology. The morphology and structure of the sagittal curves can be analyzed with a model in which each curve is represented by two arcs of a circle, tangent at the apex of the curve.[37] The landmarks are the apex of each curve and the *inflexion point,* defined as the point where the orientation of the curve changes from kyphosis to lordosis or vice versa.[37,38] The anterosuperior aspects of T1 and S1 define the proximal and distal extent of the thoracic and lumbar curves. According to this model, LL is measured between the inflexion point of the thoracic and lumbar curves proximally (T12 or L1 usually) and the S1 endplate distally, and it is the sum of the lordosis of the superior and inferior arcs above and below the apex of the curve. The angle of the inferior arc is equal to the SS and is measured from the horizontal apex (usually L4) down to S1. The lower arc, therefore, corresponds approximately to the L4-S1 angle. The angle of the superior arc has been found to have a fixed value of around 20 degrees[38,53] (Fig. 13-8).

The contribution of the L4-S1 segmental angle to the overall LL has been found to be two thirds of the total curve.[38,53,59] Theoretically, it can be assumed that in asymptomatic individuals, given the strong correlation between PI and SS (and between SS and the lower arc of the lumbar curve), PI directly influences the morphology of the lumbar spine, especially its distal part.

---

*References 23, 25, 30, 51, 56, 58.

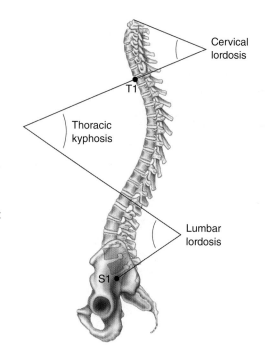

Fig. 13-8 Construction of the sagittal curves according to Berthonnaud's model. (Adapted from Roussouly P, Berthonnaud E, Dimnet J. [Geometrical and mechanical analysis of lumbar lordosis in an asymptomatic population: proposed classification] Rev Chir Orthop Reparatrice Appar Mot 89:632-639, 2003.)

Normal Variation in Spinopelvic Alignment

The variability of the shape of the pelvis and consequently of SS and their direct relation with the morphology of the lower arc of the lumbar spine may explain the characteristic sagittal profiles observed as a consequence of the changes of orientation of the pelvis. Roussouly and colleagues[38,60] proposed a classification system describing the morphology of the lumbar curves in relation to the pelvic orientation. Four types of lumbar curves have been proposed based on the values of SS and the position of the apex of the curve (Fig. 13-9).[38,51,60]

- Type 1: The SS angle is less than 35 degrees and the PI is low. The inflexion point is at L3-4. LL is short and low. TK starts from the L3 level and is long. The length ratio of TK/LL is 80:20.
- Type 2: The SS angle is less than 35 degrees and the PI is low. The inflection point is at the L1-2 level. The length ratio of TK/LL is 60:40. The lumbar curve has the appearance of a flat back.
- Type 3: The SS angle is between 35 degrees and 45 degrees, and the PI is within the normal range. This is generally considered normal overall alignment. The inflection point is at T12-1. The ratio TK/LL is almost 50:50. The spine is well balanced. This is the most common type of spine morphology, present in about 85% of the population.
- Type 4: The SS angle is greater than 45 degrees, and PI is very high. The inflection point is at T9-10. The lordotic curve is longer than the kyphotic curve. A reversed 20:80 split of TK/LL ratio is present.

All four types of curves represent normal variations that reflect the variability of the pelvic parameters.

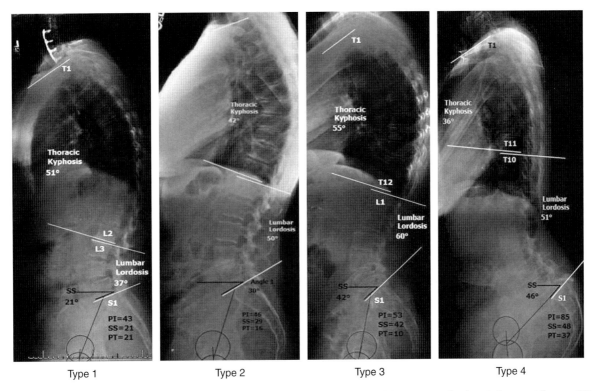

Type 1   Type 2   Type 3   Type 4

Fig. 13-9 Examples of the four types of spinal morphology, as described by Roussouly. (*PI*, Pelvic incidence; *PT*, pelvic tilt; *SS*, sacral slope.)

Spinopelvic Parameters and Predisposition for Lumbar Spine Pathology

The role of PI with degenerative spine disease has been extensively studied. The relationship of high PI with isthmic-type spondylolisthesis is well documented.[13,44,61-63] There is also strong evidence that a high PI is an independent risk factor of the development of degenerative spondylolisthesis.[9,64,65] A high PI has been associated with a high magnitude of curvature in patients with adult spinal deformity.[66] The need for a greater restoration of LL required in adult spinal deformity patients with high PI has been associated with higher risk of postoperative proximal junctional failure.[11,67,68]

A predisposition for degenerative progression based on the morphology of the lumbar spine has been suggested.[38] A type 1 curve has a short LL and very little space for the spinous processes (kissing spinous processes). This type of lordosis has been associated with higher risk of facet hyperpressure and L5 spondylolysis by a "nutcracker" effect. A type 2 curve is a flat back with low PI. The orientation of the discs is horizontal, which increases the risk of early disc degeneration and central disc herniation from increased loads transferred to the center of the disc space (Fig. 13-10). A type 4 curve, present in individuals with high PI and SS, has been associated with risk of L5 isthmic and degenerative spondylolisthesis[38] (Fig. 13-11).

Knowledge of the normal variation of the sagittal curvatures of the spine is important especially when planning surgical treatment. The distinction between a normal type 2 curve (normal flat back) from a type 4 curve with progressive degeneration, both with low lordosis, is important to appreciate and can be identified in the values of the pelvic parameters. A type 2 curve has a low PI and PT, whereas loss of lordosis in a type 4 curve is present despite high PI and abnormally high PT (see Fig. 13-11).

AGING AND COMPENSATORY MECHANISMS

Aging is associated with loss of LL, progressive kyphosis, and anterior displacement of the SVA.[23,69] A similar situation exists in the presence of chronic low back pain and degenerative lumbar pathology.[9,25,64]

The ability to correct sagittal malalignment depends not only on the PI but also on the entirety of the spine curvatures and the lower extremities position. The most common compensatory mechanisms recognized are the following:

- Pelvic retroversion or PT increase is recognized as one of the most common mechanisms of sagittal malalignment compensation and is dependent on the values of PI. The higher the value of PI the higher the ability to obtain pelvic retroversion. This mechanism is limited at its endpoint by hyperextension of the hips. An increase in PT is not economic for posture and gain, and is associated with significant disability.[15]
- Segmental hyperextension in the lumbar and thoracolumbar spine is a very common and efficient compensatory mechanism to increase local lordosis, but it also increases the risk of degeneration and segmental retrolisthesis because of the increased loads transferred in the posterior elements.
- Hypokyphosis of the thoracic spine limits the anterior translation of the C7PL. This mechanism is limited by the rigidity/degeneration of the thoracic spine and is more frequently noted in young individuals with flexible spines (Fig. 13-12).
- Cervical hyperlordosis is common with increased sagittal imbalance and allows maintenance of horizontal gaze in cases of severely increased SVA.
- Knee flexion is an attempt to decrease the forward translation of C7PL. It is usually the last compensatory mechanism to present after all others have failed and is the least economic for stance and gait. It is present in cases of severe sagittal imbalance and can be evaluated with the femoral obliquity angle (FOA).[70]

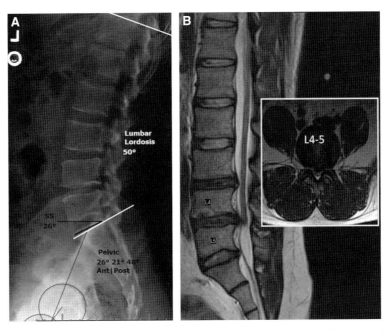

Fig. 13-10   This lateral lumbar radiograph and sagittal and axial MRI of a 23-year-old man with central disc herniation demonstrate a type 2 spine.

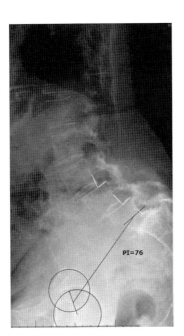

Fig. 13-11   This lateral lumbar view of a 65-year-old woman shows a high PI that predisposed her to a multilevel spondylolisthesis. (*PI*, Pelvic incidence.)

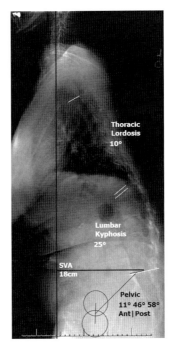

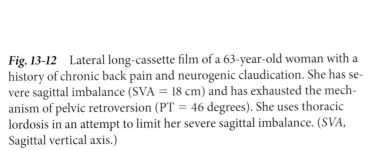

Fig. 13-12   Lateral long-cassette film of a 63-year-old woman with a history of chronic back pain and neurogenic claudication. She has severe sagittal imbalance (SVA = 18 cm) and has exhausted the mechanism of pelvic retroversion (PT = 46 degrees). She uses thoracic lordosis in an attempt to limit her severe sagittal imbalance. (*SVA*, Sagittal vertical axis.)

Understanding of the compensatory mechanisms is critical when planning adult spinal deformity reconstructive surgery. The distinction of a normal global sagittal balance from a normal-compensated balance requires recognition of the compensatory mechanisms present that preserve alignment in a normal but noneconomic position.

SPINOPELVIC PARAMETERS IN PLANNING TREATMENT FOR LUMBAR SPINE DEGENERATIVE DISEASE

Proper sagittal and coronal alignment after spine surgery are critical to achieve favorable HRQOL outcomes.[7,8,71] Correction of the C7-CSVL distance to less than 4 cm has been the traditional goal for correction of coronal imbalance. SVA is the most common parameter used to assess sagittal alignment. The goal of correction is an SVA of less than 5 cm, given the favorable correlation with HRQOL scores.[7] Recently Lafage et al[15] reported a more accurate correlation of the T1 SPI with HRQOL scores, as compared with SVA. Negative correlations with HRQOL scores were reported for SVA larger than 5 cm, PT increase, and PI-LL mismatch.[15,72] Thresholds for disability (ODI higher than 40) for these three key parameters were calculated to be SVA greater than 47 mm, PI-LL greater than 11 degrees, and PT larger than 22 degrees.[73]

Schwab et al[73] published a comprehensive classification of adult spinal deformity that was based on the three key parameters that correlated strongly with disability. Four coronal curves and three sagittal modifiers—PI-LL mismatch, SVA, and PT—were included. The coronal curves were based on the location of the apex (thoracic [T], thoracolumbar [TL], and double [D]), all with a minimum coronal Cobb angle of 30 degrees, and a fourth type with no (N) curve or with a coronal Cobb angle of less than 30 degrees. The three sagittal modifiers, PI-LL mismatch, SVA, and PT, were graded according to their severity as 0, +, or ++. Improvement of at least one grade of the sagittal modifiers was correlated with meaningful, clinical, significant HRQOL outcome improvements.[74]

Several formulas predicting ideal sagittal alignment after pedicle subtraction osteotomy (PSO) surgery have been proposed. Initially, only regional alignment was considered (Kim et al,[75] LL $\geq$ TK + 20 degrees); however, more recent formulas by Schwab et al[4] (LL $\geq$ PI − 10 degrees) and Rose et al[76] (LL + PI +TK $\leq$ 45 degrees) included pelvic parameters in light of the recognized role of the pelvis to regulate sagittal alignment. The inability to predict PT correction has been related to postoperative sagittal malalignment. Lafage et al[77,78] proposed and validated a formula that accurately predicted postoperative PT and SVA based on preoperative spinopelvic parameters.

Ondra et al[79] suggested a trigonometric method to calculate the PSO angle of correction needed to restore sagittal alignment, but it did not account for spinopelvic parameters. In the presence of severe sagittal imbalance with increased PT angles, normalization of PT required greater angular corrections than Ondra's technique predicted.[80] Le Huec et al[81] described a method (full-balance compensated index [FBI]) to calculate the amount of correction needed to correct C7PL to a desired position with a PSO, taking into account the presence of compensatory mechanisms (PT and hip flexion) (Fig. 13-13). More recently, Protopsaltis et al[29] proposed the TPA as a more useful tool to assess and plan surgical reconstruction of ASD. This novel angular parameter is not influenced by postural compensatory mechanisms, use of a walker when standing, or even the sitting position, and it can be useful as a preoperative planning tool with a target TPA of less than 14 degrees (Fig. 13-14).

When reconstructive surgery is planned, the reciprocal changes that occur in the unfused spinal segments and the risk of proximal junctional failure require special consideration. Several studies have reported a decreased risk of proximal junctional kyphosis and distal adjacent-segment degeneration after long fusions for deformity correction.[67,82-86] Several authors have recently reported on the negative impact of the postoperative increase of TK, older age, and greater preoperative sagittal alignment and higher PI occurring with proximal junctional failures.[67,87-91] Greater correction of LL was recently reported as an independent

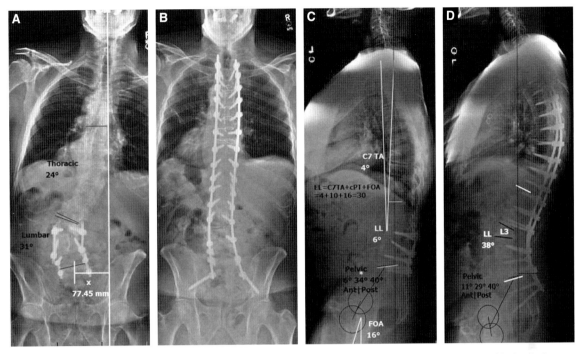

Fig. 13-13   This patient had preoperative coronal imbalance (larger than 7 cm) and compensated balanced sagittal alignment (SVA normal and PT high). The FBI technique calculates the amount of LL required using the formula LL = C7TA + cPT + FOA. In this case an asymmetrical PSO was performed, but PT was incompletely corrected. **A** and **B,** Preoperative and postoperative AP views. **C** and **D,** Preoperative and postoperative lateral views. (*C7TA,* C7 translation angle; *cPT,* compensatory pelvic tilt [if the preoperative PT is greater than 25 degrees, then the cPT = 10 degrees]; *FOA,* femoral obliquity angle.)

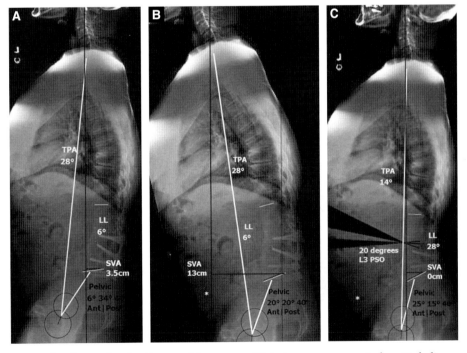

Fig. 13-14   **A,** Lateral radiograph of a 63-year-old woman with balance-compensated sagittal alignment. The SVA is in the normal range, but PT (pelvic retroversion) is very high. **B,** Reoriented radiograph reveals how this patient would stand without compensation. Notice that TPA is not affected by decreasing pelvic tilt to normal. **C,** Altered radiograph revealing how a PSO at L3 with a 20-degree wedge attains the alignment goals (SVA = 0, PT = 15, PI-LL = 12). (*LL,* Lumbar lordosis; *PSO,* pedicle subtraction osteotomy; *SVA,* sagittal vertical axis; *TPA,* T1 pelvic angle.)

risk factor for failure, implying that patients with higher PI that require greater LL corrections are at risk for proximal junctional failures, as reported previously.[11,67,68,87] Smith et al[89] found no difference in early proximal junctional failure independent of the correction of preoperative sagittal imbalance. In light of the risk of proximal junctional failure, the question that remains unanswered is whether a complete restoration of sagittal alignment is necessary in older patients with compensatory mechanisms, or whether achieving a goal of improved but less than normal LL is adequate to gain clinical benefit.

PREOPERATIVE PLANNING

CORONAL PLANE CONSIDERATIONS

The presence and cause of coronal imbalance needs to be assessed preoperatively. Preoperative coronal imbalance (more than 5 cm) and severe lateral listhesis (larger than 6 mm) have been associated with disability, but the presence of sagittal imbalance is the most reliable predictor of clinical symptoms.[7] In cases of combined coronal and sagittal deformity, correction of sagittal alignment parameters correlate with improved HRQOL outcomes.[21,74,92]

Preoperative clinical and radiographic examinations are important for diagnosis and prevention of imbalance. Prediction of coronal alignment after scoliosis correction in adults is difficult, because the rigidity of the spine is more difficult to assess. Postoperative coronal imbalance has been reported to persist in about 15% of deformity patients.[92] The magnitude of the coronal curves in adults is less affected by prone positioning, but coronal balance is usually fully restored.[93] Long, standing films in the early postoperative period are necessary to determine the need for further adjustments.[94]

The cause of pelvic obliquity in the setting of an adult deformity must be thoroughly assessed. Leg-length discrepancy is the most common cause of pelvic obliquity, often present with an associated lumbar compensatory curve. Pelvic obliquity can, alternatively, be part of a mechanism of compensation of a coronal imbalance caused by a scoliotic curve, in which the patient stands with one knee bent. With the former condition, treatment should focus on leg-length discrepancy directly, whereas the latter requires correction of scoliosis (Fig. 13-15).

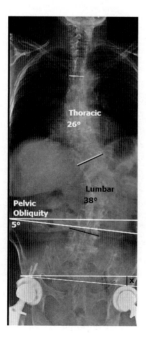

Fig. 13-15   This patient had degenerative scoliosis and pelvic obliquity secondary to leg-length discrepancy ($x = 2$ cm) after bilateral total hip arthroplasties.

SAGITTAL PLANE CONSIDERATIONS

Sagittal alignment can be analyzed preoperatively in three steps.[95,96]

Step One

The first step in the analysis of sagittal alignment is to determine the patient's global sagittal alignment using one of the global radiographic parameters described. SVA and T1 SPI are the most common radiographic parameters used; however, the newer TPA may be of great value in this situation. SVA values of less than 5 cm or T1 SPI of less than 0 degrees is considered within the normal range. The TPA, which incorporates the PT and has a normal value of less than 15 degrees, can be very helpful when planning reconstructive surgery and can help to prevent PT undercorrection. C7PL/SFD and SSA are also very reliable measures.

Step Two

The second step is the recognition of compensatory mechanisms. PT increase is the most common compensatory mechanism. The normal values of PT are obtained from studies in the young asymptomatic population; therefore age changes should be considered. PT values of more than 22 degrees have been correlated with significant disability.[15] Attention should be paid to identify the presence of additional compensatory mechanisms present as thoracic hypokyphosis or segmental retrolisthesis. The presence of knee flexion indicates noncompensated severe sagittal imbalance.

Based on the presence or absence of compensatory mechanisms, global sagittal alignment can be classified as normal, normal-compensated, and abnormal (sagittal imbalance). Normal global balance without the presence of compensatory mechanisms is a normal economic situation. Normal-compensated balance and global sagittal imbalance are noneconomic conditions that might require treatment (Figs. 13-16 and 13-17).

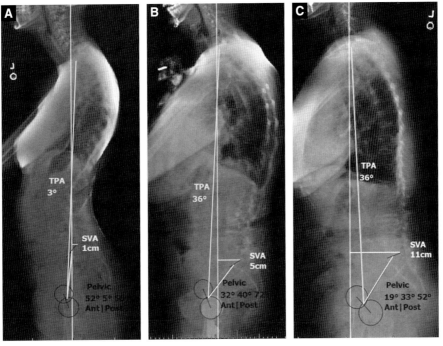

Fig. 13-16 Balanced, balanced-compensated, and imbalanced sagittal alignment. Sagittal vertical alignment *(SVA)* is normal in the first two cases and increased in the last. The T1 pelvic angle *(TPA)* is normal in the balanced condition and increased in the balanced-compensated and sagittal imbalanced situation.

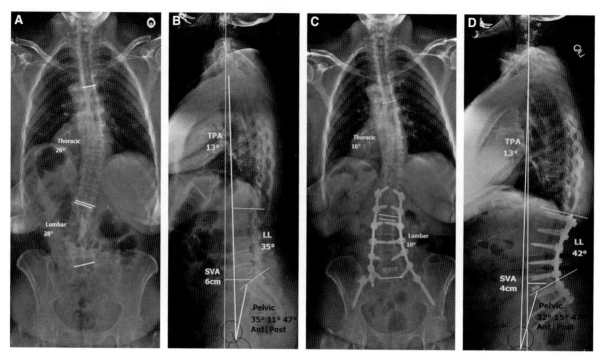

Fig. 13-17   **A** and **B,** Preoperative views of a patient with severe lumbar spinal stenosis and an increased sagittal vertical axis *(SVA)*. Pelvic tilt *(PT)* and T1 pelvic angle *(TPA)* were normal. Symptoms were relieved with forward flexion. **C** and **D,** Treatment included decompression and posterior instrumented fusion from L2 to the pelvis. *(LL,* Lumbar lordosis.)

Step Three

The third step in preoperative analysis of sagittal alignment is to calculate the amount of LL required to restore a normal, economic sagittal alignment based on the value of PI. Knowledge of the PI allows surgeons to determine the changes needed to obtain corrected values for spinopelvic parameters. The amount of LL correction required to restore sagittal alignment is determined with consideration of the following factors:

- The PI-LL mismatch (LL = PI ± 10). "The higher the value of PI, the higher the LL required" is a rule that should always be respected. With a high PI, the LL can be slightly less than the PI; with middle PI values, LL should equal PI; and with a low PI, LL should be slightly higher than the PI.
- The normal contribution of each lumbar segment to overall LL. L4-S1 lordosis contributes to two thirds of the overall LL, whereas the proximal arc of LL is usually stable (approximately 20 degrees). This distribution of lordosis should be restored when possible.
- Recognition of the morphology of the original lumbar curvature. This is helpful to prevent overcorrection or undercorrection.

These three steps should be followed regardless of the type of pathology. The goals of surgery should be to restore global balance (SVA less than 5 cm), to correct the PI-LL mismatch, and to normalize the values of PT.

TREATMENT OPTIONS WHEN TREATING LUMBAR DEFORMITY

Multiple techniques have been described for surgical correction of sagittal alignment.[48,97-101] The choice of the surgical technique will depend on the amount of correction required, the existing patient comorbidities, the flexibility of the spine, and the experience of the surgeon. The amount of LL correction that can be obtained varies with the different techniques available.

Simple rod cantilever techniques allow some LL correction in addition to the LL improvement from simple positioning on the operating table (Fig. 13-18). LL improvement with posterior *interbody cages* is about 5 to 10 degrees per level. Placement of lordotic cages anteriorly in the disc space with additional cantilever rod compression is necessary to achieve a better result. Anterior lumbar interbody cages often achieve corrections of up to 15 degrees per level (Fig. 13-19). *Modified Smith-Petersen or Ponte osteotomies* (SPOs) can achieve about 10 degrees of LL per level but require a flexible anterior disc space.

PSO is used in cases of severe sagittal imbalance that require greater corrections, up to 30 to 40 degrees, but it is associated with a high complication rate.[99,100,102] This is most commonly performed at L3, but can be performed above or below this level if required. Most commonly, the osteotomy site heals, but a posterior pseudarthrosis and subsequent rod failure are common if the discs above and below the osteotomy are intact (Fig. 13-20). One solution to this problem is to perform a posterior lumbar interbody fusion/ transforaminal lumbar interbody fusion (PLIF/TLIF) below the osteotomy and include the superior endplate and disc above in the PSO technique.[103]

Some authors advocate placement of one or two additional rods across the osteotomy site to increase rigidity. An asymmetrical PSO can be performed when coronal and sagittal deformities coexist and in the case of a failed lumbar fusion with associated sagittal imbalance. A PSO performed at the level of the nonunion can correct both the nonunion and sagittal imbalance.[103]

Rod contouring is important when sagittal alignment is corrected and should be carefully planned for the desired postoperative alignment. Rods should be bent to appropriately match the shape of the spine based on the values of PI. Pelvic fixation has been associated with better control of sagittal alignment and decreased postoperative sagittal decompensating phenomena.[104-106]

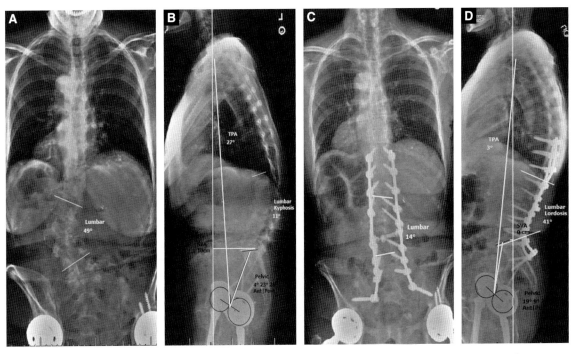

Fig. 13-18   Radiographs of a 78-year-old woman with chronic back pain, lumbar spinal stenosis and neurogenic claudication. **A,** A preoperative AP radiograph showed lumbar degenerative scoliosis of 49 degrees. **B,** The lateral film revealed sagittal imbalance (sagittal vertical axis = 10 cm, T1 pelvic angle = 27 degrees, pelvic tilt = 23 degrees, and very low pelvic incidence of 28 degrees). **C and D,** Sagittal alignment was corrected with patient positioning on the operating table, facetectomies, and a cantilever rod technique. Patients with low PI are at risk for overcorrection.

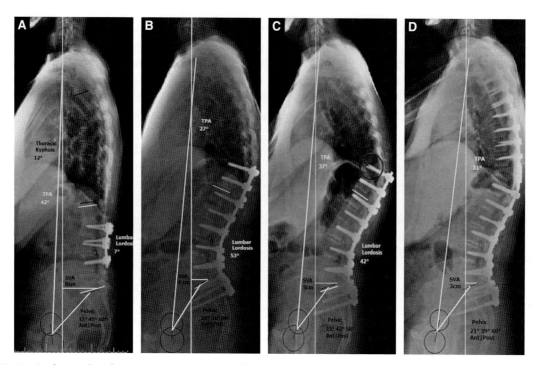

Fig. 13-19   Radiographs of a patient with iatrogenic flat back with associated sagittal imbalance. **A** and **B,** The patient was treated with anterior lumbar interbody fusion (ALIF) at two levels. LL was corrected from 7 degrees of kyphosis to 53 degrees of lordosis and PT was partially corrected. **C,** The patient developed an early UIV compression fracture at T11 *(red oval)* that was treated conservatively for 2 years. **D,** She is shown after revision that involved extension of the fusion to the upper thoracic spine. (*TPA,* T1 pelvic angle; *UIV,* upper instrumented vertebra.)

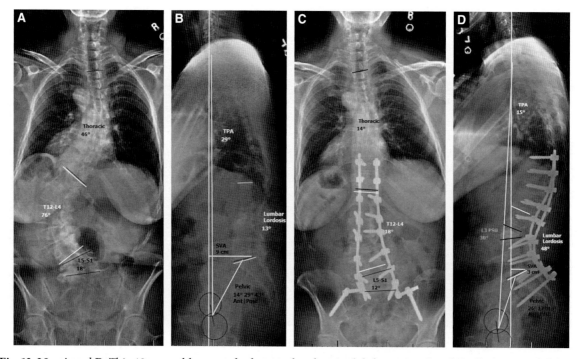

Fig. 13-20   **A** and **B,** This 48-year-old woman had coronal and sagittal deformities. **C** and **D,** She was treated with a pedicle subtraction osteotomy at L3 and had significant improvement of both coronal and sagittal plane deformities.

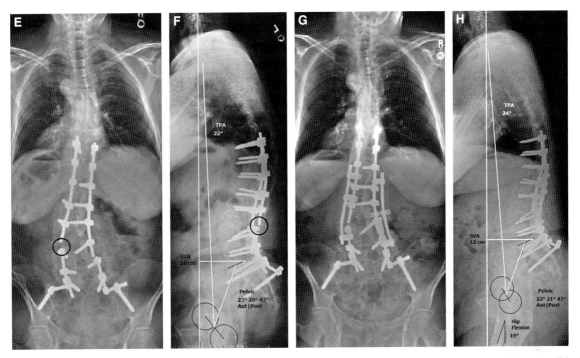

Fig. 13-20, cont'd **E** and **F,** At the 6-month postoperative visit, she presented with a left-sided rod fracture *(black circle)* around the PSO site with associated sagittal decompensation. **G** and **H,** She is shown after revision in which two additional rods were placed across the rod fracture site. *(TPA,* T1 pelvic angle.)

CONCLUSION

Spinopelvic parameters play a critical role in the regulation and maintenance of a normal economic and balanced upright position. Global radiographic parameters and spinopelvic relationships should always be considered during assessment of sagittal alignment. Long-cassette films from the head to the femurs are indispensable and should be taken with the patient standing whenever possible. Intraoperative long-cassette films are useful to assess the sagittal and coronal plane changes that occur with simple patient positioning on the table and to determine the need for additional correction.

Coronal alignment should be very carefully analyzed when adult spinal deformity surgery is planned, because persistent or worsening imbalance can occur. When pelvic obliquity is present, its cause should be assessed both clinically and radiographically. A limb-length discrepancy associated with pelvic obliquity may be the cause of an identified lumbar scoliotic curve and should be not be managed with spine surgery.

The three key parameters that strongly correlate with HRQOL are global sagittal alignment, PT, and PI-LL mismatch. Global sagittal alignment is often assessed by distance of the SVA off of the posterior corner of the S1 endplate. However, it is prone to magnification errors and misunderstanding, because it does not include effects of spinopelvic relationships. TPA and SSA are alternatives that include pelvic measures. Better control of postoperative PT may better improve sagittal alignment and HRQOLs and decrease the reciprocal proximal junctional changes. Correction of the PI-LL mismatch, adjusted according to the PI values and age, is critical for a more physiologic restoration of spinopelvic relations.

To assess sagittal alignment, global sagittal balance is measured using the SVA or the more recent angular measurements of T1 SPI and TPA. When these parameters are normal and no compensatory mechanisms are present, the sagittal alignment is defined as *balanced*. If pelvic retroversion (high PT) is present, it must be considered during preoperative planning. Last, the amount of lordosis required to restore a more normal economic sagittal balance must be calculated based on the PI, which is the foundation of spinopelvic alignment.

REFERENCES

1. Mac-Thiong JM, Labelle H, Berthonnaud E, et al. Sagittal spinopelvic balance in normal children and adolescents. Eur Spine J 16:227-234, 2007.

2. Rajnics P, Templier A, Skalli W, et al. The importance of spinopelvic parameters in patients with lumbar disc lesions. Int Orthop 26:104-108, 2002.

3. Schwab F, Lafage V, Boyce R, et al. Gravity line analysis in adult volunteers: age-related correlation with spinal parameters, pelvic parameters, and foot position. Spine 31:E959-E967, 2006.

4. Schwab F, Lafage V, Patel A, et al. Sagittal plane considerations and the pelvis in the adult patient. Spine 34:1828-1833, 2009.

5. Smith JS, Shaffrey CI, Berven S, et al; Spinal Deformity Study Group. Improvement of back pain with operative and nonoperative treatment in adults with scoliosis. Neurosurgery 65:86-93; discussion 93-94, 2009.

6. Tanguay F, Mac-Thiong JM, de Guise JA, et al. Relation between the sagittal pelvic and lumbar spine geometries following surgical correction of adolescent idiopathic scoliosis: a preliminary study. Stud Health Technol Inform 123:299-302, 2006.

7. Glassman SD, Berven S, Bridwell K, et al. Correlation of radiographic parameters and clinical symptoms in adult scoliosis. Spine 30:682-688, 2005.

8. Schwab F, Patel A, Ungar B, et al. Adult spinal deformity-postoperative standing imbalance: how much can you tolerate? An overview of key parameters in assessing alignment and planning corrective surgery. Spine 35:2224-2231, 2010.

9. Barrey C, Jund J, Noseda O, et al. Sagittal balance of the pelvis-spine complex and lumbar degenerative diseases. A comparative study about 85 cases. Eur Spine J 16:1459-1467, 2007.

10. Boulay C, Tardieu C, Hecquet J, et al. Sagittal alignment of spine and pelvis regulated by pelvic incidence: standard values and prediction of lordosis. Eur Spine J 15:415-422, 2006.

11. Gottfried ON, Daubs MD, Patel AA, et al. Spinopelvic parameters in postfusion flatback deformity patients. Spine J 9:639-647, 2009.

12. Jackson RP, Peterson MD, McManus AC, et al. Compensatory spinopelvic balance over the hip axis and better reliability in measuring lordosis to the pelvic radius on standing lateral radiographs of adult volunteers and patients. Spine 23:1750-1767, 1998.

13. Labelle H, Roussouly P, Berthonnaud E, et al. The importance of spino-pelvic balance in L5-s1 developmental spondylolisthesis: a review of pertinent radiologic measurements. Spine 30(6 Suppl):S27-S34, 2005.

14. Labelle H, Roussouly P, Chopin D, et al. Spino-pelvic alignment after surgical correction for developmental spondylolisthesis. Eur Spine J 17:1170-1176, 2008.

15. Lafage V, Schwab F, Patel A, et al. Pelvic tilt and truncal inclination: two key radiographic parameters in the setting of adults with spinal deformity. Spine 34:E599-E606, 2009.

16. Lafage V, Schwab F, Skalli W, et al. Standing balance and sagittal plane spinal deformity: analysis of spinopelvic and gravity line parameters. Spine 33:1572-1578, 2008.

17. Legaye J, Duval-Beaupère G, Hecquet J, et al. Pelvic incidence: a fundamental pelvic parameter for three-dimensional regulation of spinal sagittal curves. Eur Spine J 7:99-103, 1998.

18. Dubousset J. Importance de la vertèbre pelvienne dans l'équilibre rachidien. Application à la chirurgie de la colonne vertébrale chez l'enfant et l'adolescent. In Villeneuve P, ed. Pied Équilibre et Rachis. Paris, France: Frison-Roche, 1998.

19. Marks MC, Stanford CF, Mahar AT, et al. Standing lateral radiographic positioning does not represent customary standing balance. Spine 28:1176-1182, 2003.

20. Vedantam R, Lenke LG, Bridwell KH, et al. The effect of variation in arm position on sagittal spinal alignment. Spine 25:2204-2209, 2000.

21. Ploumis A, Liu H, Mehbod AA, et al. A correlation of radiographic and functional measurements in adult degenerative scoliosis. Spine 34:1581-1584, 2009.

22. Dubousset J. Three-dimensional analysis of the scoliotic deformity. In Weinstein SL, ed. The Pediatric Spine: Principles and Practice. New York: Raven Press, 1994.

23. Gelb DE, Lenke LG, Bridwell KH, et al. An analysis of sagittal spinal alignment in 100 asymptomatic middle and older aged volunteers. Spine 20:1351-1358, 1995.

24. Hammerberg EM, Wood KB. Sagittal profile of the elderly. J Spinal Disord Tech 16:44-50, 2003.

25. Jackson RP, McManus AC. Radiographic analysis of sagittal plane alignment and balance in standing volunteers and patients with low back pain matched for age, sex, and size. A prospective controlled clinical study. Spine 19:1611-1618, 1994.

26. McLean IP, Gillan MG, Ross JC, et al. A comparison of methods for measuring trunk list. A simple plumbline is the best. Spine 21:1667-1670, 1996.

27. Jackson RP, Simmons EH, Stripinis D. Coronal and sagittal plane spinal deformities correlating with back pain and pulmonary function in adult idiopathic scoliosis. Spine 14:1391-1397, 1989.

28. Legaye J, Hecquet J, Marty C, et al. Equilibre sagittal du rachis. Relations entre bassin et courbures rachidiennes sagittales en position debout. Rachis 5:215-216, 1993.

29. Protopsaltis T, Schwab F, Bronsard N, et al. The T1 pelvic angle (TPA), a novel radiographic measure of global sagittal deformity, accounts of both pelvic retroversion and truncal inclination and correlates strongly with HRQOL. Presented at the Forty-eighth Annual Meeting of the Scoliosis Research Society, Lyon, France, Sept 2013.

30. Roussouly P, Gollogly S, Noseda O, et al. The vertical projection of the sum of the ground reactive forces of a standing patient is not the same as the C7 plumb line: a radiographic study of the sagittal alignment of 153 asymptomatic volunteers. Spine 31:E320-E325, 2006.

31. Mac-Thiong JM, Roussouly P, Berthonnaud E, et al. Sagittal parameters of global spinal balance: normative values from a prospective cohort of seven hundred nine Caucasian asymptomatic adults. Spine 35:E1193-E1198, 2010.

32. Barrey C. Equilibre sagittal pelvi-rachidien et pathologies lombaires dégénératives. Etude comparative à propos de 100 cas. Thèse de Médecine. Université Claude Bernard, Lyon, France, 2004.

33. Le Huec JC, Saddiki R, Franke J, et al. Equilibrium of the human body and the gravity line: the basics. Eur Spine J 20(Suppl 5):558-563, 2011.

34. Berge C. Heterochronic processes in human evolution: an ontogenetic analysis of the hominid pelvis. Am J Phys Anthropol 105:441-459, 1998.

35. Skoyles JR. Human balance, the evolution of bipedalism and dysequilibrium syndrome. Med Hypotheses 66:1060-1068, 2006.

36. Duval-Beaupère G, Schmidt C, Cosson P. A Barycentremetric study of the sagittal shape of spine and pelvis: the conditions required for an economic standing position. Ann Biomed Eng 20:451-462, 1992.

37. Berthonnaud E, Dimnet J, Roussouly P, et al. Analysis of the sagittal balance of the spine and pelvis using shape and orientation parameters. J Spinal Disord Tech 18:40-47, 2005.

38. Roussouly P, Berthonnaud E, Dimnet J. [Geometrical and mechanical analysis of lumbar lordosis in an asymptomatic population: proposed classification] Rev Chir Orthop Reparatrice Appar Mot 89:632-639, 2003.

39. Mac-Thiong JM, Berthonnaud E, Dimar JR II, et al. Sagittal alignment of the spine and pelvis during growth. Spine 29:1642-1647, 2004.

40. Marty C, Boisaubert B, Descamps H, et al. The sagittal anatomy of the sacrum among young adults, infants, and spondylolisthesis patients. Eur Spine J 11:119-125, 2002.

41. Mangione P, Gomez D, Senegas J. Study of the course of the incidence angle during growth. Eur Spine J 6:163-167, 1997.

42. Tardieu C, Bonneau N, Hecquet J, et al. How is sagittal balance acquired during bipedal gait acquisition? Comparison of neonatal and adult pelves in three dimensions. Evolutionary implications. J Hum Evol 65:209-222, 2013.

43. Legaye J. Influence of age and sagittal balance of the spine on the value of the pelvic incidence. Eur Spine J. 2014 Feb 9. [Epub ahead of print]

44. Hresko MT, Labelle H, Roussouly P, et al. Classification of high-grade spondylolistheses based on pelvic version and spine balance: possible rationale for reduction. Spine 32:2208-2213, 2007.

45. Van Royen BJ, De Gast A, Smit TH. Deformity planning for sagittal plane corrective osteotomies of the spine in ankylosing spondylitis. Eur Spine J 9:492-498, 2000.

46. Van Royen BJ, Toussaint HM, Kingma I, et al. Accuracy of the sagittal vertical axis in a standing lateral radiograph as a measurement of balance in spinal deformities. Eur Spine J 7:408-412, 1998.

47. Mac-Thiong JM, Roussouly P, Berthonnaud E, et al. Age- and sex-related variations in sagittal sacropelvic morphology and balance in asymptomatic adults. Eur Spine J 20(Suppl 5):572-577, 2011.

48. Boseker EH, Moe JH, Winter RB, et al. Determination of "normal" thoracic kyphosis: a roentgenographic study of 121 "normal" children. J Pediatr Orthop 20:796-798, 2000.

49. Bernhardt M, Bridwell KH. Segmental analysis of the sagittal plane alignment of the normal thoracic and lumbar spines and thoracolumbar junction. Spine 14:717-721, 1989.

50. Hardacker JW, Shuford RF, Capicotto PN, et al. Radiographic standing cervical segmental alignment in adult volunteers without neck symptoms. Spine 22:1472-1480; discussion 1480, 1997.

51. Roussouly P, Gollogly S, Berthonnaud E, et al. Classification of the normal variation in the sagittal alignment of the human lumbar spine and pelvis in the standing position. Spine 30:346-353, 2005.

52. Vialle R, Levassor N, Rillardon L, et al. Radiographic analysis of the sagittal alignment and balance of the spine in asymptomatic subjects. J Bone Joint Surg Am 87:260-267, 2005.

53. Stagnara P, De Mauroy JC, Dran G, et al. Reciprocal angulation of vertebral bodies in a sagittal plane: approach to references for the evaluation of kyphosis and lordosis. Spine 7:335-342, 1982.

54. Roussouly P, Gollogly S, Berthonnaud E, et al. Sagittal alignment of the spine and pelvis in the presence of L5-s1 isthmic lysis and low-grade spondylolisthesis. Spine 31:2484-2490, 2006.

55. During J, Goudfrooij H, Keessen W, et al. Toward standards for posture. Postural characteristics of the lower back system in normal and pathologic conditions. Spine 10:83-87, 1985.

56. Korovessis PG, Stamatakis MV, Baikousis AG. Reciprocal angulation of vertebral bodies in the sagittal plane in an asymptomatic Greek population. Spine 23:700-704; discussion 704-705, 1998.

57. Vaz G, Roussouly P, Berthonnaud E, et al. Sagittal morphology and equilibrium of pelvis and spine. Eur Spine J 11:80-87, 2002.

58. Jackson RP, Kanemura T, Kawakami N, et al. Lumbopelvic lordosis and pelvic balance on repeated standing lateral radiographs of adult volunteers and untreated patients with constant low back pain. Spine 25:575-586, 2000.

59. Janik TJ, Harrison DD, Cailliet R, et al. Can the sagittal lumbar curvature be closely approximated by an ellipse? J Orthop Res 16:766-770, 1998.

60. Roussouly P, Nnadi C. Sagittal plane deformity: an overview of interpretation and management. Eur Spine J 19:1824-1836, 2010.

61. Labelle H, Roussouly P, Berthonnaud E, et al. Spondylolisthesis, pelvic incidence, and spinopelvic balance: a correlation study. Spine 29:2049-2054, 2004.

62. Labelle H, Mac-Thiong JM, Roussouly P. Spino-pelvic sagittal balance of spondylolisthesis: a review and classification. Eur Spine J 20(Suppl 5):641-646, 2011.

63. Mac-Thiong JM, Wang Z, de Guise JA, et al. Postural model of sagittal spino-pelvic alignment and its relevance for lumbosacral developmental spondylolisthesis. Spine 33:2316-2325, 2008.

64. Barrey C, Jund J, Perrin G, et al. Spinopelvic alignment of patients with degenerative spondylolisthesis. Neurosurgery 61:981-986; discussion 986, 2007.

65. Aono K, Kobayashi T, Jimbo S, et al. Radiographic analysis of newly developed degenerative spondylolisthesis in a mean twelve-year prospective study. Spine 35:887-891, 2010.

66. Hong JY, Suh SW, Modi HN, et al. Correlation of pelvic orientation with adult scoliosis. J Spinal Disord Tech 23:461-466, 2010.

67. Maruo K, Ha Y, Inoue S, et al. Predictive factors for proximal junctional kyphosis in long fusions to the sacrum in adult spinal deformity. Spine 38:E1469-E1476, 2013.

68. Cho KJ, Suk SI, Park SR, et al. Risk factors of sagittal decompensation after long posterior instrumentation and fusion for degenerative lumbar scoliosis. Spine 35:1595-1601, 2010.

69. Kobayashi T, Atsuta Y, Matsuno T, et al. A longitudinal study of congruent sagittal spinal alignment in an adult cohort. Spine 29:671-676, 2004.

70. Obeid I, Hauger O, Aunoble S, et al. Global analysis of sagittal spinal alignment in major deformities: correlation between lack of lumbar lordosis and flexion of the knee. Eur Spine J 20(Suppl 5):681-685, 2011.

71. Hori T, Kawaguchi Y, Kimura T. How does the ossification area of the posterior longitudinal ligament progress after cervical laminoplasty? Spine 31:2807-2812, 2006.

72. Schwab FJ, Blondel B, Bess S, et al; International Spine Study Group. Radiographical spinopelvic parameters and disability in the setting of adult spinal deformity: a prospective multicenter analysis. Spine 38:E803-E812, 2013.

73. Schwab F, Ungar B, Blondel B, et al. Scoliosis Research Society–Schwab adult spinal deformity classification: a validation study. Spine 37:1077-1082, 2012.

74. Smith JS, Klineberg E, Schwab F, et al; International Spine Study Group. Change in classification grade by the SRS–Schwab Adult Spinal Deformity Classification predicts impact on health-related quality of life measures: prospective analysis of operative and nonoperative treatment. Spine 38:1663-1671, 2013.

75. Kim YJ, Bridwell KH, Lenke LG, et al. An analysis of sagittal spinal alignment following long adult lumbar instrumentation and fusion to L5 or S1: can we predict ideal lumbar lordosis? Spine 31:2343-2352, 2006.

76. Rose PS, Bridwell KH, Lenke LG, et al. Role of pelvic incidence, thoracic kyphosis, and patient factors on sagittal plane correction following pedicle subtraction osteotomy. Spine 34:785-791, 2009.

77. Lafage V, Bharucha NJ, Schwab F, et al. Multicenter validation of a formula predicting postoperative spinopelvic alignment. J Neurosurg Spine 16:15-21, 2012.

78. Lafage V, Schwab F, Vira S, et al. Spino-pelvic parameters after surgery can be predicted: a preliminary formula and validation of standing alignment. Spine 36:1037-1045, 2011.

79. Ondra SL, Marzouk S, Koski T, et al. Mathematical calculation of pedicle subtraction osteotomy size to allow precision correction of fixed sagittal deformity. Spine 31:E973-E979, 2006.

80. Schwab F, Lafage V, Shaffrey CI, et al. Preoperative pelvic parameters must be considered to achieve adequate sagittal balance after lumbar osteotomy. Presented at the Eighteenth International Meeting on Advanced Spine Techniques, Scoliosis Research Society, Copenhagen, Denmark, July 2011.

81. Le Huec JC, Leijssen P, Duarte M, et al. Thoracolumbar imbalance analysis for osteotomy planification using a new method: FBI technique. Eur Spine J 20(Suppl 5):669-680, 2011.

82. Kim YJ, Bridwell KH, Lenke LG, et al. Proximal junctional kyphosis in adult spinal deformity after segmental posterior spinal instrumentation and fusion: minimum five-year follow-up. Spine 33:2179-2184, 2008.

83. Yagi M, Akilah KB, Boachie-Adjei O. Incidence, risk factors and classification of proximal junctional kyphosis: surgical outcomes review of adult idiopathic scoliosis. Spine 36:E60-E68, 2011.

84. Yagi M, King AB, Boachie-Adjei O. Incidence, risk factors, and natural course of proximal junctional kyphosis: surgical outcomes review of adult idiopathic scoliosis. Minimum 5 years of follow-up. Spine 37:1479-1489, 2012.

85. Harding IJ, Charosky S, Vialle R, et al. Lumbar disc degeneration below a long arthrodesis (performed for scoliosis in adults) to L4 or L5. Eur Spine J 17:250-254, 2008.

86. Kumar MN, Baklanov A, Chopin D. Correlation between sagittal plane changes and adjacent segment degeneration following lumbar spine fusion. Eur Spine J 10:314-319, 2001.

87. Annis P, Lawrence BD, Spiker WR, et al. Predictive factors for APJF after adult deformity surgery with the UIV in the thoracolumbar (TL) spine. Abstract presented at the Annual Meeting of the Lumbar Spine Research Society, Chicago, IL, May 2014.

88. Lafage V, Ames C, Schwab F, et al; International Spine Study Group. Changes in thoracic kyphosis negatively impact sagittal alignment after lumbar pedicle subtraction osteotomy: a comprehensive radiographic analysis. Spine 37:E180-E187, 2012.

89. Smith MW, Annis P, Lawrence BD, et al. Early proximal junctional failure in patients with preoperative sagittal imbalance. Evid Based Spine Care J 4:163-164, 2013.

90. Darrel S, Brodke PA, Brandon D, et al. Early proximal junctional failures in patients older than 55 years with deformity. Presented at the Twentieth International Meeting on Advanced Spinal Technologies, Scoliosis Research Society, Vancouver, BC, Canada, July 2013.

91. Hostin R, McCarthy I, O'Brien M, et al; International Spine Study Group. Incidence, mode, and location of acute proximal junctional failures following surgical treatment for adult spinal deformity. Spine. 2012 Sep 13. [Epub ahead of print]

92. Daubs MD, Lenke LG, Bridwell KH, et al. Does correction of preoperative coronal imbalance make a difference in outcomes of adult patients with deformity? Spine 38:476-483, 2013.

93. Daubs MD, Lawrence BD, Annis P, et al. The contribution of intraoperative patient positioning to overall correction of coronal and sagittal deformity in adults. Presented at the Nineteenth International Meeting on Advanced Spine Techniques, Scoliosis Research Society, Instanbul, Turkey, July 2012.

94. Ames CP, Smith JS, Scheer JK, et al. Impact of spinopelvic alignment on decision making in deformity surgery in adults: a review. J Neurosurg Spine 16:547-564, 2012.

95. Barrey C, Roussouly P, Perrin G, et al. Sagittal balance disorders in severe degenerative spine. Can we identify the compensatory mechanisms? Eur Spine J 20(Suppl 5):626-633, 2011.

96. Roussouly P, Pinheiro-Franco JL. Biomechanical analysis of the spino-pelvic organization and adaptation in pathology. Eur Spine J 20(Suppl 5):609-618, 2011.

97. Berven SH, Deviren V, Smith JA, et al. Management of fixed sagittal plane deformity: results of the transpedicular wedge resection osteotomy. Spine 26:2036-2043, 2001.

98. Bradford DS, Schumacher WL, Lonstein JE, et al. Ankylosing spondylitis: experience in surgical management of 21 patients. Spine 12:238-243, 1987.

99. Bridwell KH, Lewis SJ, Edwards C, et al. Complications and outcomes of pedicle subtraction osteotomies for fixed sagittal imbalance. Spine 28:2093-2101, 2003.

100. Daubs MD, Prokopis A, Brandon D, et al. Perioperative complications of pedicle subtraction osteotomy. Neurosurg Focus 34:A1-A38, 2013.

101. Halm H, Metz-Stavenhagen P, Zielke K. Results of surgical correction of kyphotic deformities of the spine in ankylosing spondylitis on the basis of the modified arthritis impact measurement scales. Spine 20:1612-1619, 1995.

102. Camargo FP, Cordeiro EN, Napoli MM. Corrective osteotomy of the spine in ankylosing spondylitis. Experience with 66 cases. Clin Orthop Rel Res 157-167, 1986.

103. Qian BP, Qiu Y, Wang B, et al. Pedicle subtraction osteotomy through pseudarthrosis to correct thoracolumbar kyphotic deformity in advanced ankylosing spondylitis. Eur Spine J 21:711-718, 2012.

104. Harimaya K, Mishiro T, Lenke LG, et al. Etiology and revision surgical strategies in failed lumbosacral fixation of adult spinal deformity constructs. Spine 36:1701-1710, 2011.

105. Tsuchiya K, Bridwell KH, Kuklo TR, et al. Minimum 5-year analysis of L5-S1 fusion using sacropelvic fixation (bilateral S1 and iliac screws) for spinal deformity. Spine 31:303-308, 2006.

106. Tumialan LM, Mummaneni PV. Long-segment spinal fixation using pelvic screws. Neurosurgery 63:183-190, 2008.

14

Considerations and Pitfalls in Spinopelvic Fixation Techniques: Evidence From the Literature and Recommendations

Cliff B. Tribus

Spinal deformity patients present numerous challenges to surgeons. One of these is the decision of whether or not to cross the lumbosacral junction. The L5-S1 disc space is at a biomechanical disadvantage, because it is adjacent to the pelvis. The large lever arm of the pelvis makes immobilization of this lowest disc space exceedingly difficult. These challenges are magnified when the planned surgical construct extends proximally into the upper lumbar or thoracic spine. In these longer constructs, simple pedicle screws at S1 often prove insufficient to stabilize the L5-S1 disc space enough to promote fusion. The need to extend instrumentation into the lower sacrum or the ilium becomes readily apparent in this patient group.[1-9] This chapter provides a brief history of spinopelvic fixation and indications. Various accepted techniques and biomechanical considerations are presented. Finally, complications of iliosacral fixation are discussed.

EVOLUTION OF TECHNIQUE

In 1982 Luque[8] reported on 65 consecutive patients with scoliosis whose cause was idiopathic (25 patients) or polio (40 patients). In this work he presented his description of segmental instrumentation and sublaminar wires. He also described the L-rod technique in which prebent bars were placed either into the ala of the ilium or immediately inferior to the posterior superior iliac spine (PSIS) of the iliac crest. This appears to be the precursor to the Galveston technique described by Allen and Ferguson.[10]

In 1984 Allen and Ferguson[10] presented in *Spine* their experience with 44 patients requiring pelvic fixation. Their series of patients was treated at the University of Texas Medical Branch in Galveston, Texas; hence the technique was called the *Galveston technique*. Their study dated from April 1978 to October 1982. The authors credited Luque, who had initiated the L-rod instrumentation system. The authors developed their technique and reported that best results occurred with a rod that was longer than 6 cm, completely interosseous within the ilium, and within 1.5 cm of the sciatic notch.[11] Since that time, modern instrumentation techniques and biomechanical studies have better delineated the parameters for pelvic fixation. Allen and Ferguson correctly identified the length of the fixation as being a critical issue. Ultimately, their construct combining smooth rods with iliac fixation to a thoracolumbar construct of rods and sublaminar wires was replaced with much more rigid transpedicular fixation in the thoracolumbar spine and threaded screws in the ilium. Their innovation should not be discounted, however. They refined a system that incorporated lumbosacral fixation into the ilium.

In 1991 Boachie-Adjei et al[1] reported on 22 patients treated with the Galveston technique, which consisted of fixation into the pelvis and a Luque construct proximally. They promoted the idea of anterior multilevel discectomy and fusion without instrumentation followed by posterior instrumentation in a staged technique. With this refined technique they reduced their pseudarthrosis rate, reporting a fusion rate of 77%, and maintained lumbar lordosis by avoiding distraction.

In 1992 McCord et al[12] presented their widely referenced work on biomechanical analysis of lumbosacral fixation (Fig. 14-1). They used an in vitro calf model to test 10 standard lumbosacral spine fixation systems. Their stated goals were to determine whether or not newly evolved pedicle screw systems provided biomechanical advantage over the Harrington technique of distraction hooks into the sacrum or the previously described Luque fixation technique. Their constructs included a control, S1 pedicle fixation, fixation in S2, and fixation spanning the sacroiliac joint into the ilium. Their work showed the superiority of iliac fixation. Triangulation of pedicle screws showed biomechanical superiority, and extension of screws down to S2 added a biomechanical advantage. Yet it was the iliac screws that substantially increased stability across the L5-S1 disc space. The authors described the "pivot point," which is a point at the posterior aspect of the L5-S1 disc. Any instrumentation in the sacrum or ilium has a superior biomechanical advantage if the tip of the instrumentation extends anterior to this pivot point. This was particularly true with iliac screws. This study also proved to be fairly pivotal in the conversion of Harrington distraction constructs and Luque rectangular constructs to become little more than historical entities.

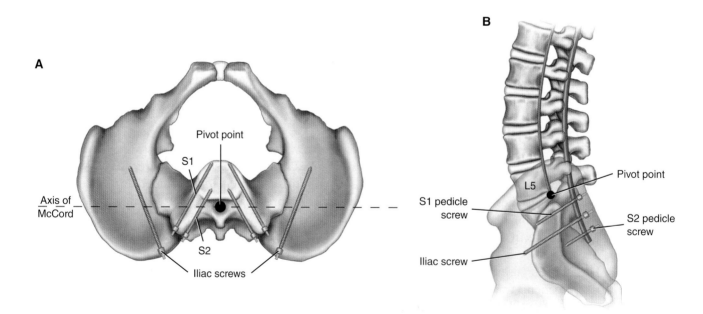

Fig. 14-1 **A,** Axial and **B,** lateral views show the pivot point described by McCord et al. (Adapted from McCord DH, Cunningham BW, Shono Y, et al. Biomechanical analysis of lumbosacral fixation. Spine 17[8 Suppl]:S235-S243, 1992.)

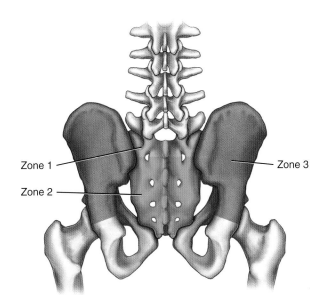

Fig. 14-2   Sacroiliac zones 1, 2, and 3, as described by O'Brien et al. (Adapted from O'Brien MF, Kuklo TR, Lenke LG. Sacropelvic instrumentation: anatomic and biomechanical zones of fixation. Semin Spine Surg 16:76-90, 2004.)

In 2004 O'Brien et al[13,14] further refined our understanding of iliosacral fixation techniques. Based on this biomechanical study, they described fixation zones of the iliosacrum. Zone 1 is the S1 level of the sacrum. Zone 2 refers to the rest of the sacrum and zone 3 is the ilium (Fig. 14-2). As instrumentation is added to each successive zone, the fixation strength increases.

INDICATIONS

Extension of instrumentation to the distal sacrum or ilium should be considered in the following clinical situations:
- A fusion to the sacrum with proximal extension to L2 or above. This can be performed as a primary operation in an adult deformity patient, to link a previous thoracolumbar fusion to the sacrum, or to treat a previous pseudarthrosis of L5-S1 below a long fusion[1-9] (Figs. 14-3 and 14-4).
- A high-grade spondylolisthesis[15] (Fig. 14-5)
- A sagittal imbalance with flat-back syndrome requiring an osteotomy[1-9] (Fig. 14-6)
- Planned correction of pelvic obliquity[1-9]
- A sacral fracture below a lumbar fusion[16]
- Resection of a sacral tumor[17]

The common denominator of each of these diagnoses is the inordinate amount of biomechanical stress at the L5-S1 level either because of the long constructs involved or the reduction forces inherent in the deformity correction.

The addition of an interbody fusion at L5-S1 through an anterior approach or a posterior interbody approach is strongly supported particularly in the adult population. Whereas biomechanical studies do not show that the addition of an anterior interbody grafting adds much to the strength of the construct, the additional exploitation of surface area for fusion mass and restoration of the anterior column at this challenging level make it well worth the additional surgical insult.[15,18] In 2010 Lee et al[19] reported on the critical length of fusion requiring additional fixation to the ilium to prevent nonunions of the lumbosacral junction. They presented their data on 327 patients, 47 of whom had nonunions at the L5-S1 junction. They showed union rates of greater than 87% from L3 to the sacrum, 92% from L4 to the sacrum, and 96% from L5 to the sacrum. When fusions were extended above L3, the fusion rate was less than 65%. A reasonable interpretation of these data is to add iliac fixation for fusion to the sacrum from L2 or above.

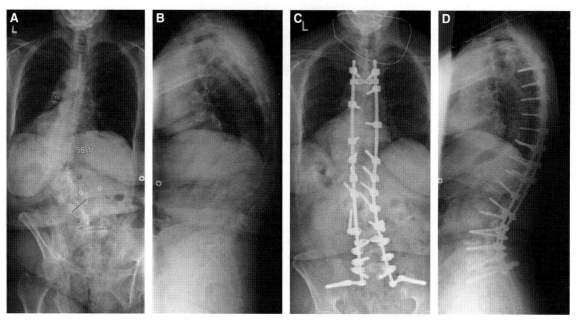

Fig. 14-3　**A** and **B,** Preoperative AP and lateral radiographs of a patient with kyphoscoliosis. **C** and **D,** Postoperative AP and lateral radiographs of the same patient after thoracic to iliac crest instrumentation.

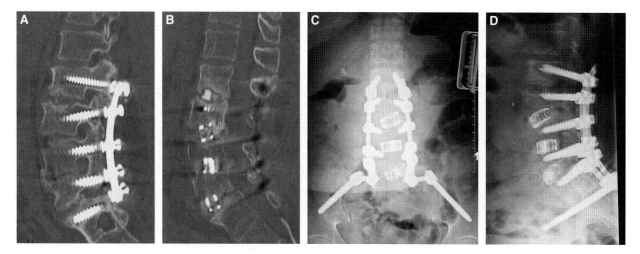

Fig. 14-4　**A** and **B,** Preoperative sagittal CT scans of a patient with L2-3 and L5-S1 pseudarthrosis. **C** and **D,** Postoperative AP and lateral radiographs of the same patient after revision pseudarthrosis repair and iliac fixation.

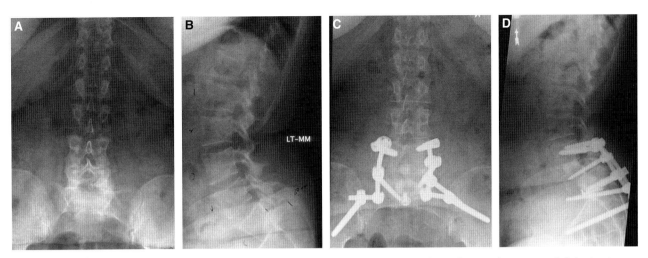

Fig. 14-5 **A** and **B,** Preoperative AP and lateral radiographs of a patient with grade III isthmic spondylolisthesis. **C** and **D,** Postoperative AP and lateral radiographs of the same patient after anterior-posterior L4-S1 posterior spinal fusion with iliac fixation.

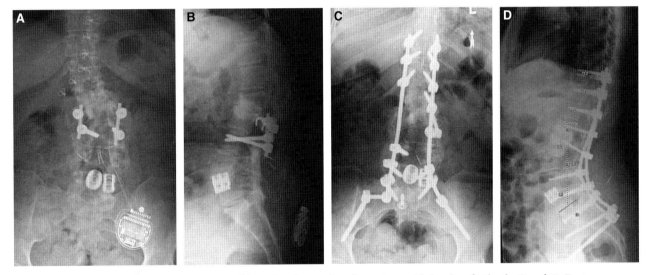

Fig. 14-6 **A** and **B,** Preoperative AP and lateral radiographs of a patient with lumbar flat back. **C** and **D,** Postoperative AP and lateral radiographs of the same patient after an osteotomy and reconstruction with iliac screws.

OPTIONS FOR ILIOSACRAL FIXATION

S1 SCREWS

S1 screws are the most common modern form of sacral fixation. Pseudarthrosis rates are higher, however, with longer constructs; therefore additional fixation is indicated. In 2002 Lehman et al[20] reported on the biomechanics of S1 screw positioning. Tricortical fixation was presented as being strongest, followed by bicortical and unicortical fixation.

S1 AND S2 SCREWS

The addition of S2 fixation points improves sacral fixation strength, but only minimally. Divergence of the S2 screws proximally and laterally into the sacral ala provides the best S2 fixation points. The relative advantage of this technique is that the sacroiliac joint is not violated. However, the anterior projection of the S1 and S2 screws does not pass anteriorly enough to cross the pivot point described by McCord; thus fixation options that include the ilium provide added biomechanical advantage. Additionally, the use of S1 and S2 screws particularly with available sacral plate systems substantially reduces the surface area available for fusion mass.[21] Vascular injury can result from penetration of the anterior cortex with S1 and S2 screws.

INTRASACRAL RODS

Jackson and McManus[22] first described intrasacral rods. These devices share both the advantages and disadvantages of S2 screws in that they spare the sacroiliac joint but remain dorsal to the pivot point. Technically the rod penetrates the posterior sacral cortex at the level of S2 and passes laterally to the sacral foramina, remaining within the sacrum without penetrating the anterior cortex. The rods are smooth and lack the fixation of iliac screws, but preservation of the posterior cortex provides resistance to failure in flexion.

ILIOSACRAL SCREWS

Iliosacral screws are technically challenging. They are placed from a starting point lateral to the PSIS and are directed across the sacroiliac joint through the S1 pedicles. The advantage is the ability to capture four cortices. However, biomechanically they are not as strong as iliac screws; they cross the sacroiliac joint and are more challenging to place.

ILIAC BARS

Iliac bars involve placement of a single or double rod through each PSIS posterior to the sacrum. The spinal rod is then cross-connected to the iliac bar. The sacroiliac joint is crossed, and the fixation remains posterior to the pivot point. However, in situations such as tumor resections, sacral bars can be useful in a surgeon's armamentarium.

ILIAC SCREWS

Iliac screws have largely replaced the Galveston technique as the strongest construct to fix long, instrumented fusions to the iliosacrum. The increased modularity of modern systems and further understanding of iliac anatomy has simplified their use.[18,23-25] The sacroiliac joint is spanned, and this is of clinical consequence, but if performed appropriately, fixation anterior to the pivot point can be obtained. Hardware prominence of iliac screws can result in a clinical problem and should be anticipated when choosing a staring point for the screws. Pelvic anatomy may obviate the possibility of placing bilateral iliac screws. A unilateral screw can alternatively be placed, resulting in similar biomechanics.[26]

Several authors have written about iliac screw length and trajectory. In 2001 Berry et al[23] delineated two lines of trajectory for iliac screws starting from the PSIS. The first directs the screw toward the superior border of the acetabulum. In the second trajectory, the screw is directed from the PSIS toward the anterior superior iliac spine. This line resulted in minimal screw length of up to 110 mm in adults and 90 mm in teenagers. In 2010 Tian et al[24] showed that a screw of up to 135 mm in males and 110 mm in females can be placed along this trajectory. Placement of iliac screws of at least 100 mm in length should be possible in most adults; the goal is a minimum screw length of 80 mm in males and 70 mm in females. The important concept is to confirm that the screw length runs anterior to the pivot point, does not enter the acetabulum, and remains entirely within bone.

In the traditional open technique of iliac screw placement, the PSIS is the starting point. Aggressive rongeuring of the PSIS allows the starting point to be recessed and limits hardware prominence. Fluoroscopy can facilitate placement of a pedicle finder between the inner and outer table of the ilium. Alternatively, the outer table of the ilium can be exposed, providing a palpable reference point and access to bone graft and facilitating palpation of the sciatic notch. Rough parameters for a trajectory are 25 degrees laterally and 30 degrees caudally. Probing for cortical violations should be performed. Tapping is done, especially in strong bone, and the screw is placed. Radiographic confirmation that the sciatic notch and acetabulum have not been violated is critical. Screws are connected to the lumbosacral construct either directly to the rod or through extenders. This construct has the relative advantage of spanning the sacroiliac joint rather than crossing it directly (Fig. 14-7).

Variations on starting points for iliac screws have been developed to serve a variety of purposes, for example, to prevent hardware prominence, to facilitate connectivity to the lumbosacral construct, or to make minimally invasive techniques more user friendly. The starting point for these techniques is generally moved medially.

In 2010 Kebaish[27] introduced S2-alar (S2AI) screws. The starting point of S2 allows a much lower profile to the head of the screw and better alignment with the S1 screw for ease of rod connection. It has also proved technically feasible with a percutaneous approach.[28] The starting point for the S2AI screw is inferior and lateral to the S1 foramina, with a trajectory of 45 degrees to the floor and 20 to 30 degrees caudal. Fluoroscopy is helpful. The major disadvantage of S2AI screws is that they directly penetrate the sacroiliac joint. This disadvantage may prove to be of little clinical consequence[29] (Fig. 14-8).

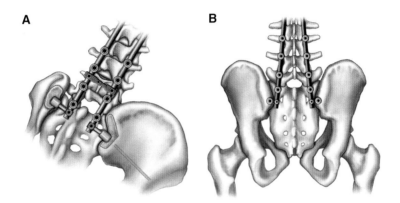

Fig. 14-7 **A,** Oblique and **B,** AP images demonstrate the iliac screw fixation technique. A notched starting point in the posterior superior iliac spine is extended to connect the iliac screw to the rod.

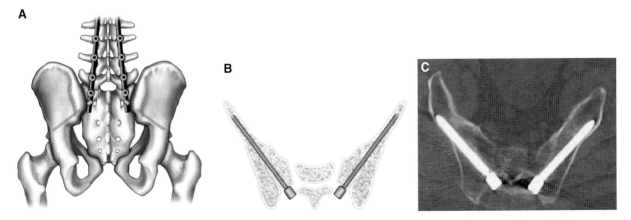

Fig. 14-8 **A,** AP and **B,** axial images demonstrate placement of S2AI screws. **C,** An axial CT scan shows S2AI screws crossing the sacroiliac joint. (**C,** Courtesy of Khaled M. Kebaish, MD.)

A four-rod technique that employs two pairs of iliac screws has been described. A linked, four-rod technique has been shown to be more rigid than a linked, two-rod technique. A four-rod technique is more complicated than a two-rod technique, yet it may have usefulness in sacral tumor reconstructions or in patients in whom sacral fixation is otherwise compromised.[17,30]

COMPLICATIONS OF ILIAC SCREW FIXATION

Cho et al[2] reported an overall failure rate of lumbopelvic fixation of 34.3% in their series of 67 patients who received S1 screws and iliac screws in a long construct. Risk factors included larger pelvic incidence, undercorrection of lumbar lordosis, and sagittal balance. The absence of anterior column support at L5-S1 was not a statistically significant risk factor.

Loosening of iliac screws is a common complication of iliac fixation. In the Cho series,[2] five patients had iliac screw halos, and each of these patients had an improved ODI score. Unlike pedicle screw loosening elsewhere in the spine, this finding does not mean that pseudarthrosis or even a clinical problem is present. Loosening of iliac screws is likely a reflection of the continued motion through the sacroiliac joint placing stress on the iliac fixation. Sacral pain can be present with iliac fixation in the setting of loose or well-fixed iliac screws. Pain can be relieved by removal of the iliac screws, but it is recommended that this be delayed until at least 1 year after the index procedure. Hardware prominence of the iliac screws can also be corrected by late hardware removal and has a higher predictability of favorable outcome. Unrecognized acetabular violation will have catastrophic consequences for the affected hip joint and should be vigilantly ruled out before leaving the operating room.

CONCLUSION

Iliosacral fixation is an important technique for spinal surgeons. The various constructs differ in ease of placement, strength, and complications. The categories striate nicely into constructs that remain completely within the sacrum and those that cross the sacroiliac joint and exploit the ilium. Surgeons must decide which construct is appropriate for their patients and execute the procedure with awareness of efficacy, efficiencies, and complications.

REFERENCES

1. Boachie-Adjei O, Dendrinos GK, Ogilvie JW, et al. Management of adult spinal deformity with combined anterior-posterior arthrodesis and Luque-Galveston instrumentation. J Spinal Disord 4:131-141, 1991.
2. Cho W, Mason JR, Smith JS, et al. Failure of lumbopelvic fixation after long construct fusions in patients with adult spinal deformity: clinical and radiographic risk factors: clinical article. J Neurosurg Spine 19:445-453, 2013.
3. Devlin VJ, Asher MA. Biomechanics and surgical principles of long fusions to the sacrum. Spine State Art Rev 10:515-544, 1996.
4. Kostuik JP, Hall BB. Spinal fusions to the sacrum in adults with scoliosis. Spine 5:489-500, 1983.
5. Kostuik JP. Spinopelvic fixation. Neurol India 53:483-488, 2005.
6. Kuklo TR, Bridwell KH, Lewis SJ, et al. Minimum 2-year analysis of sacropelvic fixation and L5-S1 fusion using S1 and iliac screws. Spine 26:1976-1983, 2001.
7. Luque ER, Cardoso A. Segmental correction of scoliosis with rigid internal fixation, preliminary report. Orthop Trans 1:136-137, 1977.
8. Luque ER. The anatomic basis and development of segmental spinal instrumentation. Spine 7:256-259, 1982.
9. Tsuchiya K, Bridwell KH, Kuklo TR, et al. Minimum 5-year analysis of L5-S1 fusion using sacropelvic fixation (bilateral S1 and iliac screws) for spinal deformity. Spine 31:303-308, 2006.

10. Allen BL Jr, Ferguson RL. The Galveston technique of pelvic fixation with L-rod instrumentation of the spine. Spine 9:388-395, 1984.

11. Allen BL Jr, Ferguson RL. The Galveston experience with L-rod instrumentation for adolescent idiopathic scoliosis. Clin Orthop Relat Res 229:59-69, 1988.

12. McCord DH, Cunningham BW, Shono Y, et al. Biomechanical analysis of lumbosacral fixation. Spine 17(8 Suppl):S235-S243, 1992.

13. O'Brien MF, Kuklo TR, Blanke KM, et al, eds. Spinal Deformity Study Group Radiographic Measurement Manual. Memphis, TN: Medtronic Sofamor Danek, 2004.

14. O'Brien MF, Kuklo TR, Lenke LG. Sacropelvic instrumentation: anatomic and biomechanical zones of fixation. Semin Spine Surg 16:76-90, 2004.

15. Molinari RW, Bridwell KH, Lenke LG, et al. Complications in the surgical treatment of pediatric high-grade, isthmic dysplastic spondylolisthesis. A comparison of three surgical approaches. Spine 15:1701-1711, 1999.

16. Klineberg E, McHenry T, Bellabara C, et al. Sacral insufficiency fractures caudal to instrumented posterior lumbosacral arthrodesis. Spine 33:1806-1811, 2008.

17. Shen FH, Harper M, Foster WC, et al. A novel "four-rod technique" for lumbopelvic reconstruction: theory and technical considerations. Spine 31:1395-1401, 2006.

18. Lebwohl NJ, Cunningham BW, Dmitriev A, et al. Biomechanical comparison of lumbosacral fixation techniques in a calf spine model. Spine 27:2312-2320, 2002.

19. Lee CS, Chung SS, Choi SW, et al. Critical length of fusion requiring additional fixation to prevent nonunion of the lumbosacral junction. Spine 35:E206-E211, 2010.

20. Lehman RD, Kulkot TR, Anderson RC, et al. Advantages of pedicle screw fixation directed into the apex of the sacral promontory over bicortical fixation: a biomechanical analysis. Spine 27:806-811, 2002.

21. Park YS, Kim HS, Baek SW, et al. Lumbosacral fixation using the diagonal S2 screw for long fusion in degenerative lumbar deformity: technical note involving 13 cases. Clin Orthop Surg 5:225-229, 2013.

22. Jackson RP, McManus AC. The iliac buttress. A computed tomographic study of sacral anatomy. Spine 18:1318-1328, 1993.

23. Berry JL, Stahurski T, Asher MA. Morphometry of the supra sciatic notch intrailiac implant anchor passage. Spine 26:E143-E148, 2001.

24. Tian X, Li J, Sheng W, et al. Morphometry of iliac anchorage for transiliac screws: a cadaver and CT study of the Eastern population. Surg Radiol Anat 32:455-462, 2010.

25. Tis JE, Helgeson M, Lehman RA, et al. A biomechanical comparison of different types of lumbopelvic fixation. Spine 34:E866-E872, 2009.

26. Tomlinson T, Chen J, Upasani V, et al. Unilateral and bilateral sacropelvic fixation result in similar construct biomechanics. Spine 33:2127-2133, 2008.

27. Kebaish KM. Sacropelvic fixation: techniques and complications. Spine 35:2245-2251, 2010.

28. O'Brien JR, Matteini L, Yu WD, et al. Feasibility of minimally invasive sacropelvic fixation: percutaneous S2 alar iliac fixation. Spine 35:460-464, 2010.

29. Sponseller PD, Zimmerman R, Ko PS, et al. Low profile pelvic fixation using S2 alar iliac (S2AI) fixation in the pediatric population improves results at two-year minimum follow-up: paper #86. Spine: Affiliated Society Meeting Abstracts 10:114, 2009.

30. Kelly BP, Shen FH, Schwab JS, et al. Biomechanical testing of a novel four-rod technique for lumbo-pelvic reconstruction. Spine 33:E400-E406, 2008.

PART III

Biomechanics of Spinal Deformity and Effects of Spinal Instrumentation

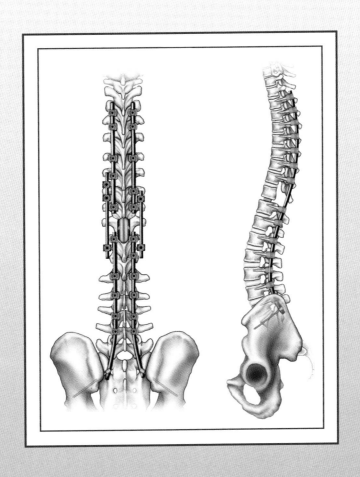

15

Materials and Biomaterials Used for Spinal Deformity Correction

Adam Lindsay ▪ *Eric Otto Klineberg*

Albee[1] developed spinal fusion surgery in 1911 for the management of Pott's disease. He placed a tibial implant to stabilize and stop the spread of spinal tuberculosis. It is now used for the correction of many different pathologies. Fractures, dislocations, neoplastic disruptions, kyphosis, spondylolisthesis, intervertebral disc disease, and scoliosis are some of the spinal abnormalities that are treated with spinal fusion. For a fusion to occur, both biological and mechanical stability must be achieved. Spinal implantation allows surgeons to provide stability needed for fusion and restoration of normal spinopelvic alignment. This is a much broader spectrum than Albee first envisioned.

Spinal deformity correction today relies on the same principles: controlled realignment and maintenance and an osseous union. Spinal instrumentation plays a significant role and has seen major advances in the past 50 years. In 1962 Harrington[2] developed the first spinal instrumentation, consisting of steel rods and internal fixation that used hooks with distraction (Fig. 15-1). The system was beautifully simple and used a single rod to correct scoliosis across multiple spinal levels. In polytrauma patients, the Harrington method can provide a quick and stable three-point fixation when combined with a rod sleeve. Although this sys-

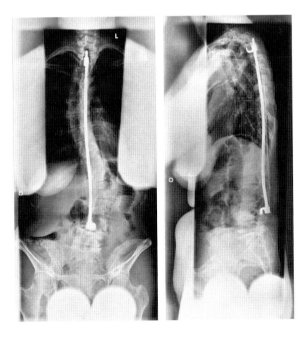

Fig. 15-1 The Harrington single rod for the correction of coronal scoliosis with a typical flat-back deformity.

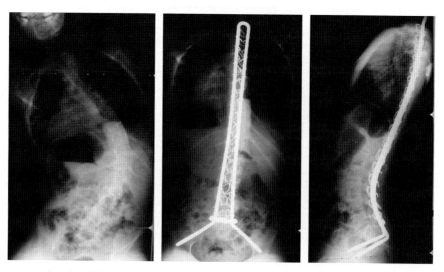

Fig. 15-2   A Luque rod and sublaminar rods were placed in this patient to correct neuromuscular scoliosis. The stainless steel rod is a single rod that has been contoured and fixed to the spine with sublaminar wires and intraosseous pelvic fixation.

tem had inherent complications, including a high rate of pseudarthroses formation, caudal sacral hook dislodgement, and flat-back syndrome at the lumbar spine, it is the basis from which many other systems have evolved.

During the decades after the introduction of Harrington's first rod instrumentation, the Galveston technique was developed for spinal deformity correction. Allen and Ferguson[3] reported enhanced lumbosacral stability of the Luque rod[4] when the distal end of the rod was fixed intraosseously to the pelvis (Fig. 15-2). They described improved operative outcomes and less frequent component failure when more than 6 cm of the L-rod was inserted into the ilium. Rapid developments of new techniques, metals, and implant choices over the past 50 years offer surgeons a variety of options for spinal deformity correction. Both adult and pediatric spinal curvature corrections have been implemented with rods, screws, wires, hooks, and interbody cage systems, which were developed in an effort to promote fusion and correct deformity.[5]

The goal of this chapter is to familiarize readers with the most recent and widely used materials and biomaterials in adult spinal deformity surgery. We discuss the relative strengths and weaknesses of the most common spinal deformity materials that are used for implants and of interbody fusion options. Considerable variability exists between instrumentation, surgical approach, and unique device specifications.

IMPLANTS

The consensus in both the literature and in clinical practice is that no single material is best. Surgeons must rely on the clinical context and past experience to guide their choice of materials that are best suited for the ideal outcome.[6] Examples of these important considerations include: preoperative bone density and quality, the number of levels to be fused, the vector of injury or traumatic disruption of anatomy, the surrounding structures (including soft tissue damage), the immune status of the patient, and the anticipated mechanical stress to be placed on materials during fusion. Each patient's biology and ability to achieve a spinal fusion are critical. All implants and material choices will fail if union does not occur.

Options for fusionless devices are evolving. Interest is growing in the treatment of degenerative cervical and lumbar disease with total disc arthroplasty, and results are variable.[7,8] New options exist for the management of pediatric scoliosis. Early-onset scoliosis is commonly managed with growing rods that are changed often; however, new magnetic rods allow lengthening in situ.[9,10] New technology for patients with adolescent idiopathic scoliosis involves the use of anterior tethering and staples to guide growth to correct scoliosis before or in lieu of fusion.[11,12] Large animal models have shown vertebral tethers to be effective in creating[13] and correcting idiopathic scoliosis.[14] Tethers provide a dynamically stable yet corrective system to modulate spinal scoliosis. They are particularly useful for correcting large curvature defects.[15] Although clinical data are minimal and comprise a description by Crawford and Lenke[16] of two pediatric patients with no complications, they offer an exciting new possibility for fusionless correction of idiopathic spinal scoliosis, particularly in patients who are at high risk of progression. Finally, new materials with memory (nitinol) can be used to gradually correct scoliosis after fixation in the spine.[17]

BIOMECHANICS

The general properties of materials used for spinal surgery include Young's modulus, stress, strain, and strength versus stiffness. Most implants, cages, and wires are composed of metallic components. Stress (defined as force per unit area) and strain (defined as the amount of deformation a material undergoes compared with its initial size and shape) of a material need to be considered[18] (Fig. 15-3). A material under stress will undergo deformation, either plastic or elastic. Elastic deformation is characterized by a material's ability to return to its original length. Plastic deformation instead indicates when a material is permanently held in the shape it has following the force application. The point at which linear elastic deformation is surpassed and then progresses to plastic deformation is known as the *yield point*. Stress and strain are proportional until the yield point is reached. After this point, given both linear and angular forces on the fusion materials, materials' respective abilities to undergo plastic or elastic deformation will differ.[18,19] The strength of a material is then governed by how quickly it reaches the yield point.

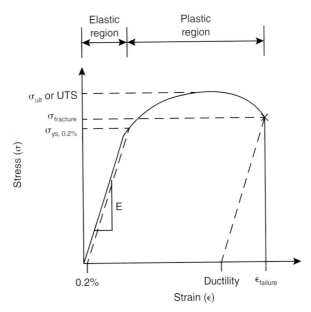

Fig. 15-3 A standard stress-strain curve. *Ductility* is the plastic strain at failure. The *area under the curve* is material toughness. (*E*, Modulus of elasticity, or Young's modulus; σ_{ult} *or UTS*, ultimate tensile strength [highest stress reached]; σ, stress in pounds per square inch; $\sigma_{fracture}$, strength at fracture; $\sigma_{ys, 0.2\%}$, offset yield strength; ε, the corresponding strain [unitless]; $\varepsilon_{failure}$, strain at failure.) (Adapted from Lucas GL, Cooke FW, Friis E, eds. A Primer of Biomechanics. New York: Springer-Verlag, 1999.)

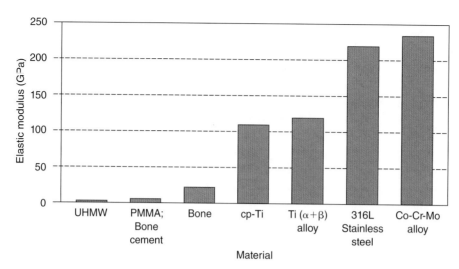

Fig. 15-4   Elastic modulus of some materials commonly used in orthopedic surgeries. (*Co-Cr-Mo,* Cobalt-chromium-molybdenum; *cp-Ti,* commercially pure titanium; *GPa,* gigapascals; *PMMA,* polymethylmethacrylate; *Ti* (α + β), titanium (alpha-type + beta-type); *UHMW,* ultrahigh molecular weight.) (Republished with permission of Taylor and Francis Group LLC Books, from Biomaterials in Orthopedics, Yaszemski MJ, Trantolo DJ, Lewandrowski KU, Hasirci V, Altobelli DE, Wise DL, 2004, pp 41-62; permission conveyed through Copyright Clearance Center, Inc.)

The *modulus of elasticity* (Young's modulus) is defined as a constant of deformability of a material; that is, the elastic properties of a material, given a linear compression or stretching force. It is by definition the ratio of stress to strain and a measure of the stiffness of a material. Simply stated, stress is the force applied to a material, strain is the material's response measured as a change in length compared with the original length, and the elastic (Young's) modulus is the amount of force resistance of the material. In a stress-strain curve, Young's modulus is the slope of the curve under the elastic region of the curve: the steeper the curve, the stiffer the material. At the proportional limit, the proportional increase in stress versus strain is exceeded, and deformation begins.

Biomechanical evaluation of the materials listed in Fig. 15-4 includes their respective strength, stiffness, and modulus properties.[20,21] Surgeons should consider these properties in combination with the clinical parameters when choosing a material or materials.

STEEL

Steel has been a prolific and long-standing material used in spinal fusion. Surgical steel has proved to be a reliable and incredibly strong material for orthopedic surgeries for more than 50 years. Its role in spinal surgery has diminished over the past two decades in large part because of the availability of more radiologic and clinically favorable materials.[22] However, because of the aging population and reduction in mortality associated with spinal surgery, the opportunities for steel implants are still numerous and relevant for discussion.

Stainless surgical steel is a ferruginous alloy composed mainly of iron with chromium, nickel, magnesium, molybdenum, and carbon.[23] Combinations of materials adjust the corrosive or modulus of steel with only minor changes to its overall biomechanical properties. Its construction is fairly simple and relatively inexpensive, compared with other materials. The nickel component plays a role in hypersensitivity reactions. A small subset of patients may have a true allergic reaction to nickel and require allergy testing or the use of a different material.[24]

Table 15-1 Comparison of Physical and Mechanical Properties of Various Implant Materials and Natural Bone

Properties	Natural Bone	Magnesium	Ti Alloy	CoCr Alloy	Stainless Steel	PEEK
Density (g/cm³)	1.8-2.1	1.74-2.0	4.4-4.5	8.3-9.2	7.9-8.1	1.3
Elastic modulus (GPa)	3-20	41-45	110-117	230	189-205	3.6
Compressive yield strength (MPa)	130-180	65-100	758-1117	450-1000	170-310	172
Fracture toughness (MPa m^½)	3-6	15-40	55-115	N/A	50-200	23.6 (at 90° C)

Adapted from Staiger MP, Pietak AM, Huadmai J, et al. Magnesium and its alloys as orthopedic biomaterials: a review. Biomaterials 27:1728-1734, 2006.
CoCr, Cobalt chromium; *g/cm*, grams per centimeter; *GPa*, gigapascal; *MPa*, megapascal; *N/A*, not applicable; *PEEK*, polyetheretherketone; *Ti*, titanium.

Steel has a very high modulus of elasticity and a high yield point[25,26] (Table 15-1). This property makes it an excellent choice for holding the spine in a fixed position. However, it requires greater strength to deform the rod for proper contouring and more mobilization of the spine to the rod. Once deformed, steel has low ductility and maintains the shape of the bend. This can help a surgeon gain the correction desired, but it significantly stresses the bone-implant interface. Careful consideration of bone density is critical when a decision is made to use steel anchors.

Metal implants can corrode over time. Significant attention has been given to the metal ions that leach into a patient's bloodstream. Therefore corrosion of the primary rigid materials used in fusion surgery need to be considered preoperatively.[27] Surgical steel, compared with other materials, has shown increased corrosion in in vivo and in vitro studies.[27-29] Interestingly, when Serhan et al[29] evaluated galvanized fusion materials from cadaver spines in normal saline solution, they found that steel underwent significantly more corrosion. Surgical steel is considered inferior to both titanium and cobalt chrome (CoCr) in this regard.

Surgical steel has significant imaging characteristics. As with each metal implant discussed in this chapter, artifact generation during MRI or CT can have substantial clinical implications. Steel fares relatively poorly compared with other implants because of its increased ferrous content.[22] Indeed, the artifact created on radiologic imaging with surgical steel are substantially greater than newer spine surgery materials, including other metals.

Despite the drawbacks of surgical steel, it has three distinct advantages. First, it is one of the most rigid materials; therefore it is the least likely to fracture or fail under strain. Second, because of its long-standing use, highly customized steel materials can be obtained fairly easily. Finally, it is the least expensive of all the surgical materials mentioned in this chapter.

TITANIUM

Titanium (Ti), or more recently Ti-Al-vanadium alloy, is one of the most prolific materials used in orthopedic surgery. Spinal surgery is not an exception, and Ti use has expanded from a supplemental material to the mainstay of spinal implants. It is used in cages, rods, and screws. In any venue where metal is applied as a support, Ti has been heavily studied with good results.[6,30] We will discuss some of the recent data that do and do not support the use of Ti implants.

Ti and its alloys are five times as stiff as cortical bone and approximately half as stiff as CoCr and steel.[26,31] Although this characteristic allows greater stress distribution to adjacent surfaces, it predisposes them to elastic deformation from significant stressors. Surgeons familiar with Ti rods will note that immediately on release from bending, they have a peculiar rebound effect. Often, this necessitates overbending Ti rods to achieve the appropriate curvature, which is not required with other metallic implants. This intraoperative phenomenon is attributed to change within the bent region, but the material remains stable in the unbent region.[32] Further, Ti rods are particularly sensitive to notching or surface scratching.[31] Ti-based alloys create a layer of corrosion resistance, but surface scratching or notching will compromise the oxide layer and increase corrosion.[33] Ti is also known to be especially susceptible to wear when in contact with ultrahigh-molecular-weight polyethylene because of poor shear strength and increased corrosion via the same mechanism seen in notching, although this is reduced with ionic treatment of the metal.[34-36]

Despite the drawbacks of Ti, it is used prevalently in adult spinal reconstruction. The most often mentioned clinical quality of Ti is the lack of interference with common imaging studies. Given the alloy composition of many Ti-based implants, it is safe to use in MRI scans, which are most valuable for identifying and preserving neural structures. Although older studies contributed to the general knowledge about titanium's safety and superior imaging[37] in MRI, newer publications further establish radiologic advantages of Ti over newer metals.[38]

Biomechanically and biophysically, Ti is a considerably ductile material (especially compared with steel and CoCr). However, this provides multiple surgical advantages. First, Ti implants have greater yield strength (see Table 15-1)—the strength before the material fails—because it allows more plastic deformation before failure. In essence, the lower elastic modulus of Ti implants allows greater distribution of load to surrounding vertebral bodies, which confers a protective effect on the implant itself. These properties of Ti are especially helpful in preventing difficulties with adjacent fracture of adjacent vertebral segments proximal and distal to the construct.

Additionally, Ti provides an excellent strength/weight ratio. Ti alloys further advance this benefit by stabilizing the materials. As seen with surgical steel, the choice of material in surgery depends in part on its ability to be manipulated before insertion. Ti is advantageous in that, unlike other metals, its ductility allows surgeons to curve and adjust the fixtures to patient-specific anatomy with relative ease. Usually, the rod needs to be bent so that its curvature is more than that of the final desired curvature because of ductility. The biomechanical properties of Ti provide compelling evidence for its use, and these reasons are further bolstered by its clinical properties.

Surgeons must always consider the material properties that affect patient outcomes. Ti has been shown to provide excellent long-term stability. Of particular interest to surgeons is the resistance Ti instruments have to biofilm development.[6,39] Given the consequences of postoperative infections, including revision surgery, reimplantation, intravenous antibiotics, and prolonged or additional hospitalizations, Ti has become the material of choice in patients who have an ongoing infection or are at considerable risk for developing one.

Many patients with surgical metal implants inquire about their ability to pass through airport metal detectors when traveling. Recently, Chinwalla and Grevitt[40] evaluated sensitivity of spinal implants to metal detectors. They compared known spinal reconstruction patients' reactivity to both archway and handheld metal detectors. Archway detectors did not detect up to 215 g of Ti, but handheld devices detected all types of metal. Because of heightened security at most airports, it is critical that patients have appropriate documentation.

COBALT CHROME

CoCr implant use in spinal fusion is relatively new. Although its biomechanical properties are similar to those of surgical steel, literature to support its use as a stand-alone material is relatively sparse. CoCr has been most often used in spinal rods, because it makes these instruments stronger, compared with Ti, with similar imaging characteristics.[38,41,42]

CoCr is second only to Ti with regard to corrosion. Nevertheless, CoCr instrumentation has come under scrutiny because of the amount of ion leeching that develops with normal corrosion of the material. Recent publications in major medical journals have discussed a disturbing correlation between cobalt ions from hip prostheses and the development of dilated cardiomyopathy.[43,44] Suggestions have been made that any type of instrumentation containing cobalt present in patients with heart failure should prompt the analysis of blood cobalt. However, careful meta-analyses have shown that only under rare conditions should a physician suspect significant systemic effects of cobalt.[45] The threshold for adverse effect of metallic ions is a blood cobalt concentration of 300 μ/L. A recent review concluded that polycythemia is the most sensitive indicator of systemic disease, but clinical evaluation is warranted if cardiac, endocrine, or hematologic symptoms are noted in implant patients. Finally, early chelation with diethylenetriamine pentaacetic acid (DTPA) has been recommended for cobalt radionuclide chelation, although dimercaptosuccinic acid (DMSA), ethylenediaminetetraacetic acid (EDTA), and N-acetylcysteine are also effective.[45,46] Clinical monitoring and early chelation have been suggested to reduce progression of disease; however, no formal guidelines on chelation therapy have been established.

CoCr has advantages and disadvantages in terms of its material strength. It is more ductile than steel and has an increased yield strength compared with Ti (see Table 15-1); however, CoCr implants can cause unintended bone damage.[47] Surgeons should strongly consider the extent of osteoporosis in patients with a kyphotic or scoliosed spine, because the rigidity of the rod will challenge the bone-screw interface.[33] Additionally, the total failure strength of CoCr implants is not yet known, but studies have shown it to be heavily resistant to fatigue.[42] Further cadaveric and animal models are needed to quantify the forces that cause the material to fail.

CoCr is significantly better than steel for imaging, but it is inferior to Ti in this regard, particularly near the cobalt implant. In a recent study comparing imaging artifacts of CoCr and Ti, Ahmad et al[41] found artifacts on axial T1- and T2-weighted MRI to be approximately 3.5 mm smaller in patients with Ti instrumentation. They evaluated 15 patients via postoperative MRI (6 with CoCr, 9 with Ti) who underwent lumbar spinal fusion. Blinded radiologists then measured and quantified the amount of artifact noted with each material. Although CoCr implants generated a significantly greater artifact size, the authors found no difference in visualization of the spinal canal. These findings are promising, because although CoCr may mildly disrupt local soft tissue evaluation, it may not affect radiologic identification of canal obstruction.

NITINOL

Nitinol is a nickel-Ti alloy that is relatively new to spinal instrumentation. Interest in nitinol is driven largely by its unique biomechanical properties. That is, nitinol has superelasticity, allowing the metal to retain shape memory.[48,49] It has high resistance to kinking or plastic deformation, providing exceptional stability while maintaining physiologic load-bearing capabilities. This may allow a rod that has been manufactured with a curve to continue to exert corrective force after placement. Additional correction can occur with time, or with growth. Nitinol is largely used in cardiovascular stents, kink-resistant guide wires, and tools employed in minimally invasive surgeries. It is beginning to be used more frequently in spinal rod systems and locking mechanisms.[50] It has proved effective as a staple material in the correction of moderate idiopathic pediatric scoliosis.[51] The prebent staple is placed parallel to the endplate, but it will attempt to regain its shape and exert the corrective force on the spinal growth plates and therefore modulate the growth of the spinal column. Further, ninitol is relatively well tolerated (most likely because of the Ti component) and has been shown to evoke little local inflammatory responses by host tissue in animal studies.[52] The obvious drawbacks are the risk for development of hypersensitivity reactions to nickel alloy.

POLYETHERETHERKETONE POLYMER RODS

Despite the advantages of metals, the pressures that they place on the vertebral spine can be detrimental to adjacent spinal segments. Despite the application of more flexible and dynamic systems that redistribute load (for example, the Dynesys system [Zimmer, Inc., Warsaw, IN]), adjacent-level disease and fracture remain a significant problem for deformity surgeons.[53,54] As recently as 2007, semirigid instrumentation made from synthetic polymers such as polyetheretherketone (PEEK) have surfaced as an alternative.[55] With an elastic modulus between those of cancellous and cortical bone but substantially lower than that of Ti (see Table 15-1), PEEK rods provide a minimal amount of motion along the spinal segment. This in turn provides more evenly distributed load sharing, and potentially reduces adjacent-segment degeneration, strain to the pedicle screws, and construct failure particularly in osteoporotic bone. Indeed, PEEK systems have been described as a good alternative for treating a moderately degenerate suboptimal disc.[6,56,57]

Compared biomechanically with metal systems, PEEK systems have shown increased durability, strength, stability, and overall biomechanical profile.[55-57] They are radiolucent, usually with contrast agent to identify breakages; therefore visualization of structures on CT and MRI is optimal. This advantage makes detection of rod failure difficult with conventional imaging modalities such as radiography or CT, because the rods are radiolucent. PEEK rod systems more closely mimic physiologic load displacement loads to the anterior column, primarily as a result of their relatively low elastic modulus. This reduces stress on the bone-screw interface.[58,59] Though physiologically superior, the systems are not flawless, however, and they are susceptible to fracture.

The primary disadvantages of PEEK systems are their cost and limited use in multilevel spinal fusion. At this time, they are considerably more expensive than all other available rod materials, including Ti alloys. PEEK rods are not used for deformity surgery, because they cannot be easily manipulated or contoured for patient-specific correction. Currently, they are only used in limited (one-level or two-level) fusions. The contour of PEEK rod systems cannot be adjusted to fit a patient's specific anatomy; therefore they are useless when larger spinal distances must be spanned for correction.

SUBLAMINAR WIRES AND CABLES

Sublaminar wires can be used at the apical curve for deformity correction and provides a greater ability to regain kyphosis, compared with pedicle screw–only constructs.[54,60-62] Wire-only techniques, as first described by Luque,[61] are rarely used; however, hybrid wire-rod and wire–pedicle screw constructs are still employed. Sublaminar wire anchor points are usually placed in the thoracic spine to improve kyphosis by drawing the spine to the precontoured rods (see Fig. 15-2). Sublaminar wiring has a variety of drawbacks, most notably poor control of the spine in the axial plane, which typically requires thoracoplasty for cosmesis, rather than vertebral derotation. Additionally, the placement of sublaminar wires has the potential to cause substantial neurologic damage, and although it has proved safe through multiple studies, it requires surgical expertise.[60,62]

Stainless steel was the original wire material used for spinal surgery but has fallen out of favor recently for two reasons. It has galvanized properties that make it incompatible with Ti implants,[29] and it creates excess imaging artifacts on CT and MRI. Pure Ti is not used as a sublaminar wire material, because it is easily stretched and fractured during tightening, given its biomechanical properties. CoCr and Ti alloy wires instead provide the compatibility and tensile strength necessary for appropriate stabilization. CoCr wires have been approved by the FDA for spinal corrective surgery as recently as 2005, despite long-standing use in hip surgery.[33] Cluck and Skaggs[60] found CoCr wires to be superior to stainless steel wires in tension and load to failure cycles. CoCr alloy wire's ductile properties, they noted, allow the wires to be tightened and retightened multiple times with a substantially lower rate of failure. Despite the learning curve for the use of CoCr sublaminar wires in corrective surgery, they can provide a safe and reliable method of curve correction, particularity at the apex of the kyphosis.

SUBLAMINAR TETHERS

Sublaminar wires have the disadvantage of breaking and cutting through porous bone, and they can be technically challenging to place and manipulate. To combat these problems, sublaminar tethers have been developed. They use the same biomechanical principles for sublaminar fixation but can be tightened and retightened with little risk of fatigue failure. They are typically composed of nylon or other braided material for excellent strength and allow a broader surface area of contact along the lamina to prevent pullout. Additionally, unlike metal wires, they are not subject to fatigue failure or fracture during application.

INTERBODY DEVICES

In contrast to the extravertebral support provided by the Harrington rod technique or the Galveston technique, surgeons may choose to perform anterior discectomy and release to promote anterior fusion. These interbody devices are varied and provide immediate anterior support and correction[63] (Fig. 15-5). From a mechanical perspective, anterior interbody insertion shields axial stress while minimizing shearing and torsional bending.[6] The biomechanical properties of rod systems contribute to cage material selection. However, interbody fusion for spinal correction has the distinct advantage that bone grafts can be used alongside other biomaterials.[6,33,56,64]

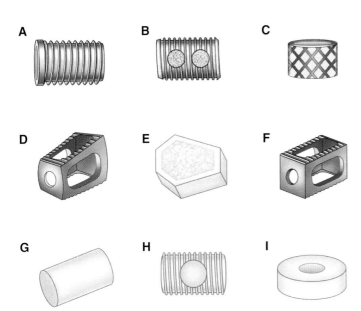

Fig. 15-5 Lumbar interbody fusion devices. **A,** Ray cylindrical threaded fusion cage. **B,** Bagby and Kuslich (BAK) cylindrical threaded fusion cage (Spine-Tech, Inc., Minneapolis, MN). **C,** Surgical titanium mesh. **D,** Tapered (lordotic) fusion cage. **E,** Iliac crest autograft or allograft bone. **F,** Carbon fiber fusion cage. **G,** Nonthreaded femoral cortical bone dowel. **H,** Threaded femoral cortical bone dowel. **I,** Femoral ring allograft. The devices shown in **E, G, H,** and **I** are derived from biologic materials. (Adapted from Devlin VJ, Pitt DD. The evolution of surgery of the anterior spinal column. Spine 12:493-528, 1998.)

Although the interbody approach does not inherently require interbody devices, the addition of supporting structures has shown improvements in construct stiffness. Interbody cages can be combined with single- or double-rod systems to increase stability and for anterior-only correction. Fricka et al[65] found that although a dual-rod anterior system provided superior flexion-extension and torsional stiffness, it did not improve lateral bending stiffness. They concluded that adding a second rod may be helpful to obtain the initial lordosis, but it does not impart additional stiffness to the overall construct.

Drawbacks to anterior implantation with cages are largely related to cost and surgical morbidity. Anterior instrumentation requires substantial familiarity with the approach in the thoracolumbar region.[6,56,63,66] Potential complications include damage to the great vessels and to the mediastinal and gastrointestinal structures in the thoracic and lumbar spine, respectively. An access surgeon may be required for patients with particularly difficult pathology.

Polyetheretherketone Interbody Cages

Synthetic interbody cages can be made in any specific shape, and they maintain consistent load-bearing capabilities. They can be combined with fixation devices and screws for immediate stabilization. They are resistant to fracture or deformation based on their biomechanical properties.[33,55] Additionally, they do not transmit disease or require complex sterilization techniques. Threaded interbody fusion devices have been in use for over 15 years with favorable results.[67] Anterior load-bearing devices made from different metals or synthetic polymer increase construct stiffness and decrease the incidence of posterior implant failure.[68] Recent changes to cage coatings, alloys, and bone-metal-protein combinations have further enhanced the clinical and biomechanical outcomes in spinal fusion. The implants themselves will never be incorporated into the body but can be used to manipulate the spine and to provide stability for fusion to occur either within or around them. The finer details of spinal fusion are out of the scope of this chapter; however, one of the distinct advantages of anterior cage constructs is their improved spinal segment fusion. They may be filled with autologous bone (most commonly from the preceding corpectomy), which in turn leads to improved fusion. More impressively, when combined with osteoinductive materials such as rhBMP-2, PEEK cages have excellent fusion properties, often achieving or exceeding fusion rates of 80%.[69]

PEEK cages, as with PEEK rod systems, are superior in their imaging qualities and load sharing.[70] As discussed previously, they provide a more physiologic load-bearing material in both a posterior construct and an interbody device. However, PEEK cages have a few practical advantages over metal-alloy constructs. Similar to bone but unlike alloy devices, PEEK cages can be drilled for revision and correction. PEEK implants have the distinct advantage of relatively easy removal, whereas metal implants are a considerably more complex surgical obstacle. In the cervical spine, PEEK implants been shown to be superior to titanium implants in maintaining cervical interspace height.[71] PEEK and Ti are often combined to optimize the load-bearing properties of these materials.

Osseointegration and fusion are paramount to the long-term viability of inserted graft. PEEK systems have a unique disadvantage in that they often fail to integrate with host bone, and thus limit incorporation of the graft. Recently, Han et al[72] sought to overcome these biocompatibility limitations by coating the PEEK materials with Ti. Interestingly, they found that low-temperature electron-beam coating of PEEK materials with Ti markedly improved the biocompatibility—as measured by bone-implant contact—of PEEK screws both in vivo and in vitro. They noted that osteoblast cellular responses can be up to twofold more in Ti-covered screws, compared with uncovered materials. The drastic improvement in biocompatibility has led manufacturers to begin coating their cages with Ti in an effort to draw surgeons back to PEEK implants for fusion.

Titanium Interbody Cages

Titanium and Ti alloys have a vastly improved stiffness modulus and superior imaging, compared with surgical steel.[61] Although their imaging interference is not as ideal as that of PEEK systems, they provide more consistent mechanical support. Polly et al[73] used a simulated single-level spinal fusion model to evaluate the biomechanical supplementation that titanium interbody cages provided. They compared interbody cage positioning (anterior, posterior, or middle) and posterior rod diameter (4 or 5 mm) and the resulting effect on construct stiffness, interbody cage strain, and intracage pressure under compressive flexural loading. They made two important biomechanical conclusions: (1) the addition of a titanium interbody cage provided additional construct stiffness if positioned in the anterior position and (2) as the cage was moved from the posterior to the anterior position, strain on the posterior rods decreased. Compared with bone grafts, however, Ti has inferior osteogenic properties; these can be corrected when the cage construct is combined with bone stimulating products or grafts. Ti cages can be modified to incorporate screws for immediate stabilization. Finally, Ti is superior to other graft materials (PEEK in particular) in that it is more readily overgrown by host bone and far less costly to manufacture. Surface etching and modification in Ti alloy materials widen this disparity and correlates well with osseous integration.[74]

The use of titanium cages as fixation adjuncts in anterior and posterior fusion has been scrutinized. In a randomized clinical trial comparing the use of femoral ring allograft versus titanium cages in circumferential lumbar fusions, allograft showed an improved clinical outcome.[75] In 78 patients with similar demographics, ODI, VAS for back and leg pain, and SF-36 results were significantly improved at the 26-month follow-up. The authors described titanium as inferior clinically and less cost effective. Additionally, because Ti cages are often filled with either osteogenic materials or cancellous/cortical bone mixtures, they are extremely difficult to remove or modify once the graft has fused.[76]

A recent study evaluating the biomechanical properties of fibular versus Ti grafts, however, revealed no significant differences in the stiffness of these materials.[77] Using isolated cadaver vertebrae, T11-12 and L2-3 were fused, underwent corpectomy, and either one of two Ti cages were installed and secured. Stiffness was measured under flexion, extension, and lateral left and right bending. The authors found no difference in stiffness between materials. Though these reports provide valuable biomechanical information, the variability in overall strength of the graft that is dependent on muscular and soft tissue involvement should be considered.

Carbon Fiber Interbody Cages

Carbon fiber implants contain a similar modulus to bone, and reinforcement with PEEK enhances resistance to deformation with prolonged strain.[78] Bone has an elastic modulus of approximately 20 GPa, and traditional polymer-based implants may exceed this by 20- to 30-fold.[79] Coating of PEEK with carbon fiber reduces this discrepancy, allowing more even distribution of loads to adjacent structures, thus reducing patent bone and component damage.

One drawback of carbon fiber–PEEK implants stems from the inherent hydrophobicity of the materials themselves. Bone apposition is limited at the bone-implant surface because of resultant fibrous tissue placement at the bone-implant interface. Devine et al[80] sought to limit this by coating the carbon fiber–PEEK screws with Ti to prevent this complication. They found significant bone apposition and removal torque improvements with the coated materials. Coating with more biocompatible materials may also improve cage incorporation, but this has yet to be tested.

BIOABSORBABLE POLYMER IMPLANTS

Bioabsorbable implants are an attractive alternative to traditional bone or metallic cages. They can facilitate progressive loading as the resorption process continues.[81] There is, however, concern that resorption through phagocytosis creates additional inflammatory tissue. These cages, or spacers, can be filled with autologous bone grafts for improved results. Coe[82] described impressive fusion rates (96.8%) using operative cylindrical bioabsorbable polymer spacers manufactured with a 70:30 copolymer of poly-L-lactide and D,L-lactide (Hydrosorb, Medtronic Sofamor Danek, Memphis, TN) and packed with iliac crest autograft bone. The fusion rates were recorded after the known life expectancy of the material. This seemingly offers another alternative to bone grafts and may provide an implantable device void of metallic ions.

Unfortunately, polymer implants have an unpredictable and often intense inflammatory response. Böstman et al[83] described a nonspecific foreign body reaction to implanted biodegradable rods that manifested as sterile sinus drainage and giant cell development at the implant site. Frost et al[84] recently reviewed cases and described extensive osteolysis at the 1-year follow-up. Despite the sparse clinical data on these materials, concern about the predictability of resorption and inflammatory response has led many companies to abandon the production of these cages.

CORTICAL ALLOGRAFT

Allograft (homologus) or autograft (autologous) bone material has been traditionally used in the interbody space in spinal fusion. Placement of this graft stimulates osteogenesis, resulting in new bone tissue. The resulting mineralization—and thus fusion—allows greater load and physiologic stress bearing; hence it is used throughout the spine. Even more impressive is the variety of sources that can stimulate osteogenesis. Bone, fat, and muscle have been shown to have osteogenic stem cells and progenitor cells capable of promoting fusion.[6,85,86] Donor site morbidity associated with harvesting autologous bone is often considered the limiting factor in the use of this biologic material.[6,87]

The composition of each of the bone grafts has many advantages and disadvantages. The biomechanical properties of each will be briefly discussed as they pertain to the comparison of autologous versus cadaveric bone graft materials. In general, a graft achieves load-bearing capacity after complete biologic incorporation, which is intimately related to biologic and mechanical properties of the graft-host interface.[33] Only a small amount of original graft survives because of limited nutrient delivery, and other physiologic abnormalities will alter the relative strength of the graft itself.[88]

Autologous bone grafts have fairly obvious immunoneutral properties, giving them a distinct advantage in promoting fusion. They can easily be removed for revision and augmented with additional biocompatible materials. Autologous cortical bone is often used as a strut in anterior lumbar interbody fusion or as bone-wire constructs in cervical spinal fusion.[88] Cortical bone implants obviously have an improved rate of biocompatibility with surrounding spinal tissues, but this comes at a biomechanical cost.[5,89,90] Cortical bone has both a lower Young's modulus—thus a lower resistance to loads before reaching yield strength—and decreased stiffness, compared with alloy and polymer materials. Therefore cortical bone grafts will reach a point of plastic deformity sooner than other materials (see Figs. 15-3 and 15-4).

Compared with other bone graft materials, the main mechanical advantage of cortical bone is superior mechanical strength at the time of insertion. In anterior interbody approaches, this is of paramount importance. However, unlike bioabsorbable materials, which hold strength despite absorption, or metallic materials, which fail to absorb at all, cortical bone has repeatedly demonstrated loss of mechanical strength over a period of 12 to 24 months. Increased porosity of the graft occurs mainly in the first 2 years via the phenomenon of *creeping substitution,* wherein osteoblastic appositional bone reconstruction occurs along existing channels, which is prolonged in cortical bone.[88] At 2 years the loss in strength plateaus, and the physical integrity of the graft normalizes.[88] Logically, mechanical strength loss is inversely associated with graft patency. To maximize the incorporation of the bone graft while minimizing the loss of strength from creeping substitution, cortical bone is often combined with cancellous bone.

Attempts at combining cortical and cancellous bone are common. Cancellous percentages remain consistently at approximately 59% of the graft, regardless of wedge size.[90] Unfortunately, these combinations are often considerably variable in their mechanical strength and may depend on harvest site, surgical manipulation, and initial bone health.[33,90] As an example, Takeda[90] showed that grafts from the anterior iliac crest provided increased mechanical support compared with grafts from the posterior crests. Similarly, the compression strength of fibular grafts significantly exceeds that of rib grafts.[89]

Allograft is appealing, because it allows incorporation, can be easily manipulated, and has no donor morbidity. It is similar but not equal to autograft, however. The sterilization process substantially decreases the overall mechanical compression strength in these grafts.[91] Irradiation and freeze-drying have both been shown to have a dose-dependent, deleterious effect on the time to microfracture and mechanical resistance to loads. Cornu et al[92] provided the explanation that the sterilization process inadvertently lowers a graft's ability to absorb and distribute stress and in turn makes the material more brittle.[33] Even with more-recent sterilization techniques that spare the compression stress of allograft bones,[91] they are still often considered inferior mechanically because of increased time to fusion with host bone.

CONCLUSION

Spinal surgeons have many options when choosing appropriate materials and biomaterials for spinal deformity correction. Certainly there is no right implant for every case, and each implant needs to be tailored to the patient and to the surgical procedure. New products and new material combinations are available and offer surgeons more choices and more complexity. In the future, new material combinations are sure to emerge, and their effectiveness and cost effectiveness will determine their adoption.

REFERENCES

1. Albee HF. Transplantation of a portion of the tibia into the spine for Pott's disease. A preliminary report 1911. Clin Orthop Relat Res 460:14-16, 2007.
2. Harrington PR. Treatment of scoliosis correction and internal fixation by spine instrumentation. J Bone Joint Surg Am 44:591-610, 1962.
3. Allen BL Jr, Ferguson R. The Galveston technique of pelvic fixation with L-rod instrumentation of the spine. Spine 9:388-394, 1984.
4. Luque ER. Segmental spinal instrumentation for correction of scoliosis. Clin Orthop Relat Res 163:192-198, 1982.
5. Moshirfar A, Rand FF, Sponseller PD, et al. Pelvic fixation in spine surgery: historical overview, indications, biomechanical, relevance, and current techniques. J Bone Joint Surg Am 87(Suppl 2):89-106, 2005.
6. Herkowitz HN, Garfin SR, Eismont FJ, et al, eds. Rothman-Simeone The Spine: Expert Consult, vol 1. Philadelphia: Elsevier, 2011.
7. Blumenthal S, McAfee PC, Guyer RD, et al. A prospective, randomized, multicenter Food and Drug Administration investigational device exemptions study of lumbar total disc replacement with the CHARITE artificial disc versus lumbar fusion. I. Evaluation of clinical outcomes. Spine 30:1565-1575, 2005.
8. Pickett GE, Mitsis DK, Sekhon LH, et al. Effects of a cervical disc prosthesis on segmental and cervical spine alignment. Neurosurg Focus 17:1-35, 2004.
9. Akbarnia BA, Cheung K, Noordeen H, et al. Next generation of growth-sparing techniques: preliminary clinical results of a magnetically controlled growing rod in 14 patients with early-onset scoliosis. Spine 38:665-670, 2013.

10. Yue JJ, Bertagnoli R, McAfee PC, et al, eds. Motion Preservation Surgery of the Spine: Advanced Techniques and Controversies. Philadelphia: Elsevier, 2008.

11. Guille JT, D'Andrea LP, Betz RR. Fusionless treatment of scoliosis. Orthop Clin North Am 38:541-545, 2007.

12. Newton PO, Farnsworth CL, Faro FD, et al. Spinal growth modulation with an anterolateral flexible tether in an immature bovine model: disc health and motion preservation. Spine 33:724-733, 2008.

13. Roth AK, Bogie R, Jacobs E, et al. Large animal models in fusionless scoliosis correction research: a literature review. Spine J 13:675-688, 2013.

14. Braun JT, Akyuz E, Udall H, et al. Three-dimensional analysis of 2 fusionless scoliosis treatments: a flexible ligament tether versus a rigid-shape memory alloy staple. Spine 31:262-268, 2006.

15. Braun JT, Akyuz E, Ogilvie JW, et al. The efficacy and integrity of shape memory alloy staples and bone anchors with ligament tethers in the fusionless treatment of experimental scoliosis. J Bone Joint Surg Am 87:2038-2051, 2005.

16. Crawford CH III, Lenke LG. Growth modulation by means of anterior tethering resulting in progressive correction of juvenile idiopathic scoliosis: a case report. J Bone Joint Surg Am 92:202-209, 2010.

17. More RB, Sanders JO, Sanders AE. Nitinol spinal instrumentation and method for surgically treating scoliosis. U.S. Patent No. 5,290,289. Mar 1, 1994.

18. Lucas GL, Cooke FW, Friis E, eds. A Primer of Biomechanics. New York: Springer-Verlag, 1999.

19. Tamarin Y, ed. Atlas of Stress-Strain Curves, ed 2. Metals Park, OH: ASM International, 2002.

20. Ashman RB, Birch JG, Bone LB, et al. Mechanical testing of spinal instrumentation. Clin Orthop Relat Res 227:113-125, 1988.

21. Niinomi M, Tomokazu H, Shigeo N. Material characteristics and biocompatibility of low rigidity titanium alloys for biomedical applications. In Yaszemski MJ, Trantolo DJ, Lewandrowski KU, et al, eds. Biomaterials in Orthopedics. New York: Marcel-Dekker, 2004.

22. Rudisch A, Kremser C, Peer S, et al. Metallic artifacts in magnetic resonance imaging of patients with spinal fusion: a comparison of implant materials and imaging sequences. Spine 23:692-699, 1998.

23. Disegi JA, Eschbach L. Stainless steel in bone surgery. Injury 31:D2-D6, 2000.

24. Pavan A, Williams JG, eds. Fracture of Polymers, Composites and Adhesives, vol 27. Philadelphia: Elsevier, 2000.

25. Yaszemski MJ, ed. Biomaterials in Orthopedics. Boca Raton, FL: CRC Press, 2013.

26. Staiger MP, Pietak AM, Huadmai J, et al. Magnesium and its alloys as orthopedic biomaterials: a review. Biomaterials 27:1728-1734, 2006.

27. Cahoon JR, Holte RN. Corrosion fatigue of surgical stainless steel in synthetic physiological solution. J Biomed Mat Res 15:137-145, 1981.

28. Heller JG, Shuster JK, Hutton WC. Pedicle and transverse process screws of the upper thoracic spine: biomechanical comparison of loads to failure. Spine 24:654-658, 1999.

29. Serhan H, Slivka M, Albert T, et al. Is galvanic corrosion between titanium alloy and stainless steel spinal implants a clinical concern? Spine J 4:379-387, 2004.

30. Niinomi M. Mechanical biocompatibilies of titanium alloys for biomedical applications. J Mech Behav Biomed Mat 1:30-42, 2008.

31. Dick JC, Bourgeault CA. Notch sensitivity of titanium alloy, commercially pure titanium, and stainless steel spinal implants. Spine 26:1668-1672, 2001.

32. Nakai M, Niinomi M, Zhao X, et al. Self-adjustment of Young's modulus in biomedical titanium alloys during orthopaedic operation. Mater Let 65:688-690, 2011.

33. Benzel EC. Spine Surgery: Techniques, Complication Avoidance, and Management (Expert Consult-Online), ed 3. Philadelphia: Elsevier, 2012.

34. Semlitsch M. Titanium alloys for hip joint replacements. Clin Mater 2:1-13, 1987.

35. Xiong D, Zhan G, Zhongmin J. Friction and wear properties of UHMWPE against ion implanted titanium alloy. Surf Coat Technol 201:6847-6850, 2007.

36. McKellop HA, Röstlund TV. The wear behavior of ion-implanted Ti-6A1-4V against UHMW polyethylene. J Biomed Mater Res 24:1413-1425, 1990.

37. Rupp R, Ebraheim NA, Savolaine ER, et al. Magnetic resonance imaging evaluation of the spine with metal implants. General safety and superior imaging with titanium. Spine 18:279-385, 1993.

38. Trammell TR, Flint K, Ramsey CJ. A comparison of MRI and CT imaging clarity of titanium alloy and titanium alloy with cobalt-chromium-alloy pedicle screw and rod implants in the lumbar spine. J Bone Joint Surg Am 94:1479-1483, 2012.

39. Zhao L, Chu PK, Zhang Y, et al. Antibacterial coatings on titanium implants. J Biomed Mater Res B Appl Biomat 91:470-480, 2009.

40. Chinwalla F, Grevitt MP. Detection of modern spinal implants by airport metal detectors. Spine 37:2011-2016, 2012.

41. Ahmad FU, Sidani C, Fourzali R, et al. Postoperative magnetic resonance imaging artifact with cobalt-chromium versus titanium spinal instrumentation: presented at the 2013 Joint Spine Section Meeting. Clinical article. J Neurosurg Spine 19:629-636, 2013.

42. Nguyen TQ, Buckley JM, Ames C, et al. The fatigue life of contoured cobalt chrome posterior spinal fusion rods. Proc Inst Mech Eng H 225:194-198, 2011.

43. Zeh A, Planert M, Siegert G, et al. Release of cobalt and chromium ions into the serum following implantation of the metal-on-metal Maverick-type artificial lumbar disc (Medtronic Sofamor Danek). Spine 32:348-352, 2007.

44. Allen LA, Ambardekar AV, Deveraj KM, et al. Clinical problem-solving. Missing elements of the history. New Engl J Med 370:559-566, 2014.

45. Paustenbach DJ, Galbraith DA, Finley BL. Interpreting cobalt blood concentrations in hip implant patients. Clin Toxicol 52:98-112, 2014.

46. Devlin JJ, Pomerleau AC, Brent J, et al. Clinical features, testing, and management of patients with suspected prosthetic hip-associated cobalt toxicity: a systematic review of cases. J Med Toxicol 9:405-415, 2013.

47. Scheer JK, Tang JA, Deviren V, et al. Biomechanical analysis of cervicothoracic junction osteotomy in cadaveric model of ankylosing spondylitis: effect of rod material and diameter. Presented at the American Society of Mechanical Engineers 2010 Summer Bioengineering Conference, Naples, FL, June 2010.

48. Duerig TW, Pelton A, Stöckel D. An overview of nitinol medical applications. Mater Sci Eng A273:149-160, 1999.

49. Sanders JO, Sanders AE, More R, et al. A preliminary investigation of shape memory alloys in the surgical correction of scoliosis. Spine 18:1640-1646, 1993.

50. Yeung K, Lu WW, Luk KD, et al. Mechanical testing of a smart spinal implant locking mechanism based on nickel-titanium alloy. Spine 31:2296-2303, 2006.

51. Lavelle WF, Samdani AF, Cahill PJ, et al. Clinical outcomes of nitinol staples for preventing curve progression in idiopathic scoliosis. J Pediatr Orthop 31(1 Suppl):S107-S113, 2011.

52. Rhalmi S, Charette S, Assad M, et al. The spinal cord dura mater reaction to nitinol and titanium alloy particles: a 1-year study in rabbits. Eur Spine J 16:1063-1072, 2007.

53. Lafage V, Ames C, Schwab F, et al. Changes in thoracic kyphosis negatively impact sagittal alignment after lumbar pedicle subtraction osteotomy: a comprehensive radiographic analysis. Spine 37:E180-E187, 2012.

54. Mitsunaga LK, Klineberg EO, Gupta MC. Laminoplasty techniques for the treatment of multilevel cervical stenosis. Adv Orthop. 2012 Mar 6. [Epub ahead of print]

55. Kurtz SM, Devine JN. PEEK biomaterials in trauma, orthopedic, and spinal implants. Biomaterials 28:4845-4869, 2007.

56. DeWald RL, Arlet V, Carl AL, et al, eds. Spinal Deformities: The Comprehensive Text. New York: Thieme Medical Publishers, 2003.

57. Mavrogenis AF, Vottis C, Triantafyllopoulos G, et al. PEEK rod systems for the spine. Eur J Orthop Surg Traumatol. 2014 Feb 2. [Epub ahead of print]

58. Bono CM, Kadaba M, Vaccaro AR. Posterior pedicle fixation-based dynamic stabilization devices for the treatment of degenerative diseases of the lumbar spine. J Spinal Disord Tech 22:376-383, 2009.

59. Gornet MF, Chan FW, Coleman JC, et al. Biomechanical assessment of a PEEK rod system for semi-rigid fixation of lumbar fusion constructs. J Biomech Eng 133:081009, 2011.

60. Cluck MW, Skaggs DL. Cobalt chromium sublaminar wires for spinal deformity surgery. Spine 31:2209-2212, 2006.

61. Luque ER. Segmental spinal instrumentation of the lumbar spine. Clin Orthop Relat Res 203:126-134, 1986.

62. Girardi FP, Boachie-Adjei O, Rawlins BA. Safety of sublaminar wires with Isola instrumentation for the treatment of idiopathic scoliosis. Spine 25:691-695, 2000.

63. Devlin VJ, Pitt DD. The evolution of surgery of the anterior spinal column. Spine 12:493-528, 1998.

64. Betz RR, Petrizzo AM, Kerner PJ, et al. Allograft versus no graft with a posterior multisegmented hook system for the treatment of idiopathic scoliosis. Spine 31:121-127, 2006.

65. Fricka KB, Mahar AT, Newton PO. Biomechanical analysis of anterior scoliosis instrumentation: differences between single and dual rod systems with and without interbody structural support. Spine 27:702-706, 2002.

66. Faciszewski T, Winter RB, Lonstein JE, et al. The surgical and medical perioperative complications of anterior spinal fusion surgery in the thoracic and lumbar spine in adults. A review of 1223 procedures. Spine 20:1592-1599, 1995.

67. Ray CD. Threaded titanium cages for lumbar interbody fusions. Spine 22:667-679, 1997.

68. Klemme WR, Owens BD, Dhawan A, et al. Lumbar sagittal contour after posterior interbody fusion: threaded devices alone versus vertical cages plus posterior instrumentation. Spine 26:534-537, 2001.

69. Burkus JK, Gornet MF, Dickman CA, et al. Anterior lumbar interbody fusion using rhBMP-2 with tapered interbody cages. J Spinal Disord Tech 15:337-349, 2002.

70. Cho DY, Liau WR, Lee WY, et al. Preliminary experience using a polyetheretherketone (PEEK) cage in the treatment of cervical disc disease. Neurosurgery 51:1343-1350, 2002.

71. Niu CC, Liao JC, Chen WJ, et al. Outcomes of interbody fusion cages used in 1 and 2-levels anterior cervical discectomy and fusion: titanium cages versus polyetheretherketone (PEEK) cages. J Spinal Disord Tech 23:310-316, 2010.

72. Han CM, Lee EJ, Kim HE, et al. The electron beam deposition of titanium on polyetheretherketone (PEEK) and the resulting enhanced biological properties. Biomaterials 31:3465-3470, 2010.

73. Polly DW Jr, Klemme WR, Cunningham BW, et al. The biomechanical significance of anterior column support in a simulated single-level spinal fusion. J Spinal Disord 13:58-62, 2000.

74. Wong M, Eulenberger J, Schenk R, et al. Effect of surface topology on the osseointegration of implant materials in trabecular bone. J Biomed Mater Res 29:1567-1575, 1995.

75. McKenna PJ, Freeman B, Mulholland RC, et al. A prospective, randomised controlled trial of femoral ring allograft versus a titanium cage in circumferential lumbar spinal fusion with minimum 2-year clinical results. Eur Spine J 14:727-737, 2005.

76. Liao JC, Niu CC, Chen JW, et al. Polyetheretherketone (PEEK) cage filled with cancellous allograft in anterior cervical discectomy and fusion. Int Orthop 32:643-648, 2008.

77. Cardenas RJ, Javalkar V, Patil S, et al. Comparison of allograft bone and titanium cages for vertebral body replacement in the thoracolumbar spine: a biomechanical study. Neurosurgery 66(6 Suppl Operative):314-318, 2010.

78. Steinberg EL, Rath E, Schlaifer A, et al. Carbon fiber reinforced PEEK Optima—a composite material biomechanical properties and wear/debris characteristics of CF-PEEK composites for orthopedic trauma implants. J Mech Behav Biomed Mater 17:221-228, 2013.

79. Rho JY, Ashman RB, Turner CH. Young's modulus of trabecular and cortical bone material: ultrasonic and microtensile measurements. J Biomech 26:111-119, 1993.

80. Devine DM, Hahn J, Geoffery RR, et al. Coating of carbon fiber-reinforced polyetheretherketone implants with titanium to improve bone apposition. J Biomed Mater Res B Appl Biomater 101:591-598, 2013.

81. Middleton JC, Tipton AJ. Synthetic biodegradable polymers as orthopedic devices. Biomaterials 21:2335-2346, 2000.

82. Coe JD. Instrumented transforaminal lumbar interbody fusion with bioabsorbable polymer implants and iliac crest autograft. Neurosurg Focus 16:1-9, 2004.

83. Böstman O, Hirvensalo E, Mäkinen J, et al. Foreign-body reactions to fracture fixation implants of biodegradable synthetic polymers. J Bone Joint Surg Br 72:592-596, 1990.

84. Frost A, Baquori E, Brown M, et al. Osteolysis following resorbable poly-L-lactide-co-D, L-lactide PLIF cage use: a review of cases. Eur Spine J 21:449-454, 2012.

85. Bosch P, Musgrave DS, Lee JY, et al. Osteoprogenitor cells within skeletal muscle. J Orthop Res 18:933-944, 2000.

86. Gronthos S, Franklin DM, Leddy HA, et al. Surface protein characterization of human adipose tissue-derived stromal cells. J Cell Physiol 189:54-63, 2001.

87. Younger EM, Chapman MW. Morbidity at bone graft donor sites. J Orthop Trauma 3:192-195, 1989.

88. Muschler GF, Lane JM, Dawson EG. The biology of spinal fusion. In Cotler JM, Cotler HB, eds. Spinal Fusion: Science and Technique. New York: Springer-Verlag, 1990.

89. Wittenberg RH, Moeller J, Shea M, et al. Compressive strength of autologous and allogenous bone grafts for thoracolumbar and cervical spine fusion. Spine 15:1073-1078, 1990.

90. Takeda M. Experience in posterior lumbar interbody fusion: unicortical versus bicortical autologous grafts. Clin Orthop Relat Res 193:120-126, 1985.

91. Mikhael MM, Huddleston PM, Zobitz ME, et al. Mechanical strength of bone allografts subjected to chemical sterilization and other terminal processing methods. J Biomech 41:2816-2820, 2008.

92. Cornu O, Banse X, Docquier PL, et al. Effect of freeze-drying and gamma irradiation on the mechanical properties of human cancellous bone. J Orthop Res 18:426-431, 2000.

16

Behavior of Interbody Implant Materials

Sharath Bellary ▪ *Sohaib Z. Hashmi* ▪ *Kevin Sonn* ▪ *Wellington K. Hsu*

Although conventional lumbar spine fusion surgery has historically involved the posterolateral approach, interbody fusion procedures have contributed to the evolution of arthrodesis techniques. The associated procedures include anterior lumbar interbody fusion (ALIF), posterior lumbar interbody fusion (PLIF), transforaminal lumbar interbody fusion (TLIF), and lateral interbody fusion. Lumbar interbody spine fusion principles were originally described during the 1930s and involve a total discectomy followed by instrumentation to contain bone grafts and to stabilize the fused segments.[1,2]

Interbody fixation has several advantages over posterolateral fusion. With interbody fixation, bone healing depends on compression in the disc space versus tension along the intertransverse processes. Interbody grafts bear 80% of spinal loads in compression; posterolateral grafts bear only 20% of such loads.[3] Interbody grafts can occupy up to 90% of intervertebral bony surface area, whereas posterolateral grafts typically occupy only 10% of the total surface area.[4] The interbody space is more vascularized than the posterolateral space, thereby providing greater opportunity for bony fusion.

To achieve solid, load-sustaining arthrodesis while restoring coronal and sagittal balance, selection of the appropriate interbody graft type is critical. Interbody implant materials include autograft, allograft, titanium cages, and polyetheretherketone (PEEK), bioabsorbable, and ceramic devices. This chapter will review the unique biomechanical properties and characteristics of these materials.

AUTOGRAFT

Autologous bone graft remains the standard against which graft alternatives are compared. Autograft bone provides all of the characteristics necessary for bone growth and regeneration: osteoinductive signals through growth factors, an osteoconductive matrix scaffold, osteogenic cells, and the capacity for vascularization.[5] With PLIF, an 88% fusion rate has been reported with the use of autologous corticocancellous strips and pegs alone (without supplementary fixation) at 1 year of follow-up.[6] However, iliac crest bone graft (ICBG) has disadvantages. ICBG harvest–associated complications and morbidities include deep hematoma, incisional hernia, permanent neurologic injury, vascular injury, sacroiliac joint injury, ureteral injury, permanent Trendelenburg gait, donor site fracture, deep infection, persistent donor site pain, and cosmetic dissatisfaction.[7] The most frequently reported complication is chronic donor site pain, which has been reported to be as high as 60% at 2 years of follow-up.[8] However, more recent studies suggest that chronic autograft harvest site pain has been overestimated. In a cross-sectional clinical study, Howard et al[9] studied harvest site pain intensity and severity in 112 patients who had posterior lumbar fusion followed by either autograft ICBG or recombinant human bone morphogenic protein-2 (rhBMP-2) and no graft harvest, with a mean follow-up duration of 41 months (range 6 to 211 months). The authors concluded that the incidence of pain over the iliac crest was similar for both groups of patients. In addition to the associated complications, the harvest procedure can increase surgical time and blood loss. Iliac crest can be in limited supply and have variable performance in high-risk individuals.

ALLOGRAFT

Allogenic bone graft is the most common nonautologous graft material used during spine surgery. Mineralized allograft bone primarily provides osteoconductivity. It has low osteoinductive and osteogenic capacities, because osteoprogenitor cells are lost during tissue processing and transplantation. This alternative can be used as a stand-alone or supplemental treatment or as a graft extender during interbody fusion. Allograft bone can be used as a structural cortical allograft with a femoral ring or bone dowel to provide substantial structural stability that is suitable for interbody arthrodesis[10,11] (Fig. 16-1). Particulate cancellous allograft has been packed inside interbody spacers or cages.[12,13] Corticocancellous allografts combine both of these bone types and can be more quickly integrated into a fusion site as a result of the larger surface area of cancellous bone, compared with stand-alone cortical constructs.[10,11] Although allograft chiefly provides osteoconductive potential with minimal osteogenic capacity, bony incorporation along the sites of compression is often seen.

Allograft bone poses the potential risk of disease transmission from the donor tissue. To minimize this risk, the American Association of Tissue Banks established guidelines that are required for all accredited tissue banks. All tissue banks must also uphold the U.S. Food and Drug Administration guidelines for allograft tissue transplantation.[14] Serologic testing includes evaluation for antibodies to HIV, hepatitis B surface antigen, syphilis rapid plasma reagent and fluorescent treponemal antibody, hepatitis C virus, and human T-cell lymphocyte virus 1.[14] With proper donor evaluation and tissue processing, there have been no reports of bacterial disease transmission and only one case of viral disease transmission of HIV from 1994 to 2007.[15] The risk of HIV transmission in screened allograft bone has been estimated at 1 in 1.6 million.[16]

Several characteristics determine the mechanical strength of individual allografts. Corticocancellous graft fabrication with cuts perpendicular to the long axis and closer to the ends of long bones results in the strongest compressive strength.[17] Because bone mineral density decreases in adults, donor age is an important consideration during bone harvest. To maintain sufficient compressive strength of the allograft, harvesting from male donors who are less than 55 years old and female donors who are less than 45 years old has been suggested.[14] Each harvest location has unique mechanical properties. Mechanical compression tests of allografts have demonstrated the greatest strength in the femoral cortical rings followed by fibular, posterior tricortical iliac, anterior iliac crest, and rib grafts in descending order of force to failure[18,19] (Table 16-1). Brantigan et al[20] investigated the clinical mechanical properties of allograft bone processed for PLIF. The authors found no significant difference in compressive mechanical strength between allograft prepared by freeze-drying, air-drying, ethylene oxide sterilization, or incubation at 37° C for 1 week before testing.[20]

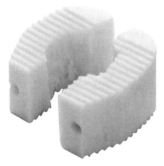

Fig. 16-1   Cortical allograft interbody device. (Image provided by Medtronic Sofamor Danek USA.)

Table 16-1 Biomechanical Failure Load and Stiffness Properties of Allografts Used in Lumbar Interbody Fusion

Allograft Location	Failure Load (kN)	Stiffness (kN)
Femur	45 ± 18	42.4 ± 6.9
Fibula	13.9 ± 3.8	26.5 ± 6.4
Iliac crest (zones 1, 2, and 3)	5.5 ± 1.8	9.3 ± 4.1

From Rao S, McKellop H, Chao D, et al. Biomechanical comparison of bone graft used in anterior spinal reconstruction: freeze-dried demineralized femoral segments versus fresh fibular segments and tricortical iliac blocks in autopsy specimens. Clin Orthop Relat Res 289:131-135, 1993.
kN, Kilonewtons.

Clinical evidence that compares allograft with autograft is scarce. Dennis et al[21] performed ALIF of 40 levels in 31 patients using either structural autologous bone, allograft, or a combination of autograft and allograft ICBG. They measured disc space preoperatively, immediately postoperatively, and an average of 29 months postoperatively. The authors found no significant difference between groups for disc space height at a mean of 29.6 months (range 7 to 54 months), and the overall fusion rate was 68%. Similarly, Loguidice et al[22] performed ALIF in 85 patients for painful disc disruption or symptomatic pseudarthrosis. The authors reported an overall fusion rate of 80%, with no significant difference in fusion rates between the autologous and allogenic graft groups.

Cancellous allograft has been used in combination with other structural graft implants. In a recent randomized trial, Putzier et al[23] performed circumferential (anterior interbody with posterior instrumentation and fixation) monosegmental lumbar fusion in two groups using either cancellous allograft or iliac crest autograft inside a PEEK cage in 44 patients. Significantly lower radiographic fusion rates at 6 months of follow-up were reported in the allograft group, compared with the autograft group; however, fusion rates were equivalent at 12 months. Because of the slower rate of bony incorporation with allograft, posterior fixation has been recommended to supplement allograft during ALIF.[12,24] Pradhan et al[25] performed a prospective cohort study with 36 patients undergoing ALIF with the use of femoral ring allografts. The pseudarthrosis rate was reported to be as high as 26% with either ICBG or bone morphogenic protein 2 (BMP-2) inside structural allograft.

Barnes et al[26] performed a retrospective review of 49 PLIF patients in whom either allograft cylindrical threaded cortical bone dowels or allograft impacted wedges were placed. The authors found a 13.6% rate of permanent nerve root injury in the group with cylindrical threaded cortical bone dowels and a 0% rate in the group with impacted wedges ($p = 0.049$). Although the fusion rates were similar, the authors concluded that clinical outcomes were significantly better with the use of impacted wedges. Allograft spacers that are contoured with a sawtooth pattern and a wedge shape have also been used successfully.[24] Arnold et al[27] performed a prospective nonrandomized study of 89 patients undergoing PLIF with sawtooth-contoured cortical allograft spacers with posterior pedicle fixation. A radiographic fusion rate of 98% was found at 12 and 24 months of follow-up. The authors reported a graft-related complication rate of 1.6%.

Allograft implants can be effective for interbody lumbar fusion procedures when they are used in appropriate clinical situations. The use of modern standardized harvest procedures with thorough sterilization techniques virtually negates the risk of potential disease transmission. Structural allograft implants—especially when used in combination with posterior instrumentation—provide immediate mechanical strength, which results in fusion rates that are comparable to those obtained with autograft implants. Cancellous allograft implants used in PLIF procedures should be combined with additional fixation to achieve acceptable fusion rates.

TITANIUM

Interest in the use of titanium in orthopedic implants has rapidly expanded since the 1950s, when Branemark first reported the osseointegration phenomenon that the substance demonstrated.[28] Titanium has many properties that make it attractive for use as an interbody implant, such as corrosion and wear resistance and a high elastic modulus. Currently, commercially pure titanium (CP Ti) grade 4 (ASTM F67) and titanium grade 5 (Ti6Al4V; ASTM F136) are the most commonly used titanium alloys in orthopedics. One important biomechanical advantage is that the Young's modulus of elasticity of titanium alloys used in orthopedics is reported to be between 100 and 120 GPa, which is more similar to that of bone at 12 to 25 GPa, compared with other metals[29-32] (Table 16-2). Titanium has also been shown to induce BMP-2, BMP-4, BMP-7, alkaline phosphatase, and osteocalcin expression in osteoprogenitor cells in vitro, and it increases the degree of cellular maturation and differentiation, compared with that seen in cells grown on a PEEK surface.[33] This osteoinductive property of titanium makes it attractive for use within a confined region such as a disc space, because PEEK may form a fibrous connective tissue interface that allows micromotion and thus prevents implant stability. Titanium also creates a good osteoconductive surface on which osteoblasts can adhere and thrive.[34]

Surface modifications have been proposed as additional mechanisms to increase the attractiveness of titanium as an implant material. Chemical surface alterations such as calcium ion implantation and hydroxyapatite (HA) coating have increased calcium phosphate content and bony integration at the implant interface.[35-38] Oxides that form on the surface of the implant are resistant to reaction with the chloride ions that naturally occur in the blood and the interstitial fluid.[35] The plasma coating of titanium and its alloys with HA to a depth of 200 μ has been shown to increase the bond strength of the implant interface by 8 to 20 MPa.[39-41] However, calcium ion implantation to a depth of as little as 10 μ has resulted in an increase in calcium phosphate content at the implant interface.[35]

Mechanical surface modifications such as increased surface porosity and grit blasting have demonstrated increased surface area and allowed bony ingrowth into the implant, and they have promoted an osteogenic and angiogenic microenvironment[38,42,43] (Fig. 16-2). Surface modification of this type is typically between 1000 and 1600 nm deep. Osteoprogenitor cells and intracellular fluid have been shown to readily penetrate pores with a size of at least 100 μ. Titanium that has a porosity of 40% has an elastic modulus experimentally measured to be 3.5 GPa, which is nearly identical to that of cortical bone.[44] Both chemical and mechanical surface modifications have trade-offs in practical use. Chemical treatment of the titanium surface decreases wear and corrosion resistance.[35,36] Grit blasting and surface porosity decrease the stiffness of the implant at the interface, which negatively affects material's wear resistance.[43,45] Of the different titanium alloys, Ti6Al4V showed the highest resistance to corrosion across a number of environments in vitro.[46]

Although titanium offers strong, early fixation because of its relative stiffness, stress shielding by the interbody implant can lead to eventual subsidence. Reported fusion rates for titanium interbody implants have generally been good,[47-51] although implant subsidence was often noted.[47,50] The degree of subsidence is variable and may depend on the location in the spine and the position of the implant, with subsidence and fusion rates being inversely correlated.[47] Another critical factor is the bone mineral density of the patient.[52] Although subsidence in the cervical spine is often present, clinical complications are rare.[49]

Table 16-2 Elastic Modulus, Yield Strength, and Ultimate Strength of Various Biomaterials

Material	Elastic Modulus (GPa)	Yield Strength (MPa)	Ultimate Strength (MPa)
Cortical bone	12 to 25	170	205
Trabecular bone	0.1	3.4	15 to 20
Titanium	100 to 120	692	785
Polyetheretherketone	3.6	90 to 100	110 to 200
Cobalt-chrome	220 to 230	921	1024
Stainless steel (316)	205 to 210	170 to 750	465 to 950
Ceramic	25 to 80	2 to 20	20 to 25

This table includes data from references 28-32, 67, 95, and 103-107.
GPa, Gigapascals; *MPa*, megapascals.

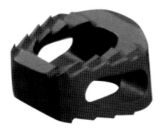

Fig. 16-2 Titanium cervical implant. (Image courtesy of TrueMed Group, LLC/ARZZT International, Medical Division, www.arzzt.com.)

Implant subsidence can depend on a number of factors. Grant et al[53] demonstrated that the posterolateral region of the endplate ring is twice as strong as the center of the endplate. Others confirmed this finding by showing that the highest load to failure occurred in the posterolateral areas just anterior to the pedicles. Titanium cages placed in this area have shown more physiologic load transfer and higher loads to failure in biomechanical studies, although the results were not significant.[54-56] Cage width has been shown to be inversely correlated with subsidence rates; however, implant subsidence of up to 2 mm occurred in up to 76.7% of patients with single, wide, stand-alone cages in their lumbar spines.[57,58] With paired, narrow titanium cages, subsidence rates were shown to depend on the space between the implants. An interdevice distance of 6 mm resulted in a subsidence rate of 41.0%, whereas an interdevice distance of 2 mm resulted in a subsidence rate of 85.7%.[56] Implant subsidence can be detrimental to lumbar fusion. With titanium interbody implants, closer evaluation is recommended to identify these problems.

Because titanium has demonstrated more MRI-friendly artifact characteristics, compared with other metals (for example, cobalt-chromium and stainless steel), postoperative imaging with MRI produces better resolution.[59-62] In in vitro studies, the MRI artifact was dependent on the geometry of the implant, with a more cylindrical shape producing better results.[63] Despite this, high-quality MRI images of the spine that display the neural structures are still possible to obtain, and orthogonal plain radiographs can be used to evaluate new bone formation.[61,63,64]

POLYETHERETHERKETONE

PEEK is a high-temperature thermoplastic polymer comprising an aromatic backbone with ketone and ether functional groups. This structure makes the material stable at temperatures of more than 300° C, resistant to degradation, and stronger than many metals.[65] PEEK has a Young's modulus of elasticity similar to that of cortical bone (see Table 16-2), which promotes optimal stress distribution between the spacer and the adjunctive local bone graft.[66,67] Biomechanically this allows a more ideal load-sharing construct that leads to improved bony incorporation and fusion (Wolff's law). Stresses on the endplates are also reduced, which potentially results in less subsidence, compared with other implants (for example, titanium).[67]

Because PEEK has no integrative properties, an implant itself will not be incorporated into the host bone. Osteoinductive materials are used either outside or inside of the cage to form the bony fusion that provides biomechanical stability. Synthetic PEEK cages are available in various sizes and shapes to accommodate the patient's anatomy (Fig. 16-3, A). PEEK was first employed in spinal fusion in April 1989.[68] Since then these implants have been very well studied in the lumbar interbody setting. These cages have been shown to demonstrate excellent fusion rates that range from 95% to 100% for ALIF, TLIF, and PLIF (all with posterior pedicle screw fixation).[66,69-71] In contrast with allograft implants, PEEK cages have been clinically shown to reliably achieve and maintain long-term disc height and lordotic angle.[66,69-71] For example, McAfee et al[70] reported no cases of subsidence when using PEEK for TLIF in a series of 120 patients treated for spondylolisthesis. Wan et al[71] compared PEEK cages packed with local cancellous autograft and femoral ring allografts in ALIF with long posterior stabilization for spinal deformity on 83 levels (30 femoral ring allografts and 53 PEEK cages) in 48 patients. The minimum follow-up was 7.5 months and the mean follow-up was 17.3 months. Foraminal height and segmental lordosis were similar, but PEEK cages better maintained these measurements[71] (Table 16-3). Higher fusion rates were seen with PEEK at 3 months (42% versus 20%), 6 months (79% versus 51%), 12 months (96% versus 72%), and at final follow-up (95% versus 84%). Conversely, Cutler et al[66] reported no significant difference in lordotic angle between PEEK and femoral cortical allograft and no subsidence with PEEK devices, compared with 2 cases of subsidence out of 21 operations with femoral cortical allograft in TLIF.

Difficulty with determining the solidity of a spinal fusion remains a major problem when radiopaque implants are used. The visualization of cage interspace bone bridging on plain radiographs is crucial for the confirmation of successful fusion.[72,73] This decision can have a significant impact on the management of patients with residual pain after interbody fusion.[73] Unlike titanium, PEEK cages are radiolucent, and they greatly enhance the visualization of bony healing with plain radiographic techniques.[73] PEEK cages show less artifact on CT scans and MRI, compared with metal implants, thus facilitating further evaluation of fusion success.

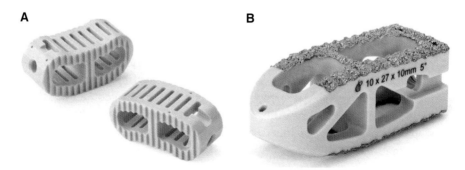

Fig. 16-3   **A,** Polyetheretherketone interbody implant device. (© Solvay. All rights reserved except advertising.) **B,** Polyetheretherketone interbody device with porous titanium coating. (Image courtesy of Spinal Elements®, Inc.)

Table 16-3 Comparison of Polyetheretherketone Versus Femoral Ring Allograft in Anterior Lumbar Interbody Fusion With Long Posterior Stabilization

Treatment	Femoral Ring Allograft L4-L5	Femoral Ring Allograft L5-S1	Polyetheretherketone L4-L5	Polyetheretherketone L5-S1
Total levels	16	14	26	27
Disc height increase immediately after surgery (mm)	3.5	3.5	3.8	3.7
Disc height increase at final follow-up (mm)	1.7	1.9	2.9	2.7
Foraminal height increase immediately after surgery (mm)	1.8	0.9	1.8	1.4
Foraminal height increase at final follow-up (mm)	1.3*	0.3*	1.0	0.8
Segmental lordosis increase immediately after surgery (degrees)	3.0	3.8	5.3	4.7
Segmental lordosis increase at final follow-up (degrees)	0.3*	0.3*	4.3	1.3*

Measurements are averages in relation to preoperative values.
*Nonsignificant increase, compared with preoperative measurement.

Modern PEEK cage alterations have overcome the chemical and biologic inertness of PEEK, which limits its long-term stability.[65,74] Consequently, various modifications such as HA composite, beta-tricalcium phosphate composite, plasma treatment, titanium alloy, HA coating, titanium coating, and three-dimensional porous coating have been explored to improve the bioactivity and osseointegration of implants.[65,74] Although many of these composites have demonstrated enhanced bioactivity, in some cases the biomechanical properties of PEEK have been compromised by these formulations.[65] For example, combining PEEK with greater amounts of HA significantly increases the modulus of elasticity, decreases tensile strength, and increases fatigue damage.[65,75]

As a result of these drawbacks, surface modifications have been explored to improve osseointegration without compromising implant strength and toughness. Studies exploring the various coating modifications have demonstrated promising results in vitro and in animal models.[65,74,76-79] Zhao et al[74] found improved cell adhesion and the greater expression of markers of osteogenic differentiation (runt-related transcription factor 2 [Runx2], alkaline phosphatase, and collagen type I alpha1 chain [Col1a1]) when PEEK was coated with a porous, three-dimensional sulfonated surface, compared with standard PEEK. In a rat femur model, PEEK with a three-dimensional coated surface demonstrated increased bone volume and improved pushout strength.[74] Suska et al[77] found improved bone-implant contact in HA-coated PEEK, compared with uncoated PEEK in rabbit femur and tibia models. Titanium-coated PEEK (see Fig. 16-3, B) has increased cell proliferation and differentiation in vitro and bone-implant contact in a rabbit tibia model.[78] Because noncoated PEEK implants cannot be incorporated into the bony surface, a fibrous tissue layer forms around the cage[80]; this potentially leads to implant loosening, and it may provide a niche for bacterial growth.[81] Concern about biofilm and bacterial growth on PEEK has recently been expressed in response to the ease of colonization found in vitro.[82,83] Gorth et al[83] found greater biofilm formation and bacterial counts on PEEK, compared with titanium and silicon nitride. Despite the low incidence of infection, various surface modifications are being explored[81] to minimize bacterial colonization of PEEK and associated morbidities that can occur with infection after spine surgery.[84,85]

Fusion rates with PEEK cages depend on the bone graft substitutes used, which include allograft, autograft, ceramics, and growth factors. BMP-2, which has been approved by the U.S. Food and Drug Administration for use with the titanium LT-Cage lumbar tapered infusion device (Medtronic Sofamor Danek, Memphis, TN) only in ALIF,[86] has also been used in off-label applications with PEEK. Although the evidence-based literature suggests that Infuse (Medtronic Sofamor Danek), which contains the rhBMP-2 molecule, is the most potent bone graft substitute on the market,[87] case series demonstrate a high incidence of complications if this product is not used judiciously and correctly.[88] A systematic review found the following complications of lumbar fusions with the use of BMP-2: resorption/osteolysis (44%), cage migration (27%), neutralizing antibodies against rhBMP-7 (26%), subsidence (25%), elevated response to bovine type I collagen (16%), radiculitis (11%), heterotopic bone formation (8%), hematoma (4%), and wound complications (2%).[89] The incidence of complications has not been shown to correlate with the dose used.[89] Nevertheless, many surgeons believe that overdosing with BMP-2 can lead to significant ramifications.

PEEK provides an inert, safe, and structurally sound spacer. A central, open space provides the structural support needed to prevent a loss of disc height, and it allows the placement of local autograft or biologic substitute to promote fusion. PEEK cages offer the advantages of achieving and maintaining disc height and lordotic angle (where titanium excels and allograft can fall short) while simultaneously optimizing the biomechanical load for fusion and accommodating the bone graft to provide optimal biology for osseous fusion. The main characteristic of PEEK that requires improvement is osseointegration at the bone-implant interface.

CERAMICS

Ceramic implants were initially produced to be osteoconductive and biodegradable substitutes for bone graft.[90,91] Ceramics used in orthopedics are biocompatible crystalline materials and can be made from a wide range of materials such as silicon nitrade, tricalcium phosphate (TCP), HA, calcium sulfate, and collagen. Ceramics are simple to produce, bioinert, and easy to sterilize. Most often ceramic scaffolds are used in a granular form as bone graft extenders, but structural interbody implants are available[90,92,93] (Fig. 16-4). The most commonly used materials in orthopedics are tricalcium phosphate and HA, which are used either individually or in combination. Ceramic implants can be constructed to mimic the material properties of bone, depending on material processing and porosity[94,95] (see Table 16-2). Ceramics vary markedly in the material properties. For instance, TCP and HA are highly brittle ceramics and cannot withstand

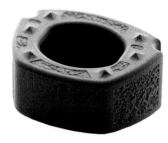

Fig. 16-4   Ceramic interbody device. (Valeo® C Interbody Fusion Device, courtesy of Amedica Corporation.)

much deformation before failure. Conversely, silicon nitride is an extremely strong and tough ceramic, and can withstand stresses that would result in the failure of plastics and many metals. For spinal fusion applications, ceramics are generally used in conjunction with rigid fixation devices (for example, plates and screws) until they can be incorporated into bone. TCP and HA are eventually biodegraded by the host tissue, but silicon nitride remains as a permanent interbody. Close follow-up is required to ensure that these implants have not fractured or resorbed, which can result in motion at the fusion site.

Ceramics have been shown to be osteoconductive,[96,97] with the capability of bony ingrowth into the implant and an interface strength of up to 10 MPa.[98] They are also amenable to surface modifications with bioactive compounds such as rhBMP-2 to enhance bony incorporation.[91,99] Few studies have investigated the use of these interbody implants. In the largest case series to date, Stanislaw et al[100] showed good or satisfactory outcomes at 6 months in 78.5% of PLIF cases that involved the use of ceramic interbody implants, although long-term follow-up and subsidence rates are not available. The CAncellous Structured Ceramic Arthrodesis Device (CASCADE) trial is currently investigating the effectiveness of ceramic versus PEEK cages for anterior cervical discectomy and fusion surgeries.[92] This clinical trial will evaluate the clinical outcomes and fusion rates at 2 years of follow-up. A total of 100 patients will be randomized into two groups, and the extent of fusion will be determined with plain radiographs and CT scans. Patients will receive either a ceramic cage filled with cancellous structured ceramic or a PEEK interbody device filled with bone graft material. No exogenous growth factors will be used in this trial.

The potential advantages of ceramics are attractive. Because these implants are radiopaque,[101] plain radiographs can be used to evaluate resorption and new bone replacement.[102] Ceramics do not cause the imaging artifacts typically seen with metallic implants; therefore the evaluation of fusion with MRI or CT may be superior to that obtained from patients with metallic implants.[61,62,92,100-102] The use of CT without artifact in patients with ceramic implants may also allow clinicians to better evaluate pseudarthrosis, compared with results in patients with metallic interbody spacers.

CONCLUSION

Lumbar interbody arthrodesis was initially developed to improve stability, fusion rates, and sagittal plane correction in patients with spinal segmental instability. The current indications have evolved to include the treatment of spinal deformity, segmental instability, and discogenic low back pain. As modern techniques for interbody fusion improve with minimally invasive procedures, the demand for appropriate graft implants will increase. Current popularly used interbody grafts include allograft spacers, titanium cages, PEEK interbody spacers, and ceramic implants either as stand-alone grafts or in combination with graft alternatives or instrumented fixation. More high-level studies that investigate existing and developing graft options are necessary to evaluate clinical applicability, advantages, disadvantages, and associated complications. Spine surgeons will then have a greater understanding of graft options and be better able to choose appropriately from among the clinical parameters available to them.

REFERENCES

1. Tay BB, Berven S. Indications, techniques, and complications of lumbar interbody fusion. Semin Neurol 22:221-230, 2002.
2. Wiltfong RE, Bono CM, Charles Malveaux WMS, et al. Lumbar interbody fusion: review of history, complications, and outcome comparisons among methods. Curr Orthop Pract 23:193-202, 2012.
3. Wang JC, Mummaneni PV, Haid RW. Current treatment strategies for the painful lumbar motion segment: posterolateral fusion versus interbody fusion. Spine 30(16 Suppl):S33-S43, 2005.

4. Mummaneni PV, Haid RW, Rodts GE. Lumbar interbody fusion: state-of-the-art technical advances. Invited submission from the Joint Section Meeting on Disorders of the Spine and Peripheral Nerves, March 2004. J Neurosurg Spine 1:24-30, 2004.

5. Khan SN, Cammisa FP Jr, Sandhu HS, et al. The biology of bone grafting. J Am Acad Orthop Surg 13:77-86, 2005.

6. Lin PM, Cautilli RA, Joyce MF. Posterior lumbar interbody fusion. Clin Orthop Relat Res 180:154-168, 1983.

7. Myeroff C, Archdeacon M. Autogenous bone graft: donor sites and techniques. J Bone Joint Surg Am 93:2227-2236, 2011.

8. Dimar JR II, Glassman SD, Burkus JK, et al. Two-year fusion and clinical outcomes in 224 patients treated with a single-level instrumented posterolateral fusion with iliac crest bone graft. Spine J 9:880-885, 2009.

9. Howard JM, Glassman SD, Carreon LY. Posterior iliac crest pain after posterolateral fusion with or without iliac crest graft harvest. Spine J 11:534-537, 2011.

10. Bauer TW, Muschler GF. Bone graft materials. An overview of the basic science. Clin Orthop Relat Res 371:10-27, 2000.

11. Stevenson S, Horowitz M. The response to bone allografts. J Bone Joint Surg Am 74:939-950, 1992.

12. Sarwat AM, O'Brien JP, Renton P, et al. The use of allograft (and avoidance of autograft) in anterior lumbar interbody fusion: a critical analysis. Eur Spine J 10:237-241, 2001.

13. Yu CH, Wang CT, Chen PQ. Instrumented posterior lumbar interbody fusion in adult spondylolisthesis. Clin Orthop Relat Res 466:3034-3043, 2008.

14. Ehrler DM, Vaccaro AR. The use of allograft bone in lumbar spine surgery. Clin Orthop Relat Res 371:38-45, 2000.

15. Mroz TE, Joyce MJ, Lieberman IH, et al. The use of allograft bone in spine surgery: is it safe? Spine J 9:303-308, 2009.

16. Costain DJ, Crawford RW. Fresh-frozen vs. irradiated allograft bone in orthopaedic reconstructive surgery. Injury 40:1260-1264, 2009.

17. Chen D, Kummer FJ, Spivak JM. Optimal selection and preparation of fresh frozen corticocancellous allografts for anterior interbody lumbar spinal fusion. J Spinal Disord 10:532-536, 1997.

18. Chau AM, Xu LL, Wong JY, et al. Current status of bone graft options for anterior interbody fusion of the cervical and lumbar spine. Neurosurg Rev 37:23-37, 2014.

19. Rao S, McKellop H, Chao D, et al. Biomechanical comparison of bone graft used in anterior spinal reconstruction. Freeze-dried demineralized femoral segments versus fresh fibular segments and tricortical iliac blocks in autopsy specimens. Clin Orthop Relat Res 289:131-135, 1993.

20. Brantigan JW, Cunningham BW, Warden K, et al. Compression strength of donor bone for posterior lumbar interbody fusion. Spine 18:1213-1221, 1993.

21. Dennis S, Watkins R, Landaker S, et al. Comparison of disc space heights after anterior lumbar interbody fusion. Spine 14:876-878, 1989.

22. Loguidice VA, Johnson RG, Guyer RD, et al. Anterior lumbar interbody fusion. Spine 13:366-369, 1988.

23. Putzier M, Strube P, Funk JF, et al. Allogenic versus autologous cancellous bone in lumbar segmental spondylodesis: a randomized prospective study. Eur Spine J 18:687-695, 2009.

24. Janssen ME, Lam C, Beckham R. Outcomes of allogenic cages in anterior and posterior lumbar interbody fusion. Eur Spine J 10(Suppl 2):S158-S168, 2001.

25. Pradhan BB, Bae HW, Dawson EG, et al. Graft resorption with the use of bone morphogenetic protein: lessons from anterior lumbar interbody fusion using femoral ring allografts and recombinant human bone morphogenetic protein-2. Spine 31:E277-E284, 2006.

26. Barnes B, Rodts GE Jr, Haid RW Jr, et al. Allograft implants for posterior lumbar interbody fusion: results comparing cylindrical dowels and impacted wedges. Neurosurgery 51:1191-1198; discussion 1198, 2002.

27. Arnold PM, Robbins S, Paullus W, et al. Clinical outcomes of lumbar degenerative disc disease treated with posterior lumbar interbody fusion allograft spacer: a prospective, multicenter trial with 2-year follow-up. Am J Orthop 38:E115-E122, 2009.

28. Navarro M, Michiardi A, Castaño O, et al. Biomaterials in orthopaedics. J R Soc Interface 5:1137-1158, 2008.

29. Goel VK, Ramirez SA, Kong W, et al. Cancellous bone Young's modulus variation within the vertebral body of a ligamentous lumbar spine—application of bone adaptive remodeling concepts. J Biomech Eng 117:266-271, 1995.

30. Rho JY, Tsui TY, Pharr GM. Elastic properties of human cortical and trabecular lamellar bone measured by nanoindentation. Biomaterials 18:1325-1330, 1997.

31. Hoffmeister BK, Smith SR, Handley SM, et al. Anisotropy of Young's modulus of human tibial cortical bone. Med Biol Eng Comput 38:333-338, 2000.

32. ASTM International. ASTM F136 - 13. Standard specification for wrought titanium-6aluminum-4vanadium ELI (extra low interstitial) alloy for surgical implant applications (UNS R56401), 2003. Available at *www.astm. org/Standards/F136.htm.*

33. Olivares-Navarrete R, Gittens RA, Schneider JM, et al. Osteoblasts exhibit a more differentiated phenotype and increased bone morphogenetic protein production on titanium alloy substrates than on poly-ether-ether-ketone. Spine J 12:265-272, 2012.

34. Oliveira DP, Palmieri A, Carinci F, et al. Osteoblasts behavior on chemically treated commercially pure titanium surfaces. J Biomed Mater Res A 102:1816-1822, 2014.

35. Hanawa T. Metal ion release from metal implants. Mater Sci Eng C Mater Biol Appl 24:745-752, 2004.

36. Liu XC, Chu PK, Ding C. Surface modification of titanium, titanium alloys, and related materials for biomedical applications. Mater Sci Eng Mater Biol Appl R 47:49-121, 2004.

37. Chen D, Bertollo N, Lau A, et al. Osseointegration of porous titanium implants with and without electrochemically deposited DCPD coating in an ovine model. J Orthop Surg Res 6:56, 2011.

38. Svehla M, Morberg P, Zicat B, et al. Morphometric and mechanical evaluation of titanium implant integration: comparison of five surface structures. J Biomed Mater Res 51:15-22, 2000.

39. Liu X, Poon RWY, Kwok SCH, et al. Plasma surface modification of titanium for hard tissue replacements. Surface and Coatings Technology 186:227-233, 2004.

40. Khor KA, Yip CS, Cheang P. Ti-6Al-4V/hydroxyapatite composite coatings prepared by thermal spray techniques. J Therm Spray Technol 6:109-115, 1997.

41. Zheng X, Huang M, Ding C. Bond strength of plasma-sprayed hydroxyapatite/Ti composite coatings. Biomaterials 21:841-849, 2000.

42. Gittens RA, Olivares-Navarrete R, McLachlan T, et al. Differential responses of osteoblast lineage cells to nanotopographically-modified, microroughened titanium-aluminum-vanadium alloy surfaces. Biomaterials 33:8986-8994, 2012.

43. Gittens RA, Olivares-Navarrete R, Cheng A, et al. The roles of titanium surface micro/nanotopography and wettability on the differential response of human osteoblast lineage cells. Acta Biomater 9:6268-6277, 2013.

44. Rubshtein AP, Trakhtenberg I, Makarova EB, et al. Porous material based on spongy titanium granules: structure, mechanical properties, and osseointegration. Mater Sci Eng C Mater Biol Appl 35:363-369, 2014.

45. Olivares-Navarrete R, Hyzy SL, Gittens RA, et al. Rough titanium alloys regulate osteoblast production of angiogenic factors. Spine J 13:1563-1570, 2013.

46. Okazaki Y, Gotoh E. Comparison of metal release from various metallic biomaterials in vitro. Biomaterials 26:11-21, 2005.

47. Lee JH, Jeon DW, Lee SJ, et al. Fusion rates and subsidence of morselized local bone grafted in titanium cages in posterior lumbar interbody fusion using quantitative three-dimensional computed tomography scans. Spine 35:1460-1465, 2010.

48. Pelletier M, Cordaro N, Lau A, et al. PEEK versus Ti interbody fusion devices: resultant fusion, bone apposition, initial and 26 week biomechanics. J Spinal Disord Tech. 2012 Jul 13. [Epub ahead of print]

49. Schmieder K, Wolzik-Grossmann M, Pechlivanis I, et al. Subsidence of the wing titanium cage after anterior cervical interbody fusion: 2-year follow-up study. J Neurosurg Spine 4:447-453, 2006.

50. van Jonbergen HP, Spruit M, Anderson PG, et al. Anterior cervical interbody fusion with a titanium box cage: early radiological assessment of fusion and subsidence. Spine J 5:645-649; discussion 649, 2005.

51. Antoni M, Charles YP, Walter A, et al. Fusion rates of different anterior grafts in thoracolumbar fractures. J Spinal Disord Tech. 2013 Sep 27. [Epub ahead of print]

52. Oxland TR, Lund T. Biomechanics of stand-alone cages and cages in combination with posterior fixation: a literature review. Eur Spine J 9(Suppl 1):S95-S101, 2000.

53. Grant JP, Oxland TR, Dvorak MF. Mapping the structural properties of the lumbosacral vertebral endplates. Spine 26:889-896, 2001.

54. Sohn MJ, Kayanja MM, Kilincer C, et al. Biomechanical evaluation of the ventral and lateral surface shear strain distributions in central compared with dorsolateral placement of cages for lumbar interbody fusion. J Neurosurg Spine 4:219-224, 2006.

55. Labrom RD, Tan JS, Reilly CW, et al. The effect of interbody cage positioning on lumbosacral vertebral endplate failure in compression. Spine 30:E556-E561, 2005.

56. Subach BR, Copay AG, Martin MM, et al. Anterior lumbar interbody implants: importance of the interdevice distance. Adv Orthop 2011:176497, 2011.

57. Choi JY, Sung KH. Subsidence after anterior lumbar interbody fusion using paired stand-alone rectangular cages. Eur Spine J 15:16-22, 2006.

58. Marchi L, Abdala N, Oliveira L, et al. Radiographic and clinical evaluation of cage subsidence after stand-alone lateral interbody fusion. J Neurosurg Spine 19:110-118, 2013.

59. Laakman RW, Kaufman B, Han JS, et al. MR imaging in patients with metallic implants. Radiology 157:711-714, 1985.

60. Mechlin M, Thickman D, Kressel HY, et al. Magnetic resonance imaging of postoperative patients with metallic implants. AJR Am J Roentgenol 143:1281-1284, 1984.

61. Wang JC, Yu WD, Sandhu HS, et al. A comparison of magnetic resonance and computed tomographic image quality after the implantation of tantalum and titanium spinal instrumentation. Spine 23:1684-1688, 1998.

62. Rudisch A, Kremser C, Peer S, et al. Metallic artifacts in magnetic resonance imaging of patients with spinal fusion. A comparison of implant materials and imaging sequences. Spine 23:692-699, 1998.

63. Ernstberger T, Heidrich G, Buchhorn G. Postimplantation MRI with cylindric and cubic intervertebral test implants: evaluation of implant shape, material, and volume in MRI artifacting—an in vitro study. Spine J 7:353-359, 2007.

64. Ernstberger T, Buchhorn G, Heidrich G. Magnetic resonance imaging evaluation of intervertebral test spacers: an experimental comparison of magnesium versus titanium and carbon fiber reinforced polymers as biomaterials. Ir J Med Sci 179:107-111, 2010.

65. Kurtz SM, Devine JN. PEEK biomaterials in trauma, orthopedic, and spinal implants. Biomaterials 28:4845-4869, 2007.

66. Cutler AR, Siddiqui S, Mohan AL, et al. Comparison of polyetheretherketone cages with femoral cortical bone allograft as a single-piece interbody spacer in transforaminal lumbar interbody fusion. J Neurosurg Spine 5:534-539, 2006.

67. Vadapalli S, Sairyo K, Goel VK, et al. Biomechanical rationale for using polyetheretherketone (PEEK) spacers for lumbar interbody fusion—a finite element study. Spine 31:E992-E998, 2006.

68. Brantigan JW, Steffee AD. A carbon fiber implant to aid interbody lumbar fusion. Two-year clinical results in the first 26 patients. Spine 18:2106-2107, 1993.

69. Brantigan JW, Steffee AD, Lewis ML, et al. Lumbar interbody fusion using the Brantigan I/F cage for posterior lumbar interbody fusion and the variable pedicle screw placement system: two-year results from a Food and Drug Administration investigational device exemption clinical trial. Spine 25:1437-1446, 2000.

70. McAfee PC, DeVine JG, Chaput CD, et al. The indications for interbody fusion cages in the treatment of spondylolisthesis: analysis of 120 cases. Spine 30(6 Suppl):S60-S65, 2005.

71. Wan Z, Dai M, Miao J, et al. Radiographic analysis of PEEK cage and FRA in adult spinal deformity fused to sacrum. J Spinal Disord Tech. 2012 May 24. [Epub ahead of print]

72. Cizek GR, Boyd LM. Imaging pitfalls of interbody spinal implants. Spine 25:2633-2636, 2000.

73. Diedrich O, Perlick L, Schmitt O, et al. Radiographic characteristics on conventional radiographs after posterior lumbar interbody fusion: comparative study between radiotranslucent and radiopaque cages. J Spinal Disord 14:522-532, 2001.

74. Zhao Y, Wong HM, Wang W, et al. Cytocompatibility, osseointegration, and bioactivity of three-dimensional porous and nanostructured network on polyetheretherketone. Biomaterials 34:9264-9277, 2013.

75. Abu Bakar MS, Cheng MH, Tang SM, et al. Tensile properties, tension-tension fatigue and biological response of polyetheretherketone-hydroxyapatite composites for load-bearing orthopedic implants. Biomaterials 24:2245-2250, 2013.

76. Converse GL, Conrad TL, Merrill CH, et al. Hydroxyapatite whisker-reinforced polyetherketoneketone bone ingrowth scaffolds. Acta Biomater 6:856-863, 2010.

77. Suska F, Omar O, Emanuelsson L, et al. Enhancement of CRF-PEEK osseointegration by plasma-sprayed hydroxyapatite: a rabbit model. J Biomater Appl. 2014 Feb 3. [Epub ahead of print]

78. Han CM, Lee EJ, Kim HE, et al. The electron beam deposition of titanium on polyetheretherketone (PEEK) and the resulting enhanced biological properties. Biomaterials 31:3465-3470, 2010.

79. Han CM, Jang TS, Kim HE, et al. Creation of nanoporous TiO2 surface onto polyetheretherketone for effective immobilization and delivery of bone morphogenetic protein. J Biomed Mater Res A 102:793-800, 2014.

80. Toth JM, Wang M, Estes BT, et al. Polyetheretherketone as a biomaterial for spinal applications. Biomaterials 27:324-334, 2006.

81. Rochford ET, Poulsson AH, Salavarrieta Varela J, et al. Bacterial adhesion to orthopaedic implant materials and a novel oxygen plasma modified PEEK surface. Colloids Surf B Biointerfaces 113:213-222, 2014.

82. Williams DL, Woodbury KL, Haymond BS, et al. A modified CDC biofilm reactor to produce mature biofilms on the surface of peek membranes for an in vivo animal model application. Curr Microbiol 62:1657-1663, 2011.

83. Gorth DJ, Puckett S, Ercan B, et al. Decreased bacteria activity on Si_3N_4 surfaces compared with PEEK or titanium. Int J Nanomedicine 7:4829-4840, 2012.

84. Weinstein MA, McCabe JP, Cammisa FP Jr. Postoperative spinal wound infection: a review of 2,391 consecutive index procedures. J Spinal Disord 13:422-426, 2000.

85. Beiner JM, Grauer J, Kwon BK, et al. Postoperative wound infections of the spine. Neurosurg Focus 15:E14, 2003.

86. Mulconrey DS, Bridwell KH, Flynn J, et al. Bone morphogenetic protein (RhBMP-2) as a substitute for iliac crest bone graft in multilevel adult spinal deformity surgery: minimum two-year evaluation of fusion. Spine 33:2153-2159, 2008.

87. McKay WF, Peckham SM, Badura JM. A comprehensive clinical review of recombinant human bone morphogenetic protein-2 (INFUSE Bone Graft). Int Orthop 31:729-734, 2007.

88. Carragee EJ, Hurwitz EL, Weiner BK. A critical review of recombinant human bone morphogenetic protein-2 trials in spinal surgery: emerging safety concerns and lessons learned. Spine J 11:471-491, 2011.

89. Mroz TE, Wang JC, Hashimoto R, et al. Complications related to osteobiologics use in spine surgery: a systematic review. Spine 35(9 Suppl):S86-S104, 2010.

90. Miyazaki M, Tsumura H, Wang JC, et al. An update on bone substitutes for spinal fusion. Eur Spine J 18:783-799, 2009.

91. Cunningham BW, Atkinson BL, Hu N, et al. Ceramic granules enhanced with B2A peptide for lumbar interbody spine fusion: an experimental study using an instrumented model in sheep. J Neurosurg Spine 10:300-307, 2009.

92. Arts MP, Wolfs JF, Corbin TP. The CASCADE trial: effectiveness of ceramic versus PEEK cages for anterior cervical discectomy with interbody fusion; protocol of a blinded randomized controlled trial. BMC Musculoskelet Disord 14:244, 2013.

93. Niu CC, Tsai TT, Fu TS, et al. A comparison of posterolateral lumbar fusion comparing autograft, autogenous laminectomy bone with bone marrow aspirate, and calcium sulphate with bone marrow aspirate: a prospective randomized study. Spine 34:2715-2719, 2009.

94. Wang CX. Influence of sintering temperatures on hardness and Young's modulus of tricalcium phosphate bioceramic by nanoindentation technique. Mater Charact 52:301-307, 2004.

95. Hing KA, Best SM, Bonfield W. Characterization of porous hydroxyapatite. J Mater Sci Mater Med 10:135-145, 1999.

96. Baramki HG, Steffen T, Lander P, et al. The efficacy of interconnected porous hydroxyapatite in achieving posterolateral lumbar fusion in sheep. Spine 25:1053-1060, 2000.

97. Flatley TJ, Lynch KL, Benson M. Tissue response to implants of calcium phosphate ceramic in the rabbit spine. Clin Orthop Relat Res 179:246-252, 1983.

98. Battraw GA, Szivek JA, Anderson PL. Bone bonding strength of calcium phosphate ceramic coated strain gauges. J Biomed Mater Res 48:32-35, 1999.

99. Takahashi T, Tominaga T, Watabe N, et al. Use of porous hydroxyapatite graft containing recombinant human bone morphogenetic protein-2 for cervical fusion in a caprine model. J Neurosurg 90(2 Suppl):224-230, 1999.

100. Stanislaw L, Milewski M, Bialecki J, et al. Posterior lumbar interbody fusion using ceramic implants. Ortop Traumatol Rehabil 6:282-287, 2004.

101. Heini PF, Berlemann U. Bone substitutes in vertebroplasty. Eur Spine J 10(Suppl 2):S205-S213, 2001.

102. Turner TM, Urban RM, Gitelis S, et al. Radiographic and histologic assessment of calcium sulfate in experimental animal models and clinical use as a resorbable bone-graft substitute, a bone-graft expander, and a method for local antibiotic delivery. One institution's experience. J Bone Joint Surg Am 83(Suppl 2[Pt 1]):S8-S18, 2001.

103. Kim Y. Prediction of mechanical behaviors at interfaces between bone and two interbody cages of lumbar spine segments. Spine 26:1437-1442, 2001.

104. Park JB, ed. Biomaterials: An Introduction. New York: Plenum, 1979.

105. Perilli E, Baleani M, Ohman C, et al. Structural parameters and mechanical strength of cancellous bone in the femoral head in osteoarthritis do not depend on age. Bone 41:760-768, 2007.

106. Hing KA, Best SM, Tanner KE, et al. Mediation of bone ingrowth in porous hydroxyapatite bone graft substitutes. J Biomed Mater Res A 68:187-200, 2004.

107. Hing KA, Best SM, Tanner KE, et al. Biomechanical assessment of bone ingrowth in porous hydroxyapatite. J Mater Sci Mater Med 8:731-736, 1997.

17

Biomechanical Effects of Long Constructs on Proximal Adjacent Levels: Considerations for Including or Excluding the Thoracolumbar Junction

Haruki Funao ▪ *Khaled M. Kebaish*

Long posterior spinal fusion using pedicle screws has greatly improved our ability to correct spinal deformities. However, these constructs increase the stiffness of the spine significantly and can affect the incidence of adjacent-segment pathology, such as proximal junctional kyphosis (PJK) with or without vertebral compression fracture. Spinal instrumentation immobilizes the motion segments, increasing the mechanical stresses at the adjacent levels, which may contribute to the prevalence of PJK.[1,2] PJK is most commonly defined as a proximal junctional sagittal Cobb angle of greater than 10 degrees and a postoperative kyphotic change of more than 10 degrees from the preoperative measurement.[3] The incidence of PJK has been reported in the range of 17% to 43% after adult spinal deformity surgery.[4-7] Patient presentations vary and include focal or diffuse back pain, prominence of the instrumentation, stooped forward posture, and neurologic deficit in severe cases. However, an incidental finding on radiographs is sometimes the only presentation. Most patients with PJK are not symptomatic. Several studies showed no significant differences in health-related quality of life in patients with or without PJK.[3,8] Conversely, Kim et al[5] reported that patients with PJK of more than 20 degrees reported a significantly lower self-image score on the SRS-22 questionnare. Yagi et al[9] noted that patients with symptomatic PJK had significantly lower total SRS-22 and ODI scores. Neurologic deficit is more likely to be seen in acute settings, which usually happens early postoperatively, especially in osteoporotic patients.[10,11] An acute and more severe clinical presentation of PJK has been called *proximal junctional failure* (PJF).[11-16] PJF should be distinguished from radiographic PJK. PJF is more likely to be related to structural failure and require surgical intervention. Hart et al[14] defined PJF as postoperative kyphotic change of greater than 10 degrees that is associated with one or more of the following signs: fracture of the vertebral body, posterior osseoligamentous disruption, or instrumentation pullout at the UIV. Some patients with structural failure may have shown progressive changes, which require revision surgery.[15-17]

Although most studies of PJF investigated the phenomenon in adolescent patients,[1,18-23] the potential risk for catastrophic junctional failure is higher in the adult deformity population, because they are more likely to have osteoporosis and sagittal deformities.[4,24] Several authors reported on the causes of PJK. Hollenbeck et al[1] indicated that PJK was caused by posterior ligament disruption and loss of muscular support. The potential risk factors for the development of PJK include age, female sex, low bone mineral density, the type of instrumentation, the level of UIV, thoracoplasty, combined anterior-posterior fusions, fusion to the sacrum, preoperative global sagittal imbalance, and large surgical correction of thoracic kyphosis.[3-6,10-13,17-20,23-25] Recently, the risk factors for recurrence of PJK were investigated in revision surgeries for PJK.[17] Significant risk factors for recurrence were a large segmental proximal kyphotic angle, a large preoperative thoracic kyphosis and sagittal vertical axis, and greater correction of thoracic kyphosis and sagittal vertical axis.

Biomechanical studies have demonstrated that the intervertebral discs, the supraspinous and interspinous ligaments, and the rib cage contribute most of the stability in the thoracic spine.[26-30] Few publications discuss how the occurrence of PJK is affected by ending long fusions to the sacrum in the lower thoracic versus the upper thoracic spine. Some biomechanical studies suggest that lower thoracic fusions may be less stable than those in the upper thoracic spine.[29,31,32] Methods used to lower the incidence of PJK include preservation of the supraspinous-interspinous ligament complex; the use of transverse hooks, cement augmentation, or transition rods at the proximal levels.[30,33-35]

EFFECT OF UPPER THORACIC VERSUS LOWER THORACIC/ THORACOLUMBAR FUSIONS

O'Shaughnessy et al[36] compared radiographic and clinical outcomes of patients who had an upper thoracic (UT) fusion and patients who had a lower thoracic (LT) fusion in primary adult scoliosis surgery. The incidence of radiographic PJK was higher in the LT group (18.4%) than in the UT group (10.0%), although this difference was not statistically significance. No significant differences were noted in preoperative clinical outcomes (SRS and ODI scores) between the UT and LT group, except for SRS self-image, which was lower in the LT group. The difference was not statistically significant at the final follow-up. Ha et al[37] also investigated this area. They compared the radiographic and clinical outcomes of patients whose UIV was at the proximal thoracic spine and those whose UIV was at the distal thoracic spine. The incidence of PJK was 34% in patients whose fusion ended in the lower thoracic spine and 27% in patients whose fusion ended in the upper thoracic spine. They found that a compression fracture at the UIV was more prevalent in fusions ending in the lower thoracic spine, whereas a vertebral subluxation was more prevalent in the upper thoracic spine group. They reported no significant differences in preoperative and postoperative clinical outcomes (VAS, SRS-22, SF-36, and ODI scores) between the two groups of patients. Hostin et al[15] investigated adult spinal deformity patients with acute PJF, and they divided the patients into two groups: those with PJF at the upper thoracic spine and those with PJF at the thoracolumbar region. They reported that patients with thoracolumbar PJF were significantly older than those with upper thoracic PJF. Acute failures more often occurred in patients whose fusion extended to the thoracolumbar region (66%), compared with those fused to the upper thoracic spine (34%). They suggested that thoracolumbar failures were likely caused by vertebral fractures; on the other hand, upper thoracic PJF was more likely the result of a soft tissue failure. Recurrence of PJK after revision surgery is common, with the incidence as high as 30.8%, which is similar to the incidence of PJK after the initial surgery.[17] Funao et al[17] reported on patients having revision surgeries for PJK. Patients whose procedures extended to the lower thoracic spine showed a slightly higher incidence of recurrent PJK (39%) than those whose fusion extended to the upper thoracic spine (27%). Yagi et al[38] investigated patients who underwent long posterior spinal fusion with the proximal fusion level ending below T9. They found that a lower instrumented vertebra at the sacropelvis, a larger correction of lumbar lordosis, and a UIV below the sagittal apex were significant risk factors for postoperative progressive thoracic kyphosis and global sagittal imbalance. Yagi et al[39] demonstrated that postoperative sagittal imbalance can be attributed to progressive thoracic kyphosis after pedicle subtraction osteotomy. Their study implied that the deterioration of global sagittal balance was mostly related to a progressive thoracic kyphosis in fusions ending in the lower thoracic spine.

BIOMECHANICAL CONSIDERATIONS

As mentioned previously, the intervertebral discs, supraspinous and interspinous ligaments, and rib cage contribute most of the stability in the thoracic spine. Anderson et al[26] assessed the effect of posterior skeletal dissection associated with an UIV anchor placement on adjacent motion-segment stiffness. They found that the supraspinous-interspinous ligament complex contributed about 6.6% of flexion stiffness. Total loss of flexion stiffness after resection of the posterior stabilizing structures and facet joint resection (Smith-Peterson or Ponte osteotomy) was 67.6%. They also demonstrated that hook placements at the UIV combined with a supraspinous-interspinous ligament resection decreased stiffness by 12.6%. Kretzer et al[27] showed that removal of the supraspinous-interspinous ligament complex significantly increased flexibility (35%) in the cervicothoracic junction. They suggested that this ligament complex contributed to destabilization of the proximal segment adjacent to a long fusion and hence to the occurrence of PJK. Cahill et al[30] reported that pressure in the nucleus and angular displacement were increased when the supraspinous-interspinous ligament complex was removed above the UIV. They indicated that the nucleus pressure increased by more than 50%, and the angular displacement increased by 19% to 26%.

Some studies emphasized the effect of the rib cage on the stability of the thoracic spine. Watkins et al[28] reported that the rib cage significantly increased the stability of the thoracic spine in flexion/extension, compression, lateral bending, and axial rotation. The rib cage and sternum provided 39.8% of the stiffness of the thoracic spine in flexion-extension. The sternum alone provided 29.4%. The rib cage and sternum provided 20.7% of the stiffness in axial compression, whereas the sternum alone provided 11.2%. The rib cage and sternum provided 35.4% of the stiffness in lateral bending, and the sternum alone provided 17.8%. In axial rotation, the rib cage and sternum provided 31.4% of the stiffness, whereas the sternum alone provided 13.4%. Fujimori et al[29] investigated each intervertebral and coupled motion of the thoracic spine in trunk rotation by using a three-dimensional imaging technique in 13 healthy male volunteers. They observed a significantly larger axial rotation in the middle segments than in the upper segments of the thoracic spine. They suggested that anatomic characteristics of the rib cage might affect the difference of rotational motion and stabilization between upper thoracic and midthoracic segments, because the first to seventh ribs are directly connected to the sternum, and the eighth to the tenth ribs are indirectly connected to the sternum. Another study revealed that the scapula contributes to the stability of this region of the spine.[40]

Healy et al[32] reported that pedicle screw fixation with instrumentation from T3-7 (upper to midthoracic region) reduced the range of motion in the thoracic spine by 16.3% in axial rotation, by 12.0% in flexion/extension, and by 18.4% in lateral bending. On the other hand, Lubelski et al[31] reported that pedicle screw fixation with instrumentation from T7-11 (midthoracic to lower thoracic region) reduced the range of motion in the thoracic spine by 33.3% in axial rotation, by 20.8% in flexion/extension, and by 23.4% in lateral bending. They suggested that thoracic spinal motion was more affected in lower thoracic vertebrae at the level of the floating ribs.

PROXIMAL JUNCTIONAL KYPHOSIS AND PROXIMAL JUNCTIONAL FAILURE PREVENTION

Several authors have recently investigated prophylactic methods to reduce the incidence of PJK and PJF. These techniques include the use of less rigid instrumentation such as a hook construct at the UIV[18,41] in the upper thoracic spine and careful choice of the UIV, which should have a lower kyphotic angle.[13] Some authors recommend not ending the fusion at the thoracolumbar junction (T12, L1) or in the midthoracic spine (the apex of kyphosis). Other methods include augmentation of the fixation at the UIV with sublaminar wires and offset hooks or augmentation of the vertebral segment with polymethylmethacrylate.[34] Kebaish et al[34] studied the biomechanical effect of prophylactic vertebroplasty at the proximal junction of long spinal fusion constructs. They compared the mechanical strength among three groups: a control group, a group treated with one-level prophylactic vertebroplasty at the UIV, and a group treated with two-level prophylactic vertebroplasty at the UIV and UIV+1. Prophylactic vertebroplasty at the UIV and UIV+1 significantly reduced the incidence of proximal junctional fractures in this long posterior spinal instrumentation cadaveric construct. Martin et al[42] investigated prophylactic vertebroplasty at the UIV and UIV+1 during posterior spinal fusion in 38 consecutive adult spinal deformity patients. They found that 13% of patients developed either PJK or PJF: 3 patients (8%) developed PJK and 2 patients (5%) developed PJF, which were markedly lower incidences compared with previous reports.[4-7]

A recent cadaveric study using porcine spine investigated the biomechanical effects on the transitional motion segment based on UIV anchor type in long posterior spinal fusion constructs. Thawrani et al[33] reported that transverse process hooks at the UIV provided a more gradual transition to physiologic spinal mobility than pedicle screws. Flexion-extension range of motion at the proximal motion segment in specimens with transverse process hooks at the UIV was significantly greater (21%) than in those with pedicle screws (9%). Stiffness was significantly higher (5.5 times) with pedicle screws than with transverse process hooks in flexion-extension. They concluded that the use of transverse process hooks at the UIV may decrease the incidence of progressive PJK, compared with placement of pedicle screws at the UIV. Cammarata et al[35] analyzed the biomechanics of PJK through computer simulations. They reported that preservation of more posterior proximal intervertebral elements, the use of transition rods and transverse process hooks at the UIV, and reduction of the global sagittal rod curvature decreased the biomechanical indexes that can be involved in PJK. Proximal transverse process hooks reduced the three biomechanical indexes by 26%, compared with pedicle screws at the UIV. They also found that the use of proximal transition rods with reduced proximal diameter from 5.5 to 4 mm decreased the PJK angle by 6%, and it decreased the proximal flexion force and movement by 4% and 8%, respectively. They suggested that transverse process hooks at the UIV, the use of transition rods, and reduction of the global sagittal rod curvature decreased the four biomechanical indexes that may be involved in PJK. In a finite element analysis, Cahill et al[30] demonstrated that the nucleus pressure at the level immediately cephalad to the upper instrumented vertebra (UIV) was 23% lower and the angular displacement was 18% to 19% less with placement of a transition rod, compared with a standard construct. They concluded that preservation of the supraspinous-interspinous ligament complex with the use of rods having a diameter transition at the proximal levels may prevent the development of PJK.

PATIENT EXAMPLES

LONG SPINAL FUSION TO THE LOWER THORACIC VERSUS UPPER THORACIC SPINE

This 62-year-old woman presented with a history of progressive, degenerative idiopathic scoliosis and worsening pain (Fig. 17-1, *A* and *B*). She underwent a posterior spinal fusion from T3 to the pelvis. Transverse process hooks were placed bilaterally at the UIV. No significant radiographic or clinical signs of PJK were evident on her 2-year postoperative radiographs (Fig. 17-1, *C* and *D*).

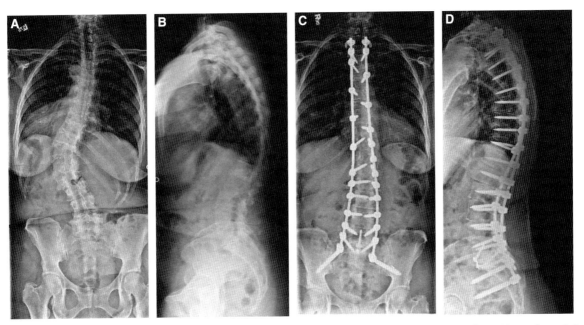

Fig. 17-1 Standing radiographs of a 62-year-old woman who had posterior spinal fusion from T3 to the pelvis. **A,** Preoperative AP and **B,** lateral views. **C,** Two-year postoperative AP and **D,** lateral views.

This 60-year-old woman presented with flat-back deformity after having posterior spinal fusion from L3 to the sacrum at another institution (Fig. 17-2, *A* and *B*). Revision posterior spinal fusion from T11 to the pelvis was performed. No significant radiographic or clinical signs of PJK were evident on her 3-year post-operative radiographs (Fig. 17-2, *C* and *D*).

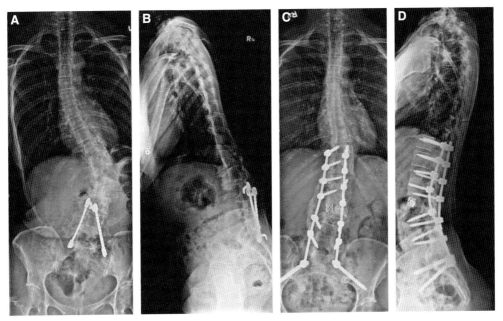

Fig. 17-2 Standing radiographs of a 60-year-old woman who underwent posterior spinal fusion from T11 to the pelvis. **A,** Preoperative AP and **B,** lateral views. **C,** Three-year postoperative AP and **D,** lateral views.

This 70-year-old woman presented with a history of rheumatoid arthritis and prior multiple surgeries. She had persistent positive sagittal malalignment and underwent posterior spinal fusion from T4 to the pelvis, followed by anterior spinal fusion from T12 to L2 with a corpectomy at L1. Pedicle screws were placed bilaterally at the UIV. The patient was diagnosed with PJK 3 months postoperatively. Her PJK and symptoms progressed (Fig. 17-3, A through C). A revision posterior spinal fusion with extension to C2 and an extended pedicle subtraction osteotomy at T4 was performed, resulting in good sagittal alignment (Fig. 17-3, D through F).

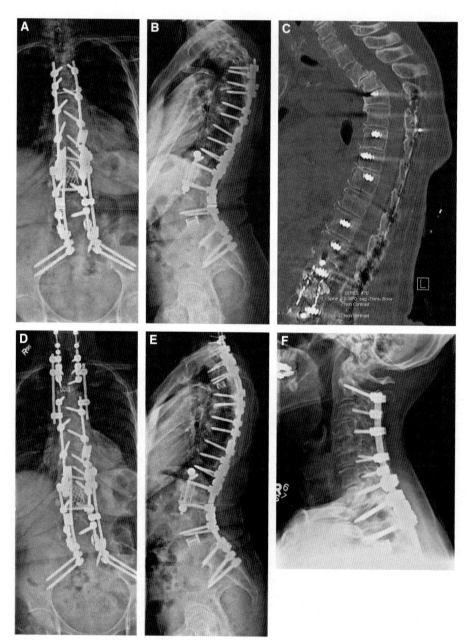

Fig. 17-3   Standing radiographs of a 70-year-old woman who developed PJK with anterolisthesis at T2-3 after combined anterior/posterior spinal fusion from T4 to the pelvis. She underwent revision posterior fusion extending to C2 with an extended PSO at T4. **A,** Preoperative AP, **B,** lateral, and **C,** CT sagittal views. **D,** Postoperative AP, **E,** lateral, and **F,** cervical lateral views.

This 73-year-old woman presented with severe low back pain and lumbar spinal stenosis symptoms. Preoperative radiographs showed lumbar scoliosis and significant sagittal malalignment (Fig. 17-4, *A* and *B*). She underwent posterior spinal fusion from T11 to the pelvis. PJK was diagnosed 2 months postoperatively (Fig. 17-4, *C* and *D*). The patient's symptoms were minimal at first; however, over time they worsened. Two years postoperatively she underwent fusion to T3 with and an extended pedicle subtraction osteotomy at T10. Good sagittal alignment was obtained (Fig. 17-4, *E* and *F*).

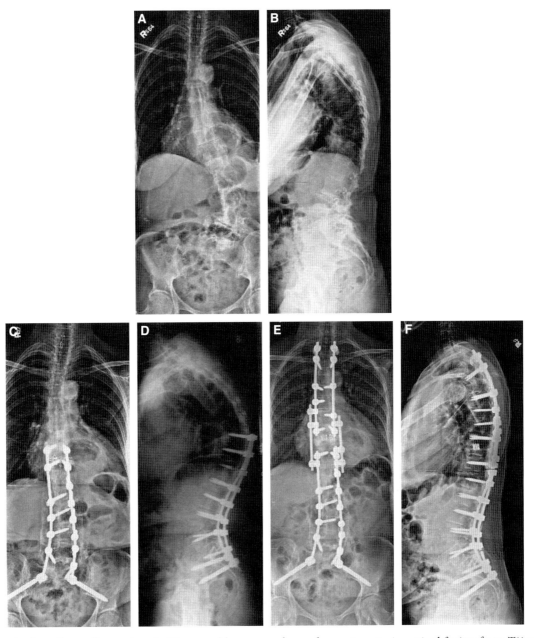

Fig. 17-4 Standing radiographs of a 73-year-old woman who underwent posterior spinal fusion from T11 to the pelvis. **A,** Preoperative AP and **B,** lateral views. **C,** Two-year postoperative AP and **D,** lateral views. **E,** Final AP and **F,** lateral views following revision spinal fusion that extended to T3 and an extended PSO at T10.

CONCLUSION

Proximal junctional kyphosis is a common postoperative complication after long posterior spinal fusion. The incidence of PJK/PJF is higher in osteoporotic and older patients. Currently there is no evidence that ending the fusion in the upper thoracic versus lower thoracic region significantly affects the incidence of PJK or PJF. PJK in the lower thoracic/thoracolumbar spine is more likely to be associated with vertebral fractures/loss of fixation, whereas PJK in the upper thoracic spine appears to be related to soft tissue failure and can have more devastating neurologic consequences. Soft tissue structures must be preserved, including the paraspinal muscles, the cephalad joint capsules, and the supraspinous-interspinous ligament complex. Prophylactic methods for reducing PJK can be effective. In the lower thoracic spine, we recommend prophylactic vertebroplasty in patients with osteoporosis or significant osteopenia. It should include the UIV and the UIV+1 and be performed at the time of surgery. In the upper thoracic spine, a less rigid construct, including the use of transverse process hooks at the UIV, can also be valuable. Transition rods and less invasive techniques that preserve the soft tissue support and prevent muscle damage can be of value, yet should warrant further investigations.

REFERENCES

1. Hollenbeck SM, Glattes RC, Asher MA, et al. The prevalence of increased proximal junctional flexion following posterior instrumentation and arthrodesis for adolescent idiopathic scoliosis. Spine 33:1675-1681, 2008.
2. Watanabe K, Lenke LG, Bridwell KH, et al. Proximal junctional vertebral fracture in adults after spinal deformity surgery using pedicle screw constructs: analysis of morphological features. Spine 35:138-145, 2010.
3. Glattes RC, Bridwell KH, Lenke LG, et al. Proximal junctional kyphosis in adult spinal deformity following long instrumented posterior spinal fusion: incidence, outcomes, and risk factor analysis. Spine 30:1643-1649, 2005.
4. Yagi M, King AB, Boachie-Adjei O. Incidence, risk factors and natural course of proximal junctional kyphosis: surgical outcomes review of adult idiopathic scoliosis. Minimum 5 years follow-up. Spine 37:1479-1489, 2012.
5. Kim YJ, Bridwell KH, Lenke LG, et al. Proximal junctional kyphosis in adult spinal deformity after segmental posterior spinal instrumentation and fusion: minimum five-year follow-up. Spine 33:2179-2184, 2008.
6. Kim HJ, Yagi M, Nyugen MS, et al. Combined anterior-posterior surgery is the most important risk factor for developing proximal junctional kyphosis in idiopathic scoliosis. Clin Orthop Relat Res 470:1633-1639, 2012.
7. Suk SI, Kim JH, Lee SM, et al. Incidence of proximal adjacent failure in adult lumbar deformity correction. Presented at the Thirty-eighth Annual Meeting of the Scoliosis Research Society, Quebec City, Canada, Sept 2003.
8. Bridwell KH, Lenke LG, Cho SK, et al. Proximal junctional kyphosis in primary adult deformity surgery: evaluation of 20 degrees as a critical angle. Neurosurgery 72:899-906, 2013.
9. Yagi M, King A, Boachie-Adjei O. Incidence, risk factors and classification of proximal junctional kyphosis: surgical outcomes review of adult idiopathic scoliosis. Spine 36:E60-E68, 2011.
10. O'Leary PT, Bridwell KH, Lenke LG, et al. Risk factors and outcomes for catastrophic failures at the top of long pedicle screw constructs: a matched cohort analysis performed at a single center. Spine 34:2134-2139, 2009.
11. Cahill DW, Etebar S. Risk factors for adjacent segment failure following lumbar fixation with rigid instrumentation for degenerative instability. J Neurosurg 90:163-169, 1999.
12. Hart RA, Prendergast MA, Roberts WG, et al. Proximal junctional acute collapse cranial to multi-level lumbar fusion: a cost analysis of prophylactic vertebral augmentation. Spine J 8:875-881, 2008.
13. Lewis SJ, Abbas H, Chua S, et al. Upper instrumented vertebra (UIV) fractures in long lumbar fusions: what are the associated risk factors? Spine 37:1407-1414, 2012.
14. Hart R, McCarthy I, Ames C, et al. Proximal junctional kyphosis and proximal junctional failure. Neurosurg Clin N Am 24:213-218, 2013.
15. Hostin R, McCarthy I, O'Brien M, et al; International Spine Study Group. Incidence, mode, and location of acute proximal junctional failures following surgical treatment for adult spinal deformity. Spine 38:1008-1015, 2013.

16. Hart R, Hostin R, McCarthy I, et al; International Spine Study Group. Development and validation of a classification system for proximal junctional failure. Presented at the Forty-seventh Annual Meeting of the Scoliosis Research Society, Chicago, IL, Sept 2012.

17. Funao H, Naef F, Kebaish K, et al. Recurrence proximal junctional kyphosis following adult spinal deformity surgery: incidence and risk factors. Presented at the Forty-ninth Annual Meeting of the Scoliosis Research Society, Anchorage, AL, Sept 2014.

18. Helgeson MD, Shah SA, Newton PO, et al. Evaluation of proximal junctional kyphosis in adolescent idiopathic scoliosis following pedicle screw, hook, or hybrid instrumentation. Spine 35:177-181, 2010.

19. Kim YJ, Bridwell KH, Lenke LG, et al. Proximal junctional kyphosis in adolescent idiopathic scoliosis following segmental posterior spinal instrumentation and fusion: minimum 5-year follow-up. Spine 30:2045-2050, 2005.

20. Kim YJ, Lenke LG, Bridwell KH, et al. Proximal junctional kyphosis in adolescent idiopathic scoliosis after 3 different types of posterior segmental spinal instrumentation and fusions: incidence and risk factor analysis of 410 cases. Spine 32:2731-2738, 2005.

21. Lee GA, Betz RR, Clements DH III, et al. Proximal kyphosis after posterior spinal fusion in patients with idiopathic scoliosis. Spine 24:795-799, 1999.

22. Rhee JM, Bridwell KH, Won DS, et al. Sagittal plane analysis of adolescent idiopathic scoliosis. The effect of anterior versus posterior instrumentation. Spine 27:2350-2356, 2002.

23. Wang J, Zhao Y, Shen B, et al. Risk factor analysis of proximal junctional kyphosis after posterior fusion in patients with idiopathic scoliosis. Injury 41:415-420, 2010.

24. Cho KJ, Suk SI, Park SR, et al. Complications in posterior fusion and instrumentation for degenerative lumbar scoliosis. Spine 32:2232-2237, 2007.

25. Kim YJ, Bridwell KH, Lenke LG, et al. Sagittal thoracic decompensation following long adult lumbar spinal instrumentation and fusion to L5 or S1: causes, prevalence, and risk factor analysis. Spine 31:2359-2366, 2006.

26. Anderson AL, McIff TE, Asher MA, et al. The effect of posterior thoracic spine anatomical structures on motion segment flexion stiffness. Spine 34:441-446, 2009.

27. Kretzer RM, Hu N, Umekoji H, et al. The effect of spinal instrumentation on kinematics at the cervicothoracic junction: emphasis on soft-tissue response in an in vitro human cadaveric model. J Neurosurg Spine 13:435-442, 2010.

28. Watkins R IV, Watkins R III, Williams L, et al. Stability provided by the sternum and rib cage in the thoracic spine. Spine 30:1283-1286, 2005.

29. Fujimori T, Iwasaki M, Nagamoto Y, et al. Kinematics of the thoracic spine in trunk lateral bending: in vivo three-dimensional analysis. Spine J 14:1991-1999, 2014.

30. Cahill PJ, Wang W, Asghar J, et al. The use of a transition rod may prevent proximal junctional kyphosis in the thoracic spine after scoliosis surgery: a finite element analysis. Spine 37:E687-E695, 2012.

31. Lubelski D, Healy AT, Mageswaran P, et al. Biomechanics of the lower thoracic spine following decompression and fusion: a cadaveric analysis. Spine J 14:2216-2223, 2014.

32. Healy AT, Lubelski D, Mageswaran P, et al. Biomechanical analysis of the upper thoracic spine after decompressive procedures. Spine J 14:1010-1016, 2014.

33. Thawrani DP, Glos DL, Coombs MT, et al. Transverse process hooks at upper instrumented vertebra provide more gradual motion transition than pedicle screws. Spine 39:E826-E832, 2014.

34. Kebaish KM, Martin CT, O'Brien JR, et al. Use of vertebroplasty to prevent proximal junctional fractures in adult deformity surgery: a biomechanical cadaveric study. Spine J 13:1897-1903, 2013.

35. Cammarata M, Aubin CE, Wang X, et al. Biomechanical risk factors for proximal junctional kyphosis: a detailed numerical analysis of surgical instrumentation variables. Spine 39:E500-E507, 2014.

36. O'Shaughnessy BA, Bridwell KH, Lenke LG, et al. Does a long-fusion "T3-sacrum" portend a worse outcome than a short-fusion "T10-sacrum" in primary surgery for adult scoliosis? Spine 37:884-890, 2012.

37. Ha Y, Maruo K, Racine L, et al. Proximal junctional kyphosis and clinical outcomes in adult spinal deformity surgery with fusion from the thoracic spine to the sacrum: a comparison of proximal and distal upper instrumented vertebrae. Neurosurg Spine 19:360-369, 2013.

38. Yagi M, Hosogane N, Okada E, et al. Factors affecting the postoperative progression of thoracic kyphosis in surgically treated adult patients with lumbar degenerative scoliosis. Spine 39:E521-E528, 2014.

39. Yagi M, Cunningham E, King A, et al. Long term clinical and radiographic outcomes of pedicle subtraction osteotomy for fixed sagittal imbalance: does level of proximal fusion affect the outcome? Minimum 5 years follow-up. Spine Deform 1:123-131, 2013.

40. Theodoridis D, Ruston S. The effect of shoulder movements on thoracic spine 3D motion. Clin Biomech 17:418-421, 2002.

41. Hassanzadeh H, Gupta S, Jain A, et al. Type of anchor at the proximal fusion level has a significant effect on the incidence of proximal junctional kyphosis and outcome in adults after long posterior spinal fusion. Spine Deform 1:299-305, 2013.

42. Martin CT, Skolasky RL, Mohamed AS, et al. Preliminary results of the effect of prophylactic vertebroplasty on the incidence of proximal junctional complications after posterior spinal fusion to the low thoracic spine. Spine Deform 1:132-138, 2013.

18

Biomechanical Effects of Long Constructs on Distal Adjacent Levels: Considerations for Including L5-S1 and Pelvic Fixation

Hamid Hassanzadeh ▪ *Philip K. Louie*
Abbas Naqvi ▪ *Junyoung Ahn* ▪ *Islam M. Elboghdady*
Khaled Aboushaala ▪ *Kern Singh*

Advancements achieved in long-construct arthrodesis of the spine are available to successfully treat adult spinal deformities. However, despite the development of new techniques to stabilize and secure long-instrumented fusions, lumbopelvic fixation remains technically challenging. The primary goal of a long-instrumented construct is to maintain global coronal and sagittal balance.[1-3] Other goals include earlier mobilization with the need for an external orthosis, decompression of the neural elements, a solid arthrodesis, prevention of deformity progression, and the minimization of potential distal adjacent-segment disease.[1-7]

Adult spines commonly have degenerative changes, compression of neural elements, relative inflexibility, less spontaneous correction, and additional medical comorbidities, compared with adolescent spines.[9] Unlike fusion in typical adolescent patients, in adults it is usually not possible to stop an instrumented fusion at L3-4 because of an element of fixed tilt and rotary subluxation at L3-4.[8,9] The caudal extent of long fusions in adult spines is controversial. Ending fusion too high (at L5) can result in distal-segment degeneration and potential future revision procedures.[1,5,10-12] However, ending fusion too low (at S1 or the pelvis) may sacrifice the remaining motion segment and lead to pseudarthrosis.* The goals of minimizing the number of spinal segments fused and preserving motion segments below the fused spinal segments are weighed against subsequent disc degeneration and possible revision surgery. Kuklo[14] suggested that attention to the resulting coronal and sagittal planes is imperative and much more important than saving fusion levels in adult patients. For many adult patients, no criteria are established regarding the caudal extent of long-instrumented spinal fusions to L5 or S1.

Strengths and concerns about current lumbopelvic fixation have been described in multiple biomechanical studies.[1,2,5,12,14-17] Maintenance of optimal coronal and sagittal balance is complicated by distal-segment disc degeneration, pseudarthrosis, and instrumentation failure. The introduction of anterior column support and pelvic fixation has improved the stability of long-instrumented fusions in adult spinal deformity.[8,9,14,18-21]

---

*References 1, 6, 9, 10, 12, 13.

LONG-INSTRUMENTED CONSTRUCT FUSION TO L5

In patients with a healthy L5-S1 disc, ending the fusion at L5 maintains lumbar motion. Several studies have examined disc disease using a modified version of a radiographic classification defined by Weiner et al.[22] According to this system, a *healthy* disc had less than 25% disc narrowing, small spur formation, minimal eburnation, no listhesis, and no gas.[1,3,4] Additionally, stopping an instrumented fusion at L5 requires a smaller-magnitude surgery. This results in fewer perioperative complications and prevents risks associated with fusions across the lumbosacral junction by decreasing operative time, blood loss, and the incidence of instrumentation complication. The increased stress on the sacroiliac (SI) joints and pseudarthrosis that occur in fusions to S1 can be prevented.[1,4-6,12,19,23]

Degeneration can progress in a healthy L5-S1 disc long after an instrumented fusion to L5 has been performed.[1] Studies have defined this change as subsequent advanced L5-sacrum disc degeneration (SAD).[3,4,11,24] Edwards et al[4] found that the development of SAD within at least 2 years of a fusion was significantly associated with a forward shift in sagittal balance and the need for revision surgery. The same group observed that younger patients were more likely to have degeneration of the L5-S1 disc after fusion to L5.[5] Younger patients may have inferior connective tissue qualities, contributing to their original spinal deformity and propensity for accelerated L5-S1 SAD. These patients may spur the process of SAD through faster return to a higher level of activity after surgery.

The L5-S1 distal-segment disc can lose lumbosacral lordosis over time, further contributing to global sagittal imbalance.[4] Brown et al[13] corrected adult scoliosis with long posterior fusions to L5. Thirty-eight percent of patients developed L5-S1 disc degeneration. The authors predicted that patients most likely to benefit from a long fusion to L5 are those with good preoperative sagittal balance, preserved lumbar lordosis, good postoperative fractional curve correction, and preserved L5-S1 disc height. Overall the incidence of distal-segment disc degeneration after fusion to L5 ranges from 38% to 73%.* Kuhns et al[3] reported that 69% of patients who received thoracolumbar deformity arthrodesis to L5 had advanced L5-S1 disc degeneration at a minimum 5-year follow-up, which was highly correlated with positive sagittal balance. Distal-segment degeneration was likely a result of decreased capacity of the patient to compensate through other mobile segments as the L5-S1 began to degenerate. All patients had healthy discs before the fusion. Eck et al[11] found that fusions short of the sacrum (to L4 or L5) were neutral, horizontal, and stable through the distal-end vertebra, but they did not have a predictable long-term result.

LONG-INSTRUMENTED CONSTRUCT FUSION TO S1

Anatomic variables that require long-instrumented fusion to S1 include severe lumbosacral pain, previous or planned decompression at L5-S1, spondylosis/spondylolysis/spondylolisthesis at L5-S1, involvement of L5 in the fractional curve with lumbosacral obliquity, advanced disc degenerative disease at L5-S1, other structural abnormalities at the L5-S1 segment, and a major fixed coronal or sagittal plane deformity.† In the absence of these anatomic variations, lumbosacral fusion has been shown to better maintain sagittal plane correction that fails with distal-segment disc degeneration. This is especially true in patients with preoperative sagittal plane imbalance. The problem of obtaining solid arthrodesis in adults having fusions to S1 has been a great challenge for many years. Pseudarthrosis rates in the literature after fusion to S1 range from 3% to 83%,[2,9,17,26-30] depending on the biomechanical supportive fixation and length of follow-up. Weistroffer et al[31] reported that 24% of patients with long fusion to the sacrum developed pseudarthrosis.

---

*References 1, 3, 5, 13, 23, 25.
†References 2-6, 10, 12, 21, 23, 24.

However, 75% of these cases were not detected until at least 2 years postoperatively. Multiple complications have been described with extension of fusion across the L5-S1 disc space. Compared with fusions that stop at L5, fusions to S1 show higher rates of SI joint arthrosis; loss of the L5-S1 motion segment, resulting in possible gait abnormalities and difficulty with perineal care; elevated intraoperative complication rates; and instrumentation failure.* Despite the risk of multiple complications, Saer et al[9] successfully performed instrumented fusions to the sacrum and reported an 88% fusion rate, with no cases of postoperative loss of lumbar lordosis.

The SI joint has been identified as an additional source of long-term complication after lumbosacral fusion. Theoretically motion still occurs across the SI joint after a solid fusion has formed across the lumbosacral junction. As the last motion segment is fused distally (L5-S1), stress may be displaced to the SI joint.[5,17] Eck et al[11] reported that none of their patients who had long-instrumented fusions to the sacrum showed clinical or radiographic signs of SI joint breakdown. Kuklo et al[16] and Tsuchiya et al[21] reported that no patients had premature sclerosis or progressive degenerative changes of the SI joint 2 years and 5 years, respectively, after fusion to S1 (and pelvic fixation). Although additional stress and strain can be placed on the SI joint after fusion across the lumbosacral junction, 5-year results showed no evidence of resultant degeneration of the joint space.

Several studies have directly compared results of patients undergoing fusions to L5 or S1. Edwards et al[4] looked at a precisely matched cohort of patients who had long-deformity fusion to L5 or S1. Although the correction of sagittal imbalance was superior in the S1 cohort, this group underwent significantly more procedures (initial and revision) and had a higher rate of medical complications and pseudarthrosis. Sixty-seven percent of the L5 cohort had radiographic evidence of advanced L5-S1 disc degeneration at the latest follow-up (mean 5.2 years). A fourth of these patients had revision extension of arthrodesis to the sacrum. However, SRS-24 functional outcomes were similar between the two groups. Cho et al[1] demonstrated a higher degree of lumbar lordosis correction in patients who underwent interbody fusion at L5-S1 than those who underwent fusion at L4-5. Fifty-eight percent of patients with fusion to L5 had developed subsequent L5-S1 disc degeneration within 2 years. No statistical difference in blood loss or operative time was observed between the two groups. Less correction was achieved with fusion to L5. This was associated with subsequent L5-S1 disc degeneration, which increased the forward shift in the sagittal C7 plumb line. Eck et al[11] extended their cohort to patients with long-instrumented fusions to L4, L5, and S1. Compared with fusions that ended in the lumbar spine, fusions to the sacrum decreased pain and increased function. Complication rates were similar between the groups.

BIOMECHANICAL CONSIDERATIONS

The anatomy and function of the L5-S1 segment is unique in comparison to the other lumbar vertebrae. L5-S1 is the largest disc and contributes to most of the flexion and extension range of motion in the lumbar spine.[33] Because the L5-S1 facet joints are sagittally orientated, lateral bending and axial rotation are minimal at this level.[33] Furthermore, this disc space is less susceptible to strain and degenerative changes because of the stabilizing features of the iliolumbar ligaments.[34] The following biomechanical factors have been described in human and animal model studies of protective and damaging forces on L5-S1 after placement of long-instrumented constructs: deep seating of L5, the effect of the construct length on distal-segment motion, and predispositions to instrumental failure.†

---

*References 1-4, 6, 9, 10, 12, 13, 24, 32.
†References 5, 7, 12-15, 17, 21, 35.

A deep-seated L5, located below the intercristal line on a standing radiograph, is thought to be protected from advanced disc degeneration; thus it is not included as part of the fusion. However, this protection has repeatedly not been shown.[5,10,11,14,36] Eck et al[11] reported that of seven patients who developed distal disc degeneration after fusion to L5, five had a deep-seated L5. Edwards et al[5] performed long fusions that stopped at L5 and observed that 55% of patients with deep seating of L5 of more than 12 mm below the intercristal line had implant loosening and loss of fixation. Among patients in whom L5 was less deep-seated (less than 12 mm), no postoperative loss of fixation was observed. The decreased ability of the L5-S1 disc to dissipate forces applied to L5 resulted in a disproportional amount of stress concentrated on the L5 bone implant.

The disc space, including those that are healthy and clinically stable before spinal fusion, is subject to abnormally large lever arms and cantilever bending forces distal to long constructs in vivo.[3,16,17] A study using porcine models investigated the effects of immobilization on facet force and lumbosacral motion.[35] Long spinal fusions (seven segments or more) increased the load and motion beneath the construct under the same total range of motion. Compared to the preoperative state, immobilization of T6-L6 demonstrated increased lumbosacral motion and facet loading at L7-S1 (120% in flexion, 243% in extension, 390% in contralateral bending, and 380% in ipsilateral bending). Both human and animal studies have revealed that the longer and more distally an instrumented fusion is extended, the higher the incidence of symptomatic degenerative changes below the level of fusion because of amplified changes in the motion pattern distally.[7,13,15,35] For patients with a fusion to S1, these large cantilever forces have resulted in several complications: loss of sacral fixation, instrumentation failure, and loss of lumbar lordosis.[14,16] Long-instrumented constructs to L5 or S1 have also been associated with instrumentation failure.[15,17,24] L5 pedicles are shorter and more cancellous, compared with those in the upper lumbar spine; therefore traditional fixation with two pedicle screws may not be adequate for long fusion.[1,37] Similarly, S1 screws are inserted into wide pedicles with less cortical bone to allow screw purchase. When they are used alone for long-construct fixation, pullout failure occurs.[17]

ANTERIOR COLUMN SUPPORT AND PELVIC FIXATION

The development of new instrumentation techniques has allowed surgeons to protect instrumented constructs and distal-adjacent segments through (1) anterior column support to increase compression stiffness at the L5-S1 junction and restore normal lumbar lordosis/sagittal alignment and (2) pelvic fixation to increase torsional stiffness at the L5-S1 junction.[1,2]

Anterior column support has been achieved with transforaminal lumbar interbody fusion (TLIF), anterior lumbar interbody support (ALIF), and posterior lumbar interbody fusion (PLIF), creating circumferential fusion.* McCord et al[39] performed a biomechanical analysis on lumbosacral segments in calves and observed maximal protection of this segment only in devices anterior to the vertebral column. Glazer et al[15] measured lumbosacral motion (flexion, extension, lateral bending, axial compression, and torsion) and found that the use of a threaded interbody fusion device best decreased motion at the L5-S1 segment. Lowest pseudarthrosis rates in revision fusion extensions to S1 occurred in patients who received an anterior graft at L4-5 and L5-S1 and instrumented fixation to both the sacrum and ilium.[18]

---

*References 2, 6, 8, 15, 16, 21, 38.

Pelvic fixation has been accomplished with iliac screws and bolts, S1–iliac screw alignment, unilateral pelvic screw fixation, S2-alar-iliac (S2AI) screw placement, and the four-rod technique.* Islam et al[18] studied revision fusion extensions to the pelvis with iliac screws or rods in patients originally receiving long-instrumented fusions for adult scoliosis. Posterior fixation alone resulted in a 53% pseudarthrosis rate, whereas iliac fixation–only resulted in a rate of 42%. However, in patients with both iliac and sacral fixation, only 21% showed pseudarthrosis at minimum 2-year follow-up after the initial fusion. Kuklo et al[16] applied bilateral iliac screws coupled with bilateral S1 screws and reported a 95% lumbosacral fusion rate. Previous iliac crest harvesting did not prevent ipsilateral iliac screw placement. At 5- to 10-year follow-ups, Tsuchiya et al[21] observed that iliac screws provided significant protection of S1 screws, as evidenced by the absence of S1 screw failure by breakage, loosening, or pullout. Emami et al[2] successfully averted future revision surgeries by applying bicortical, triangulated sacral screws with structural anterior column support at L4-5 and L5-S1 in patients with good bone stock. In patients whose bone stock was poor, they combined iliac and sacral fixation to create a stable fusion. Kim et al[38] significantly lowered pseudarthrosis rates to 24% after complete sacropelvic fixation consisting of bilateral iliac and bicortical S1 screw fixation in addition to anterior column support at L4-5 and L5-S1.

REVISION PROCEDURES

Instrumentation failure, loss of fixation, and infection are common problems that require revision. Great emphasis has been placed on revisions for pseudarthrosis after fusion to S1 and for extension of long fusions (originally to L5) to the sacropelvic region.† Precluding distal degeneration and prior revision surgery, the threshold is commonly lower for extension of a primary fusion down to the sacrum. Criteria to extend a primary fusion at L5 to S1 include increasing pain in the lumbosacral region, radiographic evidence of distal disc degeneration, coronal imbalance, and kyphotic deformity or loss of lumbar lordosis.[3,4,26,32] Edwards et al[4] observed significantly inferior SRS-24 pain scores in patients who developed distal-segment disc degeneration after a long-instrumented fusion to L5; 25% of them required revision extension to S1. Kostuik and Musha[26] examined fusion extensions to S1 in adults with degenerative changes and loss of lumbar lordosis years after receiving fusions that stopped at L4 or L5 for adolescent idiopathic scoliosis. With more rigid fixation, pseudarthrosis rates decreased to 3%. Similarly, Kuhns et al[3] noted that 69% of adults who had arthrodesis to L5 developed increasingly positive sagittal balance. Twenty-three percent of this group underwent successful fusion extension to the sacrum and regained optimal sagittal balance.

Revision procedures are generally challenging and can be associated with higher complication rates and pseudarthrosis. Fu et al[32] compared adult spinal deformity patients who received posterior fusion with sacropelvic fixation and similar patients who received a fusion that ended in the distal lumbar spine and was later extended to the pelvis. They found that the complication rates for the revision procedures, though not insignificant, were similar to those of the primary procedure. Hassanzadeh et al[42] reported similar complication rates and SRS-22 outcomes between primary and revision spinal deformity surgeries in adults. Emami et al[2] performed revision surgeries in patients with pseudarthrosis, continued sagittal deformity, and instrumentation failure after primary fusions to the sacrum. They reported that revision surgeries were as safe and effective as the primary operations.

---

*References 17, 18, 20, 31, 40, 41.
†References 2-4, 6, 12, 24, 26, 32.

PATIENT EXAMPLES

This 63-year-old man presented with a history of progressive degenerative scoliosis and worsening pain (Fig. 18-1, *A* and *B*). He underwent a posterior spinal instrumentation and fusion from L1 to L5 at an outside institution (Fig. 18-1, *C* and *D*). At the 8-month follow-up, the patient has severe back pain and right lower extremity pain and gastrocnemius weakness. MRI demonstrates a right-sided L5-S1 disc herniation with S1 nerve root impingement (Fig. 18-1, *E* and *F*).

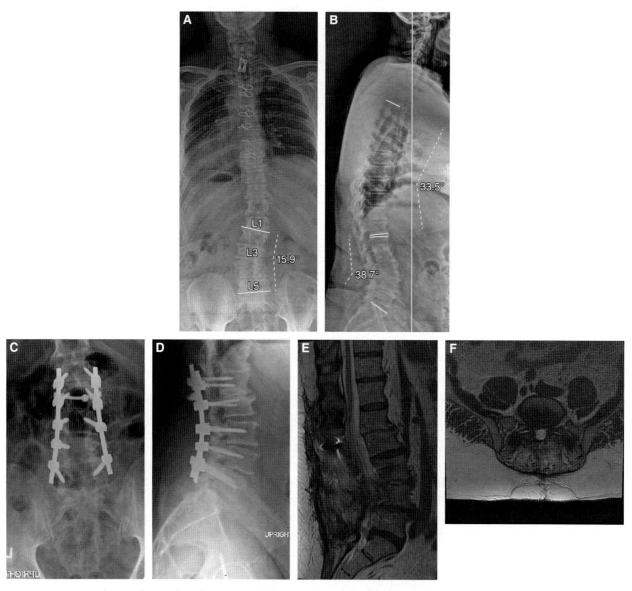

Fig. 18-1 Standing radiographs of a 63-year-old man who developed adjacent-segment degeneration at the L5-S1 level after an instrumented posterior spinal fusion from L1 to L5. **A** and **B,** Preoperative AP and lateral radiographs. **C** and **D,** Postoperative radiographs of L1-5 instrumented fusion. **E,** T2-weighted sagittal MRI demonstrates a caudally migrated extruded disc fragment with disc space collapse. **F,** T2-weighted axial MRI shows a right-sided herniated nucleus pulposus with S1 traversing nerve root impingement.

This 58-year-old woman presented with a history of idiopathic scoliosis with superimposed degenerative thoracolumbar spondylosis with worsening back pain (Fig. 18-2, *A* and *B*). She underwent posterior spinal fusion and instrumentation from T5 to L5. No significant radiographic or clinical signs of adjacent-segment degeneration are evident on her 2-year postoperative radiographs (Fig. 18-2, *C* and *D*).

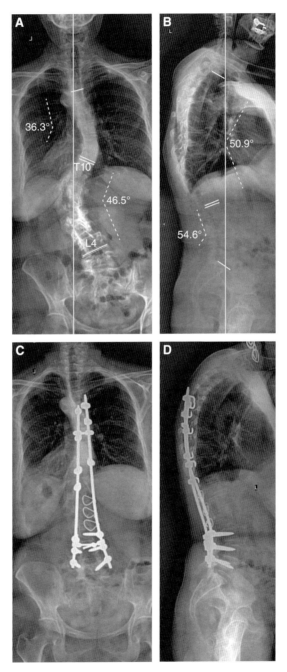

Fig. 18-2 Standing radiographs of a 58-year-old woman who underwent posterior spinal fusion from T5 to L5. **A** and **B,** Preoperative AP and lateral radiographs. **C** and **D,** Two-year postoperative AP and lateral radiographs show no evidence of adjacent-segment degeneration.

This 68-year-old woman with a history of degenerative scoliosis presented with severe low back pain and neurogenic claudication (Fig. 18-3, *A* and *B*). She underwent a multilevel laminectomy and posterior spinal fusion and instrumentation from T10 to her pelvis (Fig. 18-3, *C* and *D*).

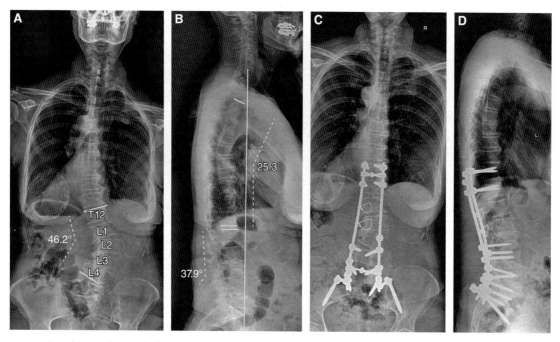

Fig. 18-3   Standing radiographs of a 68-year-old woman who had posterior spinal fusion from T10 to her pelvis. **A** and **B**, Preoperative AP and lateral radiographs. **C** and **D**, Two-year postoperative AP and lateral radiographs demonstrating resolution of scoliosis and correction of lumbar lordosis.

CONCLUSION

The distal extent of a long-instrumented fusion to correct adult spinal deformity continues to be a topic of debate. Although absolute indications exist for extending a fusion to the sacrum, considerations for stopping a fusion at L5 or S1 are less clear in patients with a healthy L5-S1 disc. In a young patient with good muscle tone and a healthy L5-S1 disc, ending the fusion at L5 may preserve the distal motion segment and reduce exposure to a larger, more complicated procedure. However, high rates of distal-segment disc degeneration have been observed after fusions to L5 in patients with a radiographically and clinically healthy L5-S1 disc. Extending a fusion to S1 has been shown to better maintain global balance in the setting of preoperative sagittal plane imbalance, while preventing subsequent degeneration and possible revision surgery at L5-S1. Risks of pseudarthrosis and increased medical complications occur as the L5-S1 motion segment is lost. Biomechanical studies performed in humans and animal models have improved fusion outcomes through the addition of anterior column support and/or pelvic fixation. These methods have strengthened the integrity of primary and revision long-instrumented fusions and their ability to correct and maintain coronal and sagittal imbalances.

REFERENCES

1. Cho KJ, Suk SI, Park SR, et al. Arthrodesis to L5 versus S1 in long instrumentation and fusion for degenerative lumbar scoliosis. Eur Spine J 18:531-537, 2009.

2. Emami A, Deviren V, Berven S, et al. Outcome and complications of long fusions to the sacrum in adult spine deformity: Luque-Galveston, combined iliac and sacral screws, and sacral fixation. Spine 27:776-786, 2002.

3. Kuhns CA, Bridwell KH, Lenke LG, et al. Thoracolumbar deformity arthrodesis stopping at L5: fate of the L5-S1 disc, minimum 5-year follow-up. Spine 32:2771-2776, 2007.

4. Edwards CC II, Bridwell KH, Patel A, et al. Long adult deformity fusions to L5 and the sacrum. A matched cohort analysis. Spine 29:1996-2005, 2004.

5. Edwards CC II, Bridwell KH, Patel A, et al. Thoracolumbar deformity arthrodesis to L5 in adults: the fate of the L5-S1 disc. Spine 28:2122-2131, 2003.

6. Polly DW Jr, Hamill CL, Bridwell KH. Debate: to fuse or not to fuse to the sacrum, the fate of the L5-S1 disc. Spine 31(19 Suppl):S179-S184, 2006.

7. Shono Y, Kaneda K, Abumi K, et al. Stability of posterior spinal instrumentation and its effects on adjacent motion segments in the lumbosacral spine. Spine 23:1550-1558, 1998.

8. Mok JM, Hu SS. Surgical strategies and choosing levels for spinal deformity: how high, how low, front and back. Neurosurg Clin N Am 18:329-337, 2007.

9. Saer EH III, Winter RB, Lonstein JE. Long scoliosis fusion to the sacrum in adults with nonparalytic scoliosis. An improved method. Spine 15:650-653, 1990.

10. Bridwell KH, Edwards CC II, Lenke LG. The pros and cons to saving the L5-S1 motion segment in a long scoliosis fusion construct. Spine 28:S234-S242, 2003.

11. Eck KR, Bridwell KH, Ungacta FF, et al. Complications and results of long adult deformity fusions down to L4, L5, and the sacrum. Spine 26:E182-E192, 2001.

12. Swamy G, Berven SH, Bradford DS. The selection of L5 versus S1 in long fusions for adult idiopathic scoliosis. Neurosurg Clin N Am 18:281-288, 2007.

13. Brown KM, Ludwig SC, Gelb DE. Radiographic predictors of outcome after long fusion to L5 in adult scoliosis. J Spinal Disord Tech 17:358-366, 2004.

14. Kuklo TR. Principles for selecting fusion levels in adult spinal deformity with particular attention to lumbar curves and double major curves. Spine 31(19 Suppl):S132-S138, 2006.

15. Glazer PA, Colliou O, Lotz JC, et al. Biomechanical analysis of lumbosacral fixation. Spine 21:1211-1222, 1996.

16. Kuklo TR, Bridwell KH, Lewis SJ, et al. Minimum 2-year analysis of sacropelvic fixation and L5-S1 fusion using S1 and iliac screws. Spine 26:1976-1983, 2001.

17. Shen FH, Mason JR, Shimer AL, et al. Pelvic fixation for adult scoliosis. Eur Spine J 22(Suppl 2):S265-S275, 2013.

18. Islam NC, Wood KB, Transfeldt EE, et al. Extension of fusions to the pelvis in idiopathic scoliosis. Spine 26:166-173, 2001.

19. Kim YJ, Bridwell KH, Lenke LG, et al. An analysis of sagittal spinal alignment following long adult lumbar instrumentation and fusion to L5 or S1: can we predict ideal lumbar lordosis? Spine 31:2343-2352, 2006.

20. Tomlinson T, Chen J, Upasani V, et al. Unilateral and bilateral sacropelvic fixation result in similar construct biomechanics. Spine 33:2127-2133, 2008.

21. Tsuchiya K, Bridwell KH, Kuklo TR, et al. Minimum 5-year analysis of L5-S1 fusion using sacropelvic fixation (bilateral S1 and iliac screws) for spinal deformity. Spine 31:303-308, 2006.

22. Weiner DK, Distell B, Studenski S, et al. Does radiographic osteoarthritis correlate with flexibility of the lumbar spine? J Am Geriatr Soc 42:257-263, 1994.

23. Horton WC, Holt RT, Muldowny DS. Controversy. Fusion of L5-S1 in adult scoliosis. Spine 21:2520-2522, 1996.

24. Fogelson JL, Krauss WE. To fuse to the sacrum or stop short: that is the question. World Neurosurg. 2013 Apr 5. [Epub ahead of print]

25. Cochran T, Irstam L, Nachemson A. Long-term anatomic and functional changes in patients with adolescent idiopathic scoliosis treated by Harrington rod fusion. Spine 8:576-584, 1983.

26. Kostuik JP, Musha Y. Extension to the sacrum of previous adolescent scoliosis fusions in adult life. Clin Orthop Relat Res 364:53-60, 1999.

27. Balderston RA, Winter RB, Moe JH, et al. Fusion to the sacrum for nonparalytic scoliosis in the adult. Spine 11:824-829, 1986.

28. Devlin VJ, Boachie-Adjei O, Bradford DS, et al. Treatment of adult spinal deformity with fusion to the sacrum using CD instrumentation. J Spinal Disord 4:1-14, 1991.

29. Grubb SA, Lipscomb HJ, Suh PB. Results of surgical treatment of painful adult scoliosis. Spine 19:1619-1627, 1994.

30. Kostuik JP, Hall BB. Spinal fusions to the sacrum in adults with scoliosis. Spine 8:489-500 1983.

31. Weistroffer JK, Perra JH, Lonstein JE, et al. Complications in long fusions to the sacrum for adult scoliosis: minimum five-year analysis of fifty patients. Spine 33:1478-1483, 2008.

32. Fu KM, Smith JS, Burton DC, et al; International Spine Study Group. Revision extension to the pelvis versus primary spinopelvic instrumentation in adult deformity: comparison of clinical outcomes and complications. World Neurosurg. 2013 Feb 21. [Epub ahead of print]

33. Yamamoto I, Panjabi MM, Crisco T, et al. Three-dimensional movements of the whole lumbar spine and lumbosacral joint. Spine 14:1256-1260, 1989.

34. Aihara T, Takahashi K, Ono Y, et al. Does the morphology of the iliolumbar ligament affect lumbosacral disc degeneration? Spine 27:1499-1503, 2002.

35. Nagata H, Schendel MJ, Transfeldt EE, et al. The effects of immobilization of long segments of the spine on the adjacent and distal facet force and lumbosacral motion. Spine 18:2471-2479, 1993.

36. Abd-El-Barr M, Groff MW. Looking through a crystal ball—the question of primarily fusing to the pelvis in adult degenerative scoliosis. World Neurosurg. 2013 Aug 3. [Epub ahead of print]

37. Kwon BK, Elgafy H, Keynan O, et al. Progressive junctional kyphosis at the caudal end of lumbar instrumented fusion: etiology, predictors, and treatment. Spine 31:1943-1951, 2006.

38. Kim YJ, Bridwell KH, Lenke LG, et al. Pseudarthrosis in long adult spinal deformity instrumentation and fusion to the sacrum: prevalence and risk factor analysis of 144 cases. Spine 31:2329-2336, 2006.

39. McCord DH, Cunningham BW, Shono Y, et al. Biomechanical analysis of lumbosacral fixation. Spine 17(8 Suppl):S235-S243, 1992.

40. Garant M. Sacroplasty: a new treatment for sacral insufficiency fracture. J Vasc Interv Radiol 13:1265-1267, 2002.

41. Kebaish KM. Sacropelvic fixation: techniques and complications. Spine 35:2245-2251, 2010.

42. Hassanzadeh H, Jain A, El Dafrawy MH, et al. Clinical results and functional outcomes of primary and revision spinal deformity surgery in adults. J Bone Joint Surg Am 95:1413-1419, 2013.

19

Implant Failure in Sagittal Plane Problems

David W. Polly, Jr.

Implants are temporary, biologic stabilizing devices that support fusion. If fusion fails and the patient is mobile, the implant will fail. The intervertebral disc of the lumbar spine is conservatively estimated to have 85 million spinal loading cycles during a 40-year period.[1,2] Life is a progressively kyphosing event. Kyphosis places a much greater load on instrumentation.[3] In addition, fixation and biologic healing are much more challenging in older patients with osteoporosis and spinal deformity, who often are taking medications such as NSAIDs, prednisone, and disease-modifying antirheumatic drugs that impair bone healing. All of these factors combined indicate that fixation failures will probably increase in frequency.

Instrumentation can be divided into two types: *anchors,* which attach to and grip the spinal elements, and *longitudinal members,* usually rods and spacers that typically are load sharing. Anchors include screws, hooks, and wires (cables and tapes). Screws can fail by loosening, breaking, or pulling out. Hooks can displace, pull out, or lose their connection with the longitudinal member. Wires, cables, and tapes can cut through the bone, break, or lose attachment. Longitudinal members include rods, plates, cables, and wires. Currently the most common longitudinal member is a rod. Rods fracture either at the points of greatest stress or at points of stress risers within a construct. Screws can fracture with significant loading and good screw purchase. Typically this occurs with inadequate anterior column support.

Interbody device settling can result in loss of correction and pseudarthrosis. Settling can occur for a variety of reasons, including inadequate cross-sectional area to support the applied load, inadequate bone stock (as is typical in osteoporosis), violation of the endplate, and improper placement. Determining adequate stiffness for a construct remains a challenge. A construct that is too stiff results in potential stress shielding of the fusion mass and may lead to a higher rate of adjacent-segment problems. A construct that is not stiff enough leads to implant failure and may cause pseudarthrosis through excessive strain on the fusion mass.

ROD FAILURE

Rod biomechanics are based on rod diameter and material. Rod stiffness is proportional to its radius to the fourth power. Rod material has a significant effect on rod stiffness: Titanium is less stiff than stainless steel and cobalt-chrome. Rod bending affects fatigue performance. Titanium is particularly notch sensitive and susceptible to failure at bend points or more typically at the point where the screw locking mechanism connects to the rod and creates a notch in the rod. Stainless steel has excellent biomechanical properties for spinal deformity correction but has poor imaging properties for both CT and MRI. Titanium has the best imaging properties, followed by cobalt-chrome and stainless steel; however, cobalt-chrome has better biomechanical and handling properties than titanium. Titanium is probably the most notch sensitive of the metals; therefore rod bending and in situ contouring are more likely to create stress risers. Stainless steel appears to be more susceptible than titanium to bacterial surface colonization. The nickel in stainless steel is more allergenic than that in titanium.

Prelordosed rods provide a higher fatigue strength than intraoperatively bent rods because of the stress relief effected during the annealing process. Isola benders (DePuy Spine, Inc., Raynham, MA), French benders, and in situ benders were used in a study conducted to determine the effect of different bending techniques on the fatigue performance of titanium alloy spinal rods assembled in vitro for a spinal verte-brectomy construct[4] (Fig. 19-1, *A* through *F*). Prelordosed rods had the most uniform curvature, followed by Isola-bent rods, French-bent rods, and those bent in situ (Fig. 19-2). The endurance limits varied for several possible reasons. The highest stress concentration for high-cycle fatigue occurred at the set screw mark (Fig. 19-3). When the rods were bent, the stress concentration at the set screw was increased depend-ing on the degree of bending at that point. The French bender marks and high bend zones were not at the same point as the set screw in the constructs studied; thus the long-term fatigue results were better (see Fig. 19-3, *C*). The Isola bender better distributed the degree of bending through the rod, so that the stress concentration at the set screw mark was actually higher versus the French bender, when the set screw was not tightened directly on the French bender mark (see Fig. 19-3, *B*). The in situ benders caused the most gouging of the rod, but these rods had an equivalent fatigue performance, compared with the Isola-bent rods (see Fig. 19-3, *D*). Maximum fatigue strength with lordosed rods can be achieved using prelordosed rods; however, rod-bending techniques that result in nonuniform bending, as with French benders, may provide superior fatigue strength compared with uniform bending techniques. This might not be true if the pedicle screws are connected to the rod at the high-bend zones.

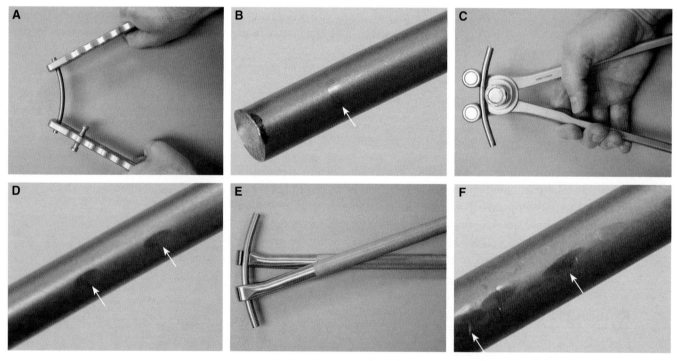

Fig. 19-1 **A,** Isola benders grip the rod at opposite ends and bend uniformly along the length. Beveled edges on the benders minimize marks on the rod. **B,** The mark from an Isola bender is slight *(arrow)*. **C,** A French bender is es-sentially a three-point bender with roller surfaces. Bends were made incrementally along the rod to achieve relative uniformity. **D,** Marks from a French bender *(arrows)* appear as oval-shaped depressions. **E,** In situ benders create a four-point bend and crisscross so that they can be used in a deep wound. Bends were made incrementally along the rod to achieve relative uniformity. **F,** Harder edges on the bender jaws create larger gouges *(arrows)* than are seen with the other benders.

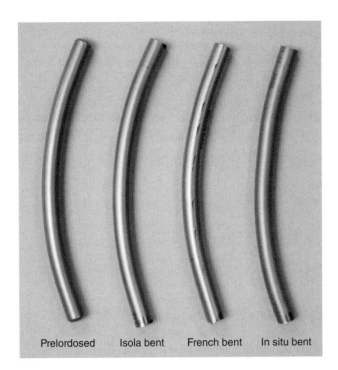

Fig. 19-2 Comparison of rod curvature.

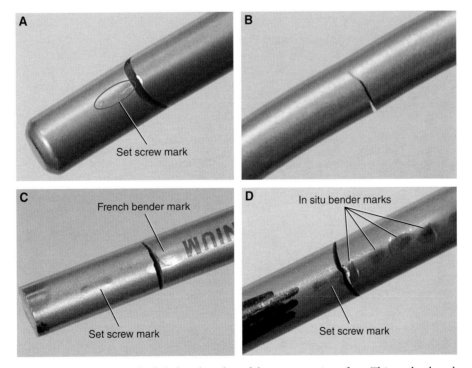

Fig. 19-3 **A,** Prelordosed rods typically failed at the edge of the set screw interface. This prelordosed rod was tested with a weak load of 420 N, where N = 625,380 cycles. **B,** Isola-bent rods usually failed at areas without obvious stress concentrations. This Isola-bent rod was tested under a peak load of 260 N, where N = 392,448 cycles. **C,** French-bent rods failed at either the bender mark or the set screw mark. This rod was tested under a peak load of 250 N, where N = 367,014 cycles. **D,** In situ–bent rods typically failed at bender marks but also at coincident bender–set screw marks. This rod was tested under a peak load of 300 N, where N = 497,673 cycles.

Continued

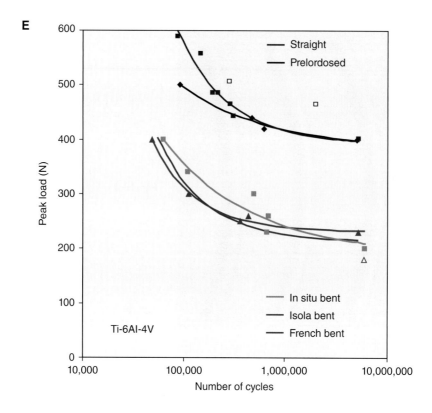

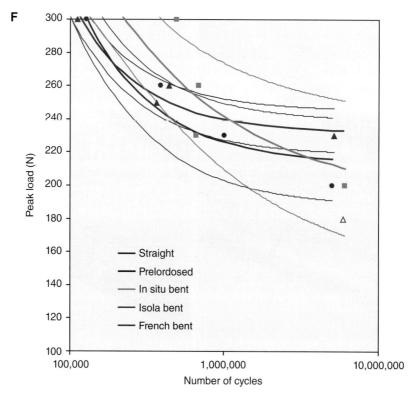

Fig. 19-3, cont'd   **E,** Prelordosed rods had a much higher endurance limit (400 N) in the vertebrectomy constructs, compared with rods bent by any of the intraoperative techniques (230 N and below). **F,** With 95% confidence limits *(thin lines)* the intraoperatively bent rods had similar fatigue curves. French-bent rods had a slightly higher endurance limit (230 N) than Isola-bent or in situ–bent rods (both 200 N).

ANCHOR FAILURE

Hooks can dislodge or pull through the bone. Dislodgement often occurred with Harrington rods, although it was never well documented in the literature. This was a mechanical result of single-endpoint nonsegmental fixation, distraction correction, and subsequent ligamentous stress relaxation. Segmental fixation, especially with the claw concept of opposing downward and upward hooks, markedly decreased the occurrence of dislodgement. Cantilever correction places significant force on hooks and can cause bony failure of either a transverse process or lamina. Hooks placed on the lamina also can have significant volumetric intrusion into the spinal canal and should not be used in patients with spinal stenosis.[5]

Screw breakage was more common with earlier screw designs and the more frequent use of posterior instrumentation without anterior column load sharing. When used for short-segment fixation of burst fractures, the breakage rates were as high as 24%.[6] Screw fracture usually occurred where the minor diameter taper ended. Other forms of loss of screw fixation include screw plowing with loss of alignment or screw pullout.[7] Screw failure at the sacrum presents particularly unique challenges. The sacrum has a thin ventral and dorsal cortical shell of bone and a center portion of vacuous cancellous bone.[8-10] Therefore, if bicortical fixation is not achieved, screws are extremely susceptible to pullout because of the large cantilever forces present at the sacrum.[11] Optimizing screw fixation at S1 requires either tricortical fixation or fixation that engages the S1 superior endplate.[12,13]

Fixation of long fusions to the pelvis requires special considerations.[14] Fixation with S1 pedicle screws alone, either with or without interbody support, places tremendous strain on the S1 screws. Typically if the fusion is longer than three to four segments, some form of iliac fixation is appropriate. Biomechanically iliac fixation is superior to other forms of adjunctive fixation, such as sacral alar screws, S2 screws, or interbody support.[15] Iliac fixation is optimized by larger screw diameters and a screw length of 80 mm or greater.[16] More recently, S2 alar iliac (S2AI) screws have become more popular. These screws should have better purchase, because they cross the dorsal cortex, the lateral sacral cortex, and the medial iliac cortex and then engage the relatively robust bone of the ilium.[11,17-20]

LATE FAILURES

More recently with the increased use of three-column osteotomies (pedicle subtraction osteotomies and vertebral column resections [VCRs]), late rod breakage is being seen.[21] Although these osteotomies represent the greatest destabilization of the spine, they allow the spinal deformity to be corrected with these techniques. Improved spinal fixation strategies have resulted in good temporary stabilization, but if an adequate fusion mass does not develop, then the rods will fatigue. This is being seen as late as 4 or 5 years after surgery (personal experience and personal communication, Lawrence G. Lenke, MD, 2013). This has led to the increasing use of more than two rods to span the gap across these types of osteotomies.

PATIENT EXAMPLES

ROD FRACTURE AFTER VERTEBRAL COLUMN RESECTION FOR SEVERE CONGENITAL ANOMALY

The destabilization associated with a VCR may require more than two rods to span an unstable gap. Biologic reconstruction of the posterior column may be needed. This 14-year-old adolescent presented with previous hemiepiphysiodesis and continued progression of deformity, with no significant pain or activity limitations (Fig. 19-4, *A* through *C*). The patient underwent posterior VCR that was complicated by a transient Brown-Séquard syndrome, which resolved completely by 6 weeks (Fig. 19-4, *D* and *E*). Eighteen months postoperatively he was involved in a strenuous physical activity and felt a pop. Radiographs showed broken rods (Fig. 19-4, *F*). CT scans showed solid fusion anteriorly but this was apparently inadequate (Fig. 19-4, *G* and *H*).

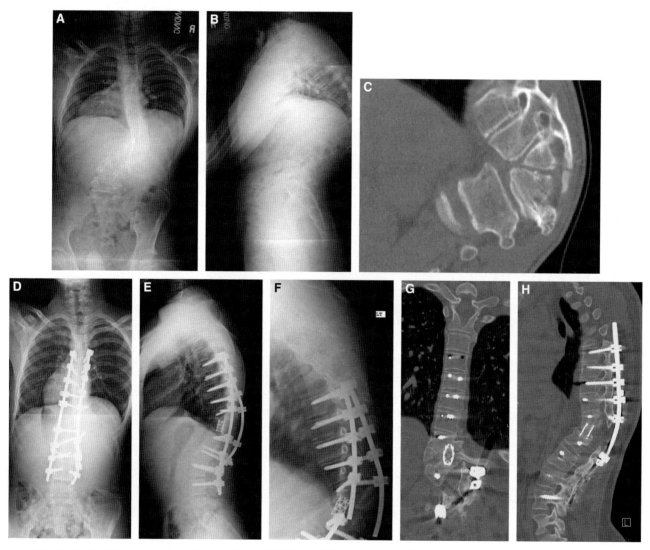

Fig. 19-4 **A-C,** Preoperative radiographs and CT showed deformity after hemiepiphysiodesis. **D** and **E,** Results after a vertebral column resection, which was complicated by a transient Brown-Séquard syndrome that resolved after 6 weeks. **F,** Radiographs revealed broken rods after a strenuous physical event. **G** and **H,** AP and lateral CT scans showed an apparently solid anterior column fusion, which was inadequate.

ROD FRACTURE IN LONG FUSION

This patient had a posterior fusion at another institution, and her most caudal screws plowed inferiorly towards the inferior endplate of the L4 vertebral body (Fig. 19-5, *A*). She healed but had to hyperextend below the fusion thereafter. After 2 years these levels wore out, and the pain was sufficient to require reintervention. Fusion was extended to the pelvis in an attempt to optimize lordosis. Although difficult to detect radiographically, the rods had fractured in three places (Fig. 19-5, *B* and *C*). The rods were titanium and had significant bends to accommodate her lordosis. They fractured at the screws where the set plugs created notching. Metallic debris stained the soft tissues at the sites of rod breakage. Revision involved a pedicle subtraction osteotomy, which resulted in improved sagittal balance, reducing stress on the distal fixation (Fig. 19-5, *D* and *E*).

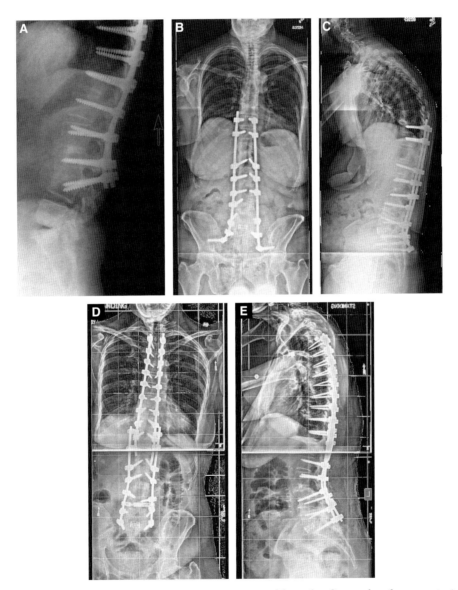

Fig. 19-5   **A,** Initial presentation. **B** and **C,** Postoperative AP and lateral radiographs after an anterior lumbar interbody fusion at L4-5 and L5-S1 with posterior reconstruction. **D** and **E,** Postoperative AP and lateral radiographs after an L3 pedicle subtraction osteotomy.

SACRAL FRACTURE AFTER ANTERIOR AND POSTERIOR FIXATION

This patient had bicortical S1 pedicle screws and an anterior plate at L5-S1, which created four anterior cortical stress risers at S1. A fracture occurred at this level. The patient developed a kyphotic deformity and healed in a kyphotic position (Fig. 19-6, *A* through *C*). She was referred for further evaluation. We decided that a sacral osteotomy was needed to adequately correct her sagittal plane alignment. Given her history of distal failure, stacked iliac screws were placed to improve fixation and correct the deformity by rotating the pelvis into alignment with the spine, rather than trying to pull the spine back to the pelvis (Fig. 19-6, *D* and *E*).

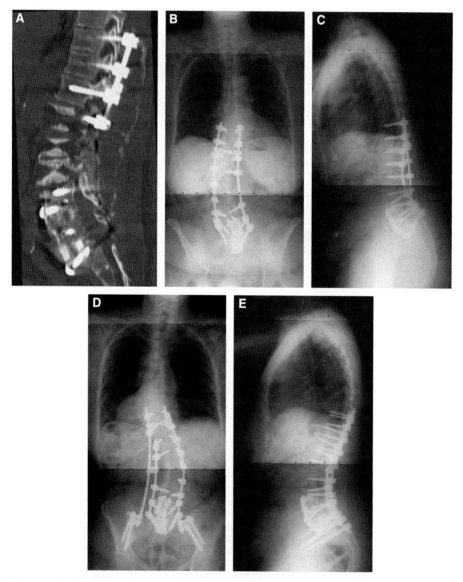

Fig. 19-6   **A,** Preoperative CT sagittal reconstruction revealed a fracture. **B** and **C,** Preoperative AP and lateral scoliosis films. **D** and **E,** Postoperative AP and lateral scoliosis films.

CONCLUSION

Failures of instrumentation occur in adult spinal deformity surgery. As older and sicker patients are treated, we can expect that failures will continue to occur. Failure types can be categorized and perhaps anticipated on a case-by-case basis. Strategies to minimize these specific failures can be applied to decrease patient-specific risks. Optimal sagittal alignment is one of these many factors.

REFERENCES

1. Kostuik JP. Intervertebral disc replacement. Experimental study. Clin Orthop Relat Res 337:27-41, 1997.
2. Cunningham BW. Basic scientific considerations in total disc arthroplasty. Spine J 4(6 Suppl):S219-S230, 2004.
3. Belmont PJ Jr, Polly DW Jr, Cunningham BW, et al. The effects of hook pattern and kyphotic angulation on mechanical strength and apical rod strain in a long-segment posterior construct using a synthetic model. Spine 26:627-635, 2001.
4. Polly DW, Slivka M, Serhan H, et al. Rod bending technique affects the fatigue performance of titanium spinal implants. Presented at the Tenth Annual International Meeting for Advanced Spine Techniques (IMAST), Rome, July 2003.
5. Polly DW Jr, Potter BK, Kuklo T, et al. Volumetric spinal canal intrusion: a comparison between thoracic pedicle screws and thoracic hooks. Spine 29:63-69, 2004.
6. Carl AL, Tromanhauser SG, Roger DJ. Pedicle screw instrumentation for thoracolumbar burst fractures and fracture-dislocations. Spine 17(8 Suppl):S317-S324, 1992.
7. McLain RF, Sparling E, Benson DR. Early failure of short-segment pedicle instrumentation for thoracolumbar fractures. A preliminary report. J Bone Joint Surg Am 75:162-167, 1993.
8. Smith SA, Abitbol JJ, Carlson GD, et al. The effects of depth of penetration, screw orientation, and bone density on sacral screw fixation. Spine 18:1006-1010, 1993.
9. Carlson GD, Abitbol JJ, Anderson DR, et al. Screw fixation in the human sacrum. An in vitro study of the biomechanics of fixation. Spine 17(6 Suppl):S196-S203, 1992.
10. Mirkovic S, Abitbol JJ, Steinman J, et al. Anatomic consideration for sacral screw placement. Spine 16(6 Suppl):S289-S294, 1991.
11. McCord DH, Cunningham BW, Shono Y, et al. Biomechanical analysis of lumbosacral fixation. Spine 17(8 Suppl):S235-S243, 1992.
12. Lehman RA Jr, Kuklo TR, Belmont PJ Jr, et al. Advantage of pedicle screw fixation directed into the apex of the sacral promontory over bicortical fixation: a biomechanical analysis. Spine 27:806-811, 2002.
13. Luk KD, Chen L, Lu WW. A stronger bicortical sacral pedicle screw fixation through the s1 endplate: an in vitro cyclic loading and pull-out force evaluation. Spine 30:525-529, 2005.
14. Orchowski J, Polly DW Jr, Klemme WR, et al. The effect of kyphosis on the mechanical strength of a long-segment posterior construct using a synthetic model. Spine 25:1644-1648, 2000.
15. Lebwohl NH, Cunningham BW, Dmitriev A, et al. Biomechanical comparison of lumbosacral fixation techniques in a calf spine model. Spine 27:2312-2320, 2002.
16. Santos ER, Sembrano JN, Mueller B, Polly DW. Optimizing iliac screw fixation: a biomechanical study on screw length, trajectory, and diameter. J Neurosurg Spine 14:219-225, 2011.
17. Chang TL, Sponseller PD, Kebaish KM, et al. Low profile pelvic fixation: anatomic parameters for sacral alar-iliac fixation versus traditional iliac fixation. Spine 34:436-440, 2009.
18. Sponseller PD, Zimmerman RM, Ko PS, et al. Low profile pelvic fixation with the sacral alar iliac technique in the pediatric population improves results at two-year minimum follow-up. Spine 35:1887-1892, 2010.
19. Cunningham BW, Sefter JC, Hu N, et al. Biomechanical comparison of iliac screws versus interbody femoral ring allograft on lumbosacral kinematics and sacral screw strain. Spine 35:E198-E205, 2010.
20. O'Brien JR, Yu W, Kaufman BE, et al. Biomechanical evaluation of S2 alar-iliac screws: effect of length and quad-cortical purchase as compared with iliac fixation. Spine 38:E1250-E1255, 2013.
21. Smith JS, Shaffrey CI, Ames CP, et al. Assessment of symptomatic rod fracture after posterior instrumented fusion for adult spinal deformity. Neurosurgery 71:862-867, 2012.

PART IV

Biologic Considerations of Spinal Fusion in Spinal Deformity

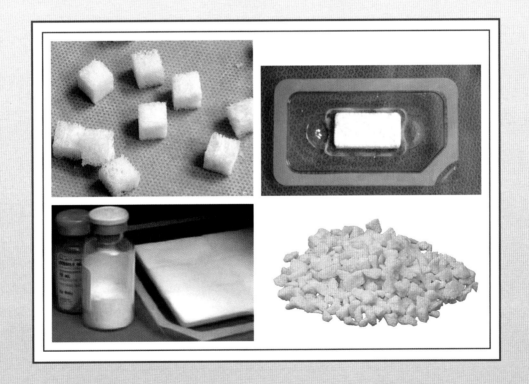

20

Host Factor Considerations

Alp Yurter ▪ *Patricia L. Zadnik* ▪ *Daniel M. Sciubba*

The surgical treatment of adult spinal deformity requires significant preoperative planning, with consideration of patient bone quality, previous surgical intervention, and global deformity. For adult patients with poor bone quality, vitamin D deficiency, osteoporosis, or metabolic bone disease, well-planned, careful medical management can optimize surgical outcomes. Intraoperative interventions, such as the off-label use of bone morphogenic protein (BMP) or off-label bone cement to reinforce surgical instrumentation, can further optimize bone growth and fusion in patients with suboptimal bone quality.[1] For patients with previous surgical intervention and subsequent instrumentation failure, proximal junctional kyphosis (PJK), or failed back surgery syndrome (FBSS), preoperative planning involves an analysis of the patient's global deformity. This chapter will review patient host factors that complicate spine surgery, including metabolic bone disease and previous spine surgery.

Numerous studies have demonstrated that poor bone quality increases the risk of instrumentation failure and subsequent deformity of global alignment.[2-7] Poor bone quality may be a product of metabolic bone disease, a term that broadly encompasses conditions characterized by abnormal osteoblast/osteoclast activity and disorganized bone remodeling. Osteoporosis is the most prevalent common metabolic bone disease,[8] resulting in 700,000 annual spinal fractures in the United States and affecting 30% of white postmenopausal women.[2] Paget's disease, the second most common metabolic bone disorder, increases with age. Postmortem analysis reveals that 3% to 3.7% of the population are afflicted with this condition at death.[8,68] Beyond metabolic bone disease, nutritional deficiencies can underlie inferior bone quality. Vitamin D plays a critical role in maintaining bone density; a deficiency of this nutrient leads to secondary hyperparathyroidism and accelerated bone loss.[9,10] Adult patients with chronic kidney disease develop metabolic insufficiencies such as secondary hyperparathyroidism and renal osteodystrophy, resulting in disordered bone mineralization. Because the density of bone directly relates to the strength of screw attachment to the spine, poor-quality bone increases the risk of screw loosening and pullout both perioperatively and postoperatively.[11-13] Microfractures of low-density bone contribute to overall, progressive deformity, which manifest as pseudarthrosis, adjacent-segment degeneration, progressive kyphosis, and/or subsequent vertebral fractures.[2,5,14]

Patients with a previous spinal deformity operation often have iatrogenic instability and deformity, which compound their original mechanism of deformity. For example, in a patient with canal stenosis from multiple osteoporotic fractures and a history of laminectomy and facetectomy, local instability from the loss of the facet joints can lead to foraminal stenosis and adjacent-facet hypertrophy. For patients with PJK above the original surgical construct, revision surgery often requires extension of instrumentation far above and below the original points of fixation. Iatrogenic deformity correction frequently necessitates removal of the original rods and pedicle screws, because bony destruction or subsidence from the interbody cage or vertebral body cages may have created new problems (see Fig. 20-2). Further, scar tissue formation can inhibit wound healing in revision surgery patients. Muscle flaps may be necessary to provide adequate closure in patients with insufficient tissue or poorly vascularized scar tissue.

Nutritional deficiency, diabetes mellitus, and obesity are systemic host factors that impair the healing process; therefore they increase the chance of postoperative complications such as infection. Nutritional deficiency can manifest in a decreased lymphocyte count and compromise the immune system. Patients with diabetes mellitus are unable to effectively utilize glucose for energy and perfuse tissues with oxygen (because of glycosylated hemoglobin and damaged microvasculature), increasing susceptibility to infection. In patients who are obese, increased surgical time, difficulty in wound closure, and fat necrosis are factors that make postoperative infection more probable.[15] Each of these host factor considerations can be managed preoperatively with careful medical therapy and close follow-up by a physician.

PREOPERATIVE PLANNING

LOW BONE MINERAL DENSITY

Before any surgical intervention for adult spinal deformity, a thorough medical and radiographic evaluation must be performed. Medical evaluation includes a dual-energy x-ray absorptiometry (DXA) study to assess bone mineral density. A DXA T-score of −1.0 to −2.5 indicates *osteopenia*, whereas a score of −2.5 or lower indicates *osteoporosis*. Patients with a DXA T-score of less than −2.5 and at least one osteoporotic fracture are classified by the World Health Organization as *severely osteoporotic*. Although osteoporosis is a known risk factor for microfractures and progressive deformity, osteopenia has also been shown to predict curve progression in adolescent scoliosis.[16] In cadaver studies, bone mineral density, as assessed by DXA, predicted bone failure with axial loading and lumbar vertebral stiffness.[17]

Mineral supplementation and pharmacologic intervention play a role in improving bone quality before surgery. In patients with advanced kidney disease or severe osteoporosis, consultation with an endocrinologist may help to identify the ideal dose, drug, and treatment schedule. Supplementation with 1200 mg of calcium per day has been shown to reduce markers of bone turnover in postmenopausal white women. Although supplementation with vitamin D is also customary, because it plays a role in bone remodeling, the same study did not demonstrate a significant effect of markers of bone turnover with vitamin D supplementation.[18] Further, treatment with bisphosphonates or recombinant parathyroid hormone can also decrease bone turnover and optimize patient bone quality preoperatively and postoperatively. Recent studies have shown that in postmenopausal women with osteoporosis who were treated with teriparatide, a recombinant parathyroid hormone, the incidence of pedicle screw loosening was significantly lower than in an untreated and bisphophonate-treated group.[19] Teriparatide reduced the risk of vertebral fracture in patients with primary osteoporosis in an observational follow-up study.[20] Animal studies support the use of teriparatide to increase the overall volume of the fusion mass as well.[21] Emerging data suggest that male patients with osteoporosis benefit from bisphosphonate treatment, with a significantly reduced risk of vertebral body fracture in the treated group.[22]

VITAMIN D DEFICIENCY AND FAILED BACK SURGERY SYNDROME

The treatment of vitamin D deficiency is critical in the preoperative stage, though frequently underestimated and neglected by spine surgeons.[23] Lack of sun exposure, inadequate nutrition, darker skin color, old age, obesity, and some medications are possible contributors to vitamin D deficiency.[24] Vitamin D levels can be assessed with a serum 25-hydroxyvitamin D screening; *normal* levels are at least 75 nmol/L (30 ng/ml), whereas 50 to 75 nmol/L (20 to 30 ng/ml) is considered *insufficient,* and less than 50 nmol/L (20 ng/ml) is *deficient*.[25] The largest vitamin D–related surgical spine study in 2013 reported an alarmingly high preoperative vitamin D deficit in 313 adult patients having spinal fusion (57% insufficient, 27% deficient).[26] Moreover, studies have linked hypovitaminosis D (less than 30 ng/ml) to FBSS.[25,27]

As a result of the paucity of spine studies investigating this host factor, vitamin D supplementation protocols vary. Stoker et al[26] suggested giving 50,000 IU of vitamin D_2 for deficient (less than 50 nmol/L or

20 ng/ml) patients for 8 weeks before surgery. Scwalfenberg[24] shared results on a series of six vitamin D–insufficient or deficient patients with chronic low back pain or failed spine surgery. The author found that patients responded most favorably to 4000 to 5000 IU/day of vitamin D_3 with respect to repletion and pain relief, though the duration of administration was not reported. In another study, Waikakul[27] gave nine patients with hypovitaminosis D and FBSS vitamin D_2 (20,000 IU/day) for 10 to 20 days to achieve normal serum levels and vitamin D_3 (600 IU/day) for maintenance. Patients had significant pain relief.

DIABETES MELLITUS AND OBESITY

An elevated preoperative serum glucose level (greater than 125 mg/dl) increases the risk of surgical-site infection, even in patients without a diabetes mellitus diagnosis. Numerous studies have found that diabetes mellitus and obesity (greater than 30 to 35 kg/m^2) independently increase the risk of infections.[15,28-32] Preoperatively, a hemoglobin A1c value should be obtained; some authors suggest a delay in elective surgery if the result exceeds 7%.[15] Patients with either or both conditions should be treated by a nutritional expert until results are acceptable. Obese patients may require a multidisciplinary team for healthy weight loss before surgery.[15]

OTHER MALNUTRITION AND IMMUNOCOMPROMISE

Numerous established markers of malnutrition should be assessed in the preoperative stage. The most common tests assess serum total lymphocyte count, prealbumin, and serum transferrin levels; less than 1500 cells/mm^3, less than 3.5 g/dl, and less than 200 mg/dl, respectively, are considered deficient and place a patient at risk for postoperative infections.[15,28,33] For example, one study found that depleted prealbumin increased the probability of developing infections such as pneumonia or urinary tract infection.[34] Nonetheless, one study of 210 neuromuscular scoliosis patients found no significant correlation between serum albumin/lymphocyte counts and deep wound infection.[35] Beyond these diagnostics, a preoperative zinc level (*deficient* is less than 95 µg/dl) can be obtained, because it correlates significantly with wound healing in orthopedic surgery. Once a deficiency is identified, nutritional consultation should begin as soon as possible.

RADIOGRAPHIC ASSESSMENT

Preoperative radiographic evaluation includes standing AP and lateral 36-inch radiographs, flexion and extension lumbar radiographs, and a CT scan to assess bone quality and fusion in patients with previous spinal surgeries. AP and lateral standing 36-inch films facilitate a deeper understanding of the global, progressive deformity, and are crucial for identifying loss of lumbar lordosis and worsening kyphosis (Fig. 20-1). Flexion and extension films highlight mobile segments of the spine and are essential for planning the extent of surgical correction.

Careful measurement of spinal parameters provides quantitative data for deformity correction. Among these measurements, the C7 plumb line, a line extending vertically from the center of the C7 vertebral body, informs surgeons of overall kyphosis in the sagittal plane and of the thoracic coronal deformity. If the line falls anterior to the posterosuperior aspect of S1, the patient has a positive sagittal balance. The central sacral vertical line, a vertical line drawn from the middle of the S1 vertebral body on a coronal radiographic view, characterizes vertebral translation and coronal imbalance. The pelvic incidence, an angle subtended by the perpendicular line to the S1 superior endplate and a line drawn from the center of the S1 superior endplate to the center of the femoral head, should be compared with the measured lumbar lordosis. Pelvic incidence–lumbar lordosis mismatch is well correlated with patient disability and can be used as a guide for surgical decision-making.[36]

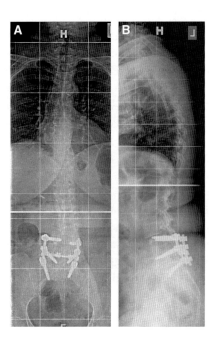

Fig. 20-1   **A,** AP and **B,** lateral standing 36-inch films.

EVOLUTION OF TECHNIQUE

Numerous operative and nonoperative techniques have been developed over the decades to treat global coronal and/or sagittal imbalance. With respect to surgical procedures, anterior spinal fusion (ASF), posterior spinal fusion (PSF), combined anteroposterior surgery (APS), Smith-Petersen osteotomy (SPO), polysegmental osteotomy, and more recently, three-column osteotomy (that is, pedicle subtraction osteotomy [PSO], and vertebral column resection [VCR]) have been employed to correct spinal deformities.[3,5,37]

GENERAL SURGICAL APPROACH

APS has been traditionally used to treat severe adult deformity.[1] However, when data began to show that anterior thoracotomy and thoracoabdominal approaches were associated with a greater complication rate, surgeons shifted toward using posterior-only approaches to correct adult spinal deformity.[1,37]

HIGH-RISK PATIENTS

To improve the fixation strength of patients with poor bone quality, particular surgical procedures have been established. Multiple-point fixation above and below the level of deformity and iliac fixation can provide stability and modest deformity correction.[2] Other techniques include sublaminar wiring, cement augmentation of pedicle screw fixation, pediculolaminar hook fixation, and the use of conical screws, expandable screws, or screws coated with polymethylmethacrylate (PMMA), hydroxyapatite, or calcium apatite.[2,7] These screw coatings are used in an off-label manner.

MINIMALLY INVASIVE PROCEDURES

Minimally invasive procedures are a late evolution of operative techniques and aim to reduce postoperative morbidity and hospitalization time. Percutaneous pedicle screw fixation, presacral lumbar interbody fusion, mini-open anterior lumbar interbody fusion, mini-open transforaminal lumbar interbody fusion, and segmental thoracolumbar-release facetectomies are examples of minimally invasive surgery techniques.[38] With respect to nonsurgical procedures, kyphoplasty is a popular treatment for osteoporotic compression fractures resulting in kyphosis. Kyphoplasty involves the percutaneous placement of an inflatable balloon tamp (approved by the FDA in 1998) within the fractured vertebral body. Inflation of the balloon restores vertebral body height and corrects kyphosis. When the balloon is deflated, the resultant cavity is injected with PMMA.[39] Numerous clinical trials confirm the analgesic potency and vertebral height restoration of kyphoplasty for osteoporotic fractures, although no evidence of global correction is seen.[40,41] The latest minimally invasive techniques combine preexisting minimally invasive procedures such as pedicle screw placement followed by vertebroplasty (a procedure similar to kyphoplasty that involves cement injection without the use of a kyphosis-rectifying balloon).[42]

ADVANTAGES AND DISADVANTAGES

ANTERIOR-ONLY APPROACH

The advantages of ASF include direct decompression of retropulsed bony fragments, which is especially relevant in fracture-susceptible patients with poor bone quality, reconstruction of a stable anterior spinal column, and preservation of posterior structures. Disadvantages include the possibility of insufficient stabilization and the need for additional posterior reinforcement. Furthermore, adjacent vertebral collapse is a notable postoperative development in patients with low bone mineral density. In these patients, ASF can result in insufficient long-term global sagittal and coronal balance.[5] Anterior approaches carry a high risk of pulmonary function compromise and are associated with additional operating time, anesthesia, and morbidity/complications.[1,14] Moreover, during revision surgery, reapproach may be complicated by severe tissue adhesion, which significantly increases the risk of major organ and vessel damage.[5]

ANTEROPOSTERIOR APPROACH

A combined approach involves anterior release and fusion followed by posterior instrumentation and fusion and has been previously associated with increased fusion rates and superior deformity correction. For example, anterior lumbar interbody fusion can complement a posterior approach to maximize lordosis and fuse the levels most prone to pseudarthrosis. However, AP procedures have high morbidity and complication rates inherent to the anterior approach, and these are magnified by the greater degree of invasiveness.[1]

POSTERIOR-ONLY APPROACH

Modern posterior-only techniques typically involve the use of pedicle screws and osteotomy, because PSF alone does not provide sufficient stabilization.[1,14] Osteotomy is a single-stage surgery that corrects the deformity at the apex, creates compressive forces at the site of bone resection, and provides maximal deformity correction.[14] Moreover, although the procedure is demanding and requires meticulous attention to detail, it offers superior sagittal correction and results in less operating time, blood loss, and postoperative morbidity than APS.[14] Because the posterior approach is overall safer and less invasive, some authors believe it is well suited for the elderly population.[14] The need to carefully manipulate neural structures is a notable disadvantage.[14] Osteotomies, especially more invasive, three-column procedures, are far from harmless; in some cases they have been associated with high rates of major complications and blood loss, especially VCR.[3] Similar to the anterior approach, long-term alignment is problematic.[5]

MINIMALLY INVASIVE TECHNIQUES

Minimally invasive surgery is an attractive option for many high-risk elderly patients with conditions such as diabetes mellitus and coronary artery disease,[43] because studies have demonstrated reduced approach-related and overall morbidity.[44] It is the latest development of adult deformity correction, and high class evidence of the benefits of minimally invasive versus open surgery is lacking.[44,45] Minimally invasive surgery is typically associated with a difficult learning curve, a unique set of technical limitations, challenges inherent to the limited workspace, and complications.[44]

Kyphoplasty is a minimally invasive technique specifically designed to treat kyphotic deformities arising from osteoporotic fractures. It provides a significant analgesic effect and improves mobility.[39] In a recent study of elderly patients with osteoporosis-induced kyphosis, kyphoplasty was superior in correcting kyphotic deformity, compared with short-segment fixation with intravertebral expandable pillars.[46] Although it can restore vertebral body height and modestly correct kyphotic angle, it cannot adequately correct sagittal imbalance.[41] Complications are rare, but they can be devastating and emergent.[39] Cement extravasation can result in invasion of the spinal canal, vena cava, lungs, heart, and kidneys.[39,46]

INDICATIONS AND CONTRAINDICATIONS

General indications for surgery include intractable mechanical pain from spinal imbalance and instability and neurologic deficit from stenosis. There is no evidence to suggest a cut-off T-score for which instrumented surgery is contraindicated; however, surgeons should consider the patient's health, age, bone quality on radiographs, DXA score, magnitude of deformity, and neurologic deficit, along with the expected length of the procedure and the need for anterior surgery.[2,14]

ANTERIOR-ONLY APPROACH

ASF is indicated for those with single-level osteoporotic vertebral collapse, because the pathology is anterior.[5,47] It may be better suited for certain regions of the spine such as the thoracolumbar junction because of the ease of access.[5] In patients with prior posterior-only fusion and substantial scar tissue, anterior-only procedures can be performed as a salvage procedure.[48] It is contraindicated in patients with poor bone quality or multiple levels of fracture, because the anterior instrumentation alone cannot sufficiently stabilize the spine.[5]

ANTEROPOSTERIOR APPROACH

APS is indicated for patients with multilevel, rigid kyphosis, because it provides a greater degree of stabilization and a superior rate of arthrodesis, compared with an anterior-only procedure. Thus patients with poor bone quality are particularly suited for this dual approach.[47] Some authors recommend APS for long fusions (above L1) to the sacrum, correction of lumbosacral obliquity, large rigid coronal plane deformity, osteoporosis, or failed fixation to S1.[49]

POSTERIOR-ONLY APPROACH

SPO is recommended when a surgeon wishes to improve lordosis by 10 degrees and deformity usually involves two or more levels. A long, smooth, rounded kyphosis (for example, Scheuermann's kyphosis), especially with prior fusion and pseudarthrosis, is ideal for SPO. Surgeons should look for a potentially mobile disc space to achieve correction. SPO can supplement PSO especially in cases of ankylosing spondylitis; surgeons should consider performing two to three SPOs. Prior failed fusions to L5 (for example, in patients with idiopathic scoliosis) that result in a 6 to 8 cm sagittal imbalance are also suited for SPO.[50,51]

PSO is recommended for cases in which a surgeon wishes to improve lordosis by 25 degrees in the thoracic spine or by 35 degrees in the lumbar spine. Indications include a short, angular kyphosis especially that seen in posttraumatic patients; severe, global, positive sagittal imbalance (more than 10 to 12 cm); and failed primary surgery involving circumferential fusion along multiple segments, which contraindicates SPO.[3,50] Other indications are severe osteoporosis with multiple fractures or spinal cord compression associated with posterior elements.[5]

VCR is a last resort procedure reserved for the most severe, fixed sagittal and coronal imbalances, especially coronal imbalances that require spinal translation for correction.[51] It is commonly indicated in patients with compensated congenital kyphosis, hemivertebra, sagittal decompensation with decompensated coronal malalignment, spondyloptosis at L5, and a resectable spinal tumor.[50] Because this procedure is the most invasive, it also has the most limited scope of indications for osteotomies, because it results in major amounts of blood loss and a high rate of complications.[3]

Minimally Invasive Techniques

Despite the paucity of evidence to define ideal candidates for minimally invasive surgery,[38] common indications are symptomatic back and leg pain that are unresponsive to conservative measures.[43] Mechanical low back pain is the most frequently cited indication by some authors; however, other general surgical indications are applicable to minimally invasive techniques, including radiculopathy, curve progression, sagittal and/or coronal imbalance with unrelenting pain, flat-back syndrome, and lumbar hyperlordosis.[43,48] Minimally invasive surgery is contraindicated for Cobb angles exceeding 90 degrees, severe comorbidities, sagittal imbalance greater than 10 cm, rigid kyphotic deformities, deformities with fused spinal segments, high-grade spondylolisthesis, and osteoporosis with a T-score of less than -2.0.[38,43] Depending on the approach, vascular anomalies and retroperitoneal fibrosis may preclude minimally invasive procedures.[38]

Kyphoplasty is indicated in the presence of intractable, intense pain around the site of osteoporotic fracture or at the level of metastases. In osteoporotic patients, conservative management should be attempted for at least 3 to 4 weeks if no need for surgical stabilization is apparent.[39] Patients should exhibit insignificant minimal sagittal imbalance; multilevel kyphoplasty can only provide very limited correction.[41] Absolute contraindications include an unmanageable bleeding disorder, pain that responds to conservative therapy, asymptomatic fracture, local or generalized infection, allergy to cement, or a tumor causing spinal cord compression.[39]

OPERATIVE TECHNIQUE

Operative techniques for deformity correction include minimally invasive approaches, foraminotomy or laminectomy for focal neurologic deficit, short- and long-construct fusion, spinopelvic fusion, lateral interbody fusion, and osteotomy. For patients with poor bone quality, the invasiveness of the approach should be customized to the deformity and potential for new bone growth. This often necessitates off-label use of common biologic agents and cements. In cadaver studies, pedicle screw augmentation with bone cements increases screw pullout strength in osteoporotic bone.[52] Further, augmentation with off-label bone cements, including PMMA, was reported in retrospective clinical studies to reduce the postoperative pain medication use in patients with degenerative scoliosis. In this same study the authors stated that augmentation with autogenous bone achieved a similar result.[53] However, in patients with poor bone quality, an equivalent outcome may not occur. The use of the largest pedicle screw that a patient's anatomy can accommodate will theoretically improve screw purchase.

Moreover, off-label use of BMP may promote fusion in osteoporotic patients, and its use is safe in a subset of deformity patients. In one large retrospective review from the Scoliosis Research Society Morbidity and Mortality Committee,[54] the authors reviewed 11,933 cases of spinal fusion with BMP and found no increase in the incidence of complications, compared with an untreated cohort for thoracolumbar and posterior cervical fusion only. However, for osteoporotic patients, most of the data supporting improved fusion are from animal models of osteoporosis.[55]

Minimally invasive techniques provide excellent outcomes for patients with adult degenerative scoliosis and can be tailored to fit each patient's deformity according to the severity of the Cobb angle and the abnormality of spinopelvic parameters. In a recent study, the authors proposed a classification system to guide decision-making in minimally invasive approaches.[38] For patients with poor bone quality or metabolic derangements contributing to poor bone quality and poor wound healing, minimally invasive techniques can reduce the wound size and limit the size of the bony defect.

For patients with severe deformity, neurologic deficit, and intractable pain, definitive surgical correction with osteotomy and long-construct fusion may be necessary. In patients with severe lumbosacral deformity, evidence suggested that sacropelvic fixation can reduce the screw pullout associated with osteoporosis.[56] In patients with fixed sagittal imbalance, PSO is an effective tool to correct the imbalance. However, specific data are not available on outcomes after osteotomy in patients with osteoporosis and metabolic bone disease. Balloon kyphoplasty can be performed in conjunction with long-construct fusion for severe deformity to restore vertebral body height in osteoporotic vertebral compression fractures.[57]

POTENTIAL COMPLICATIONS AND MANAGEMENT

SURGICAL COMPLICATIONS

In complex surgeries for spinal deformity, the potential benefits should outweigh the complications. Because age generally correlates with health status in the context of spinal deformity surgical candidates, adults typically have more complications than their younger counterparts. Poor bone quality in adults plays a major role in successful instrumentation and fusion.[58-60] Furthermore, patients over 50 years of age usually have multiple systemic diseases such as cardiovascular disease and diabetes. Older patients also exhibit a greater magnitude of degenerative changes and rigidity of the spine, which increases the difficulty of surgery.[58,59,61] Literature reviews and database studies analyzing deformity in large populations reported overall complication rates of up to 44%.[62-64] The most commonly listed complications were dural tears, wound infection, pulmonary complications (excluding pulmonary embolus), implant/radiographic complications, and neurologic deficit.[62,65] Yadla et al[63] recently reported a pseudarthrosis rate of 12.9% in 2469 patients. Unfortunately, many major complications require reoperation. In a recent review of 359 patients, Scheer et al[65] retrospectively published a revision surgery rate of 17%, with three-column osteotomy having a slightly higher rate (19%) than non-three-column osteotomy (16%).

Whether revision surgery candidates are at greater risk for complications has been recently investigated. In 2013 Hassanzadeh et al[4] retrospectively reported on the largest cohort of adult spinal deformity patients. They compared the radiographic results and functional outcomes of revision patients with those of primary surgery patients. Between the two cohorts (108 revision versus 59 primary patients), the major complication rate differed only by 1%. Moreover, neither the minor complication rate nor the reoperation rate varied significantly. Notably, the pseudarthrosis rate was 43% for the revision group and only 3% for the primary group. However, the authors speculated that this was the result of a relatively short (approximately 2 years) follow-up period. The major and minor complication rates described by Hassanzadeh et al[4] were consistent with those presented in earlier literature, suggesting that subsequent operations should not be contraindicated solely on the basis of previous failed surgeries.

MANAGEMENT OF SURGICAL COMPLICATIONS

Patients with metabolic bone disease and nutritional deficiencies are at particular risk of instrumentation failure, vertebral fracture, and pseudarthrosis. They should be treated beginning at the preoperative stage.[1,5,66,67] Behavioral modifications such as nicotine and smoking cessation should ideally take place as soon as possible and at a minimum of 8 weeks before surgery.[1] Nutritional deficiencies involving caloric, protein, calcium, and vitamin D intake need to be corrected, though the guidelines are better defined for the latter two factors.[9] According to current practice, osteoporotic patients are supplemented with 1000 to 1200 mg of calcium and 800 IU of vitamin D. Vitamin D treatment is essential, because it cures rickets, osteomalacia, and secondary hyperparathyroidism, a major pathogenic factor in elderly osteoporosis. Antiresorptive agents (for example, bisphosphonates, estrogen replacement therapy, selective estrogen-receptor modulators, or calcitonin) and anabolic agents such as parathyroid hormone can be given to improve bone mineral density and reduce fracture incidence for osteoporosis.[9] For Paget's disease, bisphosphonates, calcitonin, mithramycin, ipriflavone, and gallium nitrate can be prescribed.[68] Pharmacotherapy should be tailored to the specific metabolic bone disease.

Intraoperatively, meticulous arthrodesis technique with interbody arthrodesis at lower fusion levels can improve the chances of successful union.[1] The use of fusion-stimulating recombinant human BMP-2 can also yield significantly superior union rates, compared with iliac crest bone graft.[1] As mentioned previously, multiple-point fixation and the use of conical screws, expandable screws, pediculolaminar hook fixation, sublaminar wiring, or screws coated with PMMA, hydroxyapatite, or calcium apatite can reduce the rate of instrumentation failure.

Numerous studies document significant nutritional deficiencies in the postoperative period that are caused by the surgery-induced hypercatabolic state and significantly increase the prevalence of complications.[34,69,70] Total parenteral nutrition should be initiated once a patient is hemodynamically stable (typically 24 hours postoperatively) and terminated once oral intake is possible. Some authors adhere to the following protocol for total parenteral nutrition: 0.25 g of nitrogen/kg/day equal to 1.5 proteins/kg/day, 1 g of lipids/kg/day, and 30 kcal nonprotein/kg/day.[70] Inadequate postoperative nutrition may lead to depleted albumin, prealbumin, transferrin, and/or lymphocytes, which can increase the risk of various infections.[34,70] Moreover, antiinflammatory agents should not be given, and proper nutrition and healthy lifestyle habits should be maintained at discharge.[1]

KYPHOPLASTY COMPLICATIONS

Complications of kyphoplasty include symptomatic cement leakage, cement embolism, pulmonary embolism (PE), hematoma, neurologic impairment secondary to spinal cord compression or nerve root compression, infection, and adjacent vertebral fracture, although the overall rate is less than 2% for osteoporotic patients. Specifically, neurologic complications and PE occur at a rate of 0.03% and 0.01%, respectively.[40]

MANAGEMENT OF COMPLICATIONS RESULTING FROM KYPHOPLASTY

Cement extravasation can potentially result in some of the major complications discussed previously. It can be prevented by limiting the amount of PMMA injected. A literature review suggested injection of less than 3 to 5 ml (approximately 14% of the vertebral body volume) of PMMA into the osteoporotic vertebra.[71] In the rare event of a PE, some authors recommend no treatment aside from clinical follow-up for asymptomatic peripheral PE; however, for symptomatic or central PE, they suggest following the standard guidelines for the treatment of thrombotic PE (that is, initial heparinization followed by coumarin for 6 months).[72] Most instances of neurologic compromise, which are transient, can be managed with nerve root blocks and oral medications. Surgical decompression can be required in rare instances.[71]

PATIENT EXAMPLES

Metabolic Bone Disease With Diabetes Mellitus

This 70-year-old woman presented with an extensive history of low back pain, which began with a traumatic fall 25 years earlier. She indicated that she had an L4-5 disc "repair" after the fall and an L4-5 discectomy 2 years later. She had an L4-S1 PSF 2 years before presentation and epidural steroid injections the year before presentation. Her chief complaint at presentation was pain in her lower back that radiated from

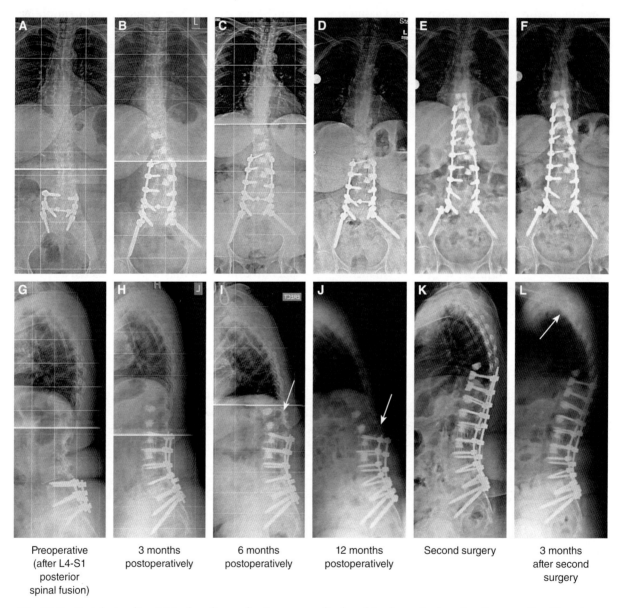

| Preoperative (after L4-S1 posterior spinal fusion) | 3 months postoperatively | 6 months postoperatively | 12 months postoperatively | Second surgery | 3 months after second surgery |

Fig. 20-2   Serial, standing 36-inch radiographs. Images are displayed in chronologic order. Preoperative films show the patient at presentation to our institution. **A-F,** AP views. **G-L,** Lateral views. **G,** Screw pullout is evident in the superior pedicle screw on the lateral view. Minimal proximal junctional kyphosis is present at the superior aspect of the construct. **B** and **H,** Three months after the index surgery, bone cement was present at multiple levels, and the construct was extended from L2 to the pelvis. **I,** Proximal junctional kyphosis was developing *(arrow).* **J,** Worsening of proximal junctional kyphosis *(arrow).* **K,** In a second surgery, the construct was extended from T10 to the pelvis. **L,** Progressive kyphosis was evident in the thoracic spine *(arrow).*

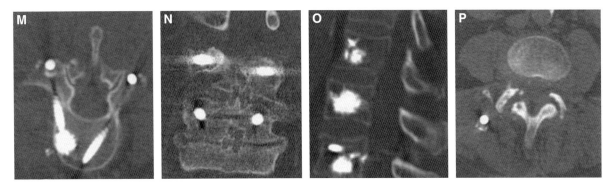

Fig. 20-2, cont'd Postoperative CT images. **M,** Cement augmentation is noted as the *bright circular structure* at the distal aspect of the left pedicle screw on axial CT. **N,** Hypodense regions representing interbody cages show subsidence and adjacent bony destruction on coronal CT. **O,** Vertebroplasty is seen on lateral CT. **P,** Unilateral facet hypertrophy is evident on axial CT.

her hips to her ankles bilaterally. The pain awoke her often from sleep. Her past medical history was significant for hypertension, smoking, osteoporosis, chronic kidney disease (baseline creatinine 2.4), and diabetes mellitus type II, requiring insulin. At presentation to our institution, imaging demonstrated proximal junctional kyphosis at L3-4, above the previous surgical construct. Loosening of spinal hardware and pseudarthrosis were seen at L4-S1. Fig. 20-2, *A* through *L,* shows serial, standing 36-inch films of her progressive deformity.

The patient was taken to the operating room for removal of L4-S1 instrumentation and L2-pelvis fusion using local allograft and off-label BMP. A decompression and laminectomy was performed at L3-4, with bone cement reinforcement of pedicle screws at L2-3 (Fig. 20-2, *M*). Pedicle screws were placed bilaterally at L2-S1 and in the bilateral pelvis. Hydroxyapatite crystals and two large BMP sponges were placed along the entire fusion from L2 to S1 to improve the likelihood of fusion. Intraoperatively we noted severe subsidence of the previous interbody cage with bony destruction (Fig. 20-2, *N*). For this reason we decided to stage the procedure, with an anterior approach 1 week later to perform L2-3 and L3-4 discectomies and to place PEEK interbody struts at L2-3 and L3-4. To offset the previous bony destruction at L2-3, vertebroplasty was performed in the L2 and L3 vertebral bodies under fluoroscopy (Fig. 20-2, *O*). Significant unilateral facet hypertrophy was noted intraoperatively (Fig. 20-2, *P*).

The patient had a complicated postoperative course with wound breakdown requiring incision and debridement followed by complex closure using bilateral paraspinous muscle flaps. Cultures from the wound grew coagulase-negative *Staphylococcus spp.* At discharge 4 weeks after surgery, she was taking antibiotics through a peripherally inserted central catheter line. She started vitamin D and calcium supplementation, and 1 year postoperatively her T-score on a DXA study was −1.5. Six months after surgery, she developed proximal junctional kyphosis. She had revision surgery requiring T10-pelvis fusion months later with off-label bone morphogenic protein and repeat bilateral paraspinous muscle flap closure (see Fig. 20-2, *E, F, K,* and *L*).

Osteoporosis

This 51-year-old woman presented with buttock and leg pain. The pain had been constant over the past several years and had been recently worsening. She had no frank weakness in either leg. Imaging showed L5-S1 spondylolisthesis with bilateral L5-S1 facet hypertrophy. The patient's preoperative DXA scan revealed severe osteoporosis (score −3.5), and she reported that a left radius fracture had failed to heal. Her past medical history was significant for a total hysterectomy at age 40. The first neurosurgeon she consulted recommended conservative surgical treatment with bilateral foraminotomies because of concerns about the patient's poor bone quality. She was referred to our institution for a second opinion.

The patient underwent preoperative treatment with teriparatide for 4 months as an off-label treatment to optimize bone quality under the supervision of an endocrinologist. We performed an instrumented arthrodesis from L5-S1 using autograft, allograft, and off-label BMP. Bilateral SPOs, total discectomies, and total facetectomies were performed at L5-S1. The pedicle screws were cannulated at L5-S1, and bone cement and screws were placed (Fig. 20-3, *A*). Carbon fiber cages (Fig. 20-3, *B*) were then placed bilaterally in the intervertebral space with local autograft and BMP to promote anterior fusion. The patient had an uncomplicated postoperative course and was discharged to outpatient rehabilitation 4 days after surgery. Six months postoperatively, she shows evidence of fusion with significant improvement of her pain symptoms.

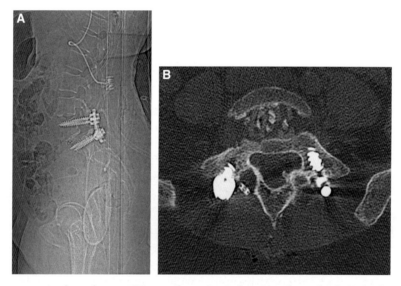

Fig. 20-3   **A,** A postoperative lateral scout CT scan shows L5-S1 fusion and interbody cage placement. **B,** The cages are best visualized on an axial CT scan.

CONCLUSION

A variety of operative treatments exist to correct global imbalances in the spine. These range from kyphoplasty and minimally invasive surgical techniques to VCR. In patients with poor bone quality, adult spinal deformity procedures should be individually tailored to ensure successful clinical outcomes. Appropriate measures must be taken at the preoperative, intraoperative, and postoperative stages to prevent instrumentation-related/radiographic failure. Recent evidence suggests that failed primary surgery is not a factor that correlates to an increased complication rate for revision surgery.

REFERENCES

1. Good CR, Auerbach JD, O'Leary PT, et al. Adult spine deformity. Curr Rev Musculoskelet Med 4:159-167, 2011.

2. DeWald CJ, Stanley T. Instrumentation-related complications of multilevel fusions for adult spinal deformity patients over age 65: surgical considerations and treatment options in patients with poor bone quality. Spine 31(19 Suppl):S144-S151, 2006.

3. Hassanzadeh H, Jain A, El Dafrawy MH, et al. Three-column osteotomies in the treatment of spinal deformity in adult patients 60 years old and older: outcome and complications. Spine 38:726-731, 2013.

4. Hassanzadeh H, Jain A, El Dafrawy MH, et al. Clinical results and functional outcomes of primary and revision spinal deformity surgery in adults. J Bone Joint Surg Am 95:1413-1419, 2013.

5. Okuda S, Oda T, Yamasaki R, et al. Surgical outcomes of osteoporotic vertebral collapse: a retrospective study of anterior spinal fusion and pedicle subtraction osteotomy. Global Spine J 2:221-226, 2012.

6. Etebar S, Cahill DW. Risk factors for adjacent-segment failure following lumbar fixation with rigid instrumentation for degenerative instability. J Neurosurg 90(2 Suppl):S163-S169, 1999.

7. Wuisman PI, Van Dijk M, Staal H, et al. Augmentation of (pedicle) screws with calcium apatite cement in patients with severe progressive osteoporotic spinal deformities: an innovative technique. Eur Spine J 9:528-533, 2000.

8. Tan LA, Kasliwal MK, Harbhajanka A, et al. Malignant degeneration of multilevel monostotic Paget's disease involving the thoracic spine: an unusual presentation. J Clin Neurosci 21:1254-1256, 2014.

9. Eriksen EF, Halse J, Moen MH. New developments in the treatment of osteoporosis. Acta Obstet Gynecol Scand 92:620-636, 2013.

10. Eastell R, Lambert H. Diet and healthy bones. Calcif Tissue Int 70:400-404, 2002.

11. Halvorson TL, Kelley LA, Thomas KA, et al. Effects of bone mineral density on pedicle screw fixation. Spine 19:2415-2420, 1994.

12. Kornblatt MD, Casey MP, Jacobs RR. Internal fixation in lumbosacral spine fusion. A biomechanical and clinical study. Clin Orthop Relat Res 203:141-150, 1986.

13. Hasegawa K, Takahashi HE, Uchiyama S, et al. An experimental study of a combination method using a pedicle screw and laminar hook for the osteoporotic spine. Spine 22:958-962; discussion 963, 1997.

14. Chang KW, Chen YY, Lin CC, et al. Apical lordosating osteotomy and minimal segment fixation for the treatment of thoracic or thoracolumbar osteoporotic kyphosis. Spine 30:1674-1681, 2005.

15. Cross MB, Yi PH, Thomas CF, et al. Evaluation of malnutrition in orthopaedic surgery. J Am Acad Orthop Surg 22:193-199, 2014.

16. Sun X, Wu T, Liu Z, et al. Osteopenia predicts curve progression of adolescent idiopathic scoliosis in girls treated with brace treatment. J Pediatr Orthop 33:366-371, 2013.

17. Hou Y, Yuan W, Kang J, et al. Influences of endplate removal and bone mineral density on the biomechanical properties of lumbar spine. PLoS One 8:e76843, 2013.

18. Aloia JF, Dhaliwal R, Shieh A, et al. Calcium and vitamin d supplementation in postmenopausal women. J Clin Endocrinol Metab 98:E1702-E1709, 2013.

19. Ohtori S, Inoue G, Orita S, et al. Comparison of teriparatide and bisphosphonate treatment to reduce pedicle screw loosening after lumbar spinal fusion surgery in postmenopausal women with osteoporosis from a bone quality perspective. Spine 38:E487-E492, 2013.

20. Sugimoto T, Shiraki M, Nakano T, et al. Vertebral fracture risk after once-weekly teriparatide injections: follow-up study of teriparatide once-weekly efficacy research (TOWER) trial. Curr Med Res Opin 29:195-203, 2013.

21. Lina IA, Puvanesarajah V, Liauw JA, et al. Quantitative study of parathyroid hormone (1-34) and bone morphogenetic protein-2 on spinal fusion outcomes in a rabbit model of lumbar dorsolateral intertransverse process arthrodesis. Spine 39:347-355, 2014.

22. Boonen S, Reginster JY, Kaufman JM, et al. Fracture risk and zoledronic acid therapy in men with osteoporosis. N Engl J Med 367:1714-1723, 2012.

23. Rodriguez WJ, Gromelski J. Vitamin D status and spine surgery outcomes. ISRN Orthopedics 2013:1-12, 2013.

24. Schwalfenberg G. Improvement of chronic back pain or failed back surgery with vitamin D repletion: a case series. J Am Board Fam Med 22:69-74, 2009.

25. Kim TH, Yoon JY, Lee BH, et al. Changes in vitamin D status after surgery in female patients with lumbar spinal stenosis and its clinical significance. Spine 37:E1326-E1330, 2012.

26. Stoker GE, Buchowski JM, Bridwell KH, et al. Preoperative vitamin D status of adults undergoing surgical spinal fusion. Spine 38:507-515, 2013.

27. Waikakul S. Serum 25-hydroxy-calciferol level and failed back surgery syndrome. J Orthop Surg 20:18-22, 2012.

28. Beiner JM, Grauer J, Kwon BK, et al. Postoperative wound infections of the spine. Neurosurg Focus 15:E14, 2003.

29. Olsen MA, Nepple JJ, Riew KD, et al. Risk factors for surgical site infection following orthopaedic spinal operations. J Bone Joint Surg Am 90:62-69, 2008.

30. Friedman ND, Sexton DJ, Connelly SM, et al. Risk factors for surgical site infection complicating laminectomy. Infect Control Hosp Epidemiol 28:1060-1065, 2007.

31. Pull ter Gunne AF, van Laarhoven CJ, Cohen DB. Surgical site infection after osteotomy of the adult spine: does type of osteotomy matter? Spine J 10:410-416, 2010.

32. Pull ter Gunne AF, Cohen DB. Incidence, prevalence, and analysis of risk factors for surgical site infection following adult spinal surgery. Spine 34:1422-1428, 2009.

33. Jevsevar DS, Karlin LI. The relationship between preoperative nutritional status and complications after an operation for scoliosis in patients who have cerebral palsy. J Bone Joint Surg Am 75:880-884, 1993.

34. Hu SS, Fontaine F, Kelly B, et al. Nutritional depletion in staged spinal reconstructive surgery. The effect of total parenteral nutrition. Spine 23:1401-1405, 1998.

35. Sponseller PD, LaPorte DM, Hungerford MW, et al. Deep wound infections after neuromuscular scoliosis surgery: a multicenter study of risk factors and treatment outcomes. Spine 25:2461-2466, 2000.

36. Schwab FJ, Blondel B, Bess S, et al. Radiographical spinopelvic parameters and disability in the setting of adult spinal deformity: a prospective multicenter analysis. Spine 38:E803-E812, 2013.

37. Good CR, Lenke LG, Bridwell KH, et al. Can posterior-only surgery provide similar radiographic and clinical results as combined anterior (thoracotomy/thoracoabdominal)/posterior approaches for adult scoliosis? Spine 35:210-218, 2010.

38. Deukmedjian AR, Ahmadian A, Bach K, et al. Minimally invasive lateral approach for adult degenerative scoliosis: lessons learned. Neurosurg Focus 35:E4, 2013.

39. Denaro V, Longo UG, Maffulli N, et al. Vertebroplasty and kyphoplasty. Clin Cases Miner Bone Metab 6:125-130, 2009.

40. Yimin Y, Zhiwei R, Wei M, et al. Current status of percutaneous vertebroplasty and percutaneous kyphoplasty: a review. Med Sci Monit 19:826-836, 2013.

41. Pradhan BB, Bae HW, Kropf MA, et al. Kyphoplasty reduction of osteoporotic vertebral compression fractures: correction of local kyphosis versus overall sagittal alignment. Spine 31:435-441, 2006.

42. Gu Y, Zhang F, Jiang X, et al. Minimally invasive pedicle screw fixation combined with percutaneous vertebroplasty in the surgical treatment of thoracolumbar osteoporosis fracture. J Neurosurg Spine 18:634-640, 2013.

43. Anand N, Baron EM. Minimally invasive approaches for the correction of adult spinal deformity. Eur Spine J 22(Suppl 2):S232-S241, 2013.

44. Bach K, Ahmadian A, Deukmedjian A, et al. Minimally invasive surgical techniques in adult degenerative spinal deformity: a systematic review. Clin Orthop Relat Res 472:1749-1761, 2014.

45. Berjano P, Lamartina C. Far lateral approaches (XLIF) in adult scoliosis. Eur Spine J 22(Suppl 2):S242-S253, 2013.

46. Hsieh JY, Wu CD, Wang TM, et al. Reduction of the domino effect in osteoporotic vertebral compression fractures through short-segment fixation with intravertebral expandable pillars compared to percutaneous kyphoplasty: a case control study. BMC Musculoskelet Disord 14:75, 2013.

47. Suk SI, Kim JH, Lee SM, et al. Anterior-posterior surgery versus posterior closing wedge osteotomy in posttraumatic kyphosis with neurologic compromised osteoporotic fracture. Spine 28:2170-2175, 2003.

48. Herkowitz HN, Sidhu KS. Lumbar spine fusion in the treatment of degenerative conditions: current indications and recommendations. J Am Acad Orthop Surg 3:123-135, 1995.

49. Berven SH, Deviren V, Mitchell B, et al. Operative management of degenerative scoliosis: an evidence-based approach to surgical strategies based on clinical and radiographic outcomes. Neurosurg Clin N Am 18:261-272, 2007.

50. Bridwell KH. Decision making regarding Smith-Petersen vs. pedicle subtraction osteotomy vs. vertebral column resection for spinal deformity. Spine 31(19 Suppl):S171-S178, 2006.

51. Bergin PF, O'Brien JR, Matteini LE, et al. The use of spinal osteotomy in the treatment of spinal deformity. Orthopedics 33:595-596, 2010.

52. Folsch C, Goost H, Figiel J, et al. Correlation of pull-out strength of cement-augmented pedicle screws with CT-volumetric measurement of cement. Biomed Tech (Berl) 57:473-480, 2012.

53. Xie Y, Fu Q, Chen ZQ, et al. Comparison between two pedicle screw augmentation instrumentations in adult degenerative scoliosis with osteoporosis. BMC Musculoskelet Disord 12:286, 2011.

54. Williams BJ, Smith JS, Fu KM, et al; Scoliosis Research Society Morbidity and Mortality Committee. Does bone morphogenetic protein increase the incidence of perioperative complications in spinal fusion? A comparison of 55,862 cases of spinal fusion with and without bone morphogenetic protein. Spine 36:1685-1691, 2011.

55. Li M, Liu X, Liu X, et al. Calcium phosphate cement with BMP-2-loaded gelatin microspheres enhances bone healing in osteoporosis: a pilot study. Clin Orthop Relat Res 468:1978-1985, 2010.

56. Shen FH, Mason JR, Shimer AL, et al. Pelvic fixation for adult scoliosis. Eur Spine J 22(Suppl 2):S265-S275, 2013.

57. Werner CM, Osterhoff G, Schlickeiser J, et al. Vertebral body stenting versus kyphoplasty for the treatment of osteoporotic vertebral compression fractures: a randomized trial. J Bone Joint Surg Am 95:577-584, 2013.

58. Bradford DS. Adult scoliosis. Current concepts of treatment. Clin Orthop Relat Res 229:70-87, 1988.

59. Lippman CR, Spence CA, Youssef AS, et al. Correction of adult scoliosis via a posterior-only approach. Neurosurg Focus 14:e5, 2003.

60. Takahashi S, Delecrin J, Passuti N. Surgical treatment of idiopathic scoliosis in adults: an age-related analysis of outcome. Spine 27:1742-1748, 2002.

61. Winter RB, Lonstein JE, Denis F. Pain patterns in adult scoliosis. Orthop Clin North Am 19:339-345, 1988.

62. Sansur CA, Smith JS, Coe JD, et al. Scoliosis research society morbidity and mortality of adult scoliosis surgery. Spine 36:E593-E597, 2011.

63. Yadla S, Maltenfort MG, Ratliff JK, et al. Adult scoliosis surgery outcomes: a systematic review. Neurosurg Focus 28:E3, 2010.

64. Weiss HR, Goodall D. Rate of complications in scoliosis surgery: a systematic review of the Pub Med literature. Scoliosis 3:9, 2008.

65. Scheer JK, Tang JA, Smith JS, et al; International Spine Study Group. Reoperation rates and impact on outcome in a large, prospective, multicenter, adult spinal deformity database: clinical article. J Neurosurg Spine 19:464-470, 2013.

66. Baron EM, Albert TJ. Medical complications of surgical treatment of adult spinal deformity and how to avoid them. Spine 31(19 Suppl):S106-S118, 2006.

67. Carl A, Kaufman E, Lawrence J. Complications in spinal deformity surgery: issues unrelated directly to intraoperative technical skills. Spine 35:2215-2223, 2010.

68. Hadjipavlou AG, Gaitanis LN, Katonis PG, et al. Paget's disease of the spine and its management. Eur Spine J 10:370-384, 2001.

69. Boachie-Adjei O, Dendrinos GK, Ogilvie JW, et al. Management of adult spinal deformity with combined anterior-posterior arthrodesis and Luque-Galveston instrumentation. J Spinal Disord 4:131-141, 1991.

70. Lalueza MP, Colomina MJ, Bago J, et al. Analysis of nutritional parameters in idiopathic scoliosis patients after major spinal surgery. Eur J Clin Nutr 59:720-722, 2005.

71. Truumees E. Vertebroplasty and kyphoplasty: complications and their management. Semin Spine Surg 20:53-66, 2008.

72. Krueger A, Bliemel C, Zettl R, et al. Management of pulmonary cement embolism after percutaneous vertebroplasty and kyphoplasty: a systematic review of the literature. Eur Spine J 18:1257-1265, 2009.

21

Biologic Options in Spinal Deformity: A Literature Review

Rahul Basho ▪ *Kenneth A. Hood* ▪ *Jeffrey C. Wang*

Since the first reported spinal fusion was performed in 1911, techniques and indications have continued to evolve. The monumental advances in spinal instrumentation have long overshadowed the incremental progress of bone graft options. Autograft was and remains the benchmark today. Concerns over donor site morbidity and availability of adequate amounts of graft have led to the search for alternatives. These requirements are heightened in deformity surgery, in which long-fusion constructs and increased biomechanical forces stress human biology. An ideal graft material has three fundamental characteristics essential to bony fusion: osteoinductivity, osteoconductivity, and osteogenesis. Many of the grafting options used today in deformity surgery have one or two of these traits and function as extenders, but none has all three. In addition, there is a paucity of deformity data on the commonly used biologics in degenerative spine: allograft, ceramics, DBM, and mesenchymal stem cells. Most of the deformity literature focuses on off-label use of recombinant human bone morphogenic protein 2 (rhBMP-2). The initial enthusiasm with its use has been tempered recently by literature that questions its safety profile and broad off-label usage. However, studies continue to emerge advocating its safety and success in improving fusion rates in spinal deformity patients.

BONE GRAFT OPTIONS

An older patient population, long-instrumentation constructs, and the need for fusion to maintain correction of deformity inherently complicate adult spinal deformity surgery. These factors combine to create the perfect scenario for pseudarthrosis development. Pseudarthrosis rates approach 24% for long instrumentation in adult spinal deformity with fusion to S1.[1] Given this high risk, the choice of bone graft is of utmost importance.

Bone grafts can be categorized based on their properties of osteogenicity, osteoinductivity, or osteoconductivity. These properties are not mutually exclusive and are to a greater or lesser extent dependent on the graft chosen. Osteogenic material directly provides cells that will produce bone, including primitive mesenchymal stem cells, osteoblasts, and osteocytes. The only bone graft option that maintains true osteogenic potential is autograft. Osteoinductive graft material contains factors that stimulate bone growth and induction of stem cells down a bone-forming lineage. The most often used bone graft options with this property are bone morphogenetic proteins, belonging to the transforming growth factor (TGF-beta) superfamily of proteins. Osteoconductive graft material provides a structural framework for bone growth. Commonly used options include autograft, allograft, DBM, and ceramics.

Autograft iliac crest bone (ICBG) is considered the bone graft option of the highest standard, against which all others are measured (Fig. 21-1). It has osteogenic, osteoinductive, and osteoconductive properties, and presents no risk of disease transmission.[2] Disadvantages include donor site pain, neurovascular injury, infection, hematoma, fracture, and bowel herniation.[3-6] In the setting of spine deformity surgery, the need for large amounts of graft may exceed the amount of ICBG that can be retrieved. Additionally, in long constructs that extend to the pelvis, harvesting ICBG can compromise fixation in this region.[2]

Allograft bone is characterized primarily by its osteoconductive properties (Fig. 21-2). In contrast to ICGB, allograft bone is not limited in quantity, decreases operative times, and prevents the potential for donor site morbidity. Disadvantages include a low risk of disease transmission. Fortunately, no cases have been reported with freeze-dried allograft.[7] Another major disadvantage is the need for processing and sterilization, which compromise mechanical strength and osteogenic and osteoinductive potential.

Allograft choices include fresh-frozen or freeze-dried cancellous chips or cortical bone. These are primarily osteoconductive and dependent on host factors for osteogenesis and osteoinduction. Fresh-frozen allograft retains its mechanical properties, whereas freeze-dried allograft can lose up to 50% of it mechanical strength.[8] Cortical allograft, for example, femoral or fibular ring, provides significant structural support, especially in compression.[9] The downside is that it incorporates slowly by periosteal new bone formation. Cancellous allograft provides substantially less mechanical strength but is incorporated much more quickly. It is more suitable for stand-alone use or as an autograft extender in areas that require less structural support such as posterolateral fusion.[10]

Ceramics are osteoconductive and available in numerous forms (Fig. 21-3). One type of ceramic used in spinal deformity surgery is coral. Marine corals have good compressive strength, low tensile strength, and low fracture toughness.[11] Microscopically, they resemble the porous structure of bone. This structure provides a scaffold for a process that closely resembles intramembranous ossification.[12,13] Potential advantages of coral ceramic include low cost and the ability to be fashioned into blocks or granules to fit specific bone voids. They have not been shown to induce an inflammatory response, and they can be sterilized, significantly reducing the risk of disease transmission.[14] Another commonly employed ceramic is tricalcium phosphate. Preparations include an injectable and a noninjectable solid. The injectable form has been shown to have four to ten times the compressive strength of cancellous bone and reaches 90% of its ultimate strength within 24 hours. Unlike other ceramics, injectable tricalcium phosphate is a true load-sharing bone graft. Its effectiveness outside of vertebroplasty is not yet known.[2] The noninjectable form has shown promise in several studies assessing fusion.[15,16] Unfortunately, a paucity of studies has been conducted on the application of ceramics in spinal deformity surgery.

BMPs are osteoinductive proteins derived from the TGF-beta superfamily that act as local signaling molecules for bone and cartilage formation. The most extensively studied is rhBMP-2 (Fig. 21-4). rhBMP-2 has garnered much attention because of study results showing higher fusion rates with its use, compared with autograft, in anterior lumber interbody fusions.[17-19] Very favorable fusion rates have also been shown in deformity surgery.[20] The major concerns with BMP are cost and potential association with malignancy, which is an unresolved problem.

DBM is allograft that has been stripped of its mineral phase, preserving only collagen and noncollagenous proteins (Fig. 21-5). The presence of BMPs, though variable, provides an osteoinductive potential.[21,22] It is available in numerous forms, including putty, gel, and sheets, and has primarily been applied as a bone graft extender. Wang et al[23] compared three commercially available DBM formulations and found significant differences in fusion rates. This variability in formulation and effectiveness is likely responsible for the lack of data supporting the use of DBM in spinal fusions.

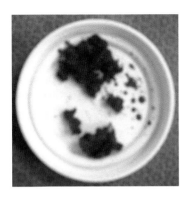

Fig. 21-1 Iliac crest autograft harvested for use in an anterior cervical fusion. This cancellous graft cannot provide structural support and is therefore placed within a PEEK interbody cage.

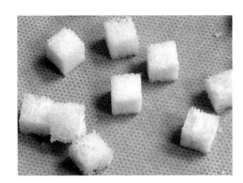

Fig. 21-2 Freeze-dried allograft bone provides structural support and is purely osteoconductive. It can be combined with autograft and placed posterolaterally in lumbar fusions.

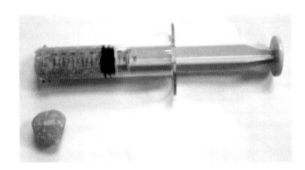

Fig. 21-3 Demineralized bone matrix is typically used as an autograft extender in posterolateral lumbar fusions. Multiple formulations exist, with varying consistencies.

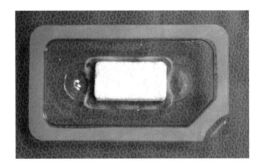

Fig. 21-4 Beta-tricalcium phosphate (Vitoss; Stryker, Kalamazoo, MI) is a purely osteoconductive ceramic that can be used as an autograft extender in posterolateral lumbar fusions. Evidence supports its efficacy as a stand-alone graft, combined with bone marrow aspirate.

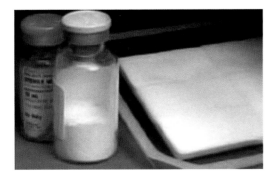

Fig. 21-5 rhBMP-2 has spawned wide, off-label usage. Recent literature indicates improved fusion rates when it is used posterolaterally and in interbody fusions within the lumbar spine. However, ideal dosing is undefined, and safety concerns persist.

LITERATURE REVIEW

The literature on the use of biologics in spinal deformity reveals clear trends. Early studies focused on the use of autograft and allograft, whereas more recent studies focused on the use of rhBMP-2. Few data are available on the use of other biologics in long-fusion constructs, likely because of the lack of reliable results in adult degenerative spine studies. It is difficult to determine the true impact of bone grafts because of variations in instrumentation, fusion techniques, surgical approaches, and patient population.

ALLOGRAFT WITH OR WITHOUT AUTOGRAFT

Early studies in adolescent idiopathic scoliosis had optimal results from the use of allograft. Dodd et al[24] compared the results in 40 patients with adolescent idiopathic scoliosis who had surgical fusion and received either femoral head allograft or iliac crest autograft. Fusion rates were excellent in both groups (100%). The allograft group had a lower rate of infection, less blood loss at surgery, and reduced postoperative pain. Such high fusion rates probably result from the favorable biology present in the pediatric population.

Much of the adult deformity literature has focused on the use of local autologous bone supplemented with allograft. Kim et al[1] evaluated pseudarthrosis rates in long-fusion constructs to the sacrum in adult spinal deformity. They retrospectively examined a cohort of 144 patients in whom long-fusion constructs were placed (five to seventeen vertebral levels, average 11.9) from 1985 to 2002 at a single institution. Because of the broad data collection period, surgical technique varied: only 88 patients had complete sacropelvic fixation, defined as anterior column support at L4-5 and L5-S1, with bilateral iliac and bicortical sacral screw fixation. Anterior fusions involved a combination of morselized rib autograft, morselized fresh-frozen allograft with or without titanium mesh cages, or femoral ring allografts. Posterior instrumentation consisted of a combination of pedicle screws, hooks, sublaminar or interspinous wires, and rods. Local bone was combined with iliac crest autograft for the posterior surgery. The pseudarthrosis rate was 24%, for which incomplete sacropelvic fixation was a risk factor.

Weistroffer et al[25] retrospectively evaluated complications in long-fusion constructs to the sacrum in a cohort of 50 patients. Most patients (47/50) had both an anterior and a posterior fusion. Curves were corrected with a combination of pedicle screws and hooks. Distal fixation was sacral in 27 patients and sacral/iliac or iliac in 23 patients. Anterior procedures involved tricortical structural allograft in the lower lumbar spine and a mixture of rib autograft and allograft in the thoracic spine. Posteriorly, a combination of allograft and autograft was placed. The authors reported a 24% pseudarthrosis rate, 75% of which did not declare itself until 2 or more years after surgery.

In a subsequent study, Kim et al[26] examined the role of modern posterior segmental instrumentation on pseudarthrosis in adult spinal deformity. The instrumentation applied was either Cotrel-Dubousset or first-generation Cotrel-Dubousset Horizon (Medtronic Sofamor Danek, Minneapolis, MN) (bilateral rods, cross-links, and a combination of hooks, intraspinous wires, sublaminar wires, and pedicle screws). A cohort of 232 patients was retrospectively reviewed. Only 81 patients had the distal extent of their fusion extended to the sacrum. Twelve patients had anterior-only fusions, 102 had posterior-only fusions, and 118 had combined anterior-posterior fusions. Autologous iliac crest bone graft was combined with local bone for the posterior surgery, and anterior graft was not specified. The pseudarthrosis rate was 17%, and distal extension of the fusion to S1 was a significant risk factor. Their previous study showed a higher pseudarthrosis rate (24%), likely because it included fusions to the sacrum.[1]

DEMINERALIZED BONE MATRIX

Data are scarce on the use of DBM in adult spinal deformity; much of it has to be extrapolated from degenerative spine literature. Cammisa et al[27] examined the role of DBM as a bone graft extender. They examined posterolateral fusions in the lumbar spine in a cohort of 120 patients who underwent one-, two-, or three-level lumbar posterolateral fusions. Each patient had autograft placed on one side and a combination of autograft and DBM on the contralateral side. Their results demonstrated low but equivalent fusion rates between the two sides, leading them to conclude that DBM was a viable option to reduce the amount of autograft necessary.

Hostin et al[28] evaluated anterior fusion rates in adult spinal deformity surgery with Healos Bone Graft Replacement (DePuy Spine, Inc., Warsaw, IN), an osteoconductive type 1 collagen–hydroxyapatite fiber matrix. Unlike allograft DBMs, Healos is derived from bovine collagen and is only osteoconductive.[29] It is combined with bone marrow aspirate to confirm osteogenic potential. In this study, Healos was combined with bone marrow aspirate and placed within carbon fiber reinforced polymer cages. Twenty-two patients had combined anterior-posterior fusions; a total of 104 anterior levels were treated. Posterior fixation included pedicle screw and rod constructs. A combination of allograft bone, Healos, and bone marrow aspirate was placed posteriorly. One year postoperatively, the overall anterior fusion rate was 95% based on radiographs, and 87% based on CT scans. Though the anterior fusion rates were high, the authors concluded that Healos was inferior to BMP with regard to fusion rates and cost.

CERAMICS

Delecrin et al[30] performed a prospective, randomized study of 58 patients in whom they compared outcomes of autograft versus a synthetic ceramic in scoliosis surgery. In 30 patients, iliac crest autograft was harvested, and in 28 patients, local bone was combined with porous biphasic calcium phosphate blocks (Triosite; Zimmer, Étupes, France). They placed posterior-only constructs, using Cotrel-Dubousset instrumentation; fusion levels were not specified. Their cohort of patients was young (range 13 to 25 years). Patients were followed for a mean of 48 months, and clinical and radiographic parameters were reported. At the final follow-up, the two groups showed no difference in correction loss of the major curve, thoracic kyphosis, or lumbar lordosis. However, a significant difference in donor site morbidity was noted, with half of the autograft group reporting continued donor site pain 6 months postoperatively. The authors concluded that calcium phosphate ceramics can show favorable results in scoliosis surgery, without the morbidity that occurs with autograft harvest. They acknowledged that their cohort of patients was young, and these results should be applied with caution to adult spinal deformity patients.

RECOMBINANT HUMAN BONE MORPHOGENIC PROTEIN 2

The discovery and use of BMPs to augment spinal fusion has ushered in an era of great hope and controversy. Articles that describe the shortcomings of initial studies performed to gain FDA approval for rhBMP-2 have raised valid concerns over its safety profile and everexpanding off-label use. Literature evaluating its off-label use in spinal deformity is positive overall, with studies indicating improved fusion rates and an acceptable complication profile.

RECOMBINANT HUMAN BONE MARROW PROTEIN 2: EFFICACY IN FUSIONS FOR ADULT SPINAL DEFORMITY

Luhmann et al[20] published the initial, single-center study evaluating the use of rhBMP-2 in adult spinal deformity patients. They evaluated 95 patient samples. (The total number of patients was 70, and 25 had anterior-posterior fusions.) The minimum follow-up was 1 year. Patient samples were divided into three groups: anterior fusions (group one, n = 46), posterior fusions (group two, n = 41), and compassionate-use fusions (group three, n = 8). rhBMP-2 was dosed as follows: 10.8 mg/level in group one, 13.7 mg/level in group two, and 28.6 mg/level in group three. A higher dose was used in group three, because it consisted of patients who had undergone prior surgeries with harvested autograft. Anterior hardware consisted of titanium mesh cages. Posterior instrumentation appeared to be pedicle screw–rod constructs, but this was not specified. Fusion rates were 96% in group one, 93% in group two, and 100% in group three. The authors reported a total of three complications: one anterior wound dehiscence, a deep wound hematoma, and one deep infection. No complications occurred in group three despite the use of high doses of rhBMP-2. The authors acknowledged that a longer follow-up was necessary to definitively determine fusion in adult spinal deformity patients.

Mulconrey et al[31] conducted a prospective study of rhBMP-2 in 98 adult spinal deformity patients who had multilevel fusions. The patients were categorized into three groups: group one had anterior spinal fusion with a titanium mesh cage filled with rhBMP-2 (average concentration of 10.9 mg/level), group two had posterolateral fusion with rhBMP-2 (average concentration of 19.8 mg/level) combined with local bone graft and tricalcium phosphate–hydroxyapatite as an extender, and group three received high-dose rhBMP-2 (average of 37.4 mg/level) on a compression-resistant matrix without autologous bone. Group three were categorized as compassionate-use patients, having had multiple prior fusion failures that involved harvested iliac crest autograft. Posterior instrumentation consisted of pedicle screw and rod constructs. All patients had a minimum radiographic follow-up of 2 years, and previously published plain radiographic fusion criteria were used.[32,33] The overall fusion rate was 95% (91% in group one, 97% in group two, and 100% in group three). No cases of hardware failure were reported; one patient required revision surgery to decompress a subfascial hematoma. The authors concluded that in multilevel fusions, rhBMP-2 eliminated the need for autograft and demonstrated excellent fusion rates. Higher doses of rhBMP-2 can produce fusion without local autograft or a bulking agent.

Maeda et al[34] directly compared ICBG to rhBMP-2 in adult spinal deformity fusions to the sacrum. The minimum follow-up was 2 years. In their cohort of 55 consecutive patients, 32 patients underwent fusion with ICBG, and 23 received rhBMP-2. The average dose was 11.6 mg/level anteriorly and 10.0 mg/level posteriorly. Differences in instrumentation were reported. In the ICBG group, 21 of 32 patients received all-pedicle-screw constructs, and 11 had hybrid hook-screw constructs. In the rhBMP-2 group, 21 of 23 patients received all-pedicle-screw constructs. The pseudarthrosis rate was 28.1% in the ICBG group versus 4.3% in the rhBMP-2 group, but this difference was not statistically significant. The only reported perioperative complication was acute tubular necrosis in a patient in the rhBMP-2 cohort; this was attributed to the use of aprotinin intraoperatively. The authors concluded that rhBMP-2 compared favorably to ICBG in terms of pseudarthrosis rates and complication profile, that aggressive local bone graft harvesting and higher all-pedicle-screw constructs in the rhBMP-2 group likely contributed to its lower pseudarthrosis rate.

Kim et al[35] performed a similar study having a 4- to 14-year follow-up, with the rationale that many nonunions in adult spinal deformity present 2 to 4 years postoperatively. They consecutively treated 63 patients: 31 received rhBMP-2 and 32 received ICBG. Instrumentation was a pedicle screw–hook hybrid construct. Anterior-posterior fusion was performed in all ICBG patients and in 23 of 31 BMP patients. The average BMP dose was 11.1 mg/level posteriorly and 30.9 mg/level anteriorly. The BMP group had a significantly lower pseudarthrosis rate (6.4% versus 28.1%). No significant difference in ODI scores was noted. Further examination of the BMP group showed a significant association between dose and pseudarthrosis: No pseudarthrosis was detected in patients who received a dose of 5 mg/level or more.

Recombinant Human Bone Marrow Protein 2: Complication Profile

Recent literature has focused less on fusion rates and more on complications from the use of rhBMP-2. Bess et al[36] performed a prospective, multicenter study of perioperative complications associated with rhBMP-2 in adult spinal deformity. Patients were divided into two groups: those who received rhBMP-2 (BMP) and those who did not (NOBMP). The minimum follow-up was 3 months. The BMP cohort was further subdivided into the following three groups based on location of BMP placement: posterior (PBMP), interbody (IBMP), and interbody and posterior spine (I+PBMP). Dosages used in this study were lower; the average posterior dose of rhBMP-2 was 2.5 mg/level, and the average interbody dose was 5 mg/level. The NOBMP group received a combination of local bone graft, allograft, and ICBG. The authors reported that BMP groups had significantly more minor and total complications per patient, but the NOBMP group had significantly more complications requiring surgery per patient. After performing a multivariate analysis, they concluded that at the previously mentioned doses, "no consistent associations existed between rhBMP-2 and major, wound, or neurological complications; superficial or deep infections; and complications requiring surgery."

Williams et al[37] evaluated 55,862 spinal fusion procedures using the Scoliosis Research Society's Morbidity and Mortality Index to determine whether BMP (rhBMP-2 and rhBMP-7) increased the incidence of perioperative complications. The authors assessed all cases of spinal fusion in which BMP was applied, including adult scoliosis. They reported that for adult scoliosis, BMP was associated with a higher overall rate of complications (13.8% versus 9.3%; $p < 0.001$). However, after the authors made adjustments for patient age and revision status, this association was no longer statistically significant. Only the use of BMP in anterior cervical procedures had a significantly higher rate of overall complications and wound infections, even after adjustment for patient age and revision status.

CONCLUSION

Evaluating all of the data before us, it becomes clear that great strides have been made in spinal deformity surgery. By revealing the biology of bone healing, we have been able to revolutionize not only deformity surgery, but spine surgery as a whole. Biologics are at the forefront of this revolution, with rhBMP-2 drawing the most interest and scrutiny. Of all the biologics discussed, it is the only one that can realistically challenge ICBG's status as the benchmark material. Recent literature has begun to define dosing and complication profiles associated with particular procedures, but questions regarding cost and safety persist. In the end, surgeons must critically evaluate the literature and apply their own clinical experience when incorporating biologics into their clinical practice.

REFERENCES

1. Kim YJ, Bridwell KH, Lenke LG, et al. Pseudarthrosis in long adult spinal deformity instrumentation and fusion to the sacrum: prevalence and risk factor analysis of 144 cases. Spine 31:2329-2336, 2006.
2. Cheng I, Oshtory R, Wildstein M. The role of osteobiologics in spinal deformity. Neurosurg Clin N Am 18:393-401, 2007.
3. Khanna G, Lewonowski K, Wood KB. Initial results of anterior interbody fusion achieved with a less invasive bone harvesting technique. Spine 31:111-114, 2006.
4. Arrington ED, Smith WF, Chambers HG, et al. Complications of iliac crest bone graft harvesting. Clin Orthop Relat Res 329:300-309, 1996.
5. Schnee CL, Freese A, Weil RJ, et al. Analysis of harvest morbidity and radiographic outcome using autograft for anterior cervical fusion. Spine 22:2222-2227, 1997.

6. Sawin PD, Traynelis VC, Menezes AH. A comparative analysis of fusion rates and donor-site morbidity for autogenetic rib and iliac crest bone grafts in posterior cervical fusion. J Neurosurg 88:255-265, 1998.

7. Tomford WW. Bone allografts: past, present and future. Cell Tissue Bank 1:105-109, 2000.

8. Berven S, Tay BK, Kleinstueck FS, et al. Clinical applications of bone graft substitutes in spine surgery: consideration of mineralized and demineralized preparations and growth factor supplementation. Eur Spine J 10(Suppl 2):S169-S177, 2001.

9. Bridwell KH, Lenke LG, McEnery KW, et al. Anterior fresh-frozen structural allografts in the thoracic and lumbar spine. Spine 20:1410-1418, 1995.

10. Knapp DR, Jones ET, Blanco JS, et al. Allograft bone in spinal fusion for adolescent idiopathic scoliosis. J Spinal Disorder Tech 18(Suppl 1):S73-S76, 2005.

11. Jarcho M. Calcium phosphate ceramics as hard tissue prosthesis. Clin Orthop Relat Res 157:259-278, 1981.

12. Chiroff RT, White EW, Weber KN, et al. Tissue ingrowth of Replamineform implants. J Biomed Mater Res 9:29-45, 1975.

13. McAndrew MP, Gorman PW, Lange TA. Tricalcium phosphate as a bone graft substitute in trauma: preliminary report. J Orthop Trauma 2:333-339, 1988.

14. White E, Shors EC. Biomaterial aspects of Interpore-200 porous hydroxyapatite. Dent Clin North Am 30:49-67, 1986.

15. Ohyama T, Kubo Y, Iwata H, et al. Beta-tricalcium phosphate as a substitute for autograft in interbody fusion cages in canine lumbar spine. J Neurosurg 97(3 Suppl):S350-S354, 2002.

16. Epstein NE. A preliminary study of the efficacy of beta tricalcium phosphate as a bone expander for instrumented posterolateral lumbar fusions. J Spinal Disord Tech 19:424-429, 2006.

17. Burkus JK, Transfeldt EE, Kitchel SH, et al. Clinical and radiographic outcomes of anterior lumbar interbody fusion using recombinant human bone morphogenetic protein-2. Spine 27:2396-2408, 2002.

18. Burkus JK, Sanhu HS, Gornet MF. Influence of rhBMP-2 on healing patterns associated with allograft interbody constructs in comparison with autograft. Spine 31:775-781, 2006.

19. Haid RW Jr, Branch CL Jr, Alexander TJ, et al. Posterior lumbar interbody fusion using recombinant human bone morphogenetic protein type 2 with cylindrical interbody cages. Spine J 4:527-538, 2004.

20. Luhmann SJ, Bridwell KH, Cheng I, et al. Use of bone morphogenetic protein-2 for adult spinal deformity. Spine 30(17 Suppl):S110-S117, 2005.

21. Petersen B, Whang PG, Iglesias R, et al. Osteoinductivity of commercially available demineralized bone matrix. Preparations in a spine fusion model. J Bone Joint Surg Am 86:2243-2250, 2004.

22. Bac HW, Zhao L, Kanim LE, et al. Intervariability and intravariability of bone morphogenetic proteins in commercially available demineralized bone matrix products. Spine 31:1299-1306, 2006.

23. Wang JC, Alanay A, Davie M, et al. A comparison of commercially available demineralized bone matrix for spinal fusion. Eur Spine J 16:1233-1240, 2006.

24. Dodd CA, Fefusson CM, Freedman L, et al. Allograft versus auto-graft bone in scoliosis surgery. J Bone Joint Surg Br 70:431-434, 1988.

25. Weistroffer JK, Perra JH, Lonstein JE, et al. Complications in long fusions to the sacrum for adult scoliosis. Spine 33:1478-1483, 2008.

26. Kim YJ, Bridwell KH, Lenke LG, et al. Pseudarthrosis in adult spinal deformity following multisegmental instrumentation and arthrodesis. J Bone Joint Surg Am 88:721-728, 2006.

27. Cammisa F, Lowery G, Garfin S, et al. Two-year fusion rate equivalency between Grafton DBM gel and autograft in posterolateral spine fusion. Spine 29:660-666, 2004.

28. Hostin R, O'Brien M, McCarthy I, et al. Retrospective study of anterior interbody fusion rates and patient outcomes of using mineralized collagen and bone marrow aspirate in multilevel adult spinal deformity surgery. J Spinal Disord. 2013 Nov 6. [Epub ahead of print]

29. Neen D, Noyes D, Shaw M, et al. Healos and bone marrow aspirate used for lumbar spine fusion: a case controlled study comparing healos with autograft. Spine 31:E636-E640, 2006.

30. Delecrin J, Takahashi S, Gouin G, et al. A synthetic porous ceramic as a bone graft substitute in the surgical management of scoliosis. Spine 25:563-569, 2000.

31. Mulconrey DS, Bridwell KH, Flynn J, et al. Bone Morphogenetic Protein (RhBMP-2) as a substitute for iliac crest bone graft in multilevel adult spinal deformity surgery. Spine 33:2153-2159, 2008.

32. Eck KR, Lenke LG, Bridwell KH, et al. Radiographic assessment of anterior titanium mesh cages. J Spinal Disord 13:501-509, 2000.

33. Lenke LH, Bridwell KH, Bullis D, et al. Results of in situ fusion for isthmic spondylolisthesis. J Spinal Disord 5:433-442, 1992.

34. Maeda T, Buchowski JM, Kim YJ, et al. Long adult spinal deformity fusion to the sacrum using rhBMP-2 versus autogenous iliac crest bone graft. Spine 34:2205-2212, 2009.

35. Kim HJ, Buchowski JM, Zebala LP, et al. RhBMP-2 is superior to iliac crest bone graft for long fusions to the sacrum in adult spinal deformity. Spine 38:1209-1215, 2013.

36. Bess S, Line B, Lafage V, et al. Does recombinant human bone morphogenetic protein-2 in adult spinal deformity increase complications and are complications associated with location of rhBMP-2 use? Spine 39:233-242, 2014.

37. Williams B, Smith J, Fu KM, et al; Scoliosis Research Society Morbidity and Mortality Committee. Does bone morphogenetic protein increase the incidence of perioperative complications in spinal fusion? A comparison of 55,862 cases of spinal fusion with and without bone morphogenetic protein. Spine 36:1685-1691, 2011.

22

Properties of Biologic Materials

Nelson Moussazadeh ▪ *Kai-Ming Fu*

Obtaining global spinal alignment is the first step in the surgical treatment of patients who have spinal deformity. Multisegment arthrodesis is an equally important long-term goal of deformity correction. Unfortunately, pseudarthrosis can be common in surgically corrected adult deformity patients[1,2] and may result in progressive pain, loss of correction, implant failure, and neurologic impairment. Patients with pseudarthrosis report lower health-related quality of life scores and many need complex revision procedures.[1,3]

Achieving successful arthrodesis over long-segment constructs is a multifactorial process. An assessment of bone density and smoking status can reveal problems that require treatment before surgery, for example, endocrinologic treatment of osteopenia and smoking cessation. Preoperative surgical planning is especially important in potentially high-risk areas (such as L5-S1). Both interbody and posterolateral fusion sites should be considered. Finally, choosing an appropriate fusion substrate is an essential part of every surgical plan that has potential long-term ramifications.

Currently, many fusion substrate options are available to deformity surgeons (Table 22-1). Choosing the best fit for a patient requires a basic understanding of bone graft incorporation and the biologic properties of the materials. *Bone graft incorporation* is defined as "the process of envelopment and interdigitation of the donor bone tissue with new bone deposited by the recipient."[4] This process occurs over several stages. The first stage is an inflammatory response, resulting in chemotaxis of host mesenchymal cells to the graft site. The second involves differentiation of these host cells into chondroblasts and osteoblasts under the influence of osteoinductive factors locally present at the host-graft interface. In the third stage, the graft undergoes revascularization and remodeling.[5,6] Bone graft material should ideally provide or be amenable to all the components for these processes (Fig. 22-1). A purely bioengineered solution should supply an osteoconductive matrix, osteoinductive factors, and osteogenic cells. In addition, a graft should offer structural support as needed. Currently, no product other than autologous bone graft can fulfill all crite-

Table 22-1 Common Bone Graft Extenders and Their Respective Properties

	Osteogenic Cells	Osteoinductive Properties	Osteoconductive Properties	Mechanical Strength
Autograft	Yes	Yes	Yes	Cortical only
Allograft	No	No	Yes	Cortical only
Demineralized bone matrix	No	Yes	Yes	No
Ceramics	No	No	Yes	Some preparations

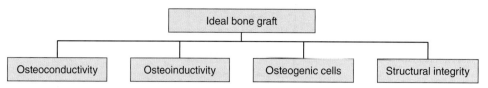

Fig. 22-1   Properties of an ideal bone graft extender.

ria perfectly. Understanding the properties of each type of fusion substrate or bone graft extender helps surgeons to plan arthrodesis procedures to achieve optimal results.

AUTOLOGOUS OPTIONS

Currently, autologous cancellous bone graft is considered the benchmark in spinal arthrodesis procedures, because it has osteoconductivity, osteoinductivity, and osteogenic cells. Cortical grafts also have structural integrity and can be used for interbody arthrodesis. Autologous bone graft does not cause allergic or immunologic reactions that can occur with a foreign graft. It is generally acceptable to patients who object to donated material for cultural or religious reasons. Autologous graft can be harvested from several sites. The most convenient means is with a surgical approach, including laminectomy or facetectomy sites. This bone may be limited in quantity and quality depending on the requirements for bone removal and the decompression techniques performed. The amount available is frequently less than that needed for long constructs, which are commonly required in deformity surgery. Although fusion rates are comparable in single-level arthrodesis between iliac crest and locally harvested autograft, the arthrodesis rate with locally harvested autograft versus iliac crest autograft for multilevel arthrodesis is a concern.[7,8] However, in adolescent deformity correction, evidence indicates that fusion rates are comparable.[9] One recent study of adults suggested similar osteogenic cell counts and osteoinductive BMP-2 production from local grafts, including laminectomy fragments and vertebral body aspirates, versus iliac crest bone fragments and aspirates.[10]

Other common sites for harvesting autograft are the ribs and the iliac crest. Ribs provide cortical and cancellous autograft. More extensive dissection posterolaterally in the thoracic spine, such as approaches for costotransversectomy, can provide access to rib tissue. Concerns with using ribs as an allograft source include potentially increased pain and the limited amount that can be harvested from each accessible donor site.

Iliac crest is a far more common source of autograft. The posterior iliac crest can be accessed through a small incision overlying the posterior superior iliac spine. Potential structures at risk include the superior gluteal artery and superior cluneal nerves; however, risk of injury can be minimized with careful planning of the incision and harvest. Alternatively, in patients treated with iliac fixation, the posterior superior iliac spine can be exposed during the iliac screw placement preparation. High-quality cortical and cancellous autograft can be harvested during this preparation, and the iliac screws can be recessed for a more comfortable placement. However, the need for iliac fixation may limit the quantity that is harvestable.

Concerns regarding iliac crest autograft include availability, especially in the quantities required for deformity operations. Many deformity procedures are revisions, and iliac crest may have previously been harvested. In addition, the harvest of iliac crest graft can be associated with added morbidity, most commonly donor site pain, infection, and hematoma.[11-14]

ALLOGRAFT OPTIONS

Allograft has been widely adopted as a bone graft extender in deformity surgery. It is readily available in sufficient quantities and avoids the morbidity of iliac crest or rib harvest. It is not associated with an increased surgical site infection rate, and the risk of transmissible disease such as human immunodeficiency virus is extremely low.[15] Multiple preparations of allograft are available. The most commonly used are freeze-dried or frozen allograft preparations. The processing for allograft removes the preponderance of antigenic burden; thus cross-matching is unnecessary. However, all preparations of allograft are immunogenic to a degree, with freeze-dried and fresh frozen allograft having less risk of antigenic response than fresh allograft.

The processing of allograft removes most osteoinductive factors and osteogenic cells. Mineralized allograft provides an osteoconductive matrix, and relies on host tissue for inductive factors and osteogenic cells. A common preparation is cancellous allograft bone chips. These are primarily used as bone graft extenders in posterolateral fusions, because they do not provide structural support. When such support is required, as in an interbody arthrodesis, cortical allograft is preferable for its mechanical strength. Fresh-frozen cortical allograft is preferable in this application, because the process of freeze-drying allografts can decrease the strength of a graft by half.[16,17]

Arthrodesis rates vary depending on the site and type of allograft used. Studies report rates of arthrodesis in both posterolateral and anterior lumbar interbody applications that are relatively comparable to reported rates for autograft.[18-21] Most studies of allograft in deformity surgery have been conducted in adolescent patients.[9,19,22] Although these reported arthrodesis rates are high, care must be taken to extrapolate the rates to the adult degenerative deformity population, in whom successful arthrodesis is more difficult to achieve. In a large study, outcomes were evaluated after allograft was used for spinal fusions in adolescents with scoliosis.[22] The authors reported a pseudarthrosis rate of 2.7% and loss of correction of 5.9%, which were comparable to historical rates with autograft.

DEMINERALIZED BONE MATRIX

Demineralized Bone Matrix (DBM) is a preparation of allograft from which the mineralized portion has been removed (Fig. 22-2). The preparation maintains some osteoconductivity, but less than that of other allograft preparations. Notably, DBM better maintains osteoinductivity of the allograft by retaining some of the growth factors, including native bone morphogenic proteins (BMPs), in small quantities. DBM does not have mechanical strength; therefore when it is used in interbody arthrodesis, the placement of a structural support such as a metal cage should be considered. DBM products come in various preparations, including putty and gels.[23]

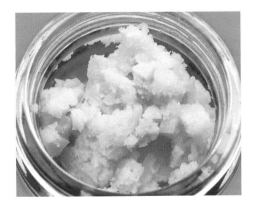

Fig. 22-2 Demineralized bone matrix. (©DOI, All rights reserved. DBX Demineralized Bone Matrix—Mix and DePuy Synthes are trademarks of DOI, or its Affiliates.)

Few studies of DBM used as a bone graft extender have been published. In single-level posterolateral fusions, arthrodesis rates comparable to those of iliac crest have been reported when DBM was used with locally harvested autograft.[24] In the largest prospective trial comparing fusion rates of posterolateral interbody fusions using autograft versus DBM-extended autograft in the same patients, Cammisa et al[25] and Tilkeridis et al[26] noted equivalent fusion rates 2 years postoperatively. In another series in which DBM was used as an interbody fusion autograft extender, posterior lumbar interbody fusion rates were equivalent at 2 years.[27]

In deformity surgery, fusion rates for DBM-only versus autograft were comparable in a study of anterior thoracic correction of idiopathic scoliosis and a retrospective study of posterolateral correction of adolescent idiopathic scoliosis.[28,29] The quality of the data on DBM is mixed and often dependent on the type of product assessed.[23,30] Most studies have evaluated short-segment arthrodesis procedures. Studies on applicability to deformity procedures have focused on adolescent idiopathic procedures. Although the osteoinductive capability with DBM is attractive, comparable effectiveness of DBM as a bone graft extender in long-segment arthrodesis has not been demonstrated.

CERAMICS

Multiple preparations of ceramic bone graft extenders and substitutes are available (Fig. 22-3). The use of ceramics as a bone graft extender or substitute is appealing in that no inflammatory response is elicited. It can be sterilized, decreasing the possibility of infectious transmission.[17,30] These products are not allografts and can be suitable to patients with cultural or religious objections to cadaveric products. All ceramic products are essentially osteoconductors with no innate osteoinductivity or osteogenic cells. They rely on host factors and cells, often derived from bone marrow aspirate. Products available include ceramics consisting of calcium sulfate, beta-tricalcium phosphate, or hydroxyapatite. Animal studies have suggested their applicability to human arthrodesis procedures.[30] However, some animal research presents contradictory results, implying limitations in the use of ceramics as bone graft extenders.[31]

Several human studies have been conducted on the effectiveness of ceramics for posterolateral arthrodesis. Hydroxyapatite appears to be the least effective ceramic bone graft extender for posterolateral arthrodesis. In a prospective randomized controlled trial in which follow-up CT and dynamic radiographs were evaluated, results suggested poor fusion in coralline hydroxyapatite plus bone marrow aspirate–extended local autograft, compared with iliac crest autograft for posterolateral arthrodesis.[32] A study designed to evaluate hydroxyapatite-bioactive glass ceramic composite as a stand-alone graft extender for this application was prematurely ended because of poor fusion rates.[33] In another study, a hydroxyapatite and collagen mixture was reported to be a more successful bone graft extender, with results equivalent to those of cancellous autograft in posterolateral arthrodesis in adult degenerative scoliosis.[34] The number of patients evaluated was small at 28, but 2-year follow-up results suggested similar pseudarthrosis rates.

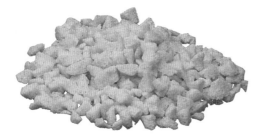

Fig. 22-3   Tricalcium phosphate ceramic granules. (©DOI, All rights reserved. chronOS Granules and DePuy Synthes are trademarks of DOI, or its Affiliates.)

Beta-tricalcium phosphate is a ceramic bone graft extender with more promising results. In single-level arthrodesis, results are comparable to those of an autograft. In a prospective randomized trial of 62 patients, no difference was reported in clinical outcome or fusion rate at 3 years.[35] However, no other comparative studies are published, and no studies have specifically assessed beta-tricalcium phosphate as an extender for multilevel deformity arthrodesis. It can be difficult to determine fusion status in patients with ceramics, because evidence indicates that bone growth may not be detectable.[36] Other ceramics have mixed or poor results in arthrodesis. For example, calcium sulfate pellets resulted in an arthrodesis rate of less than 50% at 1 year, and silicate-substituted calcium phosphate resulted in a pseudarthrosis rate that was five times higher in lumbar interbody fusions.[37,38] The choice of ceramic is therefore important in planning arthrodesis strategies.

CELL-BASED THERAPIES

One of the requirements of a successful bone graft is the presence of cells with osteogenic potential. Bone graft extenders generally do not have these cells and rely on the host to provide them. Bone marrow aspirate is easily obtained and causes relatively little morbidity. The cells obtained have osteogenic potential and have been used with bone graft extenders in attempts to achieve improved arthrodesis rates.[38] Several commercial products exist to facilitate the use of bone marrow aspirate and mesenchymal stem cells for spinal fusion procedures. However, few comparative studies support this application, and no studies to date compare its effectiveness in deformity procedures, compared with autograft.[39]

Vertebral body aspiration is a marrow-based approach postulated to improve fusion with relatively little morbidity because of its in-field availability through transpedicular cannulation. Recent studies have suggested that these samples contained osteoprogenitor cell concentrations at least equivalent to those of iliac crest aspirates, and the concentration was up to 71% more in one study.[40-42]

BONE GRAFT ENHANCERS

Achieving a solid arthrodesis in deformity surgery can be challenging. As mentioned previously, autologous grafts, especially iliac crest bone grafts, are the standard by which other bone graft extenders are compared. Pseudarthrosis rates in deformity surgery can approach 30% in some studies using autograft. Therefore interest is growing in materials that can enhance the fusion rates and improve outcomes. Materials that improve arthrodesis are considered *bone graft enhancers*. These improve the osteoinductive environment at the fusion site.

BMP is the most commonly employed bone graft enhancer. All BMPs are members of the transforming growth factor–beta superfamily and have involvement in bone formation and development. Many BMPs have been identified since their first discovery in the 1960s.[43] Recombinant human bone morphogenic protein 7 (rhBMP-7) and rhBMP-2 were approved for clinical use in limited fashion. The use of rhBMP2 has been increasing; most of these applications are off label, including posterolateral fusions.[44] Safety concerns regarding the safety profile of rhBMP-2 in off-label use have been reported.[45] Different database studies and meta-analysis reviews suggest similar complication profiles regardless of whether rhBMP-2 is used in posterolateral fusion.[46-48] The potential for an increased cancer risk has been a concern; however, results are inconclusive.[49]

The effectiveness of rhBMP-2 in achieving arthrodesis has been demonstrated in independent data reviews.[49] This improvement in arthrodesis did not correlate with improved outcomes, however.[49] It was mentioned in the discussion that rhBMP-2 may be more effective in specific patient populations such as those with adult deformity. In older patients, especially those requiring iliac fixation, fusion rates were higher when rhBMP-2 was used, compared with iliac crest bone graft.[2,14,45,50,51] Patients reported improved outcomes on the SRS-22 instrument longer than 4 years postoperatively, although other outcome measures showed no significant difference.[50] Therefore evidence indicates that fusion rates are higher in adult deformity patients when rhBMP-2 is used. The resultant evidence for improved outcomes is variable. Larger and longer prospective studies are needed to evaluate efficacy, as measured by disability and pain.

CONCLUSION

Achieving a solid fusion in deformity surgery requires a fundamental understanding of bone graft healing and the application of an appropriate graft to a properly prepared site. Pseudarthrosis is unfortunately a common occurrence in adult deformity; thus it should be discussed with the patient in preoperative counseling. Autograft is the standard against which other graft extenders, including allograft, DBM products, and ceramics, are measured. Studies evaluating the comparative effectiveness of these extenders in the adults are few and of limited quality.[19] In adolescent deformity series, most products result in reasonable fusion rates. Adolescent fusion rates tend to be higher, because these patients have more robust bone healing and strength. Therefore extrapolating these data to the adult degenerative population is difficult. Graft extenders should be chosen based on the quantity of iliac crest bone graft and local allograft available and the needs of the patient. Revision and high-risk patients may benefit from an osteoinductive enhancer; the risks and benefits need to be discussed with the patient.

REFERENCES

1. Gum JL, Carreon LY, Stimac JD, et al. Predictors of Oswestry Disability Index worsening after lumbar fusion. Orthopedics 36:e478-e483, 2013.
2. Kim YJ, Bridwell KH, Lenke LG, et al. Pseudarthrosis in long adult spinal deformity instrumentation and fusion to the sacrum: prevalence and risk factor analysis of 144 cases. Spine 31:2329-2336, 2006.
3. Bridwell KH, Baldus C, Berven S, et al. Changes in radiographic and clinical outcomes with primary treatment adult spinal deformity surgeries from two years to three- to five-years follow-up. Spine 35:1849-1854, 2010.
4. Morone MA, Boden SD, Hair G, et al. The Marshall R. Urist Young Investigator Award. Gene expression during autograft lumbar spine fusion and the effect of bone morphogenetic protein 2. Clin Orthop Relat Res 351:252-265, 1998.
5. Goldberg VM, Stevenson S. The biology of bone grafts. Semin Arthroplasty 4:58-63, 1993.
6. Zipfel GJ, Guiot BH, Fessler RG. Bone grafting. Neurosurg Focus 14:e8, 2003.
7. Sengupta DK, Truumees E, Patel CK, et al. Outcome of local bone versus autogenous iliac crest bone graft in the instrumented posterolateral fusion of the lumbar spine. Spine 31:985-991, 2006.
8. Ito Z, Imagama S, Kanemura T, et al. Bone union rate with autologous iliac bone versus local bone graft in posterior lumbar interbody fusion (PLIF): a multicenter study. Eur Spine J 22:1158-1163, 2013.
9. Violas P, Chapuis M, Bracq H. Local autograft bone in the surgical management of adolescent idiopathic scoliosis. Spine 29:189-192, 2004.
10. Sinclair S, Brodke DS, Lawrence BD. Comparing the osteogenic potential of mesenchymal stem cells isolated from multiple lumbar fusion bone graft sites. Presented at the Annual Meeting of the American Academy of Orthopaedic Surgeons, Las Vegas, NV, March 2014.
11. Arrington ED, Smith WJ, Chambers HG, et al. Complications of iliac crest bone graft harvesting. Clin Orthop Relat Res 329:300-309, 1996.
12. Banwart JC, Asher MA, Hassanein RS. Iliac crest bone graft harvest donor site morbidity. A statistical evaluation. Spine 20:1055-1060, 1995.

13. Delawi D, Dhert WJ, Castelein RM, et al. The incidence of donor site pain after bone graft harvesting from the posterior iliac crest may be overestimated: a study on spine fracture patients. Spine 32:1865-1868, 2007.

14. Kim DH, Rhim R, Li L, et al. Prospective study of iliac crest bone graft harvest site pain and morbidity. Spine J 9:886-892, 2009.

15. Tomford WW. Bone allografts: past, present and future. Cell Tissue Bank 1:105-109, 2000.

16. Berven S, Tay BK, Kleinstueck FS, et al. Clinical applications of bone graft substitutes in spine surgery: consideration of mineralized and demineralized preparations and growth factor supplementation. Eur Spine J 10(Suppl 2):S169-S177, 2001.

17. Cheng I, Oshtory R, Wildstein MS. The role of osteobiologics in spinal deformity. Neurosurg Clin N Am 18:393-401, 2007.

18. An HS, Lynch K, Toth J. Prospective comparison of autograft vs. allograft for adult posterolateral lumbar spine fusion: differences among freeze-dried, frozen, and mixed grafts. J Spinal Disord 8:131-135, 1995.

19. Fischer CR, Cassilly R, Cantor W, et al. A systematic review of comparative studies on bone graft alternatives for common spine fusion procedures. Eur Spine J 22:1423-1435, 2013.

20. Gibson S, McLeod I, Wardlaw D, et al. Allograft versus autograft in instrumented posterolateral lumbar spinal fusion: a randomized control trial. Spine 27:1599-1603, 2002.

21. Thalgott JS, Fogarty ME, Giuffre JM, et al. A prospective, randomized, blinded, single-site study to evaluate the clinical and radiographic differences between frozen and freeze-dried allograft when used as part of a circumferential anterior lumbar interbody fusion procedure. Spine 34:1251-1256, 2009.

22. Knapp DR Jr, Jones ET, Blanco JS, et al. Allograft bone in spinal fusion for adolescent idiopathic scoliosis. J Spinal Disord Tech 18 Suppl:S73-S76, 2005.

23. Aghdasi B, Montgomery SR, Daubs MD, et al. A review of demineralized bone matrices for spinal fusion: the evidence for efficacy. Surgeon 11:39-48, 2013.

24. Kang J, An H, Hilibrand A, et al. Grafton and local bone have comparable outcomes to iliac crest bone in instrumented single-level lumbar fusions. Spine 37:1083-1091, 2012.

25. Cammisa FP Jr, Lowery G, Garfin SR, et al. Two-year fusion rate equivalency between Grafton DBM gel and autograft in posterolateral spine fusion: a prospective controlled trial employing a side-by-side comparison in the same patient. Spine 29:660-666, 2004.

26. Tilkeridis K, Touzopoulos P, Ververidis A, et al. Use of demineralized bone matrix in spinal fusion. World J Orthop 5:30-37, 2014.

27. Ahn DK, Moon SH, Kim TW, et al. Demineralized bone matrix, as a graft enhancer of auto-local bone in posterior lumbar interbody fusion. Asian Spine J 8:129-137, 2014.

28. Price CT, Connolly JF, Carantzas AC, et al. Comparison of bone grafts for posterior spinal fusion in adolescent idiopathic scoliosis. Spine 28:793-798, 2003.

29. Weinzapfel B, Son-Hing JP, Armstrong DG, et al. Fusion rates after thoracoscopic release and bone graft substitutes in idiopathic scoliosis. Spine 33:1079-1083, 2008.

30. Alsaleh KA, Tougas CA, Roffey DM, et al. Osteoconductive bone graft extenders in posterolateral thoracolumbar spinal fusion: a systematic review. Spine 37:E993-E1000, 2012.

31. Miller CP, Jegede K, Essig D, et al. The efficacies of 2 ceramic bone graft extenders for promoting spinal fusion in a rabbit bone paucity model. Spine 37:642-647, 2012.

32. Korovessis P, Koureas G, Zacharatos S, et al. Correlative radiological, self-assessment and clinical analysis of evolution in instrumented dorsal and lateral fusion for degenerative lumbar spine disease. Autograft versus coralline hydroxyapatite. Eur Spine J 14:630-638, 2005.

33. Acharya NK, Kumar RJ, Varma HK, et al. Hydroxyapatite-bioactive glass ceramic composite as stand-alone graft substitute for posterolateral fusion of lumbar spine: a prospective, matched, and controlled study. J Spinal Disord Tech 21:106-111, 2008.

34. Ploumis A, Albert TJ, Brown Z, et al. Healos graft carrier with bone marrow aspirate instead of allograft as adjunct to local autograft for posterolateral fusion in degenerative lumbar scoliosis: a minimum 2-year follow-up study. J Neurosurg Spine 13:211-215, 2010.

35. Dai LY, Jiang LS. Single-level instrumented posterolateral fusion of lumbar spine with beta-tricalcium phosphate versus autograft: a prospective, randomized study with 3-year follow-up. Spine 33:1299-1304, 2008.

36. Eder C, Meissner J, Bretschneider W, et al. Analysis of a β-TCP bone graft extender explanted during revision surgery after 28 months in vivo. Eur Spine J 23(Suppl 2):157-160, 2013.

37. Nandyala SV, Marquez-Lara A, Fineberg SJ, et al. Prospective, randomized, controlled trial of silicate-substituted calcium phosphate versus rhBMP-2 in a minimally invasive transforaminal lumbar interbody fusion. Spine 39:185-191, 2014.

38. Niu CC, Tsai TT, Fu TS, et al. A comparison of posterolateral lumbar fusion comparing autograft, autogenous laminectomy bone with bone marrow aspirate, and calcium sulphate with bone marrow aspirate: a prospective randomized study. Spine 34:2715-2719, 2009.

39. Khashan M, Inoue S, Berven SH. Cell based therapies as compared to autologous bone grafts for spinal arthrodesis. Spine 38:1885-1891, 2013.

40. McLain RF, Fleming JE, Boehm CA, et al. Aspiration of osteoprogenitor cells for augmenting spinal fusion: comparison of progenitor cell concentrations from the vertebral body and iliac crest. J Bone Joint Surg Am 87:2655-2661, 2005.

41. McLain RF, Boehm CA, Rufo-Smith C, et al. Transpedicular aspiration of osteoprogenitor cells from the vertebral body: progenitor cell concentrations affected by serial aspiration. Spine J 9:995-1002, 2009.

42. Hustedt JW, Jegede KA, Badrinath R, et al. Optimal aspiration volume of vertebral bone marrow for use in spinal fusion. Spine J 13:1217-1222, 2013.

43. Urist MR. Bone: formation by autoinduction. Science 150:893-899, 1965.

44. Lad SP, Nathan JK, Boakye M. Trends in the use of bone morphogenetic protein as a substitute to autologous iliac crest bone grafting for spinal fusion procedures in the United States. Spine 36:E274-E281, 2011.

45. Carragee EJ, Hurwitz EL, Weiner BK. A critical review of recombinant human bone morphogenetic protein-2 trials in spinal surgery: emerging safety concerns and lessons learned. Spine J 11:471-491, 2011.

46. Bess S, Line BG, Lafage V, et al. Does recombinant human bone morphogenetic protein-2 use in adult spinal deformity increase complications and are complications associated with location of rhBMP-2 use? A prospective, multicenter study of 279 consecutive patients. Spine 39:233-242, 2014.

47. Singh K, Ahmadinia K, Park DK, et al. Complications of spinal fusion with utilization of bone morphogenetic protein: a systematic review of the literature. Spine 39:91-101, 2014.

48. Williams BJ, Smith JS, Fu KM, et al. Does bone morphogenetic protein increase the incidence of perioperative complications in spinal fusion? A comparison of 55,862 cases of spinal fusion with and without bone morphogenetic protein. Spine 36:1685-1691, 2011.

49. Simmonds MC, Brown JV, Heirs MK, et al. Safety and effectiveness of recombinant human bone morphogenetic protein-2 for spinal fusion: a meta-analysis of individual-participant data. Ann Intern Med 158:877-889, 2013.

50. Kim HJ, Buchowski JM, Zebala LP, et al. RhBMP-2 is superior to iliac crest bone graft for long fusions to the sacrum in adult spinal deformity: 4- to 14-year follow-up. Spine 38:1209-1215, 2013.

51. Maeda T, Buchowski JM, Kim YJ, et al. Long adult spinal deformity fusion to the sacrum using rhBMP-2 versus autogenous iliac crest bone graft. Spine 34:2205-2212, 2009.

23

Biologic Considerations in Minimally Invasive Spine Surgery

Gregory M. Mundis, Jr. ▪ *Navid R. Arandi*

The use of osteobiologics in spinal fusion surgery has increased significantly during recent years. Approximately 500,000 spinal fusion procedures are performed each year in the United States alone,[1] and nearly all require some type of bone grafting material. The goal of all spinal fusion techniques, whether they are minimally invasive or open, is to increase the chances of a solid arthrodesis at the fusion site. Autografts from the iliac crest and local bone grafts have been the historic standards for grafting materials. However, donor site morbidity, limited availability, and suboptimal mechanical integrity have shifted focus toward other viable graft alternatives.

Various alternative bone graft materials are currently available, including demineralized bone matrix (DBM), calcium-phosphate–based substitutes, autologous bone marrow, ceramics, and factor-based substitutes (bone morphogenetic protein [BMP]). The bone healing properties of an ideal bone graft substitute are entrenched in the substance's ability to promote osteogenesis (osteoblasts, osteoprogenitor cells), osteoinduction (BMP), and osteoconduction (hydroxyapatite, beta-tricalcium phosphate). Many of these materials are commonly used off label without formative supporting data, and inevitably there is a lack of understanding regarding the correct application and mechanism of action before they are used in patients.[2]

Minimally invasive spine surgery (MISS) has garnered significant press during the past two decades. Technologic advancements in combination with high perioperative complication rates, a growing elderly population, and an increased health care burden have prompted the creation of less invasive techniques to address adult spinal disorders. The role of osteobiologics has thus become critical, because many of the long-term outcomes of MISS will ultimately depend on successful arthrodesis at the fusion sites.

As surgeons, we must first understand the uses for which these graft materials have proved effective, and then we must select the correct material based on what is required from the bone graft substitute (structural support or bone production).[46] This chapter attempts to consolidate the available literature about osteobiologics in MISS and to provide a brief overview of the available grafting options and their use with various MISS surgical techniques.

THE USE OF OSTEOBIOLOGICS IN THE MINIMALLY INVASIVE SPINE SURGERY LITERATURE

A review of the MISS literature yielded a total of 43 studies[3-45] in which osteobiologics were used (Tables 23-1, 23-2, and 23-3). The studies were grouped according to the technique used for interbody fusion (lateral retroperitoneal lumbar interbody fusion [LLIF], transforaminal lumbar interbody fusion [TLIF], or posterior lumbar interbody fusion [PLIF]), with the following criteria in mind:

- The minimally invasive technique used for some or all of the patient cohort
- The sample size of the patient population (10 or more)
- The biologic material used
- The fusion and nonunion rates discovered during follow-up

Although efforts were made to include only high-quality studies, most studies of osteobiologics in MISS have considerable weaknesses. Their frequent lack of a control group in particular makes it difficult for solid conclusions to be extrapolated.

AUTOLOGOUS BONE GRAFT

Historically autologous bone graft has been considered the gold standard graft material used for spinal arthrodesis. This material possesses the three fundamental properties of an ideal bone graft: osteogenicity, osteoinductivity, and osteoconductivity. Autologous bone graft is normally collected from the iliac crest (iliac crest bone graft [ICGB]) or harvested and prepared from local bone (lamina, facet joint) during decompression procedures. Biologic properties may differ depending on the site of graft collection and whether the graft is made of cortical or cancellous bone.[2,46] Although the osteoblast content of cancellous laminar bone may be even greater than that of the iliac crest,[47] the issue of supply limitations still remains and is dependent on the number of levels decompressed. Despite its benefits, autologous bone grafting raises clinical concern with regard to associated donor site morbidity, blood loss, nerve damage, and various other complications.[2,46]

Autologous grafts (local bone, bone marrow aspirate, ICBG) were used in 33 MISS studies (see Tables 23-1, 23-2, and 23-3). Seven LLIF studies[16,21,27,32-34,43] involved the use of autologous graft in conjunction with other graft material (see Table 23-1), whereas 7 PLIF studies* exclusively made use of autologous grafting with fusion rates that ranged from 50% to 100% at the latest follow-up, despite different follow-up time points and modalities used to measure fusion rates (CT versus radiography) (see Table 23-3). All 19 TLIF studies† involved autologous graft as one of the grafting ingredients, with only 3 using autograft as the sole graft material.[29,35,36] Scheufler et al[35] were able to demonstrate a 94% fusion rate (via CT) at the follow-up in their cohort of 53 MISS TLIF patients when local bone was used as the primary graft material. Peng et al[29] showed an 80% rate of grade I fusion based on the Bridwell anterior fusion grading system at 2-year follow-up in their 29-patient cohort in which ICBG was used.[48]

Text continued on page 305

---

*References 12, 13, 17, 22, 25, 28, 40.
†References 3, 5, 10, 11, 14, 15, 18-20, 23, 24, 29, 35-38, 41, 42.

Table 23-1 Osteobiologics in Minimally Invasive Lateral Retroperitoneal Lumbar Interbody Fusion

Author	Year	Number of Patients	Follow-up Duration	Osteobiologic Material Used (number of patients)	Fusion Rates (imaging modality used to assess fusion)	Comments (implant- or fusion-related complications only [subsidence, nonunion, pseudarthrosis])
Oliveira et al[26]*	2010	15	24 mo (min)	rhBMP-2 (all)	80% achieved solid fusion at 12 mo (radiography or CT)	2 patients had additional surgeries: 1 FS caused by heterotropic bone formation treated with foraminotomy, 1 decompression procedure 1 ASD 1 asymptomatic cage subsidence
Ozgur et al[27]†	2010	62	24 mo (min)	BMP (57), autograft, and allograft	91% overall (radiography)	1 pseudarthrosis (Treatment: revision) 19% minor complication rate
Rodgers et al[32]	2010	40	3 mo (min)	DBM, allograft, autograft, and BMA (all)	Mean modified Lenke[48] fusion score of 1.1† at 12 mo (radiography or CT)	1 compression fracture at 4 wk (Treatment: vertebroplasty)
Anand et al[6]‡	2010	28	22 mo (mean)	rhBMP-2 and DBM (all)	100% at 12 mo (radiography or CT)	1 case of screw prominence (Treatment: revision) 0 pseudarthroses
Dakwar et al[9]	2010	25	11 mo (mean)	rhBMP-2 and β-TCP/HA (all)	100% radiographic fusion in 22 pt with >6 mo of follow-up (radiography or CT)	1 asymptomatic subsidence 1 asymptomatic hardware failure
Wang and Mummaneni[43]§	2010	23	13.4 mo (mean)	BMP, autograft, and allograft (all)	100% fusion at interbody levels; 71.4% fusion of posterolateral levels without interbody fusion (CT)	1 postoperative cerebrospinal fluid leak (Treatment: reexploration) 1 S1 screw pullout (Treatment: extension of the construct to the ilium)
Rodgers et al[33]	2010	66	12 mo (min)	Local bone, DBM, allograft, and BMA (all)	98.4% at 12 mo (radiography); 97% at 12 mo (CT)	6 patients had incomplete bridging bone at 12 mo (plain radiography) 1 patient with three-level LLIF showed motion (flexion-extension radiography)
Youssef et al[44]	2010	84	15.7 mo (mean)	rhBMP-2 and allograft (all)	81% solid arthrodesis at mean follow-up (radiography or CT)	2 ASDs (Treatment: 1 decompression, 1 nonoperative treatment) 1 subsidence (Treatment: nonoperative treatment) 1 VB fracture (Treatment: revision corpectomy) 1 endplate fracture (Treatment: bracing)

*Standalone cages were used in all patients; no posterior or lateral fixation was used.
†Standalone cages were used in some patients.
‡Some patients in the cohort underwent an additional minimally invasive transsacral approach for fusion at L5-S1 or L4-5.
§Some patients in the cohort underwent minimally invasive transforaminal lumbar interbody fusion in addition to lateral retroperitoneal lumbar interbody fusion.
ASD, Adjacent-segment disease; *BMA,* bone marrow aspirate; *BMP,* bone morphogenetic protein; *β-TCP,* beta-tricalcium phosphate; *CT,* computed tomography; *DBM,* demineralized bone matrix; *FS,* foraminal stenosis; *HA,* hydroxyapatite; *min,* minimum; *mo,* month or months; *pt,* patient or patients; *rhBMP-2,* recombinant human bone morphogenetic protein–2; *VB,* vertebral body; *wk,* week or weeks.

Continued

Table 23-1   Osteobiologics in Minimally Invasive Lateral Retroperitoneal Lumbar Interbody Fusion—cont'd

Author	Year	Number of Patients	Follow-up Duration	Osteobiologic Material Used (number of patients)	Fusion Rates (imaging modality used to assess fusion)	Comments (implant- or fusion-related complications only [subsidence, nonunion, pseudarthrosis])
Karikari et al[16]	2011	22	16.4 mo (mean)	BMP (17) with β-TCP/HA/collagen mix (14), femoral allograft (1), or local autograft (2)	Overall 21 of 22 pt (95.5%) who had 6 mo of follow-up demonstrated radiographic fusion (radiography or CT)	1 ASD (Treatment: vertebroplasty 3 mo postoperatively) 1 subsidence (Treatment: extension of fusion)
Caputo et al[8]¶	2013	30	14.3 mo (mean)	ACBM, MSCs, and osteoprogenitor cells (all)	112 of 127 (88.2%) LLIF levels showed bony fusion at 12 mo (CT)	1 nonunion (Treatment: revision surgery at 13 mo) 1 asymptomatic pedicle fracture (Treatment: observation) 2 anterior longitudinal ligament ruptures (Treatment: additional lateral fixation)
Tohmeh et al[39]◇	2012	40	12 mo (min)	ACBM, MSCs, and osteoprogenitor cells (all)	Complete fusion at 55 of 61 (90.2%) treated LLIF levels at 12 mo (radiography or CT)	1 potential pseudarthrosis 1 DDD (Treatment: reoperation at adjacent LLIF level)
Rodgers et al[34]	2012	44	12 mo (min)	β-TCP/HA and BMA (all)	41 of 44 (93.2%) LLIF levels achieved radiographic fusion at a mean of 17.4 mo (CT)	1 residual stenosis (Treatment: revision) 1 excision of subcutaneous lesion (thought to be graft material) at 12 mo
Anand et al[4]‡	2013	71	39 mo (mean)	rhBMP-2 and DBM (66) rhBMP-2, allograft, and DBM (34)	94.4% at 24 mo (CT)	4 pseudarthroses (Treatment: revision anteroposterior fusion ± extension to pelvis) 3 persistent stenoses (Treatment: decompression) 1 heterotropic ossification (Treatment: decompression) 1 adjacent-segment osteomyelitis (Treatment: posterior instrumented fusion) 1 ASD (Treatment: discectomy with PLIF and instrumentation) 1 PJK (Treatment: posterior instrumented fusion) 1 screw prominence (Treatment: screw removal) 20% overall complication rate

¶Some patients in the cohort underwent L5-S1 anterior lumbar interbody fusion.
◇Some patients in the cohort underwent transforaminal lumbar interbody fusion in addition to lateral retroperitoneal lumbar interbody fusion.
‡Some patients in the cohort underwent an additional minimally invasive transsacral approach for fusion at L5-S1 or L4-5.
ACBM, Allograft cellular bone matrix; *ASD,* adjacent-segment disease; *BMP,* bone morphogenetic protein; *β-TCP,* beta-tricalcium phosphate; *CT,* computed tomography; *DBM,* demineralized bone matrix; *DDD,* degenerative disc disease; *HA,* hydroxyapatite; *LLIF,* lateral retroperitoneal lumbar interbody fusion; *min,* minimum; *mo,* month or months; *MSCs,* mesenchymal stem cells; *PJK,* proximal junctional kyphosis; *pt,* patient or patients; *rhBMP-2,* recombinant human bone morphogenetic protein–2.

Author	Year	Number of Patients	Follow-up Duration	Osteobiologic Material Used (number of patients)	Fusion Rates (imaging modality used to assess fusion)	Comments (implant- or fusion-related complications only [subsidence, nonunion, pseudarthrosis])
Rodgers et al[31]†	2013	283	24 mo (min)	β-TCP/HA (24) DBM and allograft (59) DBM and cortical cancellous allograft (192) ACBM (8)	Mean modified Lenke[48] fusion score of 1.17 at 12 mo (modality of fusion assessment not specified)††	19 total complications (6.7%), with 36 (12.7%) additional surgeries performed Implant- and fusion-related complications included the following: —1 broken screw —1 rod fracture —2 adjacent segment fractures (Treatment: vertebroplasties) —21 ASDs (Treatment: adjacent level fusion —5 persistent stenoses (Treatment: decompression) —1 nonunion (Treatment: revision)
Pimenta et al[30]* (randomized controlled trial)	2013	30	36 mo (min)	Silicate and calcium phosphate ceramic (15) rhBMP-2 (15)	54% fusion in silicate and ceramic group at 12 mo (radiography or CT) 67% in rhBMP-2 group at 12 mo (radiography or CT)	3 subsidences in silicate and ceramic group 2 subsidences in rhBMP-2 group (Treatment: 1 decompression) 1 ASD in silicate and ceramic group and 3 ASDs in rhBMP-2 group (Treatment: all required revision) 1 excessive bone formation in rhBMP-2 group (Treatment: direct decompression)
Meredith et al[21]**	2013	18	14 mo (mean)	DBM (13) with BMP (9), rib (12), or ICBG (2)	94% showed radiographic fusion at mean follow-up (CT)	2 incidental durotomies (Treatment: 1 intraoperative repair, 1 revision)

†Standalone cages were used in some patients.
††Modified Lenke fusion score: *1,* consolidated; *2,* partially consolidated; *3,* not yet consolidated.
*Standalone cages were used in all patients; no posterior or lateral fixation was used.
**Lateral retroperitoneal lumbar interbody fusion was performed in the thoracic and thoracolumbar regions.
ACBM, Allograft cellular bone matrix; *ASD,* adjacent-segment disease; *BMP,* bone morphogenetic protein; β-*TCP,* beta-tricalcium phosphate; *CT,* computed tomography; *DBM,* demineralized bone matrix; *HA,* hydroxyapatite; *ICBG,* iliac crest bone graft; *min,* minimum; *mo,* month or months; *rhBMP-2,* recombinant human bone morphogenetic protein–2.

Table 23-2   Osteobiologics in Minimally Invasive Transforaminal Lumbar Interbody Fusion

Author	Year	Number of Patients	Follow-up Duration	Osteobiologic Material Used (number of patients)	Fusion Rates (imaging modality used to assess fusion)	Comments (implant- or fusion-related complications only [subsidence, nonunion, pseudarthrosis])
Mummaneni et al[23]*	2004	44	9 mo (mean)	ICBG only (19) ICBG with rhBMP-2 (21)	ICBG only group: 95% at 6 mo (radiography) ICBG with rhBMP-2 group: 95% at 6 mo (radiography)	ICBG only group: 58% donor site pain at 6 mo; 1 pseudarthrosis (Treatment: observation) ICBG with rhBMP-2 group: 2 CSF leaks, 1 potential pseudarthrosis (Treatment: observation)
Jang and Lee[14]	2005	22	19 mo (mean)	Autograft and allograft with or without ICBG (all)	92% of fusion levels showed bone union (radiography)	Subsidence at 3 sites, 1 pedicle screw failure, no reoperations performed
Schwender et al[37]	2005	49	22.6 mo (mean)	Structural allograft plus BMP, local autograft, or both (all)	100% at a min of 18 mo follow-up (radiography)	2 displaced pedicle screws (Treatment: revision) 1 graft dislodgment (Treatment: revision) 1 contralateral FS (Treatment: revision) 8.2% overall complication rate
Villavicencio et al[41]†	2005	43	20.6 mo (mean)	Local cancellous autograft or allograft, rhBMP-2, and structural allograft (all)	100% at 12 mo (CT)	2 malpositioned screws (1 required revision) 13 overall complications of MIS surgery
Anand et al[5]‡	2006	100	30 mo (mean)	Femoral allograft and ICBG (15) Femoral allograft, rhBMP-2, local autograft, and DBM (85 pt)	99% solid interbody fusion (radiography or CT)	No subsidence, screw malpositioning, or instrumentation failures
Deutsch and Musacchio[10]	2006	20	6 mo (min)	Local autograft and rhBMP-2 (all)	65% showed some degree of fusion at 6 mo (CT)	1 postoperative radiculopathy (Treatment: pedicle screw removal)
Joseph and Rampersaud[15]§	2007	33	25 mo (mean)	Local autograft with rhBMP-2 (23 pt) Local autograft without rhBMP-2 (10 pt)	Autograft with rhBMP-2 group: 91.3% at 6 mo (CT) Autograft without BMP group: 50% at 6 mo (CT)	Heterotropic ossification occurred in 20.8% of the autograft with rhBMP-2 group and 8.3% of the autograft without rhBMP-2 group Additional surgery performed in 3 patients
Scheufler et al[35]	2007	53	16 mo (mean)	Local autograft	94% at 16 mo for 46 pt with available imaging (CT)	No subsidence, implant fracture loosening, or complications reported

*This study included some patients who had open transforaminal lumbar interbody fusion.
†This study included some patients who had open transforaminal lumbar interbody fusion. However, this table only accounts for the minimally invasive spine surgery patients in the study.
‡The researchers used a technique called *cantilever transforaminal lumbar interbody fusion,* which is minimally invasive.
§This study included 10 patients who had minimally invasive posterior lumbar interbody fusion.
BMP, Bone morphogenetic protein; *CSF,* cerebrospinal fluid; *CT,* computed tomography; *DBM,* demineralized bone matrix; *ICBG,* iliac crest bone graft; *min,* minimum; *mo,* month or months; *pt,* patient or patients; *rhBMP-2,* recombinant human bone morphogenetic protein–2.

Author	Year	Number of Patients	Follow-up Duration	Osteobiologic Material Used (number of patients)	Fusion Rates (imaging modality used to assess fusion)	Comments (implant- or fusion-related complications only [subsidence, nonunion, pseudarthrosis])
Dhall et al[11]†	2008	21	24 mo (mean)	rhBMP-2 (6) Local autograft (15)	rhBMP-2 group: 100% (radiography or CT) Local autograft group: 93.3% (radiography or CT)	1 cage migration (Treatment: revision) 1 screw malposition (Treatment: revision) 2 transient L5 sensory losses 1 pseudarthrosis in local autograft group (Treatment: revision) 9.5% overall reoperation rate
Peng et al[29]	2009	29	24 mo (min)	Autograft and ICBG (all)	80% grade I per Bridwell anterior fusion grading system[48] (radiography or CT)	2 ICBG site infections (Treatment: IV antibiotics) 6.9% minor complication rate
Schizas et al[36]	2009	18	22 mo (mean)	Local autograft and ICBG (all)	No explicitly stated fusion rates No immediate postoperative instrumentation failure on CT scans	3 cases of nonunion: —2 pedicle screw loosenings 12 mo postoperatively —1 pedicle screw breakage 36 mo postoperatively 2 of 3 nonunions required revision
Mannion et al[20]¶	2011	30	7.1 mo (mean)	Local autograft and rhBMP-2 (all)	33 of 36 (92%) of the levels treated showed complete bony fusion at 7 mo (CT)	1 nonunion with cage subsidence and osteolysis (Treatment: observation) 2 heterotropic ossifications (1 TLIF, 1 PLIF) 1 case of inflammatory cysts compressing L4 nerve root with cage retropulsion (Treatment: revision)
Wang et al[42]	2010	42	26.3 mo (mean)	Local autograft (all)	No explicitly stated fusion rates	1 graft dislodgment 1 epidural hematoma 1 nonunion (not revised)
Wang et al[45]✧	2011	25	27.7 mo (mean)	Local autograft and ICBG (all)	No explicitly stated fusion rates	1 nonunion (not revised)
Lee et al[19]	2012	72	24 mo (min)	Local autograft and DBM (all)	59.4% grade I and 36.2% grade II per Bridwell interbody fusion grading system[48] at 6 mo (radiography) 97% 2 yr (95.8% follow-up rate at 6 and 12 mo)	4 asymptomatic cage migrations (6%) (not revised) 1 misplaced pedicle screw (Treatment: revision) 2 minor complications

†This study included some patients who had open transforaminal lumbar interbody fusion. However, this table only accounts for the minimally invasive spine surgery patients in the study.
¶This study included patients who had minimally invasive posterior lumbar interbody fusion at a total of four levels.
✧The researchers used minimally invasive transforaminal lumbar interbody fusion as revision surgery for patients who had previously been treated with open procedures.
CT, Computed tomography; *DBM*, demineralized bone matrix; *ICBG*, iliac crest bone graft; *min*, minimum; *mo*, month or months; *PLIF*, posterior lumbar interbody fusion; *rhBMP-2*, recombinant human bone morphogenetic protein–2; *TLIF*, transforaminal lumbar interbody fusion; *yr*, year or years.

Continued

Table 23-2   Osteobiologics in Minimally Invasive Transforaminal Lumbar Interbody Fusion—cont'd

Author	Year	Number of Patients	Follow-up Duration	Osteobiologic Material Used (number of patients)	Fusion Rates (imaging modality used to assess fusion)	Comments (implant- or fusion-related complications only [subsidence, nonunion, pseudarthrosis])
Lee et al[18]**	2012	86	25 mo (mean)	Local autograft and DBM (all)	Overall 90% (54 of 60) had grade I and II per modified Bridwell fusion grading system[48] at latest follow-up; authors considered these to be fused (and considered grades I and II to be solid fusion)	9 of 86 patients (10.5%) had complications: —4 pseudarthroses (Treatment: observation) —2 screw malpositionings (Treatment: revision) —2 deep infections (Treatment: revision) —1 extrusion of bone graft fragments (Treatment: revision)
Ammerman et al[3]	2013	23	12 mo (min)	ACBM, MSCs, osteoprogenitor cells, and local autograft (all)	91.3% of patients achieved radiographic evidence of arthrodesis at 12 mo (radiography)	2 nonunions No cases of heterotropic ossification or osteolysis
Seng et al[38]	2013	40	5 yr (min)	Local autograft and DBM (19) Autologous ICBG (13) Local autograft alone (8)	47.5% grade I Bridwell fusion score at 6 mo 87.5% grade I Bridwell fusion score at 24 mo 97.5% grade I Bridwell fusion score at 5 yr	1 case of asymptomatic cage migration 4 ASDs (1 required revision) 1 ICBG site infection (Treatment: I&D) 15% overall complication rate (includes revisions)
Nandyala et al[24] (randomized trial)	2014	52	12 mo (min)	Silicate and calcium phosphate ceramic, BMA, and local autograft (26) rhBMP-2, BMA, and local autograft (26)	Silicate and ceramic group: 46% radiographic arthrodesis at 6 mo (CT), 65% at 12 mo (CT) rhBMP-2, BMA, and autograft group: 77% radiographic arthrodesis at 6 mo (CT), 92% at 12 mo (CT)	Ceramic group: 35% pseudarthrosis rate at 12 mo; 35% (9 of 26 pt) revision rate rhBMP-2 group: 7.7% pseudarthrosis rate at 12 mo; 7.7% (2 of 26 pt) revision rate

**The researchers used a modified Bridwell fusion grading system[48]: *grade I,* fused with bony bridging and trabeculae remodeling; *grade II,* not fully bony bridged and remodeled; *grade III,* definite lucency at the top or bottom of the cage and screw; *grade IV,* definitely not fused, with false motion. *ACBM,* Allograft cellular bone matrix; *ASD,* adjacent-segment disease; *BMA,* bone marrow aspirate; *CT,* computed tomography; *DBM,* demineralized bone matrix; *I&D,* irrigation and debridement; *ICBG,* iliac crest bone graft; *min,* minimum; *mo,* month or months; *MSCs,* mesenchymal stem cells; *pt,* patient or patients; *rhBMP-2,* recombinant human bone morphogenetic protein–2; *yr,* year or years.

Table 23-3 Osteobiologics in Minimally Invasive Posterior Lumbar Interbody Fusion

Author	Year	Number of Patients	Follow-up Duration	Osteobiologic Material Used (number of patients)	Fusion Rates (imaging modality used to assess fusion)	Comments (implant- or fusion-related complications only [subsidence, nonunion, pseudarthrosis])
Joseph and Rampersaud[15]*	2007	10	25 mo (mean)	Local bone with rhBMP-2 (23) Local bone without rhBMP-2 (10)	With rhBMP-2: 91.3% fused at 6 mo (CT) Without rhBMP-2: 50% fused at 6 mo (CT)	Heterotropic ossification occurred in 20.8% of local bone with rhBMP-2 group and in 8.3% of local bone without rhBMP-2 group Additional surgery was performed in 3 patients
Park and Ha[28]	2007	32	12 mo (min)	Autologous bone (all)	96.9% fusion rate at 12 mo (radiography)	Overall complication rate: 12.5% (included 1 nonunion, 1 screw malposition, 1 cage migration, and 1 deep wound infection) 12.5% revision rate
Tsutsumimoto et al[40]	2009	10	24 mo (min)	Local autologous bone (all)	100% at 12 mo (radiography or CT)	No complications reported
Ghahreman et al[12]	2010	23	12 mo (min)	ICBG (all)	100% fusion (radiography or CT)	No complications or revisions reported for the MIS TLIF patients
Ntoukas and Muller[25]	2010	20	12 mo (min)	Local autologous bone (all)	100% solid fusion (radiography)	No revisions
Harris et al[13]	2011	30	12 mo (min)	Local autologous bone (all)	97% at 12 mo (radiography)	1 nonunion 1 DVT (Treatment: warfarin)
Kotani et al[17]	2012	43	32 mo (mean)	ICBG and autologous bone	98% fusion (radiography or CT)	No complications
Mobbs et al[22]	2012	37	11.4 mo (mean)	Autologous bone with or without allograft	No explicitly stated fusion rates	5% overall complication rate for MIS surgery No cases of nonunion

*This study included minimally invasive transforaminal lumbar interbody fusion patients and minimally invasive posterior lumbar interbody fusion patients. The transforaminal lumbar interbody fusion patients' results are presented in Table 23-2.

CT, Computed tomography; *DVT,* deep venous thrombosis; *ICBG,* iliac crest bone graft; *min,* minimum; *MIS,* minimally invasive spine; *mo,* month or months; *rhBMP-2,* recombinant human bone morphogenetic protein–2; *TLIF,* transforaminal lumbar interbody fusion.

BONE MARROW ASPIRATE AND MESENCHYMAL STEM CELLS

Bone marrow aspirate (BMA) is another form of autologous bone graft. It contains osteoprogenitor cells and growth factors that are important in cell differentiation and bone healing.[2,46] It is usually used in combination with other grafting materials (for example, ceramics) as a result of its lack of structural support. BMA can be obtained from the iliac crest or the vertebral body, and it contains osteoprogenitor cells on the order of 1 in every 5000 to 10,000 cells. To increase the concentration of osteoprogenitor cells, BMA preparation often involves centrifugation before administration.[46]

Mesenchymal stem cells (MSCs) are multipotent cells capable of differentiating into a number of different cell lineages, including bone. Traditionally MSCs are obtained from autologous BMA, but this method can yield only limited quantities of MSCs. With the correct technique, approximately 2 ml of BMA can be harvested per aspiration site; culturing can then increase the number of MSCs in BMA by more than 1 billion-fold.[46,49]

A total of seven MISS studies[3,8,24,32-34,39] described the use and outcomes of either BMA or MSCs in interbody grafting. All seven studies used BMA and MSCs in addition to other graft material. Rodgers et al[34] used BMA with a beta-tricalcium hydroxyapatite composite in 44 patients who underwent LLIF. After 17 months, radiographic fusion was observed in 93.2% of the levels (41 of 44 levels) when using CT scanning to assess arthrodesis. In a separate study, Rodgers et al[33] used BMA, DBM, and cancellous allograft in 66 patients undergoing LLIF. CT analysis showed arthrodesis at 81 of 88 levels treated (96.6%) at 12 months. MSCs were used in the form of a synthetic allograft cellular bone matrix that had been processed to retain MSCs and osteoprogenitor cells. These studies are described in more detail in the following section.

ALLOGRAFT

Allograft, which is processed cadaveric bone, is another popular graft alternative. It is available in various forms, including fresh, frozen, and freeze-dried. The processing mechanism used can be both advantageous and deleterious, because it can reduce the antigenic response of the host at the risk of decreasing osteoinductivity and osteoconductivity. The major benefit of the use of allograft lies in its abundant supply and the avoidance of complications associated with autologous graft collection.[2]

Sixteen MISS studies* involved the use of allograft as a supplementary graft material. There were two LLIF studies[8,39] and one TLIF study[3] that made use of allograft cellular bone matrix. At 1 year of follow-up, the two LLIF studies were able to demonstrate fusion on CT scans at 112 of 127 (88.2%)[8] and 55 of 61 (90.2%)[39] vertebrae levels treated (see Table 23-1). Ammerman et al[3] also used allograft cellular bone matrix with local autologous graft in their 23-patient TLIF cohort, with a 91.3% radiographic fusion rate at the 1-year follow-up (see Table 23-2).

DEMINERALIZED BONE MATRIX

DBM is another form of allograft that is produced with an acid extraction procedure that involves cortical bone. This extraction process allows the osteoinductive factors within the bone matrix to become locally available. The benefit of using DBM-based products is that they are inexpensive and available in various forms (putty, gel, strip). Various factors can influence the performance of DBM, including the quality of the donor tissue, the processing methods used, and the sterilization and storage solutions. Some studies have shown great variability in different DBMs with respect to de novo bone formation and osteogenic gene expression.[50-52] The variability of the osteoinductive potential of DBM has even been demonstrated with different batches of the same product.[53]

DBM was used only as a bone graft extender with local bone, autologous graft, allograft, and BMP in 10 MISS studies† (see Tables 23-1 and 23-2). Anand et al[6] used DBM with recombinant human BMP 2 (rhBMP-2) in their series of 28 patients undergoing LLIF; they reported solid arthrodesis as assessed by radiography in all study participants. Lee et al[19] supplemented local autologous bone graft with DBM in 72 MISS TLIF patients and were able to demonstrate grade I and II fusion according to the Bridwell fusion grading system in 95.6% of the patients.

CERAMICS

Ceramics are a group of synthetic bone graft substitutes with properties similar to those of the mineral phase of bone. They are produced with the use of a high-temperature crystal extraction process. They do not possess any osteoinductive properties, but their osteoconductive potential allows for osteoprogeni-

---

*References 3-5, 8, 14, 16, 22, 27, 31-33, 37, 39, 41, 43, 44.
†References 4-6, 18, 19, 21, 31-33, 38.

tor cell adhesion, migration, and differentiation, so they are primarily used as bone graft extenders. Examples of ceramics include hydroxyapatite, beta-tricalcium phosphate, calcium sulfate cements, coralline hydroxyapatite, and bioglass. Some of the advantages of this substance include its abundant availability, its biocompatibility and biodegradability, its structural support, and its safety for use in patients.[2,46]

Six MISS studies* involved the use of ceramics as bone graft extenders and had good fusion rates (see Tables 23-1, 23-2, and 23-3). In a randomized controlled trial that compared a silicate-substituted calcium phosphate ceramic with rhBMP-2, Pimenta et al[30] obtained a 54% fusion rate at the 12-month follow-up for 15 patients who had undergone standalone LLIF in which the ceramic was used; the fusion rate was more than 80% at 24 months after operation. In another randomized trial, Nandyala et al[24] also used silicate-substituted calcium phosphate with BMA and local autologous bone graft in 26 patients undergoing TLIF. These researchers found a 65% radiographic fusion rate at 12 months, but they also reported a 35% pseudarthrosis rate.

BONE MORPHOGENETIC PROTEIN

BMP is part of the transforming growth factor beta family, and it is involved in a number of physiologic roles, including bone healing and cartilage formation.[46] It was discovered by Urist in 1965,[54] and it has quickly become one of the most extensively used and studied bone graft substitutes. In 2002 the U.S. Food and Drug Administration officially approved the use of rhBMP-2 for single-level use in anterior lumbar interbody fusion. However, it is estimated that about 85% of rhBMP-2 use is off label.[55,56]

The efficacy of rhBMP-2 in fusion surgery has been demonstrated in a multitude of human and animal trials.[23,41,57-61] Its associated complications—retrograde ejaculation, antibody formation, graft subsidence, and ectopic bone formation—have also been well described.[15,62,63] Carragee et al[64] have even suggested an increased risk of cancer with high doses of rhBMP-2. Nevertheless, rhBMP-2 remains one of the most widely used bone graft substitutes in spinal fusion surgery.

A total of 19 MISS† studies involved the use of BMP. As a result of the wide variations in study design, length of follow-up, and fusion assessment methodology, it is difficult to assess the pearls and pitfalls of BMP use in MISS procedures. Overall fusion rates in LLIF and TLIF studies that included BMP ranged from 77% to 100% and from 65% to 100%, respectively.

CONCLUSION

The use of osteobiologics in MISS is of paramount importance to the success of the operation when fusion is the goal. There are many different factors that contribute to the selection of appropriate graft material for this type of surgery. However, the universal goal of arthrodesis has to be met with the challenges of exposure, approach, and patient factors. The limited exposure that occurs with MISS can have a positive effect and a smaller physiologic burden for healing and recovery while simultaneously involving a smaller surface area for fusion. In a similar fashion, the different approaches to the spine will result in different demands on the posterior fusion mass and fixation. For example, when minimally invasive LLIF is used, there is greater biomechanical stability because of the larger implants, and this results in an increased amount of surface area for fusion. With large anterior grafts the burden of the posterior interlaminar and intertransverse fusion is much less; it is often questioned whether this is needed at all. Patient factors that influence fusion must also be taken into account. These include smoking history, autoimmune disease,

---

*References 9, 16, 24, 30, 31, 34.
†References 4-6, 9-11, 15-16, 20-21, 23-24, 26-27, 30, 37, 41, 43-44.

osteoporosis, steroid use, age, and so on. Ultimately the surgeon must decide what combination of grafts is needed to stimulate arthrodesis by using the various osteoconductive, osteoinductive, and osteogenic materials available. The use of osteobiologics in spine surgery will continue to grow. However, with a paucity of data addressing the higher-level use of osteobiologics in MISS, we will have to continue to rely on the open spine surgery literature and expert opinion.

REFERENCES

1. Rajaee SS, Bae HW, Kanim LE, et al. Spinal fusion in the United States: analysis of trends from 1998 to 2008. Spine 37:67-76, 2012.

2. Hsu WK, Nickoli MS, Wang JC, et al. Improving the clinical evidence of bone graft substitute technology in lumbar spine surgery. Global Spine J 2:239-248, 2012.

3. Ammerman JM, Libricz J, Ammerman MD. The role of Osteocel Plus as a fusion substrate in minimally invasive instrumented transforaminal lumbar interbody fusion. Clin Neurol Neurosurg 115:991-994, 2013.

4. Anand N, Baron EM, Khandehroo B, et al. Long-term 2- to 5-year clinical and functional outcomes of minimally invasive surgery for adult scoliosis. Spine 38:1566-1575, 2013.

5. Anand N, Hamilton JF, Perri B, et al. Cantilever TLIF with structural allograft and rhBMP2 for correction and maintenance of segmental sagittal lordosis: long-term clinical, radiographic, and functional outcome. Spine 31:E748-E753, 2006.

6. Anand N, Rosemann R, Khalsa B, et al. Mid-term to long-term clinical and functional outcomes of minimally invasive correction and fusion for adults with scoliosis. Neurosurg Focus 28:E6, 2010.

7. Benglis DM, Elhammady MS, Levi AD, et al. Minimally invasive anterolateral approaches for the treatment of back pain and adult degenerative deformity. Neurosurgery 63(3 Suppl):191-196, 2008.

8. Caputo AM, Michael KW, Chapman TM, et al. Extreme lateral interbody fusion for the treatment of adult degenerative scoliosis. J Clin Neurosci 20:1558-1563, 2013.

9. Dakwar E, Cardona RF, Smith DA, et al. Early outcomes and safety of the minimally invasive, lateral retroperitoneal transpsoas approach for adult degenerative scoliosis. Neurosurg Focus 28:E8, 2010.

10. Deutsch H, Musacchio MJ Jr. Minimally invasive transforaminal lumbar interbody fusion with unilateral pedicle screw fixation. Neurosurg Focus 20:E10, 2006.

11. Dhall SS, Wang MY, Mummaneni PV. Clinical and radiographic comparison of mini-open transforaminal lumbar interbody fusion with open transforaminal lumbar interbody fusion in 42 patients with long-term follow-up. J Neurosurg Spine 9:560-565, 2008.

12. Ghahreman A, Ferch RD, Rao PJ, et al. Minimal access versus open posterior lumbar interbody fusion in the treatment of spondylolisthesis. Neurosurgery 66:296-304; discussion 304, 2010.

13. Harris EB, Sayadipour A, Massey P, et al. Mini-open versus open decompression and fusion for lumbar degenerative spondylolisthesis with stenosis. Am J Orthop (Belle Mead NJ) 40:E257-E261, 2011.

14. Jang JS, Lee SH. Minimally invasive transforaminal lumbar interbody fusion with ipsilateral pedicle screw and contralateral facet screw fixation. J Neurosurg Spine 3:218-223, 2005.

15. Joseph V, Rampersaud YR. Heterotopic bone formation with the use of rhBMP2 in posterior minimal access interbody fusion: a CT analysis. Spine 32:2885-2890, 2007.

16. Karikari IO, Nimjee SM, Hardin CA, et al. Extreme lateral interbody fusion approach for isolated thoracic and thoracolumbar spine diseases: initial clinical experience and early outcomes. J Spinal Disord Tech 24:368-375, 2011.

17. Kotani Y, Abumi K, Ito M, et al. Mid-term clinical results of minimally invasive decompression and posterolateral fusion with percutaneous pedicle screws versus conventional approach for degenerative spondylolisthesis with spinal stenosis. Eur Spine J 21:1171-1177, 2012.

18. Lee JC, Jang HD, Shin BJ. Learning curve and clinical outcomes of minimally invasive transforaminal lumbar interbody fusion: our experience in 86 consecutive cases. Spine 37:1548-1557, 2012.

19. Lee KH, Yue WM, Yeo W, et al. Clinical and radiological outcomes of open versus minimally invasive transforaminal lumbar interbody fusion. Eur Spine J 21:2265-2270, 2012.

20. Mannion RJ, Nowitzke AM, Wood MJ. Promoting fusion in minimally invasive lumbar interbody stabilization with low-dose bone morphogenetic protein-2—but what is the cost? Spine J 11:527-533, 2011.

21. Meredith DS, Kepler CK, Huang RC, et al. Extreme lateral interbody fusion (XLIF) in the thoracic and thoraco-lumbar spine: technical report and early outcomes. HSS J 9:25-31, 2013.

22. Mobbs RJ, Sivabalan P, Li J. Minimally invasive surgery compared to open spinal fusion for the treatment of degenerative lumbar spine pathologies. J Clin Neurosci 19:829-835, 2012.

23. Mummaneni PV, Pan J, Haid RW, et al. Contribution of recombinant human bone morphogenetic protein-2 to the rapid creation of interbody fusion when used in transforaminal lumbar interbody fusion: a preliminary report. Invited submission from the Joint Section Meeting on Disorders of the Spine and Peripheral Nerves, March 2004. J Neurosurg Spine 1:19-23, 2004.

24. Nandyala SV, Marquez-Lara A, Fineberg SJ, et al. Prospective, randomized, controlled trial of silicate-substituted calcium phosphate versus rhBMP-2 in a minimally invasive transforaminal lumbar interbody fusion. Spine 39:185-191, 2014.

25. Ntoukas V, Muller A. Minimally invasive approach versus traditional open approach for one level posterior lumbar interbody fusion. Minim Invasive Neurosurg 53:21-24, 2010.

26. Oliveira L, Marchi L, Coutinho E, et al. The use of rh-BMP2 in standalone extreme lateral interbody fusion (XLIF): clinical and radiological results after 24 months of follow-up. WSC J 1:19-25, 2010.

27. Ozgur B, Agarwal V, Nail E, et al. Two-year clinical and radiographic success of minimally invasive lateral trans-psoas approach for the treatment of degenerative lumbar conditions. SAS J 4:41-46, 2010.

28. Park Y, Ha JW. Comparison of one-level posterior lumbar interbody fusion performed with a minimally invasive approach or a traditional open approach. Spine 32:537-543, 2007.

29. Peng CW, Yue WM, Poh SY, et al. Clinical and radiological outcomes of minimally invasive versus open transforaminal lumbar interbody fusion. Spine 34:1385-1389, 2009.

30. Pimenta L, Marchi L, Oliveira L, et al. A prospective, randomized, controlled trial comparing radiographic and clinical outcomes between stand-alone lateral interbody lumbar fusion with either silicate calcium phosphate or rh-BMP2. J Neurol Surg A Cent Eur Neurosurg 74:343-350, 2013.

31. Rodgers JA, Gerber E, Lehman JA, et al. Clinical and radiographic outcomes in less invasive lumbar fusion: XLIF at two year follow-up. J Spine Neurosurg 2:1-6, 2013.

32. Rodgers WB, Gerber EJ, Rodgers JA. Lumbar fusion in octogenarians: the promise of minimally invasive surgery. Spine 35(26 Suppl):S355-S360, 2010.

33. Rodgers WB, Gerber E, Patterson JR. Fusion after minimally disruptive anterior lumbar interbody fusion: analysis of extreme lateral interbody fusion by computed tomography. SAS J 4:63-66, 2010.

34. Rodgers WB, Gerber E, Rodgers JA. Clinical and radiographic outcomes of extreme lateral approach to interbody fusion with B-tricalcium phosphate and hydroxyapatite composite for lumbar degenerative conditions. Int J Spine Surg 6:24-28, 2012.

35. Scheufler KM, Dohmen H, Vougioukas VI. Percutaneous transforaminal lumbar interbody fusion for the treatment of degenerative lumbar instability. Neurosurgery 60(4 Suppl 2):203-212; discussion 212-213, 2007.

36. Schizas C, Tzinieris N, Tsiridis E, et al. Minimally invasive versus open transforaminal lumbar interbody fusion: evaluating initial experience. Int Orthop 33:1683-1688, 2009.

37. Schwender JD, Holly LT, Rouben DP, et al. Minimally invasive transforaminal lumbar interbody fusion (TLIF): technical feasibility and initial results. J Spinal Disord Tech 18(Suppl):S1-S6, 2005.

38. Seng C, Siddiqui MA, Wong KP, et al. Five-year outcomes of minimally invasive versus open transforaminal lumbar interbody fusion: a matched-pair comparison study. Spine 38:2049-2055, 2013.

39. Tohmeh AG, Watson B, Tohmeh M, et al. Allograft cellular bone matrix in extreme lateral interbody fusion: preliminary radiographic and clinical outcomes. ScientificWorldJournal 2012:263637, 2012.

40. Tsutsumimoto T, Shimogata M, Ohta H, et al. Mini-open versus conventional open posterior lumbar interbody fusion for the treatment of lumbar degenerative spondylolisthesis: comparison of paraspinal muscle damage and slip reduction. Spine 34:1923-1928, 2009.

41. Villavicencio AT, Burneikiene S, Nelson EL, et al. Safety of transforaminal lumbar interbody fusion and intervertebral recombinant human bone morphogenetic protein-2. J Neurosurg Spine 3:436-443, 2005.

42. Wang J, Zhou Y, Zhang ZF, et al. Comparison of one-level minimally invasive and open transforaminal lumbar interbody fusion in degenerative and isthmic spondylolisthesis grades 1 and 2. Eur Spine J 19:1780-1784, 2010.

43. Wang MY, Mummaneni PV. Minimally invasive surgery for thoracolumbar spinal deformity: initial clinical experience with clinical and radiographic outcomes. Neurosurg Focus 28:E9, 2010.

44. Youssef JA, McAfee PC, Patty CA, et al. Minimally invasive surgery: lateral approach interbody fusion: results and review. Spine 35(26 Suppl):S302-S311, 2010.

45. Wang J, Zhou Y, Zhang ZF, et al. Minimally invasive or open transforaminal lumbar interbody fusion as revision surgery for patients previously treated by open discectomy and decompression of the lumbar spine. Eur Spine J 20:623-628, 2011.

46. Bridwell K, DeWald RL, eds. The Textbook of Spinal Surgery, vol 1, ed 3. Philadelphia: Lippincott Williams & Wilkins, 2011.

47. Defino HL, da Silva Herrero CF, Crippa GE, et al. In vitro proliferation and osteoblastic phenotype expression of cells derived from human vertebral lamina and iliac crest. Spine 34:1549-1553, 2009.

48. Bridwell KH, Lenke LG, McEnery KW, et al. Anterior fresh frozen structural allografts in the thoracic and lumbar spine. Do they work if combined with posterior fusion and instrumentation in adult patients with kyphosis or anterior column defects? Spine 20:1410-1418, 1995.

49. Muschler GF, Boehm C, Easley K. Aspiration to obtain osteoblast progenitor cells from human bone marrow: the influence of aspiration volume. J Bone Joint Surg Am 79:1699-1709, 1997.

50. Lee KJ, Roper JG, Wang JC. Demineralized bone matrix and spinal arthrodesis. Spine J 5(6 Suppl):217S-223S, 2005.

51. Peterson B, Whang PG, Iglesias R, et al. Osteoinductivity of commercially available demineralized bone matrix. Preparations in a spine fusion model. J Bone Joint Surg Am 86-A:2243-2250, 2004.

52. Bae HW, Zhao L, Kanim LE, et al. Intervariability and intravariability of bone morphogenetic proteins in commercially available demineralized bone matrix products. Spine 31:1299-1306; discussion 1307-1308, 2006.

53. Bae H, Zhao L, Zhu D, et al. Variability across ten production lots of a single demineralized bone matrix product. J Bone Joint Surg Am 92:427-435, 2010.

54. Urist MR. Bone: formation by autoinduction. Science 150:893-899, 1965.

55. Ong KL, Villarraga ML, Lau E, et al. Off-label use of bone morphogenetic proteins in the United States using administrative data. Spine 35:1794-1800, 2010.

56. Bess S, Line BG, Lafarge V, et al. Does recombinant human bone morphogenetic protein-2 use in adult spinal deformity increase complications and are complications associated with location of rhBMP-2 use? A prospective, multicenter study of 279 consecutive patients. Spine 39:233-242, 2013.

57. Gerhart TN, Kirker-Head CA, Kriz MJ, et al. Healing segmental femoral defects in sheep using recombinant human bone morphogenetic protein. Clin Orthop Relat Res 293:317-326, 1993.

58. Yasko AW, Lane JM, Fellinger EJ, et al. The healing of segmental bone defects, induced by recombinant human bone morphogenetic protein (rhBMP-2). A radiographic, histological, and biomechanical study in rats. J Bone Joint Surg Am 74:659-670, 1992.

59. Muschler GF, Hyodo A, Manning T, et al. Evaluation of human bone morphogenetic protein 2 in a canine spinal fusion model. Clin Orthop Relat Res 308:229-240, 1994.

60. Papakostidis C, Kontakis G, Bhandari M, et al. Efficacy of autologous iliac crest bone graft and bone morphogenetic proteins for posterolateral fusion of lumbar spine: a meta-analysis of the results. Spine 33:E680-E692, 2008.

61. Glassman SD, Dimar JR III, Burkus K, et al. The efficacy of rhBMP-2 for posterolateral lumbar fusion in smokers. Spine 32:1693-1698, 2007.

62. Tannoury C, An HS. Complications with the use of bone morphogenic protein-2 (BMP-2) in spine surgery. Spine J 14:552-559, 2014.

63. Cahill KS, Chi JH, Day A, et al. Prevalence, complications, and hospital charges associated with use of bone-morphogenetic proteins in spinal fusion procedures. JAMA 302:58-66, 2009.

64. Carragee EJ, Chu G, Rohatgi R, et al. Cancer risk after use of recombinant bone morphogenetic protein-2 for spinal arthrodesis. J Bone Joint Surg Am 95:1537-1545, 2013.

PART V

Isolated Considerations of Global Spinal Alignment

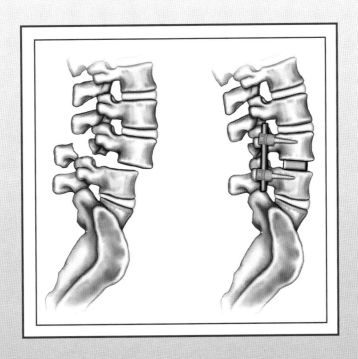

24

Spinal Alignment in the Management of Lumbar Degenerative Disc Disease

Shay Bess

Sagittal spinopelvic malalignment is an established cause of pain and disability for patients with adult spinal deformity.[1-9] However, much of the research regarding evaluation, treatment options, and outcomes for sagittal spinopelvic malalignment has focused on pediatric and adult spinal deformity. The role of sagittal spinopelvic alignment as it pertains to focal degenerative lumbar conditions is less known, as are the associated implications for treatment and outcomes. The purpose of this chapter is to review the existing data on the importance of sagittal spinopelvic alignment assessment for patients with focal lumbar degenerative disc disease (LDDD) and correlate these findings with treatment options and outcomes.

PATIENT ASSESSMENT

The techniques for evaluation of sagittal spinopelvic parameters have been thoroughly described in other chapters in this book. However, much of the theory behind the assessment of sagittal spinopelvic parameters and the supporting research pertain to patient cohorts with spinal deformity, including global malalignment and/or spondylolisthesis. Few data exist regarding the role of sagittal spinopelvic alignment in the assessment and treatment choices for patients with seemingly minimal spinal deformity. The assessment, treatment, and outcomes for patients with LDDD are controversial; therefore a comprehensive description of the clinical assessment, provocative and psychological testing, and treatment outcomes for patients with LDDD is beyond the context of this chapter.[10] However, when the reasons for pain and disability are evaluated in adults with LDDD, the sagittal spinopelvic alignment should be assessed with regard to the source of pain and the treatment options. The pelvic incidence (PI) is a morphologic parameter that is unaffected by posture or degenerative conditions of the adjacent lumbar spine. It is postulated that PI in part determines the alignment harmony for adjacent regions in the lumbar and thoracic spine.[11,12] Consequently, the PI can provide a basis for comparison between asymptomatic control subjects and symptomatic patients, and to a limited degree it can be used as a fundamental guide to assess variations in spinal alignment for patients with degenerative lumbar pathologies.

Barrey et al[11] compared the sagittal spinopelvic alignment of 85 patients with focal degenerative lumbar disorders and 154 asymptomatic control patients who had no evidence of radiographic abnormalities. Overall, the PI was similar for patients with LDDD and the controls; however, after the groups were stratified according to PI values, patients with LDDD had lower sacral slope (SS), greater pelvic tilt (PT), and decreased lumbar lordosis, compared with the control patients ($p < 0.05$). Compared with the control group, LDDD patients had global sagittal malalignment, including anterior translation of the C7 plumb line (sagittal vertical axis [SVA], which is the distance between a horizontal line from the C7 centroid and the posterior superior corner of the sacrum) and an increased C7/sacrofemoral distance (SFD) ratio (the ratio of the SVA to the SFD, which is the horizontal distance between the vertical bicoxofemoral axis and a vertical line through the posterior corner of the sacrum). The authors indicated that although the morphologic sagittal spinopelvic profiles of the LDDD patients were similar to those of the controls, patients with LDDD often had low to normal PI and consistently had reduced LL in proportion to the PI, with anterior translation of the SVA, reduction of SS, and increase in PT. Conversely, patients with degenerative spondylolisthesis had higher PI than control patients, with associated lumbar hyperlordosis that generated potentially increased stresses on the lumbar facet joints, with subsequent degenerative arthritis, incompetency of the facet joint, and resultant spondylolisthesis. The authors concluded that the painful disc in LDDD led to an antalgic posture, flattening of the lumbar spine, and the generation of anterior translation of the SVA with a compensatory increase in PT (as demonstrated by pelvic retroversion) and a decreased SS to maintain upright posture.

Although Barrey et al[11] hypothesized that the sagittal spinopelvic malalignment associated with LDDD is compensatory secondary to a painful disc, Yang et al[13] suggested that sagittal spinopelvic malalignment is the cause of LDDD and reported that Barrey et al did not use MRI to differentiate between normal and degenerative subsets within the asymptomatic control groups. Therefore patients with early LDDD might not have been identified on the radiographic analysis. With the use of radiographic imaging and lumbar MRI, Yang et al divided 160 patients into degenerative and nondegenerative groups, and they further divided the degenerative group into symptomatic and asymptomatic subgroups. The degenerative group had a lower mean PI (40.0 ± 6 degrees) than the nondegenerative group (48.7, $p < 0.05$). Additionally, the degenerative group had lower LL and SS and greater SVA and SFD values, compared with the nondegenerative group. Further analysis of the degenerative group revealed that the PI, SVA, and SFD of the symptomatic patients were similar to those of the asymptomatic group, but symptomatic patients had lower LL, lower SS, and greater PT. The authors theorized that the sagittal profile of patients with LDDD can create a biomechanical environment in the lumbar spine that predisposes to disc degeneration, including a straight lumbar spine (low LL in relation to the PI) and a vertical sacrum (high SS and high SFD).

Le Huec et al[14] proposed a cascade of sagittal malalignment in LDDD patients that often begins with loss of disc height, which decreases lumbar lordosis and moves the C7 plumb line forward. This leads to a posterior PT (pelvic retroversion and increased PT) to maintain upright posture. The authors explained that from an anatomic standpoint, the amount of compensatory pelvic rotation is limited in part by the individual pelvic morphology (PI). Therefore patients with high PI anatomically have a greater ability to maintain upright posture via pelvic retroversion (PT); however, patients with a morphologically low PI have less compensatory reserve, because the amount of compensatory PT is anatomically limited by the low PI (as indicated by the equation $PI = PT + SS$).[15,16] As the degenerative process continues, sagittal malalignment worsens, and patients develop an antalgic posture with further loss of LL (flat back), decreased SS (vertical sacrum), increased PT (retroverted pelvis), and increased SVA (forward-pitched posture). This global malalignment in turn generates more pain and potentially worsens the biomechanical environment for the lumbar disc, further accelerating disc degeneration.

SAGITTAL SPINOPELVIC ALIGNMENT AND IMPLICATIONS FOR SURGICAL TREATMENT OF LUMBAR DEGENERATIVE DISC DISEASE

Patients with LDDD can have baseline sagittal spinopelvic malalignment that predisposes to lumbar disc degeneration. Consequently, treatment options for patients with symptomatic LDDD should include correction of underlying sagittal spinopelvic malalignment. Otherwise, the baseline sagittal deformity will be maintained or potentially magnified. Korovessis et al[17] evaluated the effect of global and segmental sagittal alignment, levels of fixation, and fusion rates in 50 patients undergoing short-segment (two to four segments) posterior spinal fusion for degenerative lumbar disease, without interbody fusion. At 5.5 years postoperatively, improvement of low back pain in the study cohort correlated with sagittal alignment and fusion rates. Improvement of segmental lordosis with increased anterior deviation of the apical lumbar vertebra from the C7 plumb line correlated with improvement of global sagittal spinal alignment. Sagittal segmental alignment was not consistently improved in patients having one-level fusion, compared with patients receiving two- and three-level fusions, especially in older patients. The authors concluded that restoration of segmental alignment in patients with focal degenerative lumbar disease is critical to obtain good outcomes and may not be achievable with single-level posterior-only procedures, especially in older patients.

Interbody fusion procedures are often performed to treat LDDD. An interbody arthrodesis can help to eliminate discogenic pain sources, improve fusion rates, and restore physiologic sagittal alignment after the surgical treatment of LDDD.[18-20] Options for lumbar interbody fusion procedures include anterior lumbar interbody fusion (ALIF), lateral lumbar interbody fusion (LLIF), posterior lumbar interbody fusion (PLIF), and transforaminal lumbar interbody fusion (TLIF). Videbaek et al[21] performed a randomized trial on 148 patients with or without degenerative lumbar disease (spondylolisthesis and LDDD), who had one- and two-level posterior spinal fusion with or without ALIF. At the mean follow-up of 9.7 to 10.4 years, the ALIF group demonstrated improved segmental lordosis, compared with the group without ALIF. All other regional and global radiographic measures and clinical outcomes were similar between both groups. Improved postoperative lumbar lordosis correlated with improved clinical outcomes. Hsieh et al[22] evaluated the impact of posterior spinal fusion with ALIF versus TLIF on sagittal alignment in patients surgically treated for LDDD or spondylolisthesis. The minimum follow-up was 2 years. The mean number of levels fused was 1.4 per patient. The ALIF group showed improved postoperative lumbar lordosis, compared with the TLIF group; however, clinical outcomes were similar between both groups. Ould-Slimane et al[23] evaluated the effect of TLIF on sagittal spinopelvic parameters after single-level fusion for lumbar degenerative disorders in 45 adult patients. At the 2-year follow-up (minimum), all patients had improved sagittal spinopelvic parameters, including lumbar lordosis and PT. Improvement in postoperative SVA was not statistically significant, compared with preoperative values, although 70% of the patients who had a physiologic preoperative SVA (<5 cm) also had PT of more than 20 degrees, indicating that most patients in the study (n = 23) had findings consistent with compensated sagittal malalignment (SVA of greater than 5 cm and PT of more than 20 degrees).[14,24] Two years postoperatively, all patients had a normalized PT, and SVA was less than 5 cm. The authors emphasized the need to evaluate preoperative spinopelvic parameters using standing full-length radiographs on all patients considered for lumbar fusion procedures, regardless of the number of levels planned for fusion. These data indicate that interbody fusion combined with posterior spinal fusion for LDDD can improve sagittal alignment more effectively than posterior-only spinal fusions. Additionally, ALIF can generate greater segmental lordosis than TLIF or PLIF; however, the improvement in segmental lordosis with ALIF versus TLIF or PLIF may not correspond to improved global sagittal spinopelvic alignment. Surgeons should consider the patient-specific risks and benefits inherent to ALIF versus TLIF and PLIF procedures when considering surgery for patients with LDDD. Prior retroperitoneal abdominal surgery, morbid obesity, cardiovascular disease, pulmonary disease, and calcification of the iliac vessels and aorta are relative contraindications for ALIF procedures.[25-27] Conversely, patients with prior lumbar laminectomy can have epidural scarring that presents challenges to TLIF and PLIF approaches to the lumbar interspace and may benefit from ALIF procedures (Fig. 24-1).

The role of the shape of the interbody implant on segmental lordosis is often debated. Specifically, the controversy pertains to whether lordotic-shaped interbody cages generate greater segmental lordosis, compared with rectangular-shaped cages. Godde et al[28] evaluated the impact of cage geometry on sagittal alignment after one- and two-level PLIF procedures in 42 adult patients. The mean follow-up period was 18 months. Patients with nonlordotic (rectangular-shaped) lumbar cages demonstrated reduction in segmental lordosis, regardless of spinal segments fused (L3-4, L4-5, and L5-S1), whereas segmental lordosis improved at the fusion levels in the lordotic (wedge-shaped) cage group. SS decreased in the nonlordotic (rectangular-shaped) cage group and increased in the wedge lordotic (wedge-shaped) cage group; however, the changes

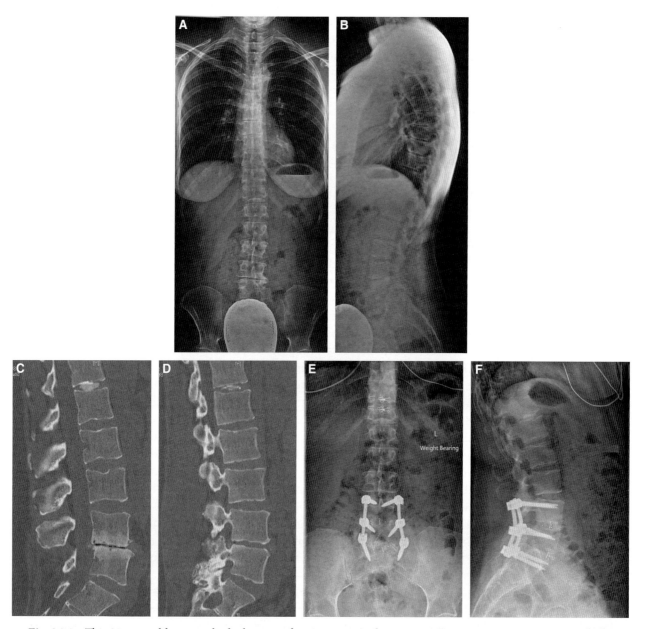

Fig. 24-1   This 37-year-old woman had a history of an L4-5, L5-S1 discectomy. She presented with L4-5 and L5-S1 degeneration with associated back and leg pain. **A** and **B,** Preoperative AP and lateral images demonstrated L4-5 and L5-S1 degeneration with associated loss of segmental lordosis and maintenance of physiologic global sagittal spinopelvic alignment. Her segmental lordosis at L4-5 was 3 degrees, lumbar lordosis was 50 degrees, pelvic incidence was 40 degrees, pelvic tilt was 10 degrees, and sagittal vertical axis was +4 mm. **C** and **D,** Preoperative sagittal reconstruction CT images revealed L4-5 lumbar disc degeneration and associated facet arthropathy at L4-5 and L5-S1. **E** and **F,** The patient was treated with L4-5 and L5-S1 posterior spinal fusion and TLIF. Two-year postoperative AP and lateral radiographs show good lumbar alignment with improvement of segmental lordosis at L4-5 and L5-S1. Segmental L4-5 lordosis is 10 degrees, and lumbar lordosis is 54 degrees.

in SS were not significantly different between groups. The authors concluded that nonlordotic (rectangular-shaped) interbody cages can decrease segmental lordosis with a resultant compensatory decrease in SS and an associated increase in PT to maintain upright posture, whereas lordotic (wedge-shaped) interbody cages can help to improve sagittal spinopelvic alignment by increasing segmental lordosis.

Lumbar disc replacement is increasingly considered a viable treatment alternative to lumbar fusion for LDDD, and appropriate patient selection criteria are critical for good outcomes. Attention to sagittal spinopelvic alignment is important to ensure good outcomes after lumbar fusion for LDDD. However, restoration of physiologic segmental sagittal alignment is substantially more feasible for fusion procedures that eliminate segmental motion, whereas lumbar disc replacement procedures depend on maintenance of postoperative segmental motion at the site of the surgically treated LDDD. Consequently, surgeons considering lumbar disc replacement for patients with LDDD need to be aware that degenerated lumbar segments can have pathologic motion secondary to degenerative changes and abnormal sagittal spinopelvic alignment, and the abnormal motion segment may not be amenable to this surgery. Pellet et al[29] evaluated the results of ALIF versus lumbar disc replacement to create an algorithm based on sagittal spinopelvic parameters to help guide surgical treatment for LDDD. The authors reported that patients with a low PI often did not require an increase in segmental lordosis to maintain physiologic sagittal alignment, especially if the L4-5 segment was considered for surgery. Therefore lumbar disc replacement was considered an appropriate treatment choice for patients who met other criteria for this procedure. However, patients with a high PI or high SS were more amenable to ALIF to restore segmental lordosis, especially if the L5-S1 segment was considered for surgery. Tournier et al[30] and Chung et al[31] reported increased segmental and total lumbar lordosis after lumbar disc replacement but no statistically significant changes in PT and SS. Lazennec et al [32] reported no change in segmental, regional, or global sagittal spinopelvic parameters 2 years after lumbar disc replacement, compared with preoperative values. Surgeons need to be aware that although this procedure can improve segmental alignment, sagittal spinopelvic malalignment will most likely not be corrected, and malaligned patients can be at risk for poor outcomes.

CONCLUSION

Sagittal spinopelvic alignment plays a critical role in the cause, assessment, and treatment of patients with LDDD. Patients with low PI may be at risk for developing LDDD, especially if an associated reduced lumbar lordosis is present, which can lead to increases in local stresses and focal degeneration. As the disc degenerates and becomes painful, patients can develop an antalgic posture, generating a postural sagittal spinopelvic malalignment with elevated SVA and a compensatory increase in PT. Then as the disc space further degenerates, the sagittal spinopelvic malalignment may become fixed. Treating physicians should assess the global spinopelvic alignment of patients with LDDD. Surgical correction of both the focal and global spinal malalignment pathologies is required for good clinical outcomes. Single-level, stand-alone, posterior-only fusion procedures may not sufficiently improve sagittal spinopelvic malalignment, especially in older patients. In this case, fusion of more than one level or an interbody fusion may be appropriate to improve segmental lordosis. Lumbar disc replacement can be a viable option for LDDD. However, patients with global sagittal spinopelvic malalignment are not good candidates for this procedure, because it does not improve regional and global sagittal spinopelvic alignment.

REFERENCES

1. Glassman SD, Bridwell K, Dimar JR, et al. The impact of positive sagittal balance in adult spinal deformity. Spine 30:2024-2029, 2005.

2. Lafage V, Schwab F, Patel A, et al. Pelvic tilt and truncal inclination: two key radiographic parameters in the setting of adults with spinal deformity. Spine 34:E599-E606, 2009.

3. Lafage V, Schwab F, Skalli W, et al. Standing balance and sagittal plane spinal deformity: analysis of spinopelvic and gravity line parameters. Spine 33:1572-1578, 2008.

4. Lafage V, Schwab F, Vira S, et al. Spino-pelvic parameters following surgery can be predicted: a preliminary formula and validation of standing alignment. Spine 36:1037-1045, 2011.

5. Lafage V, Smith JS, Bess S, et al. Sagittal spino-pelvic alignment failures following three column thoracic osteotomy for adult spinal deformity. Eur Spine J 21:698-704, 2012.

6. Scheer JK, Tang JA, Smith JS, et al. Cervical spine alignment, sagittal deformity, and clinical implications: a review. J Neurosurg Spine 19:141-159, 2013.

7. Schwab F, Lafage V, Patel A, et al. Sagittal plane considerations and the pelvis in the adult patient. Spine 34:1828-1833, 2009.

8. Schwab F, Patel A, Ungar B, et al. Adult spinal deformity-postoperative standing imbalance: how much can you tolerate? An overview of key parameters in assessing alignment and planning corrective surgery. Spine 35:2224-2231, 2010.

9. Schwab FJ, Blondel B, Bess S, et al. Radiographical spinopelvic parameters and disability in the setting of adult spinal deformity: a prospective multicenter analysis. Spine 38:E803-E812, 2013.

10. Phillips FM, Slosar PJ, Youssef JA, et al. Lumbar spine fusion for chronic low back pain due to degenerative disc disease: a systematic review. Spine 38:E409-E422, 2013.

11. Barrey C, Jund J, Noseda O, et al. Sagittal balance of the pelvis-spine complex and lumbar degenerative diseases. A comparative study about 85 cases. Eur Spine J 16:1459-1467, 2007.

12. During J, Goudfrooij H, Keessen W, et al. Toward standards for posture. Postural characteristics of the lower back system in normal and pathologic conditions. Spine 10:83-87, 1985.

13. Yang X, Kong Q, Song Y, et al. The characteristics of spinopelvic sagittal alignment in patients with lumbar disc degenerative diseases. Eur Spine J 23:569-575, 2014.

14. Le Huec JC, Charosky S, Barrey C, et al. Sagittal imbalance cascade for simple degenerative spine and consequences: algorithm of decision for appropriate treatment. Eur Spine J 20(Suppl 5):S699-S703, 2011.

15. Vaz G, Roussouly P, Berthonnaud E, et al. Sagittal morphology and equilibrium of pelvis and spine. Eur Spine J 11:80-87, 2002.

16. Roussouly P, Gollogly S, Berthonnaud E, et al. Classification of the normal variation in the sagittal alignment of the human lumbar spine and pelvis in the standing position. Spine 30:346-353, 2005.

17. Korovessis P, Repantis T, Papazisis Z, et al. Effect of sagittal spinal balance, levels of posterior instrumentation, and length of follow-up on low back pain in patients undergoing posterior decompression and instrumented fusion for degenerative lumbar spine disease: a multifactorial analysis. Spine 35:898-905, 2010.

18. Freeman BJ, Steele NA, Sach TH, et al. ISSLS prize winner: cost-effectiveness of two forms of circumferential lumbar fusion: a prospective randomized controlled trial. Spine 32:2891-2897, 2007.

19. Soegaard R, Bunger CE, Christiansen T, et al. Circumferential fusion is dominant over posterolateral fusion in a long-term perspective: cost-utility evaluation of a randomized controlled trial in severe, chronic low back pain. Spine 32:2405-2414, 2007.

20. Videbaek TS, Christensen FB, Soegaard R, et al. Circumferential fusion improves outcome in comparison with instrumented posterolateral fusion: long-term results of a randomized clinical trial. Spine 31:2875-2880, 2006.

21. Videbaek TS, Bunger CE, Henriksen M, et al. Sagittal spinal balance after lumbar spinal fusion: the impact of anterior column support results from a randomized clinical trial with an eight- to thirteen-year radiographic follow-up. Spine 36:183-191, 2011.

22. Hsieh PC, Koski TR, O'Shaughnessy BA, et al. Anterior lumbar interbody fusion in comparison with transforaminal lumbar interbody fusion: implications for the restoration of foraminal height, local disc angle, lumbar lordosis, and sagittal balance. J Neurosurg Spine 7:379-386, 2007.

23. Ould-Slimane M, Lenoir T, Dauzac C, et al. Influence of transforaminal lumbar interbody fusion procedures on spinal and pelvic parameters of sagittal balance. Eur Spine J 21:1200-1206, 2012.

24. Le Huec JC, Roussouly P. Sagittal spino-pelvic balance is a crucial analysis for normal and degenerative spine. Eur Spine J 20(Suppl 5):S556-S557, 2011.
25. Brau SA, Delamarter RB, Kropf MA, et al. Access strategies for revision in anterior lumbar surgery. Spine 33:1662-1667, 2008.
26. Brau SA, Delamarter RB, Schiffman ML, et al. Vascular injury during anterior lumbar surgery. Spine J 4:409-412, 2004.
27. Brau SA. Mini-open approach to the spine for anterior lumbar interbody fusion: description of the procedure, results and complications. Spine J 2:216-223, 2002.
28. Godde S, Fritsch E, Dienst M, et al. Influence of cage geometry on sagittal alignment in instrumented posterior lumbar interbody fusion. Spine 28:1693-1699, 2003.
29. Pellet N, Aunoble S, Meyrat R, et al. Sagittal balance parameters influence indications for lumbar disc arthroplasty or ALIF. Eur Spine J 20(Suppl 5):S647-S662, 2011.
30. Tournier C, Aunoble S, Le Huec JC, et al. Total disc arthroplasty: consequences for sagittal balance and lumbar spine movement. Eur Spine J 16:411-421, 2007.
31. Chung SS, Lee CS, Kang CS, et al. The effect of lumbar total disc replacement on the spinopelvic alignment and range of motion of the lumbar spine. J Spinal Disord Tech 19:307-311, 2006.
32. Lazennec JY, Even J, Skalli W, et al. Clinical outcomes, radiologic kinematics, and effects on sagittal balance of the 6 df LP-ESP lumbar disc prosthesis. Spine J. 2013 Nov 19. [Epub ahead of print]

25

Spinal Alignment in the Management of Isthmic Spondylolisthesis

Hubert Labelle ▪ *Jean-Marc Mac-Thiong* ▪ *Stefan Parent*

S*pondylolysis* implies a defect in the pars articularis of a vertebra. It can occur independently or in association with spondylolisthesis, defined as the forward displacement of one vertebra with respect to the adjacent caudal vertebra. Marchetti and Bartolozzi[1] have developed a classification system of spondylolisthesis (Table 25-1) that has gained increasing acceptance. Their system is based on the developmental origin versus the acquired forms of spondylolisthesis, unlike that of Wiltse et al,[2] who relied on radiologic findings. Developmental spondylolisthesis is divided into two major types (high and low dysplastic), which depend on the severity of bony dysplastic changes present on the L5 and S1 vertebrae and on the risk of further slippage. Dysplastic facet joints and spina bifida of L5 and/or S1 are common in both types, and the high dysplastic type is associated with significant lumbosacral kyphosis, a trapezoidal L5 vertebra, hypoplastic transverse processes, and sacral doming with verticalization of the sacrum. Acquired spondylolisthesis occurs secondary to trauma, surgery, a pathologic disease, or a degenerative process. The traumatic form can result from either an acute or stress fracture. Acquired traumatic spondylolisthesis secondary to a stress fracture typically occurs in young athletes and is distinct from the isthmic dysplastic type of spondylolisthesis.[3] This chapter will focus on developmental L5-S1 spondylolisthesis, which is the type that is associated with high-grade spondylolisthesis (HGS) in children, adolescents, and young adults. It is also the type associated with sagittal spinal malalignment.

Table 25-1 Marchetti and Bartolozzi's Classification of Spondylolisthesis

Developmental	Acquired
High dysplastic	Traumatic
With spondylolysis	Acute fracture
With elongated pars	Stress fracture
Low dysplastic	Postsurgical
With spondylolysis	Direct surgery
With elongated pars	Indirect surgery
	Pathologic
	Local pathology
	Systemic pathology
	Degenerative
	Primary
	Secondary

EVOLUTION OF TECHNIQUE

The traditional treatment for HGS is in situ posterolateral L5-S1 fusion with no attempt at reduction of the slip. Several publications over the past decades have reported good long-term results with this approach. In an evidence-based literature review of reduction versus in situ fusion through 2007, Transfeldt and Mehbod[4] were unable to identify Level I or II evidence on this subject. The best evidence was provided by five retrospective comparative studies (Level III). The authors were thus unable to formulate clear guidelines for treatment of HGS based on the best evidence available in the published literature.

Has anything changed over the past decade? Although the need for reduction in the surgical treatment of HGS is still debated, spinal surgeons have shifted away from performing the traditional in situ posterolateral L5-S1 fusion and toward reduction, instrumentation, and circumferential fusion. Almost all articles on HGS published in the past decade report on instrumentation with or without reduction of HGS. The only reports on in situ fusion without instrumentation are those that present long-term results of cases performed before this decade. This evolution in technique can be explained based on two factors: an improved understanding of sagittal spinopelvic alignment and improved methods of reduction, fusion, and spinopelvic fixation.

The Spine/SRS spondylolisthesis summary statement[5] for the 2005 *Spine* Focus Issue on spinopelvic alignment indicated that global sagittal plane alignment is important in both adult and pediatric patients with spondylolisthesis. In patients with high-grade developmental spondylolisthesis, this has provided a compelling rationale to reduce and realign the spondylolisthesis deformity, thus restoring global spinal balance and improving the biomechanical environment for fusion. To understand HGS, it is imperative to analyze

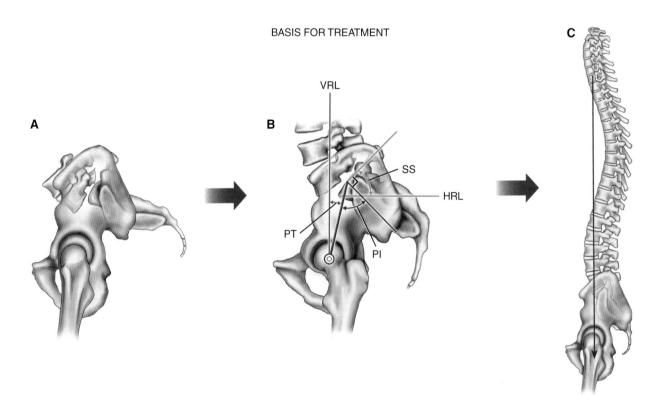

Fig. 25-1 High-grade spondylolisthesis needs to be understood within the context of **A,** local deformity, **B,** regional deformity, and **C,** global deformity. (*HRL,* Horizontal reference line; *PI,* pelvic incidence; *PT,* pelvic tilt; *SS,* sacral slope; *VRL,* vertical reference line.)

not only the local L5-S1 deformity, but also to consider the regional pelvic deformity and the global spinal deformity (Fig. 25-1). This improved knowledge has led to the development of a classification[6] based on sagittal alignment to guide patient selection for reduction versus no reduction in HGS (see Fig. 25-2). Five recent publications support this approach.[7-11]

Agabegi and Fischgrund[10] performed a recent literature review of improved methods of reduction, fusion, and spinopelvic fixation. They concluded that circumferential (360-degree) fusion is superior to postero-lateral fusion in HGS patients and results in a decreased incidence of pseudarthrosis, and solid fusion improves outcome. Most authors now recommend posterior spinopelvic fixation coupled to L5-S1 interbody support by posterior lumbar interbody fusion/transforaminal lumbar interbody fusion.[12-17]

ADVANTAGES AND DISADVANTAGES

In general, in situ L5-S1 fusion techniques have been associated with less neurologic complications than reduction, instrumentation, and circumferential fusion techniques, but these advantages occur at the expense of less improvement in sagittal alignment and a higher risk of pseudarthrosis.

A variety of fixation techniques have been recommended to achieve reduction and/or fusion and to decrease the risk of neurologic complications. These include iliac screws, iliosacral screws, custom-made cannulated screws, transsacral/transdiscal strut grafting or screws, Magerl's external fixator, sacral dome resection, Ilizarov's external fixation, and Jackson's intrasacral fixation. Unfortunately, SRS morbidity reports[18-19] demonstrate a fairly high number of complications after instrumentation with or without reduction in HGS patients. Neurologic deficits are the most common complication, ranging from 9.2% to 11.5%, and osteotomies are associated with a higher incidence of neurologic deficit.

INDICATIONS AND CONTRAINDICATIONS

The goals of surgery in high-grade developmental L5-S1 spondylolisthesis are to prevent progression, to restore global spinal alignment and normal biomechanics, and to relieve symptoms. The decision to proceed with surgical treatment can be based on the following factors:
- The degree of slip (more than 50% in a growing child or more than 75% in a skeletally mature adolescent)
- The documentation of progression beyond 30% slippage
- The persistence of functional impairment, pain, or neurologic symptoms despite appropriate non-surgical treatment
- Progressive postural deformity (cosmetic dissatisfaction) or gait abnormality

Children with HGS (Meyerding grade III or more) are usually candidates for surgery to prevent progression, regardless of symptoms. To determine whether an HGS patient should have fusion in situ or reduction, the Spinal Deformity Study Group has proposed a classification system[6] comprising six sagittal postures, developed using the radiographic measurement of slip grade and spinopelvic alignment (pelvic incidence, sacropelvic alignment, and spinal balance). The classification is based on four important characteristics that can be assessed using standing sagittal radiographs of the spine and pelvis: (1) the grade of slip (low or high), (2) the pelvic incidence (low, normal, or high), (3) spinopelvic alignment (balanced or unbalanced), and (4) the lumbosacral kyphosis (low or high). Fig. 25-2 summarizes the classification.

To classify a patient with HGS (grades III, IV, and spondyloptosis, or a slip of 50% or higher), the sagittal balance is measured by determining the sacropelvic and spinopelvic alignment using measurements of sacral slope, pelvic tilt, and the C7 plumb line. First, a patient is classified as having a balanced or an unbal-

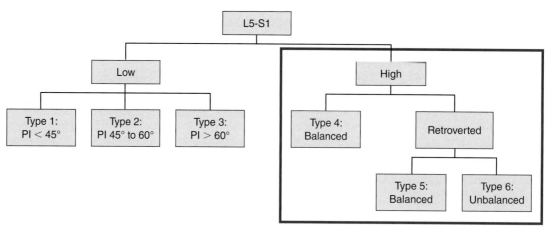

Fig. 25-2 The Spinal Deformity Study Group classification. Sagittal spinopelvic postures associated with high-grade spondylolisthesis are in the *red rectangle.*

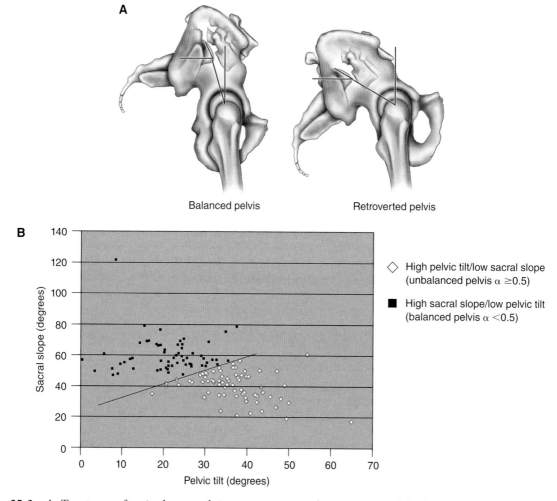

Fig. 25-3 **A,** Two types of sagittal sacropelvic posture are noted in patients with high-grade spondylolisthesis. A normal, balanced pelvis has a sacral slope angle *(red)* larger than the pelvic tilt angle *(black).* In a retroverted or unbalanced pelvis, the pelvic tilt angle *(black)* is larger than the sacral slope angle *(red).* In this type, the sacrum has a more vertical position when the patient stands. **B,** A nomogram of 133 patients with high-grade spondylolisthesis, with subgroups based on k-means cluster analysis. Groups are divided by a line of $Y = (0.844835X) + 25.021$. (**B,** From Hresko MT, Labelle H, Roussouly P, et al. Classification of high grade spondylolistheses based on pelvic version and spinal balance: possible rationale for reduction. Spine 32:2208-2213, 2007.)

anced sacropelvis using pelvic tilt and sacral slope values, as described by Hresko et al[7] (Fig. 25-3, *A*). Usually, when sacral slope is larger than pelvic tilt, the patient is classified as having a balanced pelvis. Patients whose sacral slope is lower than their pelvic tilt have an unbalanced or retroverted pelvis. Alternatively, pelvic posture can be classified more precisely using the nomogram provided by Hresko et al[7] (Fig. 25-3, *B*).

Global spinopelvic alignment is determined using a C7 plumb line. If this line falls over or behind the femoral heads, the spine is well aligned; if it lies in front of the femoral heads, the spine is considered globally malaligned. In our experience, the spine is almost always well-aligned in low-grade and high-grade spondylolisthesis patients who have a balanced sacropelvis; therefore global spinal alignment needs to be assessed predominantly in patients with high-grade deformities and an unbalanced pelvis (types 5 and 6). The three types of sagittal spinopelvic posture in HGS patients are type 4 (balanced pelvis), type 5 (retroverted pelvis with a well-aligned spine), and type 6 (retroverted pelvis with a globally malaligned spine). More recently, after it was shown that increased lumbosacral kyphosis is associated with a decrease in health-related quality of life in HGS patients,[20] two subtypes of type 5 posture were recognized.[21] These are subtype 5a, associated with a normal or low lumbosacral kyphosis (as measured by Dubousset's lumbosacral angle of 80 degrees or more), and subtype 5b, associated with a high lumbosacral kyphosis (as measured by Dubousset's lumbosacral angle of less than 80 degrees). Fig. 25-4 shows the various types of posture in HGS patients. Mac-Thiong et al[22] recently conducted a clinical assessment of this refined version of the classification system. They reported an improved and substantial intraobserver and interobserver reliability, similar to those of other currently used classifications for spinal deformity, with an overall intraobserver and interobserver agreements of 80% (kappa 0.74) and 71% (kappa 0.65), respectively.

The clinical relevance of this classification can be summarized as follows. Because PI is always much greater than normal in HGS patients, lumbar lordosis is increased to maintain the center of gravity and C7 plumb line behind the hips for a well-aligned posture. This first compensatory mechanism involves increasing

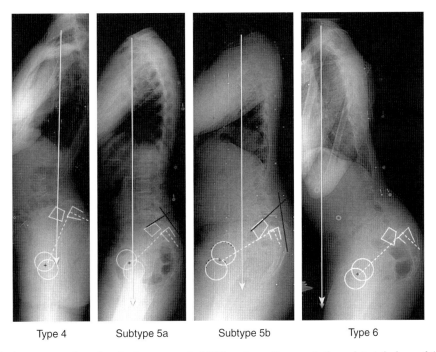

| Type 4 | Subtype 5a | Subtype 5b | Type 6 |

Fig. 25-4   Radiologic examples of sagittal postures in HGS patients. In type 4, the pelvis is balanced (the sacral slope is larger than the pelvic tilt), and the spine is balanced (the C7 plumb line *[yellow]* falls over or behind the femoral heads). In type 5, the pelvis is unbalanced, but the spine remains balanced. In subtype 5a, the lumbosacral kyphosis is normal or low, with a Dubousset's lumbosacral angle of 80 degrees or more *(red)*, whereas, in subtype 5b, the lumbosacral kyphosis is high, with a Dubousset's lumbosacral angle of less than 80 *(red)*. In type 6, both the pelvis and spine are unbalanced.

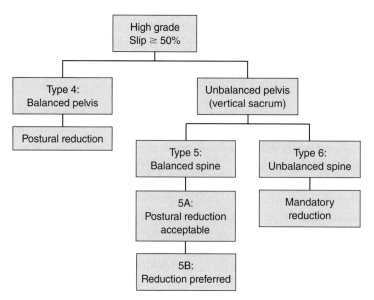

Fig. 25-5   A proposed treatment algorithm for patients with high-grade spondylolisthesis.

the intervertebral segmental lordosis and/or including more vertebrae in the lordotic segment. Every patient has a maximal attainable lumbar lordosis beyond which he or she will attempt to maintain well-aligned posture by progressive retroversion of the pelvis. This second compensation mechanism corresponds to the abnormal posture of types 5 and 6, with a retroverted pelvis and vertical sacrum. Because each patient has a fixed pelvic incidence (an anatomic parameter), SS decreases with retroversion of the pelvis, and PT increases as the sacrum becomes vertical. When the limit of these two compensation mechanisms is reached, a patient develops global sagittal truncal malalignment, most often characterized either by compensatory hip flexion or by forward leaning of the trunk with positive global sagittal alignment of the spine, or a combination of both as seen in type 6 posture. Finally, in immature subjects, increased lumbosacral kyphosis combined with anterior slipping of L5 induces higher pressure on the anterior part of the S1 growth plate, which leads to decreased growth of the anterior sacrum according to the Hueter-Volkmann law. This induces progressive rounding of the sacrum and the so-called sacral dome deformity often seen in HGS patients.

More outcome studies are needed before a definitive treatment algorithm can be established for each subtype (Fig. 25-5). It is suggested that for subjects with a type 4 spinopelvic posture, forceful attempts at reduction of the deformity may not be required. Instead, instrumentation and fusion after simple postural reduction by prone positioning of patients under anesthesia on the operating table may be all that is necessary to maintain adequate sagittal alignment, because adequate sagittal spinopelvic alignment is already present. For patients with a type 5 posture, reduction and realignment procedures should preferably be attempted. For subtype 5a, instrumentation and fusion after postural reduction can be sufficient to achieve adequate sagittal alignment, because spinal alignment is maintained and lumbosacral kyphosis is within normal limits. Reduction and realignment procedures might appear to be more needed in types 5b and 6 deformities, where sagittal alignment is severely disturbed. Although the need for reduction in the surgical treatment of L5-S1 spondylolisthesis is still debated, many studies published in the last decade support the value of this classification for the decision-making process.[7-11]

PREOPERATIVE PLANNING

On physical examination, patients with low-grade spondylolisthesis usually appear normal. With progression of the slip, patients can have an increased lumbar lordosis with a prominent abdomen and heart-shaped buttocks. The trunk can appear shortened, with the rib cage approaching the iliac crests. Patients often flex their hips and knees in an effort to compensate for the forward position of the trunk because of the anterior displacement of the body's center of gravity, resulting in a Phalen-Dickson sign.[23] A palpable step-off may be present at the lumbosacral junction. A scoliotic deformity is sometimes observed. This result is secondary to nerve root tension/compression or muscle spasm (antalgic scoliosis), asymmetrical slippage in the frontal plane (olisthetic scoliosis), or concomitant idiopathic scoliosis.

Symptomatic patients with spondylolisthesis usually have variable degrees of restricted lumbar range of motion, especially in extension. Tight hamstrings can result from the knee flexion or nerve root tension/compression, particularly at L5. Straight-leg raising and/or Lasegue's sign is usually positive in patients with L5 or S1 nerve root tension. A careful neurologic examination is critical to detect signs of nerve root compression or cauda equina syndrome.

Standing plain radiographs of the lumbosacral spine should be obtained first when spondylolisthesis is suspected. A complete radiographic investigation includes AP, lateral, right and left oblique, and Ferguson AP views centered at the lumbosacral junction. An AP view will demonstrate spina bifida occulta or dysplastic posterior elements when present. A lateral view shows spondylolisthesis and can facilitate identification of the pars defect and the anatomy of L5, the sacrum, and the pelvis. Oblique views often better reveal spondylolysis when they show the collar of the Scottish terrier dog (Scotty dog sign). A Ferguson AP view is taken parallel to the L5-S1 disc and provides a coronal view of L5 that can improve the visualization of the L5 pedicles, the transverse processes, and the sacrum. This view is also useful in evaluating the fusion mass after surgery.

In patients with spondylolisthesis, long-cassette standing PA and lateral radiographs of the spine and pelvis, including the femoral heads, are recommended to evaluate coronal and sagittal alignment. On a PA view, all associated scoliosis is noted, and the global coronal alignment is measured based on the position of the C7 plumb line in relation to the center of the upper endplate of S1. On a lateral view, the overall sagittal alignment is assessed with the location of the C7 plumb line relative to the sacrum or the femoral heads. Evaluation of the overall sagittal alignment between C7 and the femoral heads is particularly important, because a forward position of C7 is associated with poorer quality of life, particularly when C7 lies in front of the femoral heads.[24] Thoracic kyphosis and lumbar lordosis are also measured. If necessary, flexion-extension supine lateral radiographs are obtained to evaluate the translational and rotational instability of the spondylolisthetic region.

The most common method for assessing the severity of spondylolisthesis is the Meyerding classification,[25] which assigns a grade of I, II, III, or IV to slips within 25%, 50%, 75%, or 100% of the dimension of the upper endplate of S1, respectively. Grade 0 refers to spondylolysis without evidence of spondylolisthesis, whereas grade V represents spondyloptosis. The slip percentage refers to the degree of slip as a percentage of the anteroposterior diameter of the upper endplate of S1 and provides a more precise evaluation.[26] However, the technique and anatomic landmarks that are used to measure the translational severity of spondylolisthesis need to be specified. Based on our previous study,[27] we recommend measuring the translation of the posteroinferior corner of the L5 vertebral body with respect to the upper endplate of the S1 vertebral body, because it better indicates the covering of the sacral plate by the L5 vertebra (Fig. 25-6, A). Lumbosacral kyphosis should be assessed in patients who have spondylolisthesis. We have demonstrated that it is related to quality of life, especially the high-grade type.[20] Because of dysplastic or adaptative changes that occur with spondylolisthesis, different measuring techniques have been proposed. Measurement of the lumbosacral kyphosis from the upper endplate of the L5 vertebral body and the posterior border of S1 vertebral body is recommended, because lines are not drawn through dysplastic anatomy[28] (Fig. 25-6, B).

The morphology of L5, the sacrum, and the pelvis can be assessed on a lateral radiograph. Doming of the upper sacral endplate and sacral kyphosis reflect adaptive changes to the sacrum. The pelvic incidence, which is unique to each person and unaffected by position, can be used to measure the sagittal pelvic morphology. It is defined as the angle between a line perpendicular to the sacral plate and a line joining the

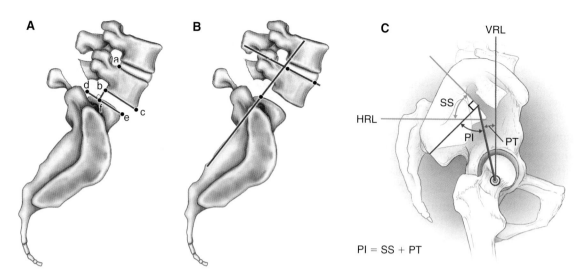

Fig. 25-6   **A,** The percentage of slip is calculated by dividing the distance of slip (the distance from *d* to *f*) by the length of the sacral plate (the distance from *d* to *e*). The result is multiplied by 100. **B,** Measurement of lumbosacral kyphosis using Dubousset's lumbosacral angle. **C,** Geometric relationships of pelvic parameters. (*a,* Postero-superior corner of L5 vertebral body; *b,* postero-inferior corner of L5 vertebral body; *c,* antero-inferior corner of L5 vertebral body; *d,* postero-superior corner of S1 vertebral body; *e,* antero-superior corner of S1 vertebral body; *f,* a perpendicular line to the sacral plate projected from point b, intersects the sacral plate at point f; *HRL,* horizontal reference line; *PI,* pelvic incidence; *PT,* pelvic tilt; *SS,* sacral slope; *VRL,* vertical reference line.)

sacral plate to the center of the axis of the femoral heads. Measurement of the sacral slope and pelvic tilt is particularly useful, because their sum corresponds to the value of the pelvic incidence (Fig. 25-6, *C*). Sacral slope is defined as the angle between the sacral endplate and the horizontal line, and pelvic tilt is the angle between a vertical line and the line joining the middle of the sacral endplate and the axis of the femoral heads. Because they are measured with respect to the horizontal plane and the vertical plane, respectively, sacral slope and pelvic tilt describe the orientation of the pelvis in the sagittal plane and not its morphology.

CT is useful to evaluate dysplasia of the posterior elements, especially if no spondylolysis is visible on plain films. It is invaluable preoperatively to assess the bony architecture of the lumbosacral junction, the available bed for posterior fusion (from the L5 transverse processes), and the degree of canal stenosis. MRI can be helpful in patients with neurologic compromise to identify the nerve roots or spinal cord at the level of the slip and to evaluate for other congenital abnormalities such as a tethered cord. In patients with HGS, a preoperative MRI is recommended to assess the neuroanatomic relations and the status of adjacent discs. Diagnosis of the degree of central spinal canal stenosis associated with an elongated L5 pars interarticularis is helpful to plan the decompression. Moreover, the status of the L4-5 and S1-2 discs will determine the need to include L4 and/or the pelvis in the fusion.

Bone scans are most useful to distinguish an acute fracture of the pars from a long-standing pars defect. They can also help to distinguish between patients with established nonunion of the defect and those in whom healing is progressing and who may benefit from immobilization. Single-photon emission computed tomography may be more accurate and sensitive than a planar bone scan.

OPERATIVE TECHNIQUE

Surgical intervention is usually reserved for patients whose symptoms do not resolve with conservative treatment and/or who show progression of the spondylolisthesis, those who have larger than a 50% slip and are symptomatic, or those whose posture and/or gait is abnormal. After a detailed and comprehensive history is taken and a physical examination performed, preoperative planning helps to determine the type of surgical intervention to tailor for a patient's specific deformity. The need for decompression is assessed with a detailed neurologic examination. We commonly perform the following three types of intervention based on the spondylolisthesis classification:

- In situ posterior fusion for low-grade spondylolisthesis (types 1, 2, and 3) with or without transforaminal lumbar interbody fusion,
- Postural reduction and fusion for HGS and a balanced pelvis (type 4) or for a retroverted pelvis and a balanced spine (type 5a), and
- Formal reduction and fusion for HGS, a retroverted pelvis, and an unbalanced spine (types 5b and 6).

Patient Positioning

Patient positioning is an important aspect of surgical treatment, because it significantly affects postural reduction of the spondylolisthesis. After general anesthesia is given, the patient is positioned prone on a radiolucent table with the hips in extension. This may close the disc space posteriorly and make it more difficult to perform a posterior-based intradiscal procedure, but it helps to correct lumbosacral kyphosis. The legs should be free and easily accessible, along with the lumbar spine and pelvis area. The surgical team should make sure that the L4-S1 area is easily visualized in the coronal and sagittal planes using fluoroscopy. Once good images have been obtained, the patient can be prepared and draped.

Incision Placement and Surgical Approach

The decision to perform a midline incision or two paracentral incisions is mainly based on the surgeon's preference and the need to perform a decompression procedure at the time of reduction and/or fusion. If surgical decompression is warranted, we usually make a single midline excision with a wide posterior exposure. For low-grade spondylolisthesis not requiring a central decompression or with foraminal stenosis, we sometimes elect to use a minimally invasive approach, with a transforaminal approach to decompress the nerve root. However, because most patients with HGS require some form of central decompression and fusion, we most commonly make a central incision.

Once the spine is widely exposed, the neural elements are decompressed as needed. If no central stenosis is present, the posterior elements are usually left in place, and pedicle screw placement can be performed. If surgical decompression is needed, we typically perform a wide posterior release that includes complete Gill fragment removal, posterior-based discectomy, and sacral dome resection occasionally, if needed for highly dysplastic deformities (Fig. 25-7). Neuromonitoring of both L5 and S1 nerve roots is usually performed with special attention to EMG activity.

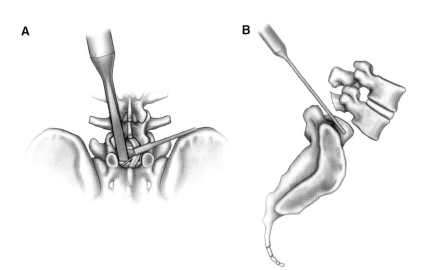

A   **B**

Fig. 25-7 Decompression, discectomy, and sacral dome resection. **A,** Careful retraction of the neural elements allows the use of an osteotome to perform a sacral dome resection, after wide disc resection. **B,** Sagittal view.

In Situ Fusion for High-Grade Spondylolisthesis

For patients who have HGS with a balanced pelvis, a well-aligned spine, and normal or low lumbosacral kyphosis (types 4 and 5a), we most frequently use a posterior-based technique with postural reduction, in situ posterolateral fusion, and screw instrumentation (Fig. 25-8, *A*). In type 4 posture, we typically place L5 and S1 bilateral screws if the L4-5 disc is normal (Fig. 25-8, *B*). In type 5a posture, we use L4, L5, and S1 bilateral pedicle screws and bilateral iliac screws (Fig. 25-8, *C*). Iliac screws are always placed to protect the S1 screws, because L5-S1 anterior support is not always provided with this procedure. Autologous iliac crest cancellous bone is always harvested, and great care is taken to decorticate both sacral alae and transverse processes. Whenever possible, the graft is inserted to connect the sacral alae and transverse processes before rods are placed to ensure optimal placement of the graft.

In patients with HGS with spondyloptosis (grade V spondylolisthesis) and a type 4 or 5 spinopelvic balance, we prefer to use a posterior-based technique that is a modification of the Bohlman procedure (Fig. 25-9, *A*). We typically instrument the L4 level with pedicle screws and iliac screws bilaterally and the S1 to L5 level with vertebral body screws (Fig. 25-9, *B*). These screws are inserted as S1 pedicle screws that protrude anteriorly into the L5 vertebral body. They are typically 60 mm in length or longer and are inserted

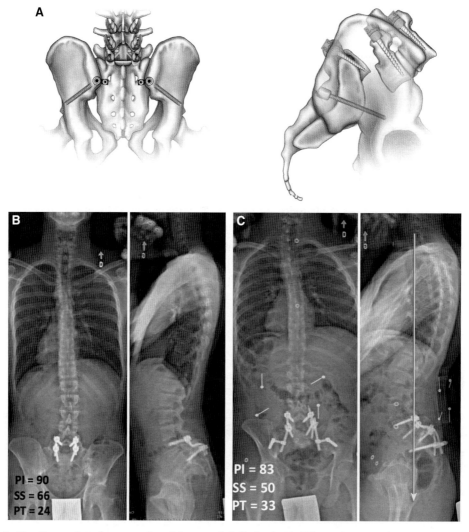

Fig. 25-8   **A,** Fixation points for types 4 and 5a spondylolisthesis. **B,** Bilateral screw placement at L5-S1 in type 4 posture with L4-5 normal disc. **C,** Bilateral pedicle and iliac screws at L4, L5, and S1 in type 5a posture.

with fluoroscopic guidance especially using the sagittal plane view to ensure proper positioning. Care must also be taken when inserting the S1 to L5 screws to prevent distraction of the space between the inferior endplate of L5 and the anterior cortex of L5. Rod contouring requires a good understanding of the local deformity and usually necessitates the use of bending irons. Iliac screws help to protect the S1 to L5 screws, because no other anterior support is present.

Formal Reduction and Fusion for High-Grade Spondylolisthesis

For patients with an unbalanced pelvis and poor global sagittal spinal alignment, we have a rationale for attempting a formal reduction to improve global spinal alignment with local reduction of the spondylolisthesis. This is performed in selected patients for whom the benefits of improved global sagittal alignment outweigh the potential risk of complications historically associated with reduction of spondylolisthesis.[18-19] After careful preoperative evaluation and planning, possible complications of reduction surgery are discussed with the patient. These include nerve root injury and postoperative motor weakness. The decision to proceed with reduction is made only after this discussion.

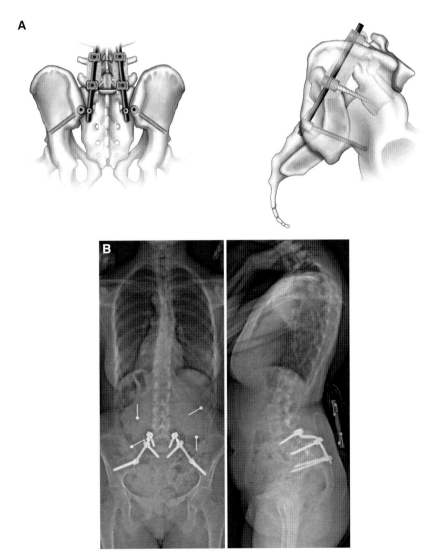

Fig. 25-9 **A,** Fixation points for spondyloptosis with a type 4 or 5 spinopelvic posture. **B,** PA and lateral radiographs of a patient with spondyloptosis and a type 5 spinopelvic posture, demonstrating the use of the fixation points shown in **A.**

The spine is exposed widely through a midline incision extending from L4 to S1. This facilitates visualization of the posterior elements and identification of the L5 pedicle, which often projects anteriorly and is difficult to readily palpate. The procedure always involves resection of the Gill fragment and wide decompression. Identification of nerve roots can be difficult especially at the L5 level, because the nerve root is often pulled forward. In extreme deformities, it may be very time consuming to identify the nerve root, but this should be done before formal reduction. In our experience, sacral dome resection is seldom indicated but can help with reduction in the case of a very rounded sacral dome. Pedicle screws are then inserted at the L5 and S1 levels, usually under fluoroscopy guidance, because the L5 pedicles are often difficult to identify. This also helps to optimally position screws especially at the S1 level, where bicortical screws are preferred, with the screws ending in the sacral promontory for added resistance to pullout forces. The disc is completely resected, and the disc space is prepared to receive an interbody cage. The posterior lumbar interbody fusion (PLIF) route is the most common trajectory, because the more lateral transforaminal lumbar interbody fusion is often not accessible in high-grade spondylolisthesis. The use of disc dilators is a very efficient way to access the intervertebral disc space, mobilize the L5 vertebral body cephalad, and decrease lumbosacral kyphosis. The disc space can be prepared using curettes and shavers, but the dilator can assist during the formal reduction.

Once the disc space is prepared and placement of pedicle screws in the pedicles of L5 and S1 is confirmed, reduction is performed (Fig. 25-10). The L5 pedicle screws should be reduction screws with or without some sort of extension tabs. We typically use an external device that connects to the screw shaft and reduces the spondylolisthesis progressively; reduction screws may also be used. In some cases, extension to L4 is warranted, but most cases end at L5. Reduction is performed gradually while the progression is assessed with fluoroscopy. Forceful reduction should not be attempted; only gentle, progressive reduction is

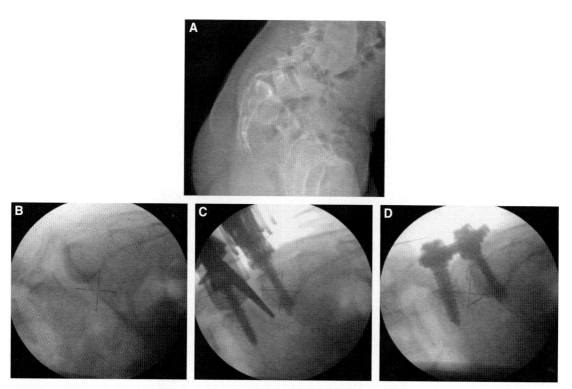

Fig. 25-10   **A,** A preoperative standing lateral radiograph shows high-grade spondylolisthesis with high lumbosacral kyphosis. **B,** Postural is reduced intraoperatively with the hips in extension. **C,** Formal reduction is performed in which the reduction apparatus is used to pull on the L5 screws, while lumbosacral kyphosis is corrected with a disc dilator. **D,** Compression has overreduced the spondylolisthesis, with an interbody cage in the L5-S1 disc space. A change in lumbosacral kyphosis is evident in **B** through **D**.

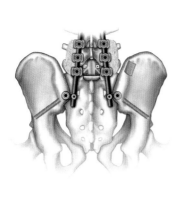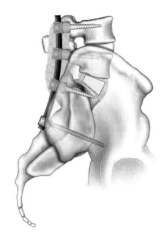

Fig. 25-11 Instrumentation for spondylolisthesis reduction with L4 and iliac screws. L4 screws may not be used if the L4 disc is normal, and the L5 pedicle screws are well anchored; iliac screws may not be used if the S1-2 disc space is narrow.

carried out. Once the desired reduction is achieved (usually less than 25% of slip), the posterior lumbar interbody fusion can be completed by inserting an appropriately sized interbody cage. Anterior placement of an interbody cage and with lordosis is usually preferred. If a preoperative MRI reveals a significant S1-2 disc space, we reinforce the construct with iliac screws to protect the S1-2 level and prevent failure at this level.[29] Once the reduction is complete, posterolateral fusion is performed using autologous iliac crest bone graft (Fig. 25-11; see Figs. 25-12 and 25-13).

POTENTIAL COMPLICATIONS AND MANAGEMENT

A recent systematic review[30] compared arthrodesis in situ and arthrodesis after reduction techniques for radiographic outcome and clinical outcome. The authors focused their analysis on eight eligible studies and compared rates of complications between the two techniques. Pseudarthrosis occurred in 9 (5.5%) of the 165 patients in the reduction group and in 18 (17.8%) of the 101 patients in the in situ group. This was highly statistically significant, and the mean risk ratio for developing a pseudarthrosis in the reduction group was 0.4. This may have occurred in part because in the in situ group, only 21% of the cases were fused with instrumentation, and all patients in the reduction group were instrumented. Based on these results, spondylolisthesis surgery either in situ or after reduction should be performed with instrumentation to decrease the risk of pseudarthrosis.

Instrumentation failure leading to revision surgery occurred in 8 of the 165 (4.8%) patients in the reduction group. These were probably related to the stresses placed on the instrumentation and nonunion. The rate of infection was similar in both groups.

One of the main arguments to favor in situ fusion versus reduction and fusion is the decreased number of neurologic complications. In the same systematic review, the rate of neurologic events was lower in the reduction group than the in situ group, but this difference was not statistically different (7.9% versus 8.9%, $p = 0.8$).[30] Neither approach had an obvious advantage of less neurologic complications. Our experience is similar; no neurologic complications have occurred in our series of patients having reduction in the past 7 years (unpublished data). Most neurologic events are characterized by sensory changes (paresthesia or dysesthesia) followed by motor nerve root injuries and cauda equina syndrome. Several cases have been reported of cauda equina syndrome after in situ fusion for HGS.[31] These were probably secondary to impingement at the dome of the sacrum or the L5 lamina. Early decompression in these cases seemed to improve neurologic recovery.

PATIENT EXAMPLES

Type 4 Spinopelvic Posture

This 19-year-old man presented with high-grade spondylolisthesis and type 4 spinopelvic posture (Fig. 25-12, *A* and *B*). In the presence of a balanced pelvis, postural reduction with posterior-only instrumentation and fusion was acceptable. Correction involved extension of the instrumentation and fusion proximally to L4, because the fusion mass remained under tension when no reduction was performed. In addition, extension of the fusion to L4 decreases the risk of pseudarthrosis with posterior-only fusion when L5 transverse processes are small, which is common in high-grade slips. Six years after surgery, follow-up radiographs show preservation of a balanced pelvis and well-aligned spine with a good fusion mass (Fig. 25-12, *C* and *D*).

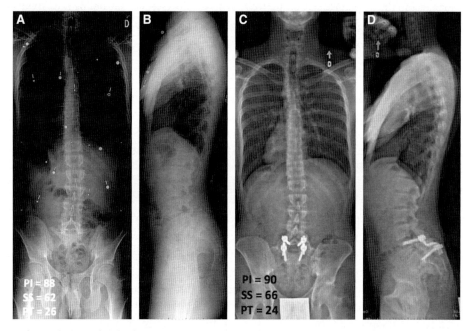

Fig. 25-12   High-grade spondylolisthesis and type 4 spinopelvic posture. **A** and **B,** This patient's preoperative anterior and lateral radiographs showed type 4 spinopelvic posture. His pelvic incidence *(PI)* was 88 degrees, sacral slope *(SS)* was 62 degrees, and pelvic tilt *(PT)* was 26 degrees. **C** and **D,** Postoperative anterior and lateral radiographs show a well-aligned spine with good fusion. His pelvic incidence is 90 degrees, sacral slope is 66 degrees, and pelvic tilt is 24 degrees.

TYPE 5A SPINOPELVIC POSTURE

This 15-year-old boy presented with an unbalanced pelvis and moderate lumbosacral kyphosis of 85 degrees, typical of high-grade spondylolisthesis and type 5a spinopelvic posture (Fig. 25-13, *A* and *B*). In this case, postural reduction with posterior-only instrumentation and fusion was acceptable. Extension of the instrumentation and fusion proximally to L4 and distally to the pelvis was preferred to maximize the fixation strength and to decrease the risk of pseudarthrosis, because no formal reduction was performed, leaving the fusion mass under tension. Five years after surgery, the patient has a well-aligned spine and a solid fusion mass (Fig. 25-13, *C* and *D*).

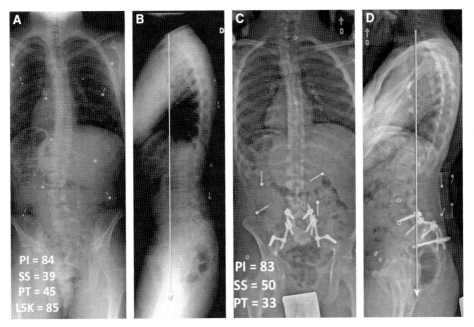

Fig. 25-13 High-grade spondylolisthesis and type 5a spinopelvic posture. **A** and **B,** This patient's preoperative anterior and lateral radiographs showed type 5a spinopelvic posture. His pelvic incidence *(PI)* was 84 degrees, sacral slope *(SS)* was 39 degrees, pelvic tilt *(PT)* was 45 degrees, and lumbosacral kyphosis *(LSK)* was 85 degrees. **C** and **D,** Postoperative anterior and lateral radiographs show a well-aligned spine with good fusion. His pelvic incidence is 83 degrees, sacral slope is 50 degrees, and pelvic tilt is 33 degrees.

Type 5b Spinopelvic Posture

This 14-year-old girl presented with an unbalanced pelvis and severe lumbosacral kyphosis (60 degrees), consistent with a type 5b spinopelvic posture (Fig. 25-14, *A* and *B*). Formal reduction of the lumbosacral kyphosis, along with posterior instrumentation and fusion, was preferred. We also performed transforaminal lumbar interbody fusion at L5-S1. We strongly recommend anterior column support when reducing spondylolisthesis to facilitate the reduction maneuver and to decrease the risk of fixation failure. Because of the significant amount of reduction achieved in this case, in addition to the normal signal in the L4-5 disc and the presence of a fused S1-2 segment on MRI, the fusion was limited to the L5-S1 segment. The patient had an uneventful postoperative course. Three years after surgery, she is asymptomatic and has no sign of pseudarthrosis or loss of reduction (Fig. 25-14, *C* and *D*).

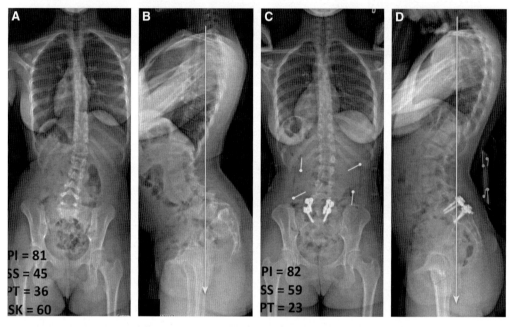

Fig. 25-14   High-grade spondylolisthesis and type 5b spinopelvic posture. **A** and **B,** This patient's preoperative anterior and lateral radiographs showed type 5b spinopelvic posture. Her pelvic incidence *(PI)* was 81 degrees, sacral slope *(SS)* was 45 degrees, pelvic tilt *(PT)* was 36 degrees, and lumbosacral kyphosis *(LSK)* was 60 degrees. **C** and **D,** Postoperative anterior and lateral radiographs show a well-aligned spine with good fusion. Her pelvic incidence is 82 degrees, sacral slope is 59 degrees, and pelvic tilt is 23 degrees.

Type 5 Spinopelvic Posture With Spondyloptosis

This 15-year-old patient had Marfan syndrome with an L5-S1 spondyloptosis (Fig. 25-15, *A*). In cases of HGS with spondyloptosis (grade V) and a type 4 or 5 spinopelvic balance, we prefer to use a posterior-based technique. This is a modification of the Bohlman procedure in which we typically instrument the L4 level with pedicle screws and iliac screws bilaterally and S1 to L5 vertebral body screws. These screws are inserted as S1 pedicle screws that protrude anteriorly into the L5 vertebral body. The patient is shown 4 years postoperatively with a well-balanced spine and solid fusion (Fig. 25-15, *B* through *D*).

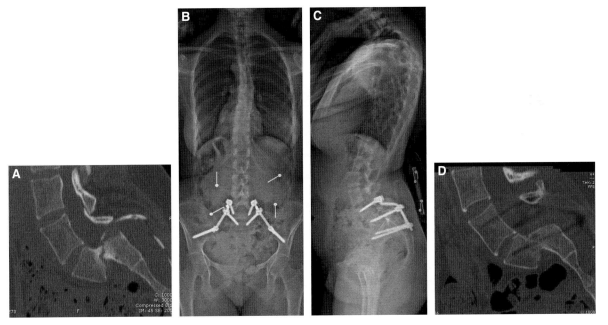

Fig. 25-15 **A,** This patient's preoperative CT scan showed almost complete listhesis of L5 over S1. **B** and **C,** Postoperative anterior and lateral radiographs demonstrate the modified Bohlman procedure with two screws extending from S1 to L5. The patient has good sagittal spinal alignment. **D,** A postoperative CT scan shows fusion between L5 and S1.

TYPE 6 SPINOPELVIC POSTURE

This 12-year-old girl presented with an unbalanced pelvis and a globally malaligned spine. She was classified as having a type 6 spinopelvic posture (Fig. 25-16, *A* and *B*). Preoperatively the patient complained of bilateral L5 radiculopathy and low back pain. She had tight hamstrings, a positive Lasegue sign bilaterally, and a typical Phalen-Dickson sign with her hips and knees flexed while standing. She was presumed to have antalgic scoliosis preoperatively, secondary to tension in L5 nerve roots. In this case, formal reduction of the spondylolisthesis with particular attention to reducing the lumbosacral kyphosis was critical. Anterior column support from transforaminal lumbar interbody fusion at L5-S1 was carried out to assist in reducing the spondylolisthesis and to ensure proper fusion at the lumbosacral junction. Posterior instrumentation and fusion was extended proximally at L4 because of the presence of L4-5 disc degeneration on the MRI. No evidence of a competent disc at S1-2 was noted. Because the reduction was almost complete, fusion to the pelvis was not required. The back pain and radiculopathy resolved postoperatively. Three years after surgery, the patient is asymptomatic with no sign of pseudarthrosis or loss of reduction (Fig. 25-16, *C* and *D*).

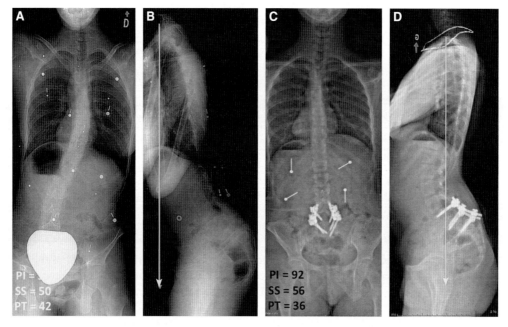

Fig. 25-16   High-grade spondylolisthesis with type 6 spinopelvic posture. **A** and **B,** This patient's preoperative anterior and lateral radiographs showed type 6 spinopelvic posture. Her pelvic incidence *(PI)* was 92 degrees, her sacral slope *(SS)* was 50 degrees, and her pelvic tilt *(PT)* was 42 degrees. **C** and **D,** Postoperative anterior and lateral radiographs show a well-aligned spine with good fusion. Her pelvic incidence is 92 degrees, sacral slope is 56 degrees, and pelvic tilt is 36 degrees.

CONCLUSION

Global sagittal plane alignment is important to consider in both adult and pediatric patients with L5-S1 high-grade developmental spondylolisthesis. The proposed classification based on sagittal alignment emphasizes that subjects with L5-S1 spondylolisthesis are a heterogenous group with various adaptations of their posture, and clinicians need to consider this during evaluation and treatment. Abnormal spinopelvic alignment alters the biomechanical stresses at the lumbosacral junction and the compensation mechanisms used to maintain an adequate posture. In patients with HGS associated with a postural abnormality, this has provided a compelling rationale to reduce and realign the spondylolisthesis deformity, thus restoring global spinal alignment and improving the biomechanical environment for fusion. A recent therapeutic Level III evidence-based review[30] supports the contention that reduction of HGS potentially improves overall spine biomechanics by correcting the local kyphotic deformity and reducing vertebral slippage, and reduction is not associated with a greater risk of developing neurologic deficits, compared with arthrodesis in situ.

REFERENCES

1. Marchetti PC, Bartolozzi P. Classification of spondylolisthesis as a guideline for treatment. In Bridwell KH, DeWald RL, Hammerberg KW, et al, eds. The Textbook of Spinal Surgery, ed 2. Philadelphia: Lippincott-Raven, 1997.
2. Wiltse LL, Newman PH, Macnab I. Classification of spondylolysis and spondylolisthesis. Clin Orthop Relat Res 117:23-29, 1976.
3. Herman MJ, Pizzutillo PD, Cavalier R. Spondylolysis and spondylolisthesis in the child and adolescent athlete. Orthop Clin North Am 34:461-467, 2003.
4. Transfeldt E, Mehbod A. Evidence-based medicine analysis of isthmic spondylolisthesis treatment including reduction versus fusion in situ for high-grade slips. Spine 32(19 Suppl):S126-S129, 2007.
5. Mardjetko S, Albert T, Andersson G, et al. Spine/SRS spondylolisthesis summary statement. Spine 30(6 Suppl):S3, 2005.
6. Labelle H, Mac-Thiong JM, Roussouly P. Spino-pelvic sagittal balance of spondylolisthesis: a review and classification. Eur Spine J 20(Suppl 5):S641-S646, 2011.
7. Hresko MT, Labelle H, Roussouly P, et al. Classification of high grade spondylolistheses based on pelvic version and spinal balance: possible rationale for reduction. Spine 32:2208-2213, 2007.
8. Mac-Thiong JM, Labelle H, Wang Z, et al. Postural model of sagittal spino-pelvic balance and its relevance for lumbosacral developmental spondylolisthesis. Spine 33:2316-2325, 2008.
9. Labelle H, Roussouly P, Chopin D, et al. Spino-pelvic alignment after surgical correction for developmental spondylolisthesis. Eur Spine J 17:1170-1176, 2008.
10. Agabegi S, Fischgrund J. Contemporary management of isthmic spondylolisthesis: pediatric and adult. Spine J 10:530-543, 2010.
11. Martiniani M, Lamartina C, Specchia N. "In situ" fusion or reduction in high-grade high dysplastic developmental spondylolisthesis (HDSS). Eur Spine J 21(Suppl 1):S134-S140, 2012.
12. DeWald CJ, Vartabedian JE, Rodts MF, et al. Evaluation and management of high-grade spondylolisthesis in adults. Spine 30(6 Suppl):S49-S59, 2005.
13. Tsuchiya K, Bridwell KH, Kuklo TR, et al. Minimum 5-year analysis of L5-S1 fusion using sacropelvic fixation for spinal deformity. Spine 31:303-308, 2006.
14. Rodriguez-Olaverri JC, Zimick NC, Merola A, et al. Comparing the clinical and radiological outcomes of pedicular transvertebral screw fixation of the lumbosacral spine in spondylolisthesis versus unilateral TLIF with posterior fixation using anterior cages. Spine 33:1977-1981, 2008.
15. Lakshmanan P, Ahuja S, Lewis M, et al. Transsacral screw fixation for high-grade spondylolisthesis. Spine J 9:1024-1029, 2009.
16. Goyal N, Wimberley DW, Hyatt A, et al. Radiographic and clinical outcomes after instrumented reduction and TLIF of mid and high-grade isthmic spondylolisthesis. J Spinal Disord Tech 22:321-327, 2009.
17. Karampalis C, Grevitt M, Shafafy M, et al. High-grade spondylolisthesis: gradual reduction using Magerl's external fixator followed by circumferential fusion technique and long-term results. Eur Spine J 21(Suppl 2):S200-S206, 2012.

18. Sansur C, Reames DL, Smith JS, et al. Morbidity and mortality in the surgical treatment of 10,242 adults with spondylolisthesis. J Neurosurg Spine 13:589-593, 2010.

19. Kasliwal M, Smith JS, Shaffrey CL, et al. Short-term complications associated with surgery for high-grade spondylolisthesis in adults and pediatric patients: a report from the Scoliosis Research Society Morbidity and Mortality Database. Neurosurgery 71:109-116, 2012.

20. Tanguay F, Labelle H, Wang Z, et al. Clinical significance of lumbosacral kyphosis in adolescent spondylolisthesis. Spine 37:304-308, 2012.

21. Dubousset J. Treatment of spondylolysis and spondylolisthesis in children and adolescents. Clin Orthop Relat Res 337:77-85, 1997.

22. Mac-Thiong JM, Duong L, Parent S, et al. Reliability of the Spinal Deformity Study Group classification of lumbosacral spondylolisthesis. Spine 37:E95-E102, 2012.

23. Phalen GS, Dickson JA. Spondylolisthesis and tight hamstrings. J Bone Joint Surg Am 43:505-512, 1961.

24. Harroud A, Labelle H, Joncas J, et al. Global sagittal balance and health-related quality of life in lumbosacral spondylolisthesis. Eur Spine J 22:849-856, 2013.

25. Meyerding HW. Spondylisthesis. Surg Gynecol Obstet 54:371-377, 1932.

26. Taillard WF. Le spondylolisthésis chez l'enfant et l'adolescent. Étude de 50 cas. Acta Orthop Scand 24:115-144, 1954.

27. Bourassa-Moreau É, Mac-Thiong JM, Labelle H. Redefining the technique for the radiological measurement of slip in spondylolisthesis. Spine 35:1401-1405, 2010.

28. Glavas P, Mac-Thiong JM, de Guise JA, et al. Assessment of lumbosacral kyphosis in spondylolisthesis: a computer assisted reliability study of six measurement techniques. Eur Spine J 18:212-217, 2008.

29. Shufflebarger HL, Geck MJ. High-grade isthmic dysplastic spondylolisthesis: monosegmental surgical treatment. Spine 30(6 Suppl):S42-S48, 2005.

30. Longo UG, Loppini M, Romeo G, et al. Evidence-based surgical management of spondylolisthesis: reduction or arthrodesis in situ. J Bone Joint Surg Am 96:53-58, 2014.

31. Shoenecker PL, Cole HO, Herring JA, et al. Cauda equina syndrome after in situ arthrodesis for severe spondylolisthesis at the lumbosacral junction. J Bone Joint Surg Am 72:369-377, 1990.

26

Spinal Alignment in the Management of Degenerative Spondylolisthesis

Robert G. Whitmore ▪ *Zoher Ghogawala*

Degenerative lumbar spondylolisthesis with spinal stenosis is a common cause of spinal morbidity and often requires operative intervention. Although surgical management of degenerative spondylolisthesis is controversial, recent evidence suggests that laminectomy with fusion is more effective than laminectomy alone. Herkowitz and Kurz[1] demonstrated that the degree of spondylolisthesis worsened in 96% of patients who underwent a laminectomy alone, compared with those who also received fusion. Revision rates are lower after laminectomy with fusion (17.1%), compared with laminectomy alone (28%, $p = 0.002$).[2] In a subanalysis of the Spine Patients Outcomes Research Trial (SPORT), patients who had grade I degenerative spondylolisthesis and a fusion had greater gain in quality-adjusted life-years, compared with those who received laminectomy alone.[3] These results were confirmed in a recent randomized controlled trial of laminectomy versus laminectomy with fusion for grade I spondylolisthesis in which fusion patients had superior outcomes and lower reoperation rates.[4]

Despite evidence in support of lumbar fusion for grade I degenerative spondylolisthesis, some patients do not have an excellent outcome after a fusion operation. Because the incidence of lumbar fusion has increased dramatically in the last few decades, with an associated increase in complications and costs, scrutiny of the poor outcomes of this procedure has grown.[5] The cost of spine care in the United States is estimated to exceed $86 billion annually, with over 300,000 spinal fusions performed each year.[6] Mean hospital charges for fusion exceed $80,000, whereas charges for decompression average $24,000.[5]

The concept of sagittal balance has emerged in recent years as a driver of superior patient outcome. Glassman et al[7] conducted a retrospective review of 752 adult spinal deformity patients between 2002 and 2003 and identified 352 patients with positive sagittal balance. A greater degree of sagittal imbalance was associated with a greater severity of patient disability, and even a mildly positive sagittal balance was poorly tolerated. In a second study of 298 spinal deformity patients, 172 without prior surgery and 126 with a previous fusion, sagittal balance was the most reliable predictor of clinical symptoms in both groups.[8]

Modern surgical techniques of lumbar fusion allow correction and restoration of sagittal balance in the treatment of degenerative spondylolisthesis. However, careful preoperative evaluation and planning are essential for overall success and durable improvement in patient outcomes.

INDICATIONS AND CONTRAINDICATIONS

Patients with degenerative spondylolisthesis who have met the criteria in Table 26-1 are appropriate surgical candidates.

PREOPERATIVE PLANNING

Measurement of sagittal balance, both preoperatively and after surgical correction of degenerative lumbar spondylolisthesis, requires an understanding of spinopelvic parameters. Spinal deformity should be assessed in relation to neutral upright spinal alignment. Plain AP and lateral radiographs are obtained of the entire spine with the patient standing and in neutral position. Cobb angles are calculated for each section of the spine: cervical lordosis (C2-7), thoracic kyphosis (T1-12), and lumbosacral lordosis (L1-S1)[9,10] (Fig. 26-1).

Pelvic alignment should be considered and can be measured by three parameters: pelvic incidence, pelvic tilt, and sacral slope. Pelvic incidence equals the sacral slope plus the pelvic tilt. Sacral slope is the angle created by a horizontal reference line and the sacral endplate. Pelvic tilt is the angle created by a vertical reference line through the midpoint between both femoral heads of the hip and a line drawn from the midpoint of the sacral endplate to the same point between the femoral heads (see Fig. 26-1).

Pelvic alignment helps to understand the global sagittal spinal alignment, which is determined either from the combination of measurements described previously or from a plumb line that extends from the midpoint of the C7 vertebral body to the dorsal rostral corner of the S1 endplate, called the *C7-S1 sagittal vertical axis* (SVA). Patients with 2 cm or more of positive sagittal balance, as measured by the SVA, are usually symptomatic.

Table 26-1 Indications and Contraindications for Surgical Intervention for Degenerative Lumbar Spondylolisthesis

Criteria Required for Lumbar Fusion	Contraindications
Clinical symptoms of lumbar spinal stenosis, lumbar radiculopathy, or increasing back pain are present, with evidence of instability at the level of spondylolisthesis.	Clinical symptoms do not follow the usual anatomic distribution related to the level of spondylolisthesis.
Symptoms are present longer than 6 to 8 weeks.	Symptoms have an acute onset and are of short duration.
Symptoms persist after conservative therapies.	Symptoms improve after physical therapy or epidural steroid injections.
Degenerative spondylolisthesis with instability or neural compression is evident radiographically (MRI and flexion-extension plain films).	Spondylolisthesis is not evident radiographically.

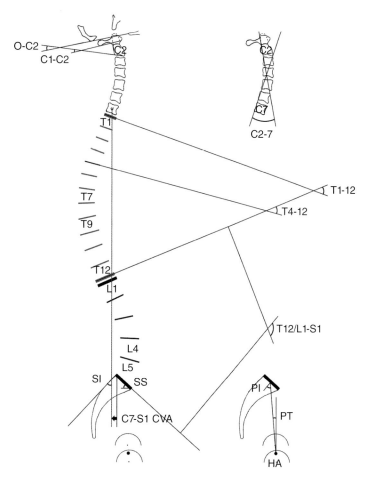

Fig. 26-1   Spinopelvic measurements on regional and global levels. (*HA,* Hip axis; *PI,* pelvic incidence; *PT,* pelvic tilt; *SI,* sacral inclination; *SS,* sacral slope.) (Printed with permission from the Mayfield Clinic.)

Surgical correction of a degenerative lumbar spondylolisthesis requires careful preoperative planning. The goal of surgery is not only correction of the neurologic compression but also realignment of the spine on a global and regional level. A recent study of patients with degenerative lumbar spondylolisthesis noted that patients with a smaller pelvic incidence required a greater restoration of lumbar lordosis, and patients with a larger pelvic incidence required a lesser degree of lordosis for an optimal outcome.[11]

OPERATIVE TECHNIQUE

Patients are positioned prone on a Jackson table (Mizuho OSI, Union City, CA) or an open frame table with either a Wilson frame attachment (Mizuho OSI) or chest and pelvic bolsters to establish normal thoracic kyphosis and lumbar lordosis. During positioning, it is important to note preoperative sagittal balance abnormalities that can necessitate additional padding of thoracic or lumbar areas to create neutral alignment (Fig. 26-2, *A*).

Fluoroscopy is usually used before the skin is incised to check the sagittal alignment and mark the skin at the correct level and entry point. When neuronavigation is available, a skin incision can be planned after completion of the navigated intraoperative CT scan. A small incision is typically made for the neuronavigation base either on the midline, with attachment to a spinous process, or on the iliac crest (Fig. 26-2, *B*).

The surgical approach selected varies according to the surgeon's preference and patient characteristics. Posterolateral fusion, with or without an interbody graft, is achieved through a traditional midline incision or in a muscle-sparing minimally invasive technique using bilateral Wiltse-type incisions.[12] In both techniques, the goal is to completely decompress the neural elements and mobilize the spondylolisthesis. This is usually accomplished by a facetectomy and/or restoration of disc height with an interbody graft

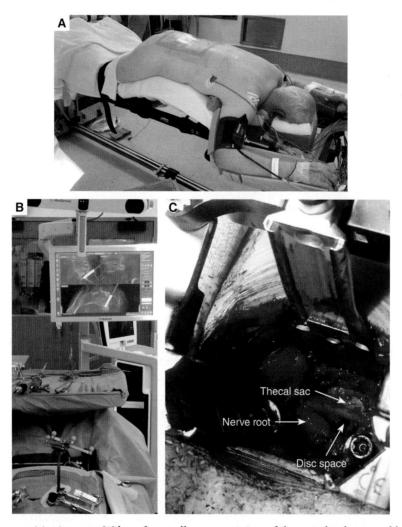

Fig. 26-2   **A,** Prone positioning on a Wilson frame allows correction of thoracic kyphosis and lumbar lordosis for spinal fusion. **B,** Navigation of spinal instrumentation using a Medtronic O-Arm Surgical Imaging System (Medtronic Sofamor Danek, Memphis, TN). The reference base is fixed into the patient's posterior superior iliac spine. A minimally invasive Medtronic Quadrant Retractor is shown. **C,** Anatomy in minimally invasive transforaminal interbody fusion includes the thecal sac, nerve root, and disc space. A Nuvasive Maximum Access Surgery (MAS) transforaminal lumbar interbody fusion (TLIF) retractor system (San Diego, CA) is shown.

(Fig. 26-2, *C*). Evidence supports the use of an interbody graft to improve clinical outcomes.[13] An interbody graft not only aids in restoration of lumbar lordosis and overall sagittal alignment, but it is also associated with a significantly higher rate of fusion: 92.6% versus 80.3%; 80.3% is the fusion rate for posterolateral fusion with pedicle screws without an interbody graft.[14]

Reduction of spondylolisthesis is controversial because of the increased risk of neurologic injury, increased blood loss, and longer procedure time. There is no level 1 evidence to indicate a difference in clinical outcomes between an in situ fusion and a slip reduction and fusion. However, the influence of sagittal balance as a long-term predictor of patient outcome suggests that efforts to surgically correct the spondylolisthesis will result in superior outcomes if the global sagittal alignment improves as a result of the correction.

After decompression of the neural elements and mobilization of spondylolisthesis, attention is focused on creation of solid arthrodesis. This is typically accomplished with autograft and/or allograft in the interbody graft and disc space and in the posterolateral recesses after careful decortication of the facet and transverse processes. Preservation of the endplate integrity is critical to ensure full restoration of foraminal height and prevent interbody graft subsidence. Various supplements to augment bone fusion such as recombinant human bone morphogenic protein is used at the surgeon's discretion. Rigid pedicle screw instrumentation is most commonly applied to support the developing bone fusion.

POTENTIAL COMPLICATIONS AND MANAGEMENT

Numerous complications can result from lumbar fusion for degenerative spondylolisthesis. One of the most common causes of neurologic injury during this procedure is insufficient mobilization and decompression of the neural elements before attempted reduction of the slip. A comprehensive knowledge of the relevant anatomy is required for safe decompression and placement of instrumentation. Neuromonitoring is often performed to improve the safety of the decompression and to assess correct placement of instrumentation. The use of neuronavigation or intraoperative CT to assess position of instrumentation can help to prevent reoperation for misplaced pedicle screws or interbody graft.

Failure to achieve fusion because of pseudarthrosis has multifactorial causes. Several technical strategies can help to promote the development of a solid bone fusion. The superior and inferior endplates of the vertebral bodies should be carefully prepared for the interbody graft. The goal is to completely remove the intervertebral disc and gently decorticate the endplate, but without frank violation of the trabecular vertebral body. Violation of the endplate often results in graft subsidence and loss of foraminal height restoration. In addition, posterolateral fusion can be achieved by a similar, careful preparation of the lateral facet and transverse processes. The bone surfaces need to be free of soft tissue and decorticated. Graft should be positioned to create a bridge between the transverse processes while contact is maintained with the lateral edge of the facet. The choice of graft (autograft versus allograft) and selection of commercially available graft substitutes can influence the likelihood of fusion and is dependent on the surgeon's preference. A discussion of this topic is beyond the scope of this chapter. With modern techniques, pseudarthrosis represents approximately 23.6% of the indication for reoperation after lumbar fusion.[2]

Deep wound infection can be as high as 11% after instrumented lumbar fusion.[15] Recently, several studies have supported the use of intraoperative vancomycin powder to reduce superficial and deep wound infection in lumbar fusion. A recent study reported a drop in the infection rate to 0.0% with the routine use of vancomycin powder for lumbar fusion.[16] Currently, we advocate routine application of vancomycin powder for all patients having an instrumented lumbar fusion.

PATIENT EXAMPLES

This 40-year-old man employed by the military had severe low back pain for almost 2 years. His symptoms had no radicular component. Conservative therapy was unsuccessful. A preoperative workup revealed a grade I degenerative spondylolisthesis at L3-4 with bilateral pars defects (Fig. 26-3, *A* and *B*). Flexion-extension films demonstrated mild movement at L3-4. He had 57 degree of lumbar lordosis, a sacral slope of 37 degrees, and pelvic incidence of 76 degrees (Fig. 26-3, *C*). A successful minimally invasive transforaminal lumbar interbody fusion was performed at L3-4 (Fig. 26-3, *D*). Postoperatively the patient has quickly resumed strenuous physical activity and has complete resolution of his preoperative symptoms (Fig. 26-3, *E*).

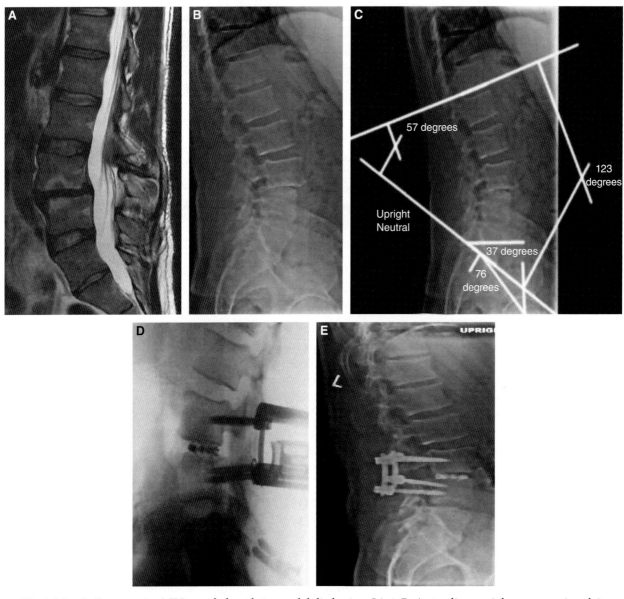

Fig. 26-3   **A,** Preoperative MRI revealed grade 1 spondylolisthesis at L3-4. **B,** A standing upright preoperative plain radiograph. **C,** Spinopelvic measurements. **D,** An intraoperative radiograph showed placement of percutaneous pedicle screws. **E,** A postoperative plain radiograph of the construct.

This 50-year-old woman presented with a history of mechanical low back pain for several years. She was working as a real estate agent and preoperatively could barely walk secondary to low back pain and left-sided radiculopathy. Preoperative imaging demonstrated a grade I degenerative spondylolisthesis at L4-5 with minimal movement on flexion-extension radiographs (Fig. 26-4, *A* and *B*). Preoperative assessment of spinopelvic parameters revealed a lumbar lordosis of 52 degrees, a lumbosacral Cobb angle of 128 degrees, and a sacral slope of 31 degrees (Fig. 26-4, *C*). She underwent a successful minimally invasive transforaminal lumbar interbody fusion. Within 6 weeks her preoperative symptoms had fully resolved, and she was working by 3 months postoperatively. One year after surgery, she is functioning very well (Fig. 26-4, *D* through *F*). Her ODI score is improved by more than 51 points. She has a solid fusion, works full time, and enjoys all activities. No specific follow-up is recommended.

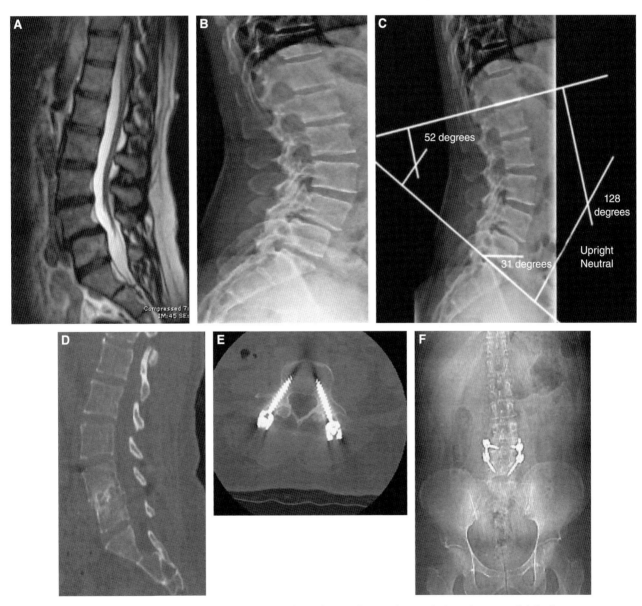

Fig. 26-4   **A** and **B,** Preoperative MRI and a standing plain radiograph revealed grade 1 spondylolisthesis at L4-5. **C,** Spinopelvic measurements. **D,** One year postoperatively, CT demonstrates robust fusion. **E,** An axial CT scan shows the position of pedicle screw instrumentation. **F,** A postoperative plain radiograph of the construct.

CONCLUSION

Restoration of sagittal balance through correction of degenerative lumbar spondylolisthesis results in excellent patient outcomes. A preoperative evaluation should include careful consideration of regional and global spinopelvic parameters. Complications can be prevented by careful surgical technique and awareness of potential problems.

REFERENCES

1. Herkowitz HN, Kurz LT. Degenerative lumbar spondylolisthesis with spinal stenosis. A prospective study comparing decompression with decompression and intertransverse process arthrodesis. J Bone Joint Surg Am 73:802-808, 1991.
2. Martin BI, Mirza SK, Comstock BA, et al. Reoperation rates following lumbar spine surgery and the influence of spinal fusion procedures. Spine 32:382-387, 2007.
3. Tosteson AN, Lurie JD, Tosteson TD, et al. Surgical treatment of spinal stenosis with and without degenerative spondylolisthesis: cost-effectiveness after 2 years. Ann Intern Med 149:845-853, 2008.
4. Ghogawala Z, Benzel E, Magge S, et al. Lumbar spinal fusion reduces risk of reoperation after laminectomy for lumbar spinal stenosis associated with grade I degenerative spondylolisthesis: initial results from the SLIP trial [abstract]. Neurosurg 67:542-543, 2010.
5. Deyo RA, Mirza SK, Martin BI, et al. Trends, major medical complications, and charges associated with surgery for lumbar spinal stenosis in older adults. JAMA 303:1259-1265, 2010.
6. Martin BI, Deyo RA, Mirza SK, et al. Expenditures and health status among adults with back and neck problems. JAMA 299:656-664, 2008.
7. Glassman SD, Bridwell K, Dimar JR, et al. The impact of positive sagittal balance in adult spinal deformity. Spine 30:2024-2029, 2005.
8. Glassman SD, Berven S, Bridwell K, et al. Correlation of radiographic parameters and clinical symptoms in adult scoliosis. Spine 30:682-688, 2005.
9. Mehta SS, Modi HN, Srinivasalu S, et al. Interobserver and intraobserver reliability of Cobb angle measurement: endplate versus pedicle as bony landmarks for measurement: a statistical analysis. Journal of pediatric orthopedics. J Pediatr Orthop 29:749-754, 2009.
10. Morrissy RT, Goldsmith GS, Hall EC, et al. Measurement of the Cobb angle on radiographs of patients who have scoliosis. Evaluation of intrinsic error. J Bone Joint Surg Am 72:320-327, 1990.
11. Hsu HT, Yang SS, Chen TY. The correlation between restoration of lumbar lordosis and surgical outcome in the treatment of low-grade lumbar degenerative spondylolisthesis with spinal fusion. J Spinal Disord Tech. 2013 Dec 11. [Epub ahead of print]
12. Wiltse LL, Bateman JG, Hutchinson RH, et al. The paraspinal sacrospinalis-splitting approach to the lumbar spine. J Bone J Surg Am 50:919-926, 1968.
13. Videbaek TS, Christensen FB, Soegaard R, et al. Circumferential fusion improves outcome in comparison with instrumented posterolateral fusion: long-term results of a randomized clinical trial. Spine 31:2875-2880, 2006.
14. Cheng L, Nie L, Zhang L. Posterior lumbar interbody fusion versus posterolateral fusion in spondylolisthesis: a prospective controlled study in the Han nationality. Int Orthop 33:1043-1047, 2009.
15. Massie JB, Heller JG, Abitbol JJ, et al. Postoperative posterior spinal wound infections. Clinical orthopaedics and related research. Clin Orthop Relat Res 284:99-108, 1992.
16. Strom R, Pacione D, Kalhorn S, et al. Lumbar laminectomy and fusion with routine local application of vancomycin powder: decreased infection rate in instrumented and non-instrumented cases. Clin Neurol Neurosurg 115:1766-1769, 2013.

27

Spinal Alignment in the Management of Lumbar Spinal Stenosis

Yiping Li ▪ Vance Fredrickson ▪ Christopher D. Baggott
Daniel K. Resnick

Lumbar spinal stenosis (LSS) has both a clinical and a radiographic definition. Clinical LSS implies a degree of radiographic LSS. However, radiographic LSS occurs frequently in asymptomatic people. Radiographic LSS is not always clearly related to clinical findings.[1,2] The reported rates for LSS surgery are increasing.[3] As scrutiny of spinal surgery increases, so must the precision in terminology and diagnosis.

A clinical diagnosis of LSS typically refers to neurogenic claudication with or without radicular pain. Symptoms are usually alleviated or reduced by sitting or bending forward. They are thought to be secondary to both mechanical compression and reduction in blood flow to the nerve roots.[4] Although neurogenic claudication is approximately 60% sensitive for radiographic spinal stenosis, it is highly specific.[5] Careful examination is needed to differentiate symptoms secondary to nerve root compression and those secondary to other pathologies.[6,7]

CLINICAL FINDINGS

Degenerative spinal stenosis, is often secondary to hypertrophy of the ligamentum flavum and hypertrophy of the facet joints.[8] The frequency at which lumbar stenosis is observed from greatest to least is as follows: L4-5, L3-4, L2-3, L5-S1, and L1-2.[9]

Clinical LSS symptoms reflect the consequences of disc degeneration and facet hypertrophy. The pathophysiology of degenerative spinal disease, initiated by disc height loss and exacerbated by abnormal segmental motion, is beyond the scope of this discussion. However, to clearly define the compressive pathology that is alleviated or reduced with flexion, we must discuss three specific aspects of the pathophysiology caused by an underlying loss of disc space height. First, the annulus fibrosus bulges in all directions as the disc desiccates over time. In the central canal, in the lateral recess, and in the neural foramina, the space allotted for the neural elements is reduced. Second, as the disc height is reduced, the ligamentum flavum buckles and is no longer held taught between the laminae, causing central and lateral recess stenosis. Third, the vertical distance between adjacent pedicles is reduced, narrowing the neural foramina. This is exacerbated by facet arthropathy, which can cause further narrowing of the lateral recess and foramina and abnormal segmental motion.

With flexion of the lumbar spine, symptomatic relief occurs through two mechanisms. First, flexion increases the interlaminar space, stretching the otherwise hypertrophied and buckled ligamentum flavum. Second, flexion of the spine moves the pedicle cephalad relative to the superior articulating process of the vertebra below, with resultant widening of the neural foramina. By the first mechanism, nerve impingement by central stenosis can be alleviated in flexion. By the second mechanism, neural foraminal stenosis can be relieved in flexion.

Symptomatically, neurogenic claudication needs to be differentiated from vascular claudication. Vascular claudication is typically exacerbated with activity and relieved with rest. Spinal flexion is not necessary to relieve symptoms because of lower extremity muscle ischemia secondary to vascular compromise. Vascular evaluation with ankle-brachial index testing can be helpful.

LSS can be complicated by concomitant spinal pathologies such as degenerative spondylolisthesis or scoliosis, which can confound the clinical findings and affect treatment and outcomes in patients with spinal stenosis.[10]

RADIOGRAPHIC FINDINGS

SPINAL STENOSIS

On cross-sectional imaging, either MRI or CT myelography, LSS is defined as narrowing of the central spinal canal, the lateral recess, or the neural foramina (in the absence of disc herniation) by the surrounding soft tissues. This is typically caused by a combination of disc bulging, facet arthropathy, and/or ligamentum flavum hypertrophy.

Myelography and MRI are the most commonly used radiographic modalities for evaluating LSS. The relationship between surrounding soft tissue structures and the spinal canal or neural foramina is best evaluated using MRI. Plain radiographs are insensitive for defining soft tissue relationships; therefore they are reserved for the assessment of spinal alignment rather than LSS. CT imaging defines the bony margins of the spinal canal. Intrathecal contrast is used with radiography or CT imaging to create a myelogram. With this technique the spinal canal and neural foramina can be assessed.

Central stenosis can be determined based on the cerebrospinal fluid (CSF) signal around the neural elements. In severe central stenosis, the CSF signal can be completely obliterated, or it can be reduced into a triangular shape if stenosis is less severe. The triangular CSF space is bordered ventrally by the intervertebral disc. This ventral compression can be exacerbated by osteophyte formation, provoked by the bulging of the annulus fibrosis. The space is bordered posterolaterally by the ligamentum flavum and facet joints. Facet arthropathy and ligamentum flavum buckling/hypertrophy can worsen posterolateral stenosis.

The lateral recess is the region ventral to the medial facet, medial to the neural foramina, and lateral to the central canal; the nerve root exits the central canal and travels caudally in the lateral recess before entering the neural foramina under the caudal pedicle. As the bypassing nerve root passes caudally in the lateral recess, a combination of ventral disc/osteophyte compression and dorsal facet/ligamentum hypertrophy can cause radicular compression.

The neural foramina can be narrowed ventrally by a bulging disc and an associated osteophyte formation. Furthermore, as the vertical distance between the pedicles is reduced with disc space collapse, the superior articulating process of the caudal vertebrae can ride higher in the neural foramina, aggravating existing facet arthropathy and ligamentum flavum hypertrophy.

Macedo et al[11] recently proposed a *sedimentation sign* on MRI for correlating imaging evidence of LSS with clinical signs of LSS. In normal supine patients, this sign is characterized by the settling of nerve roots to the posterior aspect of the spinal canal from the effect of gravity; however, in patients with symptomatic LSS, the nerve roots remain under tension and are evenly distributed within the spinal canal. The authors noted a 94% correlation of this imaging finding in patients with symptomatic LSS and a dural sac cross-sectional area of less than 80 mm^2, whereas none was observed in patients with nonspecific clinical findings of low back pain and a dural sac cross-sectional area of more than 120 mm^2. Despite encouraging results, whether the sedimentation sign facilitates the diagnosis of LSS has not been determined. Although several studies support high interobserver and intraobserver reliability, the accuracy of the sedimentation sign was only moderate and not useful to differentiate patients with clinical LSS from those with nonspecific low back pain.[11,12] Patients with severe LSS were more likely to have a positive sedimentation sign, however; therefore the imaging finding may facilitate preoperative assessment decision-making.[11 13]

Radiographic LSS occurs frequently in asymptomatic patients[14]; furthermore, patients with clinical symptoms of LSS do not always have obvious stenosis on cross-sectional imaging.[1] In a study involving asymptomatic patients with an average age of approximately 42 years, Jensen et al[15] found 7% to have spondylolisthesis, 7% to have central canal stenosis, and 7% to have neural foraminal stenosis. Boden et al[14] noted asymptomatic LSS in 21% of patients older than 60 years of age. Haig et al[1] conducted a study of patients 55 to 80 years of age, and reported asymptomatic lumbar stenosis to be present in 23% of patients. Imaging evidence of LSS was absent in 73% of patients with clinical LSS. Sirvanci et al[2] compared Oswestry Disability Index (ODI) scores and MRI findings in patients with symptomatic LSS with an average age of approximately 69 years. They found no relationship between ODI scores and the degree of LSS on imaging. Cross-sectional imaging studies are obtained with the spine in a non-load-bearing condition; therefore the studies may not have reflected the degree of neural compression that exists with load-bearing in symptomatic patients.

DEGENERATIVE SPONDYLOLISTHESIS

Spondylolisthesis is a translation of one vertebra on another. Degenerative spondylolisthesis occurs most frequently at L4-5, and is typically secondary to disc degeneration and degenerative facet disease leading to segmental instability. The collapsed disc space and lax annulus fibrosus cannot resist translational forces as effectively as healthy discs. At the lower lumbar spine, lumbar lordosis can transform axial loading forces to ventrally directed translational forces. Disc degeneration places additional stress at the facet joints and accelerates arthropathy.[16] With the vertical orientation of the lumbar facet joints, the vertebrae are predisposed to movement in the axial plane. The L5-S1 level is relatively protected from degenerative spondylolisthesis because of the alignment of the facet joints and the lumbosacral and iliolumbar ligaments, which provide additional support at this level.

DEGENERATIVE SCOLIOSIS

Scoliosis is defined as coronal curvature of more than 10 degrees. In degenerative scoliosis, degenerative changes are most frequently observed at the scoliotic apex. These changes can include facet and laminar hypertrophy and marginal osteophytosis, which may contribute to stenosis.[10,17]

INDICATIONS AND CONTRAINDICATIONS

RADIOGRAPHIC LUMBAR SPINAL STENOSIS WITHOUT CLINICAL LUMBAR SPINAL STENOSIS

Asymptomatic patients with imaging findings of LSS (as seen on CT with or without myelography or MRI) with or without spondylolisthesis and degenerative scoliosis generally do not need treatment. Typically these patients present for further evaluation after imaging findings of LSS were found incidentally. Those with evidence of spondylolisthesis and degenerative scoliosis may benefit from further follow-up to monitor spinal instability or progression of scoliosis; however, clinical outcomes are usually very favorable.[18,19]

Symptomatic Lumbar Spinal Stenosis

Patients with symptomatic LSS can benefit from some form of treatment, but surgical intervention is usually reserved for patients whose nonoperative treatment was unsuccessful, those with moderate to severe disease, and those with spinal instability.[20-24] A patient's response to nonoperative interventions depends on the severity of the disease. Approximately 20% to 40% of patients with mild to moderate clinical LSS progress to require operative intervention; however, most of those who do not progress to surgery have some amelioration of their symptoms.[25]

Standard forms of nonoperative treatment include pharmaceuticals in conjunction with exercise and physical therapy. Supplementary treatments such as traction, bracing, transcutaneous electrical nerve stimulation, and epidural steroid injections may provide some short-term symptom relief in patients with neurogenic claudication; however, evidence does not support long-term efficacy.[25-27]

Surgery for Symptomatic Lumbar Spinal Stenosis

Surgical intervention is indicated in patients with moderate or severe symptoms from LSS. Surgery is more effective than nonoperative treatment and in patients with clinical LSS who have failed a nonoperative trial. At a long-term follow-up, surgical decompression proved more effective than medical treatment especially in patients with more severe disease.[25,28-30]

Surgical Decision-Making

In patients without coexisting spondylolisthesis, deformity, or instability, decompression alone is the preferred method of treatment. No benefit has been shown in decompression with fusion as opposed to decompression alone in patients without coexisting deformity or instability.[31] The presence of significant coronal/sagittal imbalance, spondylolisthesis, or scoliosis is an indication for fusion.[20,32,33]

Spinal malalignment is associated with worsening outcomes after decompression alone in patients with LSS and directly contributes to radiculopathy, pain, and disability.[34-38] In cases of scoliosis, sagittal imbalance is more strongly correlated with pain and disability, compared with coronal imbalance; however, surgical correction of either correlates with improved outcome.[36,37,39] Decompression without fusion in patients with LSS and associated scoliosis has been associated with progression of symptoms and imaging findings of LSS.[38,40]

Decompression combined with fusion results in improved functional outcomes in patients with LSS and degenerative spondylolisthesis.[41] Degenerative spondylolisthesis can progress postoperatively after decompression without a fusion. Therefore decompression with fusion is performed in most degenerative spondylolisthesis patients.[42] Rigid instrumentation, often in the form of pedicle screws, can be used when the level of the spondylolisthesis is mobile, when regional kyphosis is present, or if radiographic instability (either overt or glacial) is seen.[41]

PREOPERATIVE PLANNING

A detailed history and physical examination are the basis for a diagnosis of clinical LSS. The information gleaned from the initial evaluation guides the decision to obtain additional detailed preoperative imaging studies for surgical planning. Patients can have symmetrical or asymmetrical low back pain and may have associated unilateral or bilateral radiculopathy. The hallmark of LSS is neurogenic claudication, often noted as burning thigh and buttocks pain that is exacerbated by standing and walking and reversed by flexion. However, associated conditions such as degenerative spondylolisthesis or degenerative scoliosis can present with more complex pain syndromes.

A detailed physical examination includes evaluation of posture, sagittal and coronal balance, and gait. Forward bending can help to detect evidence of degenerative scoliosis.[43] Palpation of the back may reveal step-offs, which are more common with high-grade spondylolisthesis.[44] Tightness of the hamstring muscles or paraspinal muscle tenderness/spasm is commonly associated with symptomatic spondylolisthesis. Hamstring and paraspinal muscle tightness can result in an abnormal gait or posture. An abnormal Romberg sign is possible, suggesting impairment of proprioceptive fibers from neurogenic claudication.[44,45]

Patients with degenerative scoliosis commonly present with axial or mechanical back pain from malalignment of the spinal column. Axial back pain typically is over the convexity of the curve because of muscle fatigue and spasm, whereas foraminal narrowing and radicular pain classically occur along the concavity of the curve.[44,46] Back pain can result from subtle spinal instability; this should alert surgeons to further evaluate alignment in the loaded condition and overall spinal balance in patients with spinal stenosis.[20]

LSS affects global spinal alignment as a result of chronic pain and postural changes from paraspinal and hamstring muscle overuse. Over time as the paraspinal and hamstring muscles endure strain and fatigue, specific compensatory mechanisms affect the interactions between disc, facets, and surrounding ligaments, facilitating spondylosis and spinal misalignment. Chronic muscle spasm and tightness in these muscles alter the normal standing position, which results in increased pain and disability.[34,35,47] Example compensatory responses include the development of spinal lordosis, pelvic retroversion, and knee flexion to maintain a standing position.[47]

The pelvis has some ability to compensate for abnormal sagittal alignment of the spine. On standing radiographs, the orientation and compensatory ability of the pelvis can be defined by the pelvic incidence, the pelvic tilt, and the sacral slope.[48] *Pelvic incidence* is defined as a fixed anatomic constant composed of the angle formed between a line perpendicular to the sacral endplate and a line joining the midpoint of the sacral endplate with the center of the femoral head. Pelvic incidence varies between individuals, representing variability between individuals in their ability to compensate for poor sagittal balance. A large pelvic incidence allows the pelvis to tilt forward or backward to accommodate an exaggerated or a reduced lumbar lordosis.

Pelvic tilt is the angle between the vertical axis and a line joining the midpoint of the sacral endplate with the center of the femoral head. This angle correlates with the degree of forward or backward rotation of the pelvis along the hips.[48] A narrower angle correlates with an anteverted pelvis and a horizontally oriented sacrum. This is associated with a hyperlordotic lumbar spine. A larger angle correlates with a retroverted pelvis and a vertically oriented sacrum. This is associated with a flat lumbar spine. A retroverted pelvis compensates for a flat lumbar spine by transmitting the axial loading forces through the hamstrings. An anteverted pelvis is seen with decreasing pelvic tilt, which transmits the loading forces directly to the femoral head, thus reducing hip and thigh muscle contraction.[47-50] Patients who compensate for a loss of lumbar lordosis with a pelvic tilt of more than about 20 degrees have symptoms of fatigue and low back pain. Lumbar lordosis within 9 degrees of the pelvic incidence reduces the need for compensatory pelvic tilting.[47-50]

Sacral slope is defined as the angle between the sacral plate and the horizontal plane. The sum of the pelvic tilt and the sacral slope is the pelvic incidence. Decreased sacral slope corresponds with a more retroverted pelvis, whereas an increased sacral slope is associated with a more anteverted pelvis. This metric is useful in understanding how axial loading can be converted into an anteriorly directed translating force at L5-S1, an important concept in spondylolisthesis at that level.

Surgeons should routinely obtain preoperative images to evaluate soft tissue structures and spinal alignment.[34,47,51] MRI provides detailed information about the relationships between the soft tissues and neural elements. CT provides a detailed evaluation of the bony anatomy. Standing, full-length, 36-inch PA and lateral scoliosis radiographs and regional AP and lateral flexion-extension radiographs allow the best evaluation of coronal and sagittal imbalances.[18] These imaging studies can serve as a baseline for monitoring curve progression in patients with degenerative scoliosis, spinal stability, or spondylolisthesis. Conventional measurements of the pelvic parameters, Cobb angle, coronal angle, plumb line, and posteroanterior translational distance are useful for decision-making.[18,44,52] Bending films are helpful for assessing the compensatory ability or flexibility of the adjacent spine. Upright imaging can be compared with supine CT or MRI to evaluate dynamic abnormal motion in the load-bearing condition.

Other factors that affect surgical planning include medical comorbidities, social factors, and patient preferences. Problems such as coronary artery disease, chronic obstructive pulmonary disease, osteoporosis, tobacco abuse, and depression can affect the clinical outcome and treatment modality offered.[53]

OPERATIVE TECHNIQUE

The mainstay of treatment for LSS is a posterior lumbar decompression through a laminectomy with or without medial facetectomy and foraminotomy. The addition of medial facetectomy or foraminotomy is dependent on the nature of a patient's symptoms and the location of neurologic compression. Open or minimally incisional techniques can be performed depending on a patient's age and medical conditions, the number of levels involved, and the location of the stenosis (central, lateral recess, or foraminal). The following is a description of a standard open multilevel decompression performed for a combination of central and lateral recess stenosis. For single-level disease or isolated foraminal disease, we prefer minimally incisional approaches (interspinous laminectomy and microforaminotomy).

PATIENT POSITIONING AND EXPOSURE

The patient is positioned prone on a Jackson table (Mizuho OSI, Union City, CA). Intravenous antibiotics are started before the skin is incised, and the patient is prepared in the usual, sterile manner. Preoperative localization with a radiopaque marker (spinal needle) helps to limit the extent of the incision.

The exposure begins with a linear skin incision over the spinous processes of interest. Next, the fascia is incised in the midline. The fascial opening can be extended cranially or caudally under the skin incision for a wider exposure (Fig. 27-1). A subperiosteal dissection is performed to expose the spinous process, lamina, and medial facet. If fusion is planned, the dissection is extended to include the entire facet (if interbody fusion is planned) or the transverse processes (if a posterolateral fusion is planned). Once the bony elements are exposed, an intraoperative radiograph is obtained to confirm the appropriate level.

DECOMPRESSION

The spinous processes are removed with a Leksell rongeur, and bone is saved if fusion is planned (Fig. 27-2, A). The laminae are thinned with a high-speed drill or Leksell rongeur (Fig. 27-2, B). A plane is developed with a Woodson or a Penfield dissector to release the superficial layer of the ligamentum flavum from the caudal end of the lamina above (Fig. 27-2, C). A deep layer of ligamentum flavum remains attached to the anterosuperior surface of the caudal lamina that is between the surgeon and the dura.[54] This layer can help to protect against dural injury during the laminectomy. Using this plane, the laminectomy is completed with Kerrison rongeurs, with careful preservation of the ligamentum flavum and epidural fat to protect the dura (Fig. 27-2, D and E). Once the laminae are removed, the ligamentum flavum and epidural fat are carefully elevated to decompress the thecal sac (Fig. 27-2, F). The ligamentum flavum requires careful dissection from the dura to prevent dural tears.

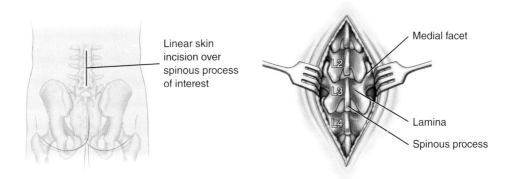

Fig. 27-1   The initial exposure.

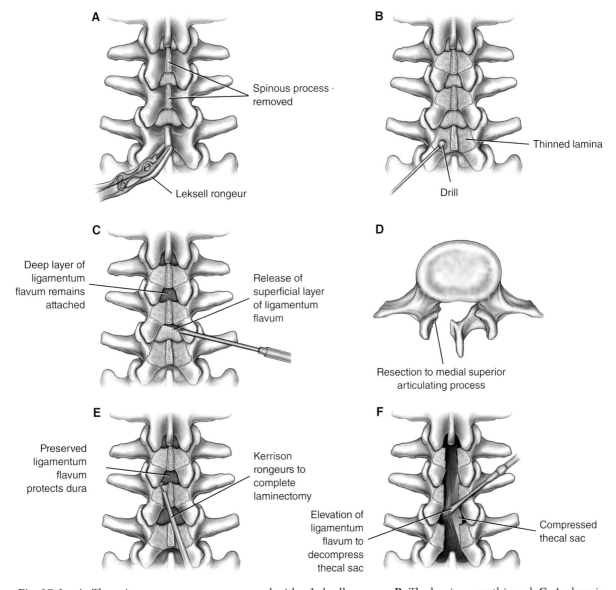

Fig. 27-2   **A,** The spinous processes are removed with a Leksell rongeur. **B,** The laminae are thinned. **C,** A plane is developed by releasing the superficial layer of the ligamentum flavum. **D,** Axial view of hemilaminectomy showing resection of medial facet to decompress lateral recess. **E,** Bone removal is completed prior to resection of ligament. **F,** The thecal sac is decompressed.

Hypertrophied ligamentum flavum and medial facet osteophytes can be resected with Kerrison punches. This process is continued until the degree of decompression is satisfactory. In general, the surgeon should be able to see over the shoulder of the nerve root to document an adequate decompression. Only up to a third of the facet is removed to prevent iatrogenic instability. If a discectomy is necessary, the nerve roots and dura can be retracted medially for this purpose.

Dural tear is a potential complication of decompression procedures and can lead to serious morbidity if it is not treated appropriately. If a dural tear occurs, herniated nerve roots are gently relocated into the thecal sac with the aid of a cottonoid. Adequate exposure of the surrounding dura is critical. Once the durotomy is sufficiently exposed, the dura can be repaired primarily with 5-0 sutures. Before the wound is closed, the repair is usually supported with fibrin glue and Gelfoam. Ventral tears (very rare in this operation) or tears that cannot be closed in a watertight fashion can be treated with Gelfoam and thrombin combined with thrombin glue. At the surgeon's discretion, a lumbar drain is placed to aid in sealing the leak.

DECOMPRESSION AND FUSION

Fusion is usually offered to patients with lumbar stenosis associated with degenerative spondylolisthesis or significant degenerative scoliosis. Fusion can be induced with a posterolateral technique (fusing the transverse processes) or an interbody technique. Anterior and lateral approaches can achieve indirect decompression of neural elements in LSS, particularly in patients with foraminal stenosis. These techniques are generally not employed for central or lateral recess stenosis.

Indirect decompression implies the use of a distraction construct to achieve a more spacious neural foramina. Most commonly, the goal is to increase the vertical distance between two vertebrae. In doing this, the pedicle of the vertebra above and the superior articulating process of the vertebra below are pulled away from each other, creating a larger neural foramina and alleviating radiculopathy. Centrally, distraction applied to the interlaminar space can reduce the compression caused by a redundant and buckled ligamentum flavum, providing a degree of central canal and lateral recess decompression. The interlaminar space can be distracted with a number of mechanisms such as intervertebral spacers, distraction forces on posterior screw-rod constructs, or interspinous spacers. Common uses of indirect decompression techniques include anterior lumbar interbody fusions, unilateral minimally invasive transforaminal lumbar interbody fusions, and coronal plane deformity correction in which the neural foramina on the concave side of the scoliosis are indirectly decompressed.[55,56]

Direct decompression techniques are used more commonly. If the pathology of LSS is from facet arthropathy or ligamentum flavum hypertrophy and resultant lateral recess or central canal stenosis, direct decompression is appropriate. Furthermore, access to the disc space for an indirect decompression and fusion may be inadequate if spondylosis if present. Removal of the hypertrophied facets and ligamentum flavum directly decompresses the spinal canal. The addition of a posterolateral fusion prevents further instability in patients with concomitant spondylolisthesis or spinal malalignment.[20,32,33]

The application of instrumentation increases the rate of fusion. The practice and choice of fusion technique need to be based on the characteristics of each patient. A patient's age, comorbidities, and degree of activity should be considered. Anatomic factors influence the choice of instrumentation. In general, a younger and healthier patient with more mobility of the spine and higher demands on the spine will do better with more aggressive surgical techniques. Conversely, older patients with comorbidities, less spinal mobility, and fewer demands on the spine will fare better with less aggressive surgical techniques.

Recently, interspinous spacers have been introduced either as stand-alone devices or for use in conjunction with conventional decompression procedures for the treatment of lumbar stenosis with or without spinal deformity. In biomedical studies, interspinous spacers have decreased the range of flexion and extension movement, increased the dimensions of the neural foramina and spinal canal, and decreased axial loading forces on the facets.[57] These devices have proved more effective than nonsurgical options in lumbar stenosis patients. However, they have not been directly compared with simple laminectomy. Furthermore, the results of nonindustry-funded studies are mixed, and we do not at present employ such devices.[58-61]

POTENTIAL COMPLICATIONS AND MANAGEMENT

WOUND INFECTION

Postoperative wound infection is a common complication after lumbar spine surgery and has an estimated incidence of 1% to 12%.[62] The risk factors associated with wound infection rates include operative time, the extent of tissue dissection, overall health, and the nutritional status of the patient.[62,63] We prefer minimally incisional approaches, which can decrease the risks of infection as a result of reduced tissue dissection and operative blood loss.[64] The addition of fusion and instrumentation in patients with spinal instability increases operative time, blood loss, and thus the risk of infection.[65] Preventative measures to reduce postoperative wound infection, including strict adherence to sterile technique and giving preoperative antibiotics, should be regularly enforced.

CEREBROSPINAL FLUID LEAKAGE

Incidental durotomy is a frequent complication of lumbar spine surgery. The reported incidence ranges from 0.5% to 18% depending on the nature of the procedure performed.[66] When durotomy is not managed properly, it can lead to persistent CSF leakage and development of an extradural arachnoid cyst, pseudomeningocele, or cutaneous fistula.[67-69] Several risk factors are associated with incidental durotomy, including female sex, older age, degenerative spondylolisthesis, and synovial cyst manipulation.

NERVE ROOT INJURY

Nerve root injury is a rare complication of surgery for spinal stenosis and is often associated with pedicle screw placement. In 1993 a survey of the American Back Society provided data on 3,939 pedicle screws in 617 cases and showed a rate of permanent nerve root injury in 14 patients (2.3% patient incidence, 0.4% screw incidence).[70] In 2011 Gautschi et al[71] published a review in which they reported a rate of nerve root irritations of 0.19% in 35,630 pedicle screws and stated that permanent nerve root injury is very rare. In 2009, results were shared from a series of 220 patients in whom three-dimensional intraoperative guidance was performed.[72] The authors reported two nerve root injuries (0.2% screw incidence and 0.9% patient incidence). Fluoroscopic and stereotactic guidance has reduced the rate of pedicle breach and screw misplacement. A 2007 meta-analysis reported improved median accuracy of in vivo lumbar pedicle screw placement with the assistance of navigation from 79% to 96.1%; complications were not reported.[73]

PATIENT EXAMPLES

This 52-year-old man had bilateral lower extremity pain when walking up inclines or steps. He had intermittent paresthesias in his right lower extremity that extended down the posterior aspect of his leg. The paresthesias and pain improved when he was supine or prone or leaning forward. He had full strength in his lower extremities. His reflexes at the patellar tendons measured 2+, and reflexes at his Achilles tendons were absent. Results of a straight-leg-raise test were negative bilaterally. He had chronic atrophic changes in his feet, but pulses in both of his feet were palpable. Preoperatively the patient demonstrated clinical and radiographic evidence of LSS with associated spondylolisthesis (Fig. 27-3, A through C). He underwent an L4-5 decompression and fusion. At his 3-month follow-up, he is well. His radicular pain and paresthesias have resolved, although he continues to have mild back pain with prolonged activity (Fig. 27-3, *D*).

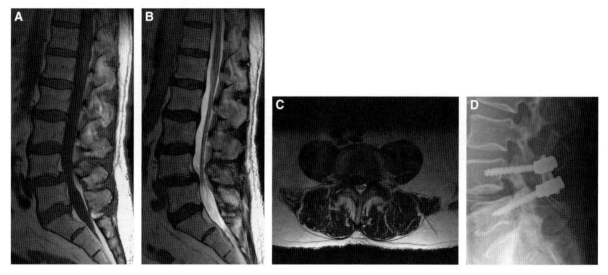

Fig. 27-3 **A-C,** This patient's preoperative MRI showed moderate to severe central and severe right lateral recess canal stenosis with spondylolisthesis of 5 mm at L4-5. **D,** A postoperative radiograph obtained after an L4-5 posterolateral fusion shows a pedicle screw fixed moment arm construct.

This 61-year-old man had a past medical history significant for a conservatively treated L4 burst fracture in 1974 that he sustained in a motorcycle accident. He had a long history of back pain; however, over the past 2 years he had increasing burning pain radiating down both of his legs to approximately the knees and sometimes slightly beyond. This pain occurred with walking approximately 100 feet. It was alleviated quickly by sitting down or lying down, and it was greatly improved by leaning forward, for example, on a shopping cart or at a workbench. The pain was present in his anterior and posterior thighs and legs, with numbness and tingling on the soles of his feet. He had no weakness, bowel or bladder problems, fevers, or chills, and no history of cancer. The patient had tried exercise therapy but no formal physical therapy. He had taken antiinflammatory medication. Pain medications dulled the pain, but his symptoms continued daily.

On examination he had good strength in his legs, with 5/5 strength in hip flexion, knee flexion, knee extension, dorsiflexion, and plantarflexion. Results of a straight-leg-raise test were negative. His reflexes were hypoactive and symmetrical at the knees and ankles. His pinprick sensation was intact. He stood in a leaned-over posture consistent with a flat back. His hips and knees were flexed. His wife stated this was how he always stood.

The patient had severe neurogenic claudication symptoms that were classic in that they were relieved by sitting or lying down or by pushing a shopping cart, and they were present in a classic distribution. His MRI scan revealed multilevel lumbar spinal stenosis, particularly at the L2-3 and L3-4 levels (Fig. 27-4, *A*). Coronal and sagittal imbalance was noted on 36-inch radiographs (Fig. 27-4, *B* and *C*). He had no significant motion in his lumbar spine on flexion-extension. Decision-making in this case was complex. The patient was counseled regarding decompression and instrumented or noninstrumented posterolateral fusion. He opted for decompression and noninstrumented fusion. Postoperatively he had significant relief from his claudication. Two years after surgery his lumbar deformity has not progressed (Fig. 27-4, *D*).

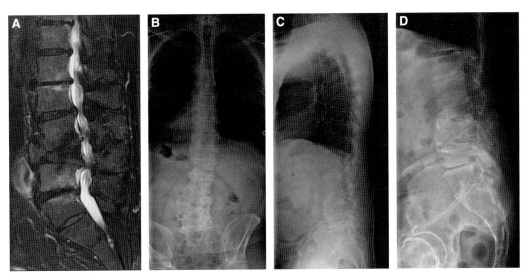

Fig. 27-4 **A,** Preoperative MRI showed an old L4 burst fracture with a posterior fragment that had retropulsed by approximately 8 mm. This resulted in moderate to severe L4-5 central canal stenosis along with multilevel degenerative disease that was worst at L2-3 and severe central canal stenosis and multilevel neural foramina stenosis that was worst at L4-5 and L5-S1. **B,** A preoperative AP radiograph showed approximately 18 degrees of convex left scoliosis of the lumbar spine from L3 through L5. **C,** A preoperative lateral radiograph revealed a positive sagittal balance associated with a flat back. **D,** Two years postoperatively a radiograph shows no change in alignment.

CONCLUSION

Surgical treatment of symptomatic LSS can improve outcomes, compared with nonsurgical treatment. Decompression alone should be considered the first-line treatment in the absence of malalignment such as degenerative scoliosis or spondylolisthesis. Fusion should be considered when stenosis coexists with scoliosis or spondylolisthesis. Instrumentation is considered if pathologic motion, instability, or iatrogenic destabilization is present.

REFERENCES

1. Haig AJ, Geisser ME, Tong HC, et al. Electromyographic and magnetic resonance imaging to predict lumbar stenosis, low-back pain, and no back symptoms. J Bone Joint Surg Am 89:358-366, 2007.
2. Sirvanci M, Bhatia M, Ganiyusufoglu KA, et al. Degenerative lumbar spinal stenosis: correlation with Oswestry Disability Index and MR imaging. Eur Spine J 17:679-685, 2008.
3. Skolasky RL, Maggard AM, Thorpe RJ Jr, et al. United States hospital admissions for lumbar spinal stenosis: racial and ethnic differences, 2000 through 2009. Spine 38:2272-2278, 2013.
4. Uesugi K, Sekiguchi M, Kikuchi S, et al. Relationship between lumbar spinal stenosis and lifestyle-related disorders: a cross-sectional multicenter observational study. Spine 38:E540-E545, 2013.
5. Turner JA, Ersek M, Herron L, et al. Surgery for lumbar spinal stenosis. Attempted meta-analysis of the literature. Spine 17:1-8, 1992.
6. Saal JA, Dillingham MF, Gamburd RS, et al. The pseudoradicular syndrome. Lower extremity peripheral nerve entrapment masquerading as lumbar radiculopathy. Spine 13:926-930, 1988.
7. Cinotti G, Postacchini F, Weinstein JN. Lumbar spinal stenosis and diabetes. Outcome of surgical decompression. J Bone Joint Surg Br 76:215-219, 1994.
8. Deyo RA, Weinstein JN. Low back pain. N Engl J Med 344:363-370, 2001.
9. Epstein NE, Maldonado VC, Cusick JF. Symptomatic lumbar spinal stenosis. Surg Neurol 50:3-10, 1998.
10. Epstein JA, Epstein BS, Jones MD. Symptomatic lumbar scoliosis with degenerative changes in the elderly. Spine 4:542-547, 1979.

11. Macedo LG, Wang Y, Battié MC. The sedimentation sign for differential diagnosis of lumbar spinal stenosis. Spine 38:827-831, 2013.

12. Tomkins-Lane CC, Quint DJ, Gabriel S, et al. Nerve root sedimentation sign for the diagnosis of lumbar spinal stenosis: reliability, sensitivity, and specificity. Spine 38:E1554-E1560, 2013.

13. Fazal A, Yoo A, Bendo JA. Does the presence of the nerve root sedimentation sign on MRI correlate with the operative level in patients undergoing posterior lumbar decompression for lumbar stenosis? Spine J 13:837-842, 2013.

14. Boden SD, Davis DO, Dina TS, et al. Abnormal magnetic-resonance scans of the lumbar spine in asymptomatic subjects. A prospective investigation. J Bone Joint Surg Am 72:403-408, 1990.

15. Jensen MC, Brant-Zawadzki MN, Obuchowski N, et al. Magnetic resonance imaging of the lumbar spine in people without back pain. New Engl J Med 331:69-73, 1994.

16. Benzel EC, Francis TB, eds. Spine Surgery: Techniques, Complication Avoidance, and Management, ed 3. Philadelphia: Elsevier, 2012.

17. Epstein JA, Epstein BS, Lavine LS. Surgical treatment of nerve root compression caused by scoliosis of the lumbar spine. J Neurosurg 41:449-454, 1974.

18. Crawford CH III, Glassman SD. Surgical treatment of lumbar spinal stenosis associated with adult scoliosis. Instr Course Lect 58:669-676, 2009.

19. Kotwal S, Pumberger M, Hughes A, et al. Degenerative scoliosis: a review. HSS J 7:257-264, 2011.

20. Caputy AJ, Spence CA, Bejjani GK, et al. The role of spinal fusion in surgery for lumbar spinal stenosis: a review. Neurosurg Focus 3:e3; discussion 1 p following e4, 1997.

21. Atlas SJ, Keller RB, Robson D, et al. Surgical and nonsurgical management of lumbar spinal stenosis: four-year outcomes from the maine lumbar spine study. Spine 25:556-562, 2000.

22. Atlas SJ, Deyo RA, Keller RB, et al. The Maine Lumbar Spine Study, Part III. 1-year outcomes of surgical and nonsurgical management of lumbar spinal stenosis. Spine 21:1787-1794; discussion 1794-1795, 1996.

23. Malmivaara A, Slatis P, Heliovaara M, et al. Surgical or nonoperative treatment for lumbar spinal stenosis? A randomized controlled trial. Spine 32:1-8, 2007.

24. Weinstein JN, Tosteson TD, Lurie JD, et al. Surgical versus nonsurgical therapy for lumbar spinal stenosis. New Engl J Med 358:794-810, 2008.

25. Watters WC III, Baisden J, Gilbert TJ, et al. Degenerative lumbar spinal stenosis: an evidence-based clinical guideline for the diagnosis and treatment of degenerative lumbar spinal stenosis. Spine J 8:305-310, 2008.

26. Tran de QH, Duong S, Finlayson RJ. Lumbar spinal stenosis: a brief review of the nonsurgical management. Can J Anaesth 57:694-703, 2010.

27. Hurri H, Slatis P, Soini J, et al. Lumbar spinal stenosis: assessment of long-term outcome 12 years after operative and conservative treatment. J Spinal Disord 11:110-115, 1998.

28. Djurasovic M, Glassman SD, Carreon LY, et al. Contemporary management of symptomatic lumbar spinal stenosis. Orthop Clin North Am 41:183-191, 2010.

29. Johnsson KE, Rosen I, Uden A. The natural course of lumbar spinal stenosis. Clin Orthop Rel Res 279:82-86, 1992.

30. Pearson A, Lurie J, Tosteson T, et al. Who should have surgery for spinal stenosis? Treatment effect predictors in SPORT. Spine 37:1791-1802, 2012.

31. Resnick DK, Choudhri TF, Dailey AT, et al. Guidelines for the performance of fusion procedures for degenerative disease of the lumbar spine. Part 10: fusion following decompression in patients with stenosis without spondylolisthesis. J Neurosurg Spine 2:686-691, 2005.

32. Detwiler PW, Marciano FF, Porter RW, et al. Lumbar stenosis: indications for fusion with and without instrumentation. Neurosurg Focus 3:e4; discussion 1 p following e4, 1997.

33. Bridwell KH, Glassman S, Horton W, et al. Does treatment (nonoperative and operative) improve the two-year quality of life in patients with adult symptomatic lumbar scoliosis: a prospective multicenter evidence-based medicine study. Spine 34:2171-2178, 2009.

34. Mac-Thiong JM, Transfeldt EE, Mehbod AA, et al. Can c7 plumbline and gravity line predict health related quality of life in adult scoliosis? Spine 34:E519-E527, 2009.

35. Glassman SD, Berven S, Bridwell K, et al. Correlation of radiographic parameters and clinical symptoms in adult scoliosis. Spine 30:682-688, 2005.

36. Smith JS, Shaffrey CI, Glassman SD, et al. Risk-benefit assessment of surgery for adult scoliosis: an analysis based on patient age. Spine 36:817-824, 2011.

37. Schwab FJ, Lafage V, Farcy JP, et al. Predicting outcome and complications in the surgical treatment of adult scoliosis. Spine 33:2243-2247, 2008.

38. Simmons ED. Surgical treatment of patients with lumbar spinal stenosis with associated scoliosis. Clin Orthop Rel Res 384:45-53, 2001.

39. Bridwell KH, Baldus C, Berven S, et al. Changes in radiographic and clinical outcomes with primary treatment adult spinal deformity surgeries from two years to three- to five-years follow-up. Spine 35:1849-1854, 2010.

40. Aebi M. The adult scoliosis. Eur Spine J 14:925-948, 2005.

41. Resnick DK, Choudhri TF, Dailey AT, et al. Guidelines for the performance of fusion procedures for degenerative disease of the lumbar spine. Part 9: fusion in patients with stenosis and spondylolisthesis. J Neurosurg Spine 2:679-685, 2005.

42. Kornblum MB, Fischgrund JS, Herkowitz HN, et al. Degenerative lumbar spondylolisthesis with spinal stenosis: a prospective long-term study comparing fusion and pseudarthrosis. Spine 29:726-733; discussion 733-734, 2004.

43. Ascani E, Bartolozzi P, Logroscino CA, et al. Natural history of untreated idiopathic scoliosis after skeletal maturity. Spine 11:784-789, 1986.

44. Simmons ED Jr, Simmons EH. Spinal stenosis with scoliosis. Spine 17(6 Suppl):S117-S120, 1992.

45. Ploumis A, Transfledt EE, Denis F. Degenerative lumbar scoliosis associated with spinal stenosis. Spine J 7:428-436, 2007.

46. Boachie-Adjei O, Gupta MC. Adult scoliosis and deformity. AAOS Instr Course Lect 48:377-391, 1999.

47. Schwab F, Patel A, Ungar B, et al. Adult spinal deformity-postoperative standing imbalance: how much can you tolerate? An overview of key parameters in assessing alignment and planning corrective surgery. Spine 35:2224-2231, 2010.

48. Legaye J, Duval-Beaupère G, Hecquet J, et al. Pelvic incidence: a fundamental pelvic parameter for three-dimensional regulation of spinal sagittal curves. Eur Spine J 7:99-103, 1998.

49. Lamartina C, Zavatsky JM, Petruzzi M, et al. Novel concepts in the evaluation and treatment of high-dysplastic spondylolisthesis. Eur Spine J 18(Suppl 1):S133-S142, 2009.

50. Boulay C, Tardieu C, Hecquet J, et al. Sagittal alignment of spine and pelvis regulated by pelvic incidence: standard values and prediction of lordosis. Eur Spine J 15:415-422, 2006.

51. Mac-Thiong JM, Roussouly P, Berthonnaud E, et al. Sagittal parameters of global spinal balance: normative values from a prospective cohort of seven hundred nine Caucasian asymptomatic adults. Spine 35:E1193-E1198, 2010.

52. Hanley EN, Phillips ED, Kostuik JP. Who should be fused? In Frymoyer JW, Ducker TB, Hadler NM, et al, eds. The Adult Spine: Principles and Practice. Philadelphia: Lippincott-Raven, 1991

53. Genevay S, Atlas SJ. Lumbar spinal stenosis. Best Pract Res Clin Rheumatol 24:253-265, 2010.

54. Olszewski AD, Yaszemski MJ, White AA III. The anatomy of the human lumbar ligamentum flavum. New observations and their surgical importance. Spine 21:2307-2312, 1996.

55. Oliveira L, Marchi L, Coutinho E, et al. A radiographic assessment of the ability of the extreme lateral interbody fusion procedure to indirectly decompress the neural elements. Spine 35(26 Suppl):S331-S337, 2010.

56. Elowitz EH, Yanni DS, Chwajol M, et al. Evaluation of indirect decompression of the lumbar spinal canal following minimally invasive lateral transpsoas interbody fusion: radiographic and outcome analysis. Minim Invasive Neurosurg 54:201-206, 2011.

57. Siddiqui M, Karadimas E, Nicol M, et al. Influence of X Stop on neural foramina and spinal canal area in spinal stenosis. Spine 31:2958-2962, 2006.

58. Zucherman JF, Hsu KY, Hartjen CA, et al. A multicenter, prospective, randomized trial evaluating the X STOP interspinous process decompression system for the treatment of neurogenic intermittent claudication: two-year follow-up results. Spine 30:1351-1358, 2005.

59. Zucherman JF, Hsu KY, Hartjen CA, et al. A prospective randomized multi-center study for the treatment of lumbar spinal stenosis with the X STOP interspinous implant: 1-year results. Eur Spine J 13:22-31, 2004.

60. Weiner BK. Letters. Re: Zucherman JF, Hsu KY, Hartjen CA, et al. A multicenter, prospective, randomized trial evaluating the X STOP interspinous process decompression system for the treatment of neurogenic intermittent claudication; two-year follow-up results. Spine 30:2846-2847, 2005.

61. Kabir SM, Gupta SR, Casey AT. Lumbar interspinous spacers: a systematic review of clinical and biomechanical evidence. Spine 35:E1499-1506, 2010.

62. Beiner JM, Grauer J, Kwon BK, et al. Postoperative wound infections of the spine. Neurosurg Focus 15:E14, 2003.

63. Wimmer C, Gluch H, Franzreb M, et al. Predisposing factors for infection in spine surgery: a survey of 850 spinal procedures. J Spinal Disord 11:124-128, 1998.

64. O'Toole JE, Eichholz KM, Fessler RG. Surgical site infection rates after minimally invasive spinal surgery. J Neurosurg Spine 11:471-476, 2009.

65. Weinstein MA, McCabe JP, Cammisa FP Jr. Postoperative spinal wound infection: a review of 2,391 consecutive index procedures. J Spinal Disord 13:422-426, 2000.

66. Takahashi Y, Sato T, Hyodo H, et al. Incidental durotomy during lumbar spine surgery: risk factors and anatomic locations: clinical article. J Neurosurg Spine 18:165-169, 2013.

67. Espiritu MT, Rhyne A, Darden BV II. Dural tears in spine surgery. J Am Acad Orthop Surg 18:537-545, 2010.

68. Hawk MW, Kim KD. Review of spinal pseudomeningoceles and cerebrospinal fluid fistulas. Neurosurg Focus 9:e5, 2009.

69. Hodges SD, Humphreys SC, Eck JC, et al. Management of incidental durotomy without mandatory bed rest. A retrospective review of 20 cases. Spine 24:2062-2064, 1999.

70. Esses SI, Sachs BL, Dreyzin V. Complications associated with the technique of pedicle screw fixation. A selected survey of ABS members. Spine 18:2231-2238; discussion 2238-2239, 1993.

71. Gautschi OP, Schatlo B, Schaller K, et al. Clinically relevant complications related to pedicle screw placement in thoracolumbar surgery and their management: a literature review of 35,630 pedicle screws. Neurosurg Focus 31:E8, 2011.

72. Nottmeier EW, Seemer W, Young PM. Placement of thoracolumbar pedicle screws using three-dimensional image guidance: experience in a large patient cohort. J Neurosurg Spine 10:33-39, 2009.

73. Kosmopoulos V, Schizas C. Pedicle screw placement accuracy: a meta-analysis. Spine 32:E111-E120, 2007.

PART VI

Specific Considerations for Operative Management of Spinal Deformity

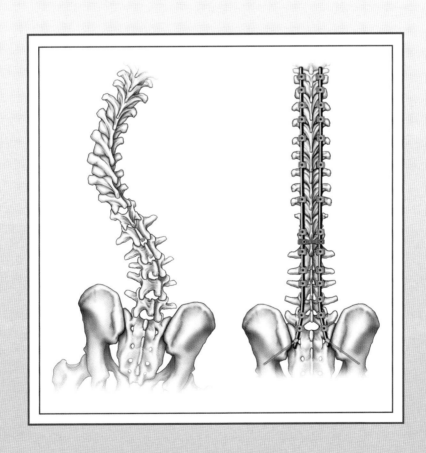

28

Spinal Alignment in the Management of Idiopathic Scoliosis

Daniel A. Baluch ▪ *Ngoc-Lam Nguyen* ▪ *Michael R. Conti Mica*
Jason W. Savage ▪ *Alpesh A. Patel*

DEFINITION AND CAUSE

Scoliosis is classically defined as a lateral curvature of the spine of more than 10 degrees in the coronal plane.[1] This simplistic definition, however, does not capture the true multiplanar involvement of the deformity. Additionally, scoliosis is a rather broad term, typically divided into three major categories. Congenital scoliosis develops in utero and is present at birth. Secondary scoliosis is a sequela of an underlying disorder such as cerebral palsy or other neuromuscular conditions. Idiopathic scoliosis, the third category, develops from an unknown cause. Adolescent idiopathic scoliosis (AIS), the topic of this chapter, is a subset of the third group that manifests during the second decade of life.

The cause of AIS is largely agreed to be multifactorial. Yagi et al[2] categorized the pathogenicity into five general theories. The neuromuscular model argues that paravertebral muscle imbalance leads to spinal curvature.[3,4] The neurohumoral concept links AIS with abnormal levels of calmodulin and melatonin.[5,6] Bone growth mismatch, with relatively stagnant posterior elements, suggests that unbalanced osseous development results in hypokyphosis and subsequent vertebral rotation.[7] The connective tissue theory postulates that deformity results from asymmetrical collagen concentrations within the intervertebral discs. The most modern and widely accepted theory is the genetic model. Scoliosis has been shown to be familial, resulting in extensive research into a molecular cause of deformity. Though many associations have been made, the cause has not been confirmed.

DEFINING SPINOPELVIC ALIGNMENT

Upright gait and posture require a harmony of vertical alignment of the head and trunk with the pelvis in which the center of mass falls in line with the femoral axis. The spine's ability to effectively position the head and trunk in space for bipedal locomotion and maintenance of horizontal gaze is dependent on the complex balance between the cervical, thoracic, lumbar, and pelvic coronal and sagittal alignment. In normal individuals, the spine is essentially straight in the coronal plane except for a subtle right thoracic convexity accommodative of the aorta. A coronal plumb line is drawn from C2 and should be within 1 cm of the midline of the sacrum.

Normative data for sagittal spinal alignment in the adolescent cohort are more variable. Reported mean thoracic kyphosis and lumbar lordosis in the pediatric population range from 38 to 44 degrees and from 48 to 64 degrees, respectively.[8,9] In general, a sagittal plumb line drawn from C7 should intersect the anterosuperior corner of the sacrum. In their study using the anterosuperior corner of the sacrum as the zero reference point, Vedantam et al[9] reported that the mean sagittal vertical axis (SVA) in asymptomatic adolescents measured −5.6 cm ± 3.5 cm, compared with a mean of −3.2 cm in asymptomatic adults. T1-spinopelvic inclination and T9-spinopelvic inclination are two measurements of global sagittal balance proposed by Duval-Beaupère et al that are gaining popularity.[10,10a] However, their clinical relevance and implications in the pediatric cohort has not been examined and is still unclear.

The principles of spinal instrumentation and fusion for AIS have changed in recent decades. Previously, the primary focus of surgical treatment was correction of the major curve in the coronal plane. Long-term outcome studies demonstrated that many of these patients developed sagittal imbalance or flat-back syndrome, leading to debilitating back pain and/or degenerative disc disease.[11,12] The risk of flat-back deformity has been shown to increase with more caudal instrumentation, especially with failure to maintain lumbar lordosis.[11,13-16] Currently, the objective of surgical management of AIS includes correction of the coronal curve or curves and restoration of regional alignment (thoracic kyphosis and lumbar lordosis) and spinopelvic parameters. The spine and pelvis should be considered associated components, because they relate to global gait and postural balance. Because pelvic tilt through the hip joints plays a crucial role in a patient's ability to compensate for sagittal imbalance and maintenance of upright posture, assessment of global spinal balance needs to include pelvic angular measurements. Dubousset coined the term *pelvic vertebra* to emphasize the importance of this concept.[10,12a]

Three important pelvic parameters have been described: pelvic incidence (PI), pelvic tilt (PT), and sacral slope (SS) (Fig. 28-1, *A* through *C*). PI is a morphologic parameter that does not change once a patient is an adult. It is defined as the angle between a line perpendicular to the sacral plate at its midpoint and a line connecting this point to the femoral heads axis. PT is defined as the angle between a vertical reference line and a line through the midpoint of the sacral plate to the axis of the femoral heads. Patients with positive sagittal imbalance compensate by retroverting the pelvis (increasing PT) (Fig. 28-1, *D*). SS is measured

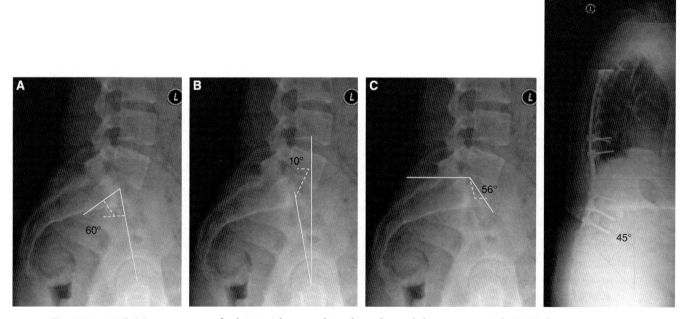

Fig. 28-1   **A-C,** Measurements of pelvic incidence, pelvic tilt, and sacral slope, respectively. **D,** Failure to restore appropriate lumbar lordosis and thoracic kyphosis leads to postoperative sagittal imbalance. This patient, who previously underwent T4-L4 posterior spinal fusion for idiopathic scoliosis, compensates for positive sagittal imbalance by increasing the pelvic tilt. (Images courtesy of Jason Savage, MD.)

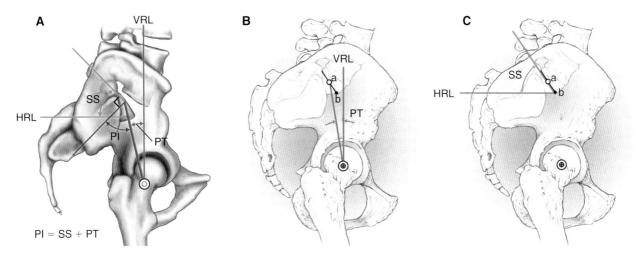

Fig. 28-2 **A,** Pelvic incidence *(PI)* is the angle subtended between two lines: one drawn from the center of the femoral heads to the midpoint of the sacral endplate *(a)* and another drawn perpendicular to the sacral endplate *(b).* **B,** The measurement of pelvic tilt *(PT).* **C,** The measurement of sacral slope *(SS). (HRL,* Horizontal reference line; *VRL,* vertical reference line.) (**B** and **C,** Courtesy of K.X. Probst/Xavier Studio, 2012; with permission.)

as the angle between a horizontal reference line and the sacral plate. According to published literature, adolescents have a mean PI of 49.1 ± 11.0 degrees, PT of 7.7 ± 8.0 degrees, and SS of 41.4 ± 8.2 degrees.[8,10]

When surgical correction is considered, a thorough knowledge of normative values provides a guideline for restoring ergonomically favorable spinopelvic alignment. Additionally, with multiple studies reporting a strong correlation between spinopelvic variables (PT, SVA, T1-spinopelvic inclination and T9-spinopelvic inclination) and health-related quality of life outcomes, understanding the complex relationship between pelvic positioning and spinal alignment is crucial for a proper diagnostic evaluation, surgical planning, and treatment of patients with AIS[10,17-22] (Fig. 28-2). Many authors have examined the interplay between the pelvis and the spine.[10,20,23-28] They have demonstrated a well-established relationship between the three previously described pelvic variables and spinal sagittal alignment parameters, whereby PI = SS + PT and LL = PI + 9 degrees (± 9 degrees). These and equations described by Lafage et al,[29] which predict that postoperative PT and SVA and are based on total LL correction to be obtained (LL = PI + 9 degrees), can be used to achieve values near established norms to maximize patient outcome. AIS is rarely associated with global malalignment (coronal and/or sagittal imbalance), because compensatory curves often restore normal posture. Unlike adult deformity in which compensatory pelvic changes (increased PT) often occur to compensate for sagittal malalignment, AIS patients commonly have normal spinopelvic parameters.

EVOLUTION OF ADOLESCENT IDIOPATHIC SCOLIOSIS SURGERY

Surgical treatment of patients with AIS has evolved substantially. Harrington[30] introduced the first generation of spinal implants for scoliosis surgery. This system exerted corrective forces through distraction of the concave side of the curve with a ratcheted bar and compression of the convex side with threaded rods and hooks. Disadvantages of Harrington instrumentation included prolonged body casting, loss of curve correction, long fusion levels, pseudarthroses, and inadequate sagittal plane correction leading to flat-back deformity.[11,12,31] Luque wires, popularized in the mid-1970s, provided segmental fixation through connection of sublaminar wires to a rod on the concavity of the curve. Deformity correction occurs through transverse traction on the periapical vertebrae as the wires are tightened, exerting corrective forces perpendicular to the axis of the rod.[31,32] In the 1980s Cotrel-Dubousset instrumentation introduced a major advancement in scoliosis surgery.[33] This system was able to produce a three-dimensional deformity correction through the concept of derotation. The use of novel hooks and lumbar pedicle screws allowed greater leverage on the vertebrae for improved correction. The use of an added device for transverse traction with Cotrel-Dubousset instrumentation, essentially acting as cross-links, further aided in deformity correction by pulling the apex of the curve toward the concavity.

Pedicle screw fixation in the thoracic spine did not gain wide acceptance early on because of concerns for neurologic and vascular injuries. Zindrick et al[34] showed that the thoracic pedicle isthmus width at T4 and T5 averaged approximately 4.5 mm and was as narrow as 2.5 mm in some specimens. Furthermore, in AIS not only are the pedicles on the concave side of the curve smaller, but the dural sac also drapes over the periapical concave vertebrae, placing it even closer to the medial wall of the pedicle.[35] However, pedicle screws have been shown to be biomechanically superior to prior forms of instrumentation.[36] Pediatric bone is more viscoelastic than that of adults, making possible placement of a screw of up to 115% of the width of the pedicle isthmus.[37] Improved fixation strength and screw purchase throughout all three columns of the spine have allowed better derotational control and curve correction in AIS patients.

INDICATIONS

NONOPERATIVE TREATMENT

Patients who present with curves smaller than 20 degrees are observed and followed every 6 months. Those with curves between 20 and 30 degrees are braced if progression of 5 degrees or more is measured between consecutive visits. Bracing is started for those who are skeletally immature (that is, Risser grade 2 or less) with curves larger than 30 degrees. If the curve apex is between T7 and L2, a thoracolumbosacral orthosis (a Boston brace) can be used. However, if the apex of the curve is above T6, a cervical extension should be included (a Milwaukee brace) for better control. Radiographs are obtained every 6 months. Approximately 50% correction should be evident on the first PA radiograph. The brace is worn until the patient is skeletally mature.

Multiple studies have shown the success of bracing compared with observation.[38,39] Recently, a prospective, multicenter study including both randomized and preference cohorts demonstrated the efficacy of bracing in patients with AIS.[40] The Bracing in Adolescent Idiopathic Scoliosis Trial (BRAIST) involved 25 institutions that evaluated skeletally immature (Risser grade 0, 1, or 2) adolescents with Cobb angles from 20 to 40 degrees. The treatment group was prescribed a thoracolumbosacral orthosis to be worn for at least 18 hours per day. Progression to 50 degrees or more was considered *treatment failure*, whereas *success* was defined as achieving skeletal maturity before reaching this amount of curvature. The trial was terminated early, because bracing was significantly more effective (72% success for bracing versus 48% success for observation).

SURGICAL INDICATIONS

The classic surgical indication is a curve of more than 50 degrees.[41,42] However, surgery is indicated for patients who fail or cannot tolerate bracing, those with curves of more than 40 degrees with thoracic lordosis, skeletally immature patients with curves from 40 to 45 degrees, or those with curves larger than 45 degrees at presentation.

Surgical goals in the treatment of AIS include obtaining and maintaining deformity correction, balancing the spine in all three planes, producing level shoulders, and minimizing the length of the construct to save motion segments.

PREOPERATIVE PLANNING

CLINICAL EVALUATION

A detailed history and physical examination are required for a diagnosis of AIS. Because AIS is a diagnosis of exclusion, a child presenting with spinal deformity provides an opportunity to reveal a previously undetected underlying condition. Family history, menarchal status, and recent growth spurts should be assessed. Caution is required with children who have back pain, because the cause can be an underlying pathologic condition.

A careful physical examination should include the dermatologic, neurologic, and musculoskeletal systems. Patients wear only their undergarments to facilitate evaluation, because an action as simple as raising the back of a shirt can alter sagittal alignment and misrepresent the true character of the deformity. Surgeons should inspect for manifestations of neurofibromatosis such as café-au-lait spots, upper and lower extremity spasticity, or evidence of an underlying tumor. Postural asymmetry is assessed in the supine and standing positions. Patients with AIS frequently manifest shoulder or waist asymmetry, rib prominence, trunk rotation, shoulder rounding, and sagittal and coronal head malalignment. Pelvic tilt should be corrected with block lifts during analysis of clinical imbalance in the coronal plane. A plumb line extended from the C7 spinous process should fall in line with the gluteal cleft. Assessment of sagittal alignment includes evaluation of forward-bending and backward-bending posture, loss of cervical and lumbar lordosis, thoracic hypokyphosis or hyperkyphosis, and hip or knee flexion postures. An Adam's forward bend test often reveals a right thoracic rib hump, which is characteristic of AIS.

RADIOGRAPHIC EVALUATION AND CLASSIFICATION

Standing 36-inch long-cassette PA and lateral radiographs are obtained. A PA view is taken with the patient's arms in a neutral, slightly abducted position, with the hips and knees extended to neutral. It should include the base of the skull and end just caudal to the lesser trochanters. A lateral film is taken of the patient in the same position; however, the arms are elevated in the sagittal plane with the humeri parallel to the floor. The breasts and gonadal region are shielded to limit radiation exposure.[43] Right and left supine side-bending films are useful for determining the flexibility of compensatory curves.[44] The Cobb angle is measured for each curve in both the coronal and sagittal planes. This angle is formed by the intersection of a line parallel to the superior endplate of the most tilted cranial end vertebra and a line parallel to the inferior endplate of the most tilted caudal end vertebra of a given curve.

The classification of AIS has evolved slowly. The original classification, described by Ponseti and Friedman,[45] was based on the number of curves and their respective apical locations. Specific curve patterns were thought to be correctible with predictable natural histories.[45] The classification system of King et al[45a] incorporated the size and flexibility of the curve pattern. Unlike the Ponseti and Friedman classification, this system guides treatment using Harrington instrumentation. However, the King system had limited applications, poor intraobserver and interobserver reliability, and potential postoperative decompensation.[46,47] Although both of these classification systems appreciated the rotational component of the deformity, neither involved the sagittal profile. The currently accepted and widely used classification described by Lenke et al[48] was the first to include the sagittal plane (Table 28-1). This system has three major components. The first consists of six curve types in the coronal plane based on the location or locations of the structural curve or curves. By definition, structural curves lack normal flexibility, as evaluated on supine side-bending radiographs. The second component, the lumbar modifier, is based on the relation of the center sacral vertical line to the lumbar apical vertebra. The sagittal thoracic modifier is the final component, which describes each curve as hypokyphotic, normal, or hyperkyphotic.[48,49]

Table 28-1   Classification of Adolescent Idiopathic Scoliosis by Lenke et al

Type	Curve Type			Curve Type
	Proximal Thoracic	**Main Thoracic**	**Thoracolumbar/ lumbar**	
1	Nonstructural	Structural (major*)	Nonstructural	Main thoracic (MT)
2	Structural	Structural (major*)	Nonstructural	Double thoracic (DT)
3	Nonstructural	Structural (major*)	Structural	Double major (DM)
4	Structural	Structural (major*)	Structural	Triple major (TM)
5	Nonstructural	Nonstructural	Structural (major*)	Thoracolumbar/lumbar (TL/L)
6	Nonstructural	Structural	Structural (major*)	Thoracolumbar/lumbar–main thoracic (TL/L-MT)

*Major = Largest Cobb measurement, always structural.
Minor = All other curves with structural criteria applied.

Structural Criteria (minor curves)

Proximal thoracic: Side-bending Cobb ≥25 degrees
        T2-5 kyphosis ≥ +20 degrees

Main thoracic: Side-bending Cobb ≥2 degrees
        T10-L2 kyphosis ≥ +20 degrees

Thoracolumbar/lumbar: Side-bending Cobb ≥25 degrees
        T10-L2 kyphosis ≥ +20 degrees

Location of Apex (SRS definition)

Curve	Apex
Thoracic	T2-11/12 disc
Thoracolumbar	T12-L1
Lumbar	L1-2 disc to L4

Modifiers

Lumbar Spine Modifier	CSVL to Lumbar Apex		Thoracic Sagittal Profile T5-12	
A	CSVL between pedicles		− (hypo)	<10 degrees
B	CSVL touches apical body or bodies		N (normal)	10-40 degrees
C	CSVL completely medial		+ (hyper)	>40 degrees

Curve type (1-6) + Lumbar spine modifier (A, B, or C) + Thoracic sagittal modifier (−, N, or +)
Classification (for example, 1B+): _____

From Lenke LG, Betz RR, Harms J, et al. Adolescent idiopathic scoliosis: a new classification to determine extent of spinal arthrodesis. J Bone Joint Surg Am 83:1169-1181, 2001.
CSVL, Center sacral vertical line; *SRS,* Scoliosis Research Society.

When planning an operation, a surgeon should evaluate each vertebra intended for instrumentation. If a CT scan is obtained, measurement of the pedicle width on axial images can help to estimate screw dimensions and trajectories. Levels that might be unsafe for pedicle screw insertion can be identified, indicating a possible need for alternative instrumentation at particular levels. Preoperative planning in this way can help to mitigate the risk of misplaced screws and neurovascular injury.[50-52]

SELECTION OF FUSION LEVELS

The selection of fusion levels in AIS patients varies substantially. Preoperative planning is of utmost importance to identify flexible versus structural curves. In general, all major and structural curves should be included in the arthrodesis, along with most lumbar modifier C curves.[48,49] Selective fusion of only the structural curves is important, because nearly 70% spontaneous correction of the compensatory curves can be expected.[53] If these principles are followed, fusion levels will generally extend from the upper end vertebra to the lower end vertebra of the structural curves; however, the goals of surgery include making the shoulders level and preserving motion segments. Therefore the choice of upper instrumented vertebra will depend largely on preoperative shoulder balance. Saving motion segments cranially is not as big a concern because of the relative rigidity of the thoracic spine. Kuklo et al[54] described the clavicle angle, which is the intersection of a tangential line from the highest aspects of both clavicles and a horizontal line. This is a reliable predictor of postoperative shoulder balance. A positive angle, which indicates left shoulder elevation, is an indication to include at least part of the proximal thoracic curve (for example, to T2) to prevent further postoperative shoulder imbalance. Conversely, the upper instrumented vertebra in a patient with left shoulder depression may be lower (for example, to T4), because correction of the structural main thoracic curve will cause compensatory correction proximally and elevation of the left shoulder. Patients with level shoulders preoperatively can be instrumented up to T3.

The distal end of a construct is often a more challenging decision, because motion segments should be spared without risking postoperative decompensation. Constructs should be as short as possible, because unfused discs in long constructs can be susceptible to degeneration and potential pain generation, although the latter is not entirely clear.[55-57] The Lenke classification is useful in helping to select the lower instrumented vertebra. Because Lenke types 3, 4, 5, and 6 include structural thoracolumbar/lumbar curves, these should be included in the fusion. In such circumstances the lower instrumented vertebra is generally the distal end vertebra. Additionally, types 1 and 2 with lumbar modifier C, in which the apical body does not touch the center sacral vertical line, should be instrumented. Conversely, type 1 and 2 curves with lumbar A or B modifiers should be excluded from the fusion unless kyphosis is greater than 20 degrees in the thoracolumbar region.[49] In these situations, the uppermost vertebra that touches the center sacral vertical line is chosen as the lower instrumented vertebra as long as it is not within the apex of the curve and the vertebra is not substantially rotated.

OPERATIVE TECHNIQUE

PATIENT POSITIONING AND EXPOSURE

Nearly all patients with AIS can be treated through a posterior approach. Those classified with Lenke 1A and Lenke 6CN AIS can be selectively approached anteriorly, whereas Lenke 5CN deformity nearly always requires an anterior approach. Neurophysiologic monitoring is performed in almost all patients.

The patient is positioned prone on a radiolucent spine table, with the abdomen hanging freely, the eyes protected from undue pressure, and all bony prominences well padded. A standard posterior incision is centered over the intended instrumented levels. Dissection is carried out laterally and subperiosteally to minimize bleeding and soft tissue injury. Once adequate exposure and hemostasis are obtained, fluoroscopy or radiography can be used to verify the appropriate vertebral levels. An inferior facetectomy is then performed with a half-inch osteotome at all but the most caudal level of the construct. This step allows better identification of pedicle screw starting points, provides a source of local autograft bone, and improves the chance the fusion.

INSTRUMENTATION

The order of instrumentation is a matter of surgeon preference; however, starting at the lower instrumented vertebra is often preferable because of the larger pedicles distally and relatively minor vertebral rotation at the end of the construct. Instrumentation then proceeds cranially. The natural progression of pedicle morphology, starting point, and trajectory guide the surgeon for the subsequent levels.

Pedicle screws can be placed using either anatomic landmarks or under fluoroscopic assistance. Suk et al[53] described their stepwise, freehand technique of placing pedicle screws in the thoracic spine. The first step involves exposure laterally to the ends of the transverse processes, followed by removal of 3 to 5 mm of the inferior facet with either an osteotome or rongeur. A 3.5 mm burr is then used to perforate the cortex for the starting point of the intended level. A gearshift is then placed through the soft cancellous bone within the pedicle for approximately 15 to 20 mm with the tip pointing laterally. It is removed and reinserted with the curve of the gearshift pointing medially, ensuring that the tip of the instrument has passed the spinal canal. A pedicle probe is then used to palpate the floor and medial, lateral, superior, and inferior bony borders of the pedicle to confirm that the walls have not been breached. A hemostat is used to mark the depth of the probe, and the pedicle screw length is measured. Next, the pathway is undertapped by 0.5 mm of the diameter of the intended screw to be inserted. The bony borders are palpated with the probe to feel the ridges of the tapped pathway and check for pedicle wall penetration. A screw with the appropriate length and diameter is then slowly advanced, maximizing the viscoelastic properties of the pediatric pedicle. Despite a 6.2% cortical penetration rate, no neurologic, visceral, or vascular complications were observed in 3204 placed screws with this procedure.

Successful pedicle screw placement in the scoliotic spine is highly dependent on the surgeon's level of experience. Pedicles in AIS are usually smaller and can have a windswept deformity, making safe insertion more challenging.[37] Fluoroscopy can facilitate identification of appropriate starting points and mitigate the risk of misplacement. Lee et al[58] described a technique that involves rotation of the C-arm. It resulted in a 2.2% medial cortex penetration rate with no neurologic or vascular complications. The C-arm is rotated in the transverse plane until the pedicles are symmetrical and a true PA view of the rotated vertebral body is obtained. Next, the endplate shadows are overlapped, and the superior and inferior endplates are made parallel to each other by adjusting the C-arm in the sagittal plane. The pedicles are then seen en face, and a radiopaque instrument can be used to identify the appropriate starting point within the pedicle. This technique of direct vertebral rotation is described in detail in the next section.

CORRECTIVE MANEUVERS

After instrumentation of the structural curve or curves, a variety of corrective maneuvers can be performed. Options include rod rotation, in situ bending, and direct vertebral rotation. Rod rotation is a good maneuver for patients with thoracic scoliosis and hypokyphosis. A rod is prebent to the desired final sagittal contour and placed into the screws on the concavity of the curvature (Fig. 28-3). If, however, the spine is hyperkyphotic, the rod is placed into the convexity. First, posteriorly and medially directed forces are applied to the rod, which is then rotated on itself with a 90-degree counterclockwise rotation, effectively correcting the coronal and sagittal deformities. This rod is then locked into the screws, and a second sagittally contoured rod is inserted on the contralateral side.

In situ rod contouring is another strategy to correct a deformity. With this technique, one rod is initially placed into the screws on the concavity of the curve, and specialized rod benders are used to correct the coronal curvature (Fig. 28-4). A rod is then added on the contralateral side, and set screws are placed to maintain correction. Alternatively, cantilever bending forces, applied first to the convex side of the curve, can be especially useful in cases of hyperkyphosis. The deformity is corrected with several adjustments before the rods are locked. While the bending forces correct the coronal deformity, pushing down on the spine simultaneously restores the appropriate sagittal alignment.

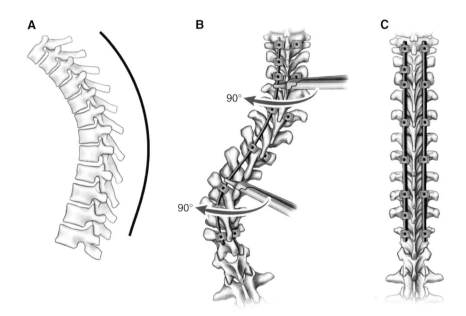

Fig. 28-3   Rod rotation maneuver. **A** and **B,** The rod is prebent to the desired final sagittal contour and placed into the screws on the concavity of the curvature. The concave rod is placed first in cases of typical thoracic hypokyphosis and rotated 90 degrees on itself to correct both the coronal and sagittal deformities. **C,** The rod is locked into the screws, and a second sagittally contoured rod is inserted on the contralateral side.

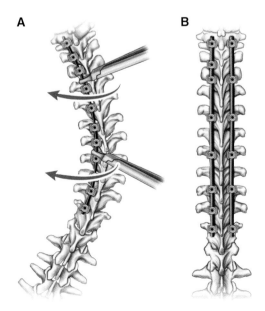

Fig. 28-4   In situ rod bending. **A,** A rod is placed into the screws on the concavity of the curve, and the specialized rod benders are used to correct the coronal deformity. **B,** A rod on the contralateral side is then inserted, and the set screws placed to maintain correction.

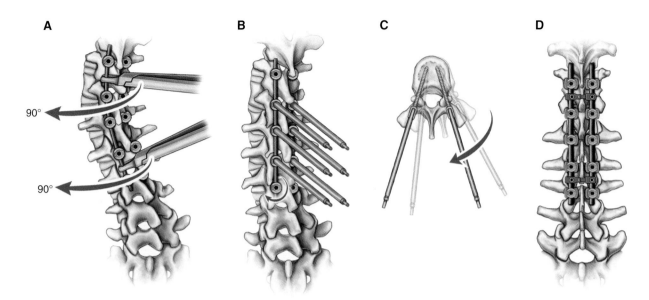

Fig. 28-5   Direct vertebral rotation is achieved by attaching multiple derotators to the periapical pedicle screws. The reduction maneuver consists of rotating the spine in the direction opposite of vertebral rotation. **A,** A precontoured rod on the concave side is derotated in the counterclockwise direction. **B** and **C,** Several screw derotators are connected to the periapical pedicle screws. The screw derotators are then turned in the direction opposite that of vertebral rotation. **D,** A concave rod is locked in place, followed by a contoured rod on the contralateral side. Cross-links are inserted to connect the two rods.

Direct vertebral rotation, described by Lee et al,[58] is a powerful technique for correcting three-dimensional deformity. The basis of this procedure is that scoliotic vertebrae are substantially rotated in the transverse plane. Additionally, pedicle screws achieve three-column fixation and transmit derotational forces that are applied posteriorly by the surgeon through the entire vertebra. By applying derotational forces in addition to rod rotation maneuvers, a surgeon is able to correct the spine in all three affected planes. First, pedicle screws are placed at each level on the concave side and at approximately every other vertebra on the convex side. A precontoured rod on the concave side is then derotated in the counterclockwise direction. Several screw derotators are connected to the periapical pedicle screws. The use of multiple derotators distributes the torque applied through several pedicles and decreases the risk of iatrogenic fracture. The screw derotators are then turned in the direction opposite of vertebral rotation (Fig. 28-5). The concave rod is locked in followed by the contoured rod on the contralateral side. Finally, cross-links are inserted to connect the two rods. If a compensatory lumbar curve is present that crosses the center sacral vertical line, the distalmost one or two lumbar screws should be derotated in the direction opposite the thoracic derotation. The authors demonstrated significantly better coronal and rotational spinal balance using this technique, compared with simple rod derotation.

ARTHRODESIS AND CLOSURE

After completion of all instrumentation and corrective maneuvers, arthrodesis is carried out. The spinous processes, excluding the end levels, are removed. Sleeves of bone are removed from the laminae with a curved osteotome. The posterior elements are decorticated with a high-speed burr. The previously harvested local autograft bone is applied to the fusion bed in addition to allograft per the surgeon's preference. Iliac crest autograft is not used if possible to minimize morbidity and to not complicate pelvic fixation, should it be necessary in the future.

A deep and superficial drain is placed, the wound closed in layers with absorbable sutures, and a sterile dressing applied. Perioperative antibiotics are continued for 24 hours. Patients are allowed to ambulate on the first postoperative day under the supervision of a physical therapist.

OPERATIVE CONSIDERATIONS

ADJUNCTIVE PROCEDURES

Several concomitant procedures are useful to either increase the flexibility of the spine and/or correct deformity. The inferior facetectomies performed during the exposure are beneficial not only for the reasons stated previously, but also to release the facet joints, which will increase the surgeon's ability to achieve the desired spinal alignment. Open or thoracoscopic anterior releases involving a discectomy and fusion can also improve the flexibility of the thoracic spine. This can be considered in severe and rigid curves of 70 degrees or more that demonstrate less than 50% correction on preoperative bending films. Anterior releases are infrequently necessary given the greater control of the vertebral column obtained with pedicle screw fixation.

A Ponte osteotomy, originally described for the treatment of thoracic hyperkyphosis, can be applied in AIS to mobilize rigid areas of the apex of the curve.[59] Although thoracic hypokyphosis is the usual sagittal plane deformity in these patients, this osteotomy can be used in less frequent cases with positive sagittal malalignment. In this procedure, the spinous processes are shortened, and the facets, ligamentum flavum, and interspinous ligaments are excised. The resulting chevron-shaped osteotomies can be increased in the craniocaudal direction and/or asymmetrically to achieve the indicated correction. Rods are placed proximally, the posterior column is shortened and compressed, and distal anchoring is carried out. Conversely, the posterior releases created by a Ponte osteotomy can help to restore appropriate sagittal alignment in a hypokyphotic spine. As the posterior bony and soft tissue restraints are released, distraction and lengthening of the posterior column will impart a kyphogenic effect on the thoracic spine.[60]

A convex rib hump can remain despite corrective maneuvers and is often a cosmetic concern in adolescents. Suk et al[53] described a thoracoplasty technique that achieves significantly better rib hump correction, compared with control groups. Through the same posterior incision, lateral dissection is carried out over the convex side beneath the fascia. Development of the interval between the iliocostalis and longissimus muscles exposes the apices of the convex ribs. After subperiosteal elevation, 4 to 5 cm of length is resected from ribs four through eight, depending on the severity of the rib hump. The remaining rib can be sutured to the transverse process or convex rod to stabilize the rib cage. The resected rib can be morselized and applied as bone graft.

SAGITTAL ALIGNMENT

Special attention should be given to the sagittal profile of the spine. Previous efforts focused primarily on coronal curve correction; however, the restoration of appropriate sagittal balance has been increasingly recognized as a critical factor for overall spine health. Thoracic hypokyphosis is the typical sagittal malalignment in AIS and is believed to result from relative anterior spinal overgrowth.[6,61-63] During deformity correction, surgeons should aim to restore normal thoracic kyphosis (20 to 40 degrees), preserve the thoracolumbar junction (T10-L2) neutral to slightly lordotic, and maintain lumbar lordosis. Procedures that decrease thoracic kyphosis will lead to further loss of lumbar lordosis.[60] Lengthening the posterior column and/or shortening the anterior column will help to appropriately balance the spine.

Multiple strategies can be employed to achieve a sagittally balanced spine. Patient positioning and an approach are the first consideration. Prone positioning on an open spine table has a lordosing effect on the thoracic spine. This is minimized by strategic bolster placement. An anterior approach with anterior spinal column compression/instrumentation has been shown to increase thoracic kyphosis more than posterior procedures.[64-66] Rhee et al[64] demonstrated a small, yet significant difference between anterior and posterior procedures (+4 degrees versus −2 degrees). The authors concluded that a properly performed procedure can correct sagittal alignment through either approach; however, the kyphogenic effect of anterior surgery should be considered in preoperative planning.

Other techniques to reduce thoracic hypokyphosis include avoiding posterior column compression and contouring the rods to the desired sagittal profile. As described previously, the flexibility of the posterior spine can be improved with Ponte-type osteotomies, with subsequent distraction and lengthening of the posterior column. Simultaneous translation on two rods, known as *ST2R*, is another method of restoring normal kyphosis. Multiple polyaxial pedicle screws with threaded extension rods are inserted and connected at a distance to two contoured titanium rods. The nuts on the threaded rods are alternatively and gradually tightened, which translates the anchored screws and vertebrae dorsally to the rods. This maneuver simultaneously improves kyphosis and reduces the coronal deformity. The authors gained an average of 27 degrees of kyphosis in patients with severe preoperative hypokyphosis (less than or equal to 10 degrees).[67]

NEUROMONITORING

The advent of rigid fixation systems has facilitated the ability to correct even the most complex spinal deformities. However, strong corrective forces pose serious risks to the integrity of neural elements. Spinal cord injury is a devastating complication of scoliosis correction surgery, with reported incidences between 0.3% to 17%.[68-72] Risk factors for neurologic injury include marked kyphosis, congenital scoliosis, preexisting neurologic impairment, and preoperative traction. Mechanisms of injury include misdirected instrumentation causing direct trauma, traction injury from overzealous correction, and cord ischemia from vessel occlusion. Surgeons have used various intraoperative techniques to monitor for impending neural injury.

The Stagnara wake-up test has been employed since the 1970s as an intraoperative tool to assess neurologic function. This test involves decreasing the level of anesthesia and instructing the patient to perform motor movements in both the upper and lower extremities. Failure to carry out specified motor tasks implies a neurologic injury. The advantages of this test are the lack of cost and its direct assessment of global neural functioning. However, the test's utility is undermined by factors related to the rehearsal process, such as the patient's understanding of the instructions, the number of times, and how recently the test was rehearsed, variable patient recall, added surgical time, and risks of complications such as inadvertent extubation, air embolism, pain, motion with loss of fixation, and false-negative and false-positive results. Hoppenfeld et al[73] described a simple and cost-effective assessment, the ankle clonus test. Ankle clonus is normally absent in an awake patient because of upper motor neuron inhibitory signals. Because patients recover from anesthesia in stages, bilateral ankle clonus can be elicited, theoretically, during the early stages of awakening, before the return of the inhibitory signals. The absence of this finding is an indicator of neurologic injury. Unfortunately, neither the wake-up test or the ankle clonus test allows real-time, continuous monitoring of spinal cord function. Furthermore, they only reflect global spinal integrity and provide no information to pinpoint the threatened spinal tracts. This lag time between injury and detection results in a missed window of opportunity for interventions that can prevent a transient insult from becoming a permanent deficit.

The drawbacks of the wake-up and ankle clonus tests have led to the development of continuous multimodal intraoperative monitoring of spinal cord function in patients having corrective scoliosis surgery. The clinical use of somatosensory evoked potentials (SSEPs) during scoliosis surgery was first described in 1977.[74] SSEPs reflect the status of the dorsal columns through monitoring of peripheral nerves, typically the posterior tibial and peroneal nerves and the ulnar nerve for the lower and upper extremities, respectively. A more modern technique involves monitoring the ventral corticospinal tracts with transcranial motor evoked potentials (TcMEPs). Together, SSEPs and TcMEPs allow real-time analysis of the integrity of dorsal and ventral spinal cord functions throughout a procedure. Kundnani et al[75] reported that neuromonitoring events occurred in 3.67% of cases of AIS surgery when both SSEPs and TcMEPs were used. The authors concluded that SSEPs are more specific and TcMEPs are more sensitive, whereas their combined potential sensitivity and specificity approaches 100%. Thuet et al[76] demonstrated that multimodal neuromonitoring detected events that led to permanent neurologic deficits in 99.6% of cases. In a more recent study evaluating intraoperative neuromonitoring events during spinal corrective surgery for idiopathic scoliosis, Buckwalter et al[77] observed a 3.6% rate of neuromonitoring changes when using both SSEPs and TcMEPs. In 86% of cases with an intraoperative neuromonitoring event, potentials returned to baseline after intervention maneuvers were performed. These and other studies have conclusively shown that multimodal intraoperative neuromonitoring accurately detects impending neurologic compromise and facilitates timely responses to protect neurologic function.[78]

POTENTIAL COMPLICATIONS AND MANAGEMENT

NEUROLOGIC INJURY

According to the latest publication from the Scoliosis Research Society morbidity and mortality database, the overall complication rate from surgery for idiopathic scoliosis is 6.3%.[72] The rate of death in children undergoing scoliosis surgery is 0.13%, with the primary cause of death stemming from respiratory complications.[78] Aside from the unlikely chance of mortality, the most serious complication of AIS surgery is the development of a new neurologic deficit. Reames et al[72] reported an overall 0.8% rate of neurologic deficits in AIS patients, with complete spinal cord injury occurring in 0.05% of the cases. Additionally, transient nerve root and incomplete cord injury occurred at rates of 0.3% and 0.4%, respectively. Fu et al[78] demonstrated that most patients with a new neurologic deficit recovered completely or partially, whereas only 5% of those affected had no recovery.

During intraoperative neuromonitoring, changes in waveform signals should alert surgeons to a potential injury. An identifiable cause should be sought and interventions initiated. Surgeons should have a preestablished algorithm for efficient and timely troubleshooting if signals change unexpectedly. Simple actions such as checking the wire connections and electrode placement, reversing excessive correction, and removing hardware can return signals to baseline. Complications related to screw malinsertion are well-documented.[79,80] When subtle maneuvers are ineffective, it may help to raise the mean arterial pressure above 80 to 90 mm Hg, correct temperature and metabolic derangements, and/or administer steroid boluses.[81] Appropriate preoperative planning and the use of pedicle screw stimulation are precautionary measures against technique-related problems.

INFECTION

Overall, the rates of surgical site infection (SSI) in AIS surgery range from 0.5% to 6.7%.[82] The most frequently isolated organisms are Staphylococcal followed by Pseudomonal species.[78] Prophylactic intrawound vancomycin powder has been shown to be effective in reducing SSIs in adult spine patients[83,84]; its utility in the pediatric population, however, has not been evaluated. SSI can be classified as superficial or deep, with reported rates of 0.5% and 0.8%, respectively.[72] The treatment and outcomes differ. Most authors recommend hardware removal for delayed, deep infections. However, the lack of consensus on the definition of delayed SSI has created controversies regarding the timing of hardware explantation.[85-88]

In general, acute, deep SSIs can be treated with aggressive irrigation and debridement with retention of hardware to prevent loss of deformity correction and potential spinal instability.[82] Removal or retention of bone graft is determined on a case-by-case basis. Such patients require long-term parenteral antibiotics for 4 to 6 weeks, followed by oral suppression for 2 to 6 months. Primary closure over drains or the use of negative pressure vacuum dressings has proved effective.[89-91] In contrast to acute infections, most surgeons agree that if arthrodesis is stable, implant removal is necessary for complete eradication of delayed SSIs.[78] These patients should be counseled regarding the risk of curve progression and the possible need for future revision surgery.[88,92,93] Most of these wounds can be closed over drains and infections eradicated with a short course of parenteral (2 to 5 days) and subsequent oral antibiotics for 7 to 14 days.[82]

PATIENT EXAMPLE

This patient was diagnosed with scoliosis at the age of 15 years. At the time of her diagnosis, the curve was approximately 18 degrees. When she was 19 years old, the curve measured 48 degrees, and 2 months later it was 59 degrees (Fig. 28-6, *A* and *B; Table* 28-2). She had mild discomfort in her back but only when lying down for long periods of time. She had no radiating pain in her lower extremities, a right trunk shift, and a large right rib prominence. The patient was scheduled for another office visit in 6 months, at which time her curve from T5-L1 measured 67 degrees, as shown on bending films (Fig. 28-6, *C* and *D*). Posterior spinal instrumentation and fusion was performed from T4-L1. Six months postoperatively the patient has started physical therapy and is doing well. She has no weakness, numbness, or radiating pain. Her postoperative radiographs show the hardware in place with no signs of loosening. Coronal and sagittal alignment are unchanged, and her curve Cobb angle is 15 degrees (Fig. 28-6, *E* and *F*; see Table 28-2).

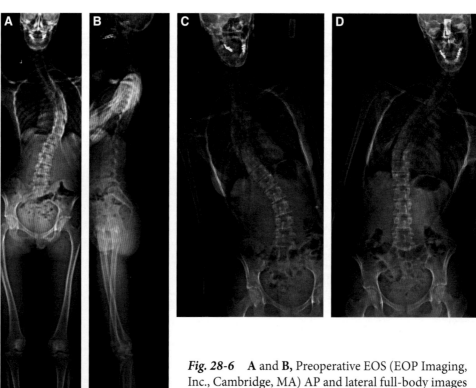

Fig. 28-6   **A** and **B,** Preoperative EOS (EOP Imaging, Inc., Cambridge, MA) AP and lateral full-body images showed a Lenke 1 main thoracic curve and a Cobb angle of 59 degrees. **C** and **D,** Preoperative bending films showed a 67-degree curvature from T5-L1.

Table 28-2 Sagittal Plane Measurements

Parameter	Preoperative Value	Postoperative Value
Sagittal vertical axis	−35 mm	−35 mm
Thoracic kyphosis T4-1 (degrees)	0	13.5
Lumbar lordosis (degrees)	36	50
Pelvic tilt (degrees)	6.4	0
Pelvic incidence (degrees)	31	31

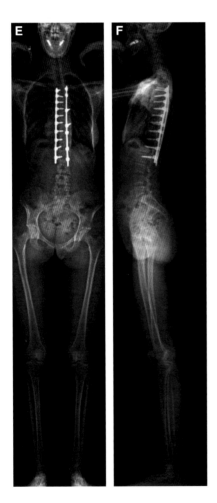

Fig. 28-6, cont'd **E** and **F,** Six-month postoperative AP and lateral EOS full-body images. Her postoperative Cobb angle is 15 degrees. (Images courtesy of Thomas Errico, MD.)

CONCLUSION

Although scoliosis is classically defined as a coronal curve larger than 10 degrees, it has become evident that the condition is truly a multiplanar deformity. Additionally, the concept of *spinopelvic balance* has revolutionized the assessment and treatment of spinal deformities. As instrumentation evolved, surgeons obtained greater control of the spine with better techniques for deformity correction. A thorough understanding of the Lenke classification will guide surgeons in differentiating structural from compensatory curves and in identifying regions of the deformity that should be included in an arthrodesis. Appreciation of the intimate relationship between the pelvis and spine, along with thoughtful preoperative planning and carefully exacted reduction techniques, should allow surgeons to restore normal spinal alignment. Appropriate spinal balance achieved in this way will maximize the chance of a successful outcome.

REFERENCES

1. Kane WJ. Scoliosis prevalence: a call for a statement of terms. Clin Orthop Rel Res 43-46, 1977.
2. Yagi M, Machida M, Asazuma T. Pathogenesis of adolescent idiopathic scoliosis. J Bone Joint Surg Reviews 2:e2, 2014.
3. Le Febvre J, Triboulet-Chassevant A, Missirliu MF. Electromyographic data in idiopathic scoliosis. Arch Phys Medicine Rehabil 42:710-711, 1961.
4. Saatok T, Dahlberg E, Bylund P, et al. Steroid hormone receptors, protein, and DNA in erector spinae muscle from scoliotic patients. Clin Orthop Relat Res 197-207, 1984.
5. Kindsfater K, Lowe T, Lawellin D, et al. Levels of platelet calmodulin for the prediction of progression and severity of adolescent idiopathic scoliosis. J Bone Joint Surg Am 76:1186-1192, 1994.
6. Machida M, Dubousset J, Imamura Y, et al. Melatonin. A possible role in pathogenesis of adolescent idiopathic scoliosis. Spine 21:1147-1152, 1996.
7. Somerville EW. Rotational lordosis; the development of single curve. J Bone Joint Surg Br 34:421-427, 1952.
8. Mac-Thiong JM, Labelle H, Berthonnaud E, et al. Sagittal spinopelvic balance in normal children and adolescents. Eur Spine J 16:227-234, 2007.
9. Vedantam R, Lenke LG, Keeney JA, et al. Comparison of standing sagittal spinal alignment in asymptomatic adolescents and adults. Spine 23:211-215, 1998.
10. Schwab F, Lafage V, Patel A, et al. Sagittal plane considerations and the pelvis in the adult patient. Spine 34:1828-1833, 2009.
10a. Duval-Beaupère G, Legaye J. Composante sagittale de la statique rachidienne (in French). Rev Rhum 71:105, 2004.
11. Lagrone MO, Bradford DS, Moe JH, et al. Treatment of symptomatic flatback after spinal fusion. J Bone Joint Surg Am 70:569-580, 1988.
12. La Grone MO. Loss of lumbar lordosis. A complication of spinal fusion for scoliosis. Orthop Clin North Am 19:383-393, 1988.
12a. Dubousset J. Importance de la vertèbre pelvienne dans l'équilibre rachidien. Application à la chirurgie de la colonne vertébrale chez l'enfant et l'adolescent. In Villeneuve P, ed. Pied Équilibre et Rachis. Paris: Frison-Roche, 1998.
13. Aaro S, Ohlen G. The effect of Harrington instrumentation on sagittal configuration and mobility of the spine in scoliosis. Spine 8:570-575, 1983.
14. Kostuik JP, Hall BB. Spinal fusions to the sacrum in adults with scoliosis. Spine 8:489-500, 1983.
15. Gottfried ON, Daubs MD, Patel AA, et al. Spinopelvic parameters in postfusion flatback deformity patients. Spine J 9:639-647, 2009.
16. Vitale MG, Colacchio ND, Matsumoto H, et al. Flatback revisited? Reciprocal loss of lumbar lordosis following selective thoracic fusion. Presented at the Forty-sixth Annual Meeting of the Scoliosis Research Society, Louisville, KY, Sept 2011.
17. Lafage V, Schwab F, Patel A, et al. Pelvic tilt and truncal inclination: two key radiographic parameters in the setting of adults with spinal deformity. Spine 34:E599-E606, 2009.
18. Schwab FJ, Smith VA, Biserni M, et al. Adult scoliosis: a quantitative radiographic and clinical analysis. Spine 27:387-392, 2002.

19. Schwab F, Dubey A, Pagala M, et al. Adult scoliosis: a health assessment analysis by SF-36. Spine 28:602-606, 2003.
20. Schwab F, Farcy JP, Bridwell K, et al. A clinical impact classification of scoliosis in the adult. Spine 31:2109-2114, 2006.
21. Glassman SD, Bridwell K, Dimar JR, et al. The impact of positive sagittal balance in adult spinal deformity. Spine 30:2024-2029, 2005.
22. Glassman SD, Berven S, Bridwell K, et al. Correlation of radiographic parameters and clinical symptoms in adult scoliosis. Spine 30:682-688, 2005.
23. Jackson RP, Peterson MD, McManus AC, et al. Compensatory spinopelvic balance over the hip axis and better reliability in measuring lordosis to the pelvic radius on standing lateral radiographs of adult volunteers and patients. Spine 23:1750-1767, 1998.
24. Labelle H, Roussouly P, Berthonnaud E, et al. The importance of spino-pelvic balance in L5-s1 developmental spondylolisthesis: a review of pertinent radiologic measurements. Spine 30:S27-S34, 2005.
25. Legaye J, Duval-Beaupère G. Sagittal plane alignment of the spine and gravity: a radiological and clinical evaluation. Acta Orthop Belg 71:213-220, 2005.
26. Schwab F, Lafage V, Boyce R, et al. Gravity line analysis in adult volunteers: age-related correlation with spinal parameters, pelvic parameters, and foot position. Spine 31:E959-E967, 2006.
27. Vialle R, Levassor N, Rillardon L, et al. Radiographic analysis of the sagittal alignment and balance of the spine in asymptomatic subjects. J Bone Joint Surg Am 87:260-267, 2005.
28. Lafage V, Schwab F, Skalli W, et al. Standing balance and sagittal plane spinal deformity: analysis of spinopelvic and gravity line parameters. Spine 33:1572-1578, 2008.
29. Lafage V, Schwab F, Vira S, et al. Spino-pelvic parameters after surgery can be predicted: a preliminary formula and validation of standing alignment. Spine 36:1037-1045, 2011.
30. Harrington PR. Treatment of scoliosis. Correction and internal fixation by spine instrumentation. J Bone Joint Surg Am 44:591-610, 1962.
31. Potter BK, Lenke LG, Kuklo TR. Prevention and management of iatrogenic flatback deformity. J Bone Joint Surg Am 86:1793-1808, 2004.
32. Luque ER. Segmental spinal instrumentation for correction of scoliosis. Clin Orthop Relat Res 163:192-198, 1982.
33. Cotrel Y, Dubousset J, Guillaumat M. New universal instrumentation in spinal surgery. Clin Orthop Relat Res 227:10-23, 1988.
34. Zindrick MR, Wiltse LL, Doornik A, et al. Analysis of the morphometric characteristics of the thoracic and lumbar pedicles. Spine 12:160-166, 1987.
35. Parent S, Labelle H, Skalli W, et al. Thoracic pedicle morphometry in vertebrae from scoliotic spines. Spine 29:239-248, 2004.
36. Hackenberg L, Link T, Liljenqvist U. Axial and tangential fixation strength of pedicle screws versus hooks in the thoracic spine in relation to bone mineral density. Spine 27:937-942, 2002.
37. O'Brien MF, Lenke LG, Mardjetko S, et al. Pedicle morphology in thoracic adolescent idiopathic scoliosis: is pedicle fixation an anatomically viable technique? Spine 25:2285-2293, 2000.
38. Nachemson AL, Peterson LE. Effectiveness of treatment with a brace in girls who have adolescent idiopathic scoliosis. A prospective, controlled study based on data from the Brace Study of the Scoliosis Research Society. J Bone Joint Surg Am 77:815-822, 1995.
39. Rowe DE, Bernstein SM, Riddick MF, et al. A meta-analysis of the efficacy of non-operative treatments for idiopathic scoliosis. J Bone Joint Surg Am 79:664-674, 1997.
40. Weinstein SL, Dolan LA, Wright JG, et al. Effects of bracing in adolescents with idiopathic scoliosis. New Engl J Med 369:1512-1521, 2013.
41. Lagrone MO, King HA. Idiopathic adolescent scoliosis: indications and expectations. In Bridwell KH, DeWald RL, eds. The Textbook of Spinal Surgery, ed 2. Philadelphia: Lippincott-Raven, 1997.
42. Edgar MA, Mehta MH. Long-term follow-up of fused and unfused idiopathic scoliosis. J Bone Joint Surg Br 70:712-716, 1988.
43. Lehman L. Scoliosis and spine imaging. Radiologic Technol 79:373-377, 2008.
44. Moe JH. Methods and technique in evaluation of idiopathic scoliosis. In The American Academy of Orthopaedic Surgeons, ed. Symposium on the Spine. St Louis: Mosby, 1969.
45. Ponseti IV, Friedman B. Prognosis in idiopathic scoliosis. J Bone Joint Surg Am 32:381-395, 1950.
45a. King HA, Moe JH, Bradford DS, et al. The selection of fusion levels in thoracic idiopathic scoliosis. J Bone Joint Surg 65-A:1302-1313, 1983.

46. Padua R, Padua S, Aulisa L, et al. Patient outcomes after Harrington instrumentation for idiopathic scoliosis: a 15- to 28-year evaluation. Spine 26:1268-1273, 2001.

47. Bridwell KH, McAllister JW, Betz RR, et al. Coronal decompensation produced by Cotrel-Dubousset "derotation" maneuver for idiopathic right thoracic scoliosis. Spine 16:769-777, 1991.

48. Lenke LG, Betz RR, Harms J, et al. Adolescent idiopathic scoliosis: a new classification to determine extent of spinal arthrodesis. J Bone Joint Surg Am 83:1169-1181, 2001.

49. Lenke LG, Betz RR, Haher TR, et al. Multisurgeon assessment of surgical decision-making in adolescent idiopathic scoliosis: curve classification, operative approach, and fusion levels. Spine 26:2347-2353, 2001.

50. Gstoettner M, Lechner R, Glodny B, et al. Inter- and intraobserver reliability assessment of computed tomographic 3D measurement of pedicles in scoliosis and size matching with pedicle screws. Eur Spine J 20:1771-1779, 2011.

51. Harasymczuk P, Kotwicki T, Koch A, et al. The use of computer tomography for preoperative planning and outcome assessment in surgical treatment of idiopathic scoliosis with pedicle screw based constructs: case presentation. Orthop Traumatol Rehabil 11:577-585, 2009.

52. Liljenqvist UR, Link TM, Halm HF. Morphometric analysis of thoracic and lumbar vertebrae in idiopathic scoliosis. Spine 25:1247-1253, 2000.

53. Suk SI, Lee CK, Kim WJ, et al. Segmental pedicle screw fixation in the treatment of thoracic idiopathic scoliosis. Spine 20:1399-1405, 1995.

54. Kuklo TR, Lenke LG, Graham EJ, et al. Correlation of radiographic, clinical, and patient assessment of shoulder balance following fusion versus nonfusion of the proximal thoracic curve in adolescent idiopathic scoliosis. Spine 27:2013-2020, 2002.

55. Bartie BJ, Lonstein JE, Winter RB. Long-term follow-up of adolescent idiopathic scoliosis patients who had Harrington instrumentation and fusion to the lower lumbar vertebrae: is low back pain a problem? Spine 34:E873-E878, 2009.

56. Kuhns CA, Bridwell KH, Lenke LG, et al. Thoracolumbar deformity arthrodesis stopping at L5: fate of the L5-S1 disc, minimum 5-year follow-up. Spine 32:2771-2776, 2007.

57. Danielsson AJ, Nachemson AL. Back pain and function 23 years after fusion for adolescent idiopathic scoliosis: a case-control study-part II. Spine 28:E373-E383, 2003.

58. Lee SM, Suk SI, Chung ER. Direct vertebral rotation: a new technique of three-dimensional deformity correction with segmental pedicle screw fixation in adolescent idiopathic scoliosis. Spine 29:343-349, 2004.

59. Geck MJ, Macagno A, Ponte A, et al. The Ponte procedure: posterior only treatment of Scheuermann's kyphosis using segmental posterior shortening and pedicle screw instrumentation. J Spinal Disord Tech 20:586-593, 2007.

60. Newton PO, Yaszay B, Upasani VV, et al. Preservation of thoracic kyphosis is critical to maintain lumbar lordosis in the surgical treatment of adolescent idiopathic scoliosis. Spine 35:1365-1370, 2010.

61. de Jonge T, Dubousset JF, Illes T. Sagittal plane correction in idiopathic scoliosis. Spine 27:754-760, 2002.

62. Deacon P, Archer IA, Dickson RA. The anatomy of spinal deformity: a biomechanical analysis. Orthopedics 10:897-903, 1987.

63. Dickson RA. The aetiology of spinal deformities. Lancet 1:1151-1155, 1988.

64. Rhee JM, Bridwell KH, Won DS, et al. Sagittal plane analysis of adolescent idiopathic scoliosis: the effect of anterior versus posterior instrumentation. Spine 27:2350-2356, 2002.

65. Muschik MT, Kimmich H, Demmel T. Comparison of anterior and posterior double-rod instrumentation for thoracic idiopathic scoliosis: results of 141 patients. Eur Spine J 15:1128-1138, 2006.

66. Sucato DJ, Agrawal S, O'Brien MF, et al. Restoration of thoracic kyphosis after operative treatment of adolescent idiopathic scoliosis: a multicenter comparison of three surgical approaches. Spine 33:2630-2636, 2006.

67. Clement JL, Chau E, Kimkpe C, et al. Restoration of thoracic kyphosis by posterior instrumentation in adolescent idiopathic scoliosis: comparative radiographic analysis of two methods of reduction. Spine 33:1579-1587, 2008.

68. MacEwen GD, Bunnell WP, Sriram K. Acute neurological complications in the treatment of scoliosis. A report of the Scoliosis Research Society. J Bone Joint Surg Am 57:404-408, 1975.

69. Diab M, Smith AR, Kuklo TR. Neural complications in the surgical treatment of adolescent idiopathic scoliosis. Spine 32:2759-2763, 2007.

70. Coe JD, Arlet V, Donaldson W, et al. Complications in spinal fusion for adolescent idiopathic scoliosis in the new millennium. A report of the Scoliosis Research Society Morbidity and Mortality Committee. Spine 31:345-349, 2006.

71. Langeloo DD, Lelivelt A, Louis Journée H, et al. Transcranial electrical motor-evoked potential monitoring during surgery for spinal deformity: a study of 145 patients. Spine 28:1043-1050, 2003.

72. Reames DL, Smith JS, Fu KM, et al. Complications in the surgical treatment of 19,360 cases of pediatric scoliosis: a review of the Scoliosis Research Society Morbidity and Mortality database. Spine 36:1484-1491, 2011.

73. Hoppenfeld S, Gross A, Andrews C, et al. The ankle clonus test for assessment of the integrity of the spinal cord during operations for scoliosis. J Bone Joint Surg Am 79:208-212, 1997.

74. Nash CL Jr, Lorig RA, Schatzinger LA, et al. Spinal cord monitoring during operative treatment of the spine. Clin Orthop Relat Res 126:100-105, 1977.

75. Kundnani VK, Zhu L, Tak H, et al. Multimodal intraoperative neuromonitoring in corrective surgery for adolescent idiopathic scoliosis: evaluation of 354 consecutive cases. Indian J Orthop 44:64-72, 2010.

76. Thuet ED, Winscher JC, Padberg AM, et al. Validity and reliability of intraoperative monitoring in pediatric spinal deformity surgery: a 23-year experience of 3436 surgical cases. Spine 35:1880-1886, 2010.

77. Buckwalter JA, Yaszay B, Ilgenritz R, et al. Analysis of intraoperative neuromonitoring events during spinal corrective surgery for idiopathic scoliosis. Spine Deform 1:434-438, 2013.

78. Fu KM, Smith JS, Polly DW, et al. Morbidity and mortality associated with spinal surgery in children: a review of the Scoliosis Research Society morbidity and mortality database. J Neurosurg Pediatr 7:37-41, 2011.

79. Suk SI, Kim WJ, Lee SM, et al. Thoracic pedicle screw fixation in spinal deformities: are they really safe? Spine 26:2049-2057, 2011.

80. Hicks JM, Singla A, Shen FH, et al. Complications of pedicle screw fixation in scoliosis surgery: a systematic review. Spine 35:E465-E470, 2010.

81. Pahys JM, Guille JT, D'Andrea LP, et al. Neurologic injury in the surgical treatment of idiopathic scoliosis: guidelines for assessment and management. J Am Acad Orthop Surg 17:426-434, 2009.

82. Li Y, Glotzbecker M, Hedequist D. Surgical site infection after pediatric spinal deformity surgery. Curr Rev Musculoskelet Med. 2012 Feb 9. [Epub ahead of print]

83. Sweet FA, Roh M, Sliva C. Intrawound application of vancomycin for prophylaxis in instrumented thoracolumbar fusions: efficacy, drug levels, and patient outcomes. Spine 36:2084-2088, 2011.

84. O'Neill KR, Smith JG, Abtahi AM, et al. Reduced surgical site infections in patients undergoing posterior spinal stabilization of traumatic injuries using vancomycin powder. Spine J 11:641-646, 2011.

85. Clark CE, Shufflebarger HL. Late-developing infection in instrumented idiopathic scoliosis. Spine 24:1909-1912, 1999.

86. Hedequist D, Haugen A, Hresko T, et al. Failure of attempted implant retention in spinal deformity delayed surgical site infections. Spine 34:60-64, 2009.

87. Richards BR, Emara KM. Delayed infections after posterior TSRH spinal instrumentation for idiopathic scoliosis: revisited. Spine 26:1990-1996, 2001.

88. Ho C, Skaggs DL, Weiss JM, et al. Management of infection after instrumented posterior spine fusion in pediatric scoliosis. Spine 32:2739-2744, 2007.

89. van Rhee MA, de Klerk LW, Verhaar JA. Vacuum-assisted wound closure of deep infections after instrumented spinal fusion in six children with neuromuscular scoliosis. Spine J 7:596-600, 2007.

90. Canavese F, Gupta S, Krajbich JI, et al. Vacuum-assisted closure for deep infection after spinal instrumentation for scoliosis. J Bone Joint Surg Br 90:377-381, 2008.

91. Rohmiller MT, Akbarnia BA, Raiszadeh K, et al. Closed suction irrigation for the treatment of postoperative wound infections following posterior spinal fusion and instrumentation. Spine 35:642-646, 2010.

92. Muschik M, Luck W, Schlenzka D. Implant removal for late-developing infection after instrumented posterior spinal fusion for scoliosis: reinstrumentation reduces loss of correction. A retrospective analysis of 45 cases. Eur Spine J 13:645-651, 2004.

93. Cahill PJ, Warnick DE, Lee MJ, et al. Infection after spinal fusion for pediatric spinal deformity: thirty years of experience at a single institution. Spine 35:1211-1217, 2004.

29

Spinal Alignment in the Management of Congenital Scoliosis

Charles I. Jones III ▪ *Richard E. McCarthy*

Congenital scoliosis is a category of spinal deformity that usually occurs as a result of an unknown cause during the first few weeks of intrauterine development. Although the condition is present at birth, the physical symptoms may not clinically manifest for months or years.[1] Scoliosis is characterized by an often-progressive primary curve driven by a focal segment of asymmetrical, atypical vertebrae resulting from failure of formation, failure of segmentation, or both. The resultant abnormality is usually described along a continuum from fully segmented hemivertebrae (formation) to fully formed vertebrae joined by a unilateral bar (segmentation). Combinations of these can occur and affect the degree of deformity and the expected rate of progression. Congenital abnormalities can occur at any level throughout the spinal column. This chapter focuses on the thoracic and lumbar regions, particularly the cervicothoracic, thoracolumbar, and lumbosacral junctions, because deformity at these locations can have more severe clinical ramifications and provide a unique challenge in treating the resultant scoliosis.[2]

CLINICAL WORKUP

The critical first step in the management of congenital scoliosis is early diagnosis. Subtle or obvious physical deformity may be the presenting complaint of parents of otherwise-normal children who have no other reason to be evaluated radiographically. In these cases, a careful history is obtained and a physical examination performed. Plain PA and lateral radiographs of the thoracolumbar spine that include the pelvis are obtained. Careful evaluation and scrutiny of imaging studies is essential to identify abnormalities and document the nature and degree of deformity. Secondary compensatory curves that develop in response to the primary congenital curve levels need to be recognized.

RADIOGRAPHIC EVALUATION

Radiographs are inspected in a stepwise fashion, beginning with a PA view. Images are carefully assessed for quality. They should include the entire area of study, be properly labeled *left* or *right,* and marked as standing, sitting, or supine. Before assessment of the spinal column, the clinician evaluates the rib cage and pelvis for symmetry, morphology, and balance. Next, each spinal level in a PA projection is checked for structural abnormality such as asymmetrical vertebral bodies, missing or additional levels, and abnormal pedicles. Curves are carefully measured to quantify magnitudes, usually using the Cobb method, with special attention to additional curves that are either unique deformities or secondary to a primary focal abnormality. For ambulatory patients, standing films are especially useful to determine coronal balance (measured in horizontal distance from a plumb line drawn through the center of S1) and pelvic obliquity, which may be underrepresented by supine radiographs. A sitting PA view is a suitable substitute for non-ambulatory or wheelchair-bound patients. In addition, left- and right-bending films facilitated by manual reduction from the examiner can provide valuable information about the relative flexibility of the deformity and help to guide corrective maneuvers. The rigidity of the curve is essential in determining surgical levels to include within a fusion construct.

Incompletely formed or segmented levels are usually best appreciated on a supine PA projection. Continuous intervertebral lateral walls with incomplete disc spaces signify unilateral bars, whereas asymmetrical pedicles with confluent adjacent disc spaces suggest hemivertebral formation. Clinicians should also be vigilant in identifying combinations of bars and hemivertebrae, because these carry the highest risk for rapid curve progression when present at the same level. Additional patterns of multiple congenital malformation such as Klippel-Feil and Jarcho-Levin syndromes and associations with appendicular malformations such as phocomelia are noted. Radiographs can reveal obvious or subtle coexistent, discrete congenital abnormalities present in multiple curves.

On a lateral projection, normal or abnormal formation of the vertebral bodies, disc spaces, and posterior elements can be seen on initial inspection. The thoracic vertebrae normally have slight wedging at each level (less than 5 degrees), whereas the superior and inferior endplates of the lumbar segments are more parallel. Diminution of the disc spaces and/or obliqueness of the rectangular body projections can result from coronal curves or spinal rotation. Cobb measurements of the thoracic and lumbar spine reveal relative hyperkyphosis or hypokyphosis of the thoracic spine (normal 20 to 40 degrees),[3] abnormal lordosis of the lumbar spine (normal approximately 25 to 45 degrees),[4] and increased angulation in the cervicothoracic and thoracolumbar segments, which are normally straight. Sagittal balance can be determined by drawing a plumb line downward from the center of the body of C7. Normally this line intersects the posterosuperior corner of the body of S1, and those that fall anterior or posterior to this point signify positive or negative sagittal balance, respectively. Similar to a PA projection, standing lateral radiographs provide more information than supine views about sagittal balance because of the spinal column's function as a dynamic tension band in supporting body weight.

COMPUTED TOMOGRAPHY EVALUATION

If the diagnosis is unclear or if a complex abnormality is present, biplanar radiography[5] or noncontrast CT of the thoracic and/or lumbar spine with orthogonal and three-dimensional reconstructions is exceptionally useful for understanding the anatomy of congenital deformity. In special circumstances, three-dimensional printing can be used to create discrete models that can be held in the hands for additional study. Some of these models can even be sterilized for intraoperative use to provide palpable assistance in determining pedicle screw placement and boundaries for resection. Because of the potential side effects of high-dose ionizing radiation on a growing patient's bony and soft tissues, every attempt should be made to minimize the need and extent of additional, advanced radiographic imaging.

MAGNETIC RESONANCE IMAGING EVALUATION

The use of MRI is growing for preoperative evaluation of spinal deformity as a tool to identify concurrent intrathecal pathologies such as Chiari malformations, syringomelia, diastomatomelia, and tethered cords, which can occur in at least 30% of patients with congenital scoliosis.[6,7] If one of these deformities is present, consultation with a neurosurgeon is recommended to determine whether correction is appropriate before or during surgical intervention, which can otherwise alter the length of the spinal cord and place a patient at additional risk for neurologic compromise.

Once a congenital scoliosis is diagnosed, the findings are correlated with a careful history and global physical examination to rule out other clinical associations, because midline defects can coexist with other patterns such as the VATER/VACTERL (vertebral anomalies, anal atresia, cardiac defects, tracheoesophageal fistula and/or esophageal atresia, renal and radial anomalies, and limb defects) syndromes. When screening modalities are warranted, they should include echocardiography, urinalysis, and renal ultrasound, because the incidence of cardiac and urologic anomalies coexistent with congenital scoliosis is 10% and 25%, respectively.[1] For patients without previous overt symptomatology whose spinal deformity is the first diagnosis, this may be the first clue to discovering serious underlying pathology, and early cardiac or renal subspecialty referral may of enormous benefit. For deformities that can cause chest wall restriction and thoracic insufficiency syndrome, early pulmonary consultation is valuable. Timely management of these entities is not only beneficial to overall patient health, but it can also help to decrease the risk for perioperative complications of deformity surgery.

TREATMENT STRATEGIES

Several treatment options are available. These depend on numerous factors, including the type and location of the deformity, patient age, degree of deformity, and the surgeon's experience with the various operative interventions. Treatment methods have evolved with advancing technology of instrumentation, most notably pedicle screw–based constructs, which have made posterior-only approaches popular among many surgeons.[8-14]

Balanced deformity that can occur in complex, adjacent abnormalities like Jarcho-Levin syndrome or opposed hemivertebrae should be carefully assessed and followed closely if nonoperative management is chosen. If thoracic development is not impeded and coronal and sagittal balance are maintained, surgical management may not be warranted if mild deformity is not progressive. However, the risks of deferring early surgery include enhanced difficulty in correcting larger, severe curves, the inherent increase in rigidity of structural curves as the spine matures, and the inability to harness remaining growth potential as adjunctive corrective therapy.

With asymmetrical focal failures of segmentation and/or formation (unilateral bars and/or hemivertebrae), progression in an immature spine is expected.[15,16] In contrast to "watchful waiting" of congenital curves in patients with mild-to-moderate idiopathic scoliosis, which has been reported to be successful,[17] bracing of progressive primary curves in congenital deformity is not usually recommended, although bracing of compensatory curves is sometimes effective. In these cases early diagnosis is critical to initiate early surgical intervention in an attempt to achieve maximum correction, to prevent development of chest malformation, to reduce the burden of the required operative procedure, to allow early treatment of flexible secondary curves, and to best use remaining growth.[18-22]

With early identification, an abnormality can be corrected with short-segment fusion as early as 2 years of age. This principle of early surgery is extremely important to maximize growth potential of an immature spine and to prevent the development of secondary changes in adjacent levels and compensatory curves. Implants can be removed 1 to 2 years after fusion to enhance spinal development and to ensure that patients are free of instrumentation during adolescence. With delay of even a few years, surgical intervention can require longer fusion and construct lengths, resulting in limited spinal motion with reduced growth potential. Although the length of a normal spinal column increases significantly from infancy to maturity, the spinal canal reaches 90% of its final diameter by 5 years of age; therefore bilateral pedicle screw constructs can safely be placed without inducing iatrogenic stenosis and root impingement.[8]

Special consideration should be given to focal defects at the cervicothoracic, thoracolumbar, and lumbosacral junctions, because they can lead to greater deformity than those occurring at midthoracic or midlumbar levels.[2] This is a result of the relatively straight, normal alignment across these transitional levels and the observation that even small angulations at these junctions can result in large alterations to a patient's coronal and/or sagittal balance. Because the thoracic and sacral spines are relatively rigid, compared with the cervical and lumbar spines, these transitional areas are critical in terms of applied stress and spinal kinematics. Inclusion of additional fusion levels might be necessary to stabilize a construct while healing occurs (to a greater degree than midlumbar or midthoracic abnormalities), at the cost of spinal motion and growth potential.

The overall theme in the approach toward treatment of congenital scoliosis is successful and complete *identification* of deformed segments and *early intervention* to *maintain* and *harness* remaining growth. Surgery can safely be performed in juvenile spines, allowing reconstruction with shorter fusion lengths usually with pedicle screw and rod instrumentation.

SURGICAL OPTIONS

The surgical option depends on the location and nature of the abnormality. Options include the following:
- Hemivertebral complete excision (vertebral column resection [VCR]) or incomplete excision (osteotomy versus decancellation with implosion)
- Bar excision/osteotomy
- Internal strut bracing with extraspinal instrumentation and thoracotomy using a vertical expandable prosthetic titanium rib (VEPTR) device (Synthes, Inc., West Chester, PA)
- Convex hemiarthrodesis in situ spinal fusion without correction for stabilization to limit progression of complex curves

VCU offers the greatest degree of three-dimensional correction.

Many authors have published series of hemivertebral excision with short-segment fusion and have demonstrated good results.[8-14] This is the preferred method of treatment for an isolated, single-level hemivertebra with or without contralateral bars. For these cases, anatomy and surgeon preference guide the approach (all posterior or combined anterior-posterior) and technique (complete resection with adjacent disc removal, intravertebral osteotomy with decancellation and preservation of the hemivertebral endplates, and/or hemiphysiodesis[23,24] versus apical-only fusion[25]).

The choice for many spinal procedures is guided by the level of deformity, the surgeon's experience/comfort, and patient-specific considerations. A thorough grasp of each patient's anatomy and functional capacity is essential in preoperative planning. For example, a patient with poor pulmonary function can be at greater risk for anterior-based procedures violating the diaphragm or pleural spaces. These patients might have a better overall result with a more posterior approach, especially if the defect is thoracic. Similarly, the extent of an operation should be tailored for each patient, because physiologic capacity can guide the extent of the procedure. When intervention is extensive because of the pathology, staging portions of the procedure in separate operative sessions or the use of preoperative traction may be appropriate.

For patients with multilevel abnormalities, surgical planning is more complex and may necessitate additional resection and reconstruction within separate or contiguous instrumentation/fusion constructs. Careful preoperative assessment of secondary curves is essential to determine whether they are structural or nonstructural and rigid or flexible. The surgical goals should include restoration of normal spinal alignment with minimization of fused segments in order to preserve as much growth as possible. However, if the pathology and the patient's goals warrant stabilization without large deformity correction, minimization of complications with simpler surgery should be considered, provided that the procedure adequately treats the problem. In these cases, surgeons should very clearly indicate the intent of the surgery by marking the extent of a fusion with small metal clips, for future reference.

Especially for young patients, thoracic and thoracolumbar spinal pathology can result in coronal and/or sagittal plane deformity that alters the normal morphology of the rib cage, thereby reducing the space available for developing lung parenchyma. The resulting *thoracic insufficiency* is a significant entity that has been shown to have a critical effect on functional capacity.[26] When the planned benefits of reconstruction through resection and fusion are outweighed by the deleterious effects on the chest with requisite spinal column shortening, rib cage expansion through a VEPTR device, with or without thoracotomy, offers an attractive option. With this technique, fusion can be limited or avoided with extraperiosteal insertion of the instrumentation, thoracoplasty, and rib cage growth can be guided by sequential lengthening of the internal splint. Scoliosis with chest wall deformity can be managed with extraspinal rib-to-rib, spine-to-rib, or pelvis-to-rib configurations.[27] This is especially helpful in respiratory comprised patients.

When an anomalous level or levels are completely excised, insertion of allograft and autograft struts can be particularly useful to fill remaining bone voids, increase the success for fusion, and provide an anterior fulcrum to obtain additional lordosis when combined with posterior compressive instrumentation. Common choices for commercially available allograft include machined cortical wedges normally used for transforaminal and posterior interbody fusions and metal cages that can be supplemented with allograft or autograft. When autograft is preferred, bone from the excised segment or an adjacent rib is frequently sufficient. Additional cortical or corticocancellous graft can be harvested from the iliac crest or ribs.

Although combined anterior and posterior approaches have historically been useful for vertebral excision,[28-33] advances in pedicle screw design and implantation technique have increased popularity of all-posterior approaches for VCR. These require increased awareness and protection of the neural elements with the use of specialized instruments (spoons, angled impactors, and square-cutting osteotomes). However, intrathoracic complications associated with the lungs, diaphragm, and great vessels are prevented, making this an attractive option. As mentioned previously, pedicle screws can safely be applied even in young children, without significant detriment to adjacent intrathecal structures. Placement of screws within young pedicles has also proved quite safe in the hands of experienced surgeons.[34]

Although screw placement is relatively safe and straightforward in normally formed and adult spines, insertion into immature and deformed anatomy presents additional challenges. For this reason, intraoperative fluoroscopy is frequently used to aid in determining starting points and screw position. Newer advances in imaging, including real-time computer navigation and intraoperative CT (O-Arm, Medtronic Sofamor Danek, Minneapolis, MN), have been very successful in improving surgeon confidence in diagnosis and management of complex abnormalities and deformed pedicles.[35] The ability to perform limited, intraoperative, three-dimensional radiographic assessment of spinal correction allows surgeons to navigate, as well as, confirm proper placement of instrumentation before closure. Needed changes can be made within the same operative setting instead of in a subsequent return to the operation after a higher-dose postoperative CT scan.

For older children in whom additional growth is not anticipated, guided-growth techniques may not be needed. Because large increases in curve magnitude caused by asymmetrical anatomy and imbalanced growth are not expected, osteotomy may be the most viable option. For kyphotic deformities, posterior convex instrumentation and compression (in the thoracic spine)[36] or multilevel facetectomy (Ponte or Smith-Petersen–type osteotomies) may be useful in reducing relatively stiff kyphosis. These osteotomies, when performed at the level of an anterior disc, can be expected to contribute 10 to 15 degrees of correction per segment. When the deformity is focal, rigid, and more severe, pedicle subtraction osteotomy can improve single-level alignment by up to 40 degrees; an osteotomy can also be performed in an asymmetrical fashion to correct both sagittal and coronal imbalance.[37-41]

Additional correction may necessitate single-level or multilevel VCR, providing the greatest improvement in alignment with increased risk for intraoperative and perioperative complications.[41-43] This procedure produces spinal instability through a three-column resection, requiring patience and vigilance during reduction to prevent dural buckling and iatrogenic neurologic injury. Anterior column reconstruction with cages and/or strut grafting is often essential, and three-rod stabilization with combined bilateral pedicle screw–rod and supplemented at times with laminar hook–rod constructs should be considered.[20] Bracing is common in the postoperative period, based on patient characteristics and confidence in the instrumentation construct.

PATIENT EXAMPLES

Unilateral Fully Segmented Hemivertebrae at the Thoracolumbar Junction

This 15-month-old boy was referred for scoliosis and kyphosis at the thoracolumbar junction with a focal abnormality at L1 on PA and lateral radiographs. When the boy was 1 year old, his mother noted a small gibbus deformity; however, radiographs at that time did not indicate a specific abnormality. His past medical, surgical, and family histories were unremarkable. A physical examination revealed a slight gibbus deformity at the thoracolumbar junction. His neurologic function was normal for his age in all four extremities, and no other deformities were noted. Careful assessment of his standing radiographs revealed a right-sided incompletely formed L1, resulting in a fully segmented hemivertebra with preserved adjacent discs. This caused a left-sided 42-degree curve at the thoracolumbar junction, a compensatory 27-degree right-sided curve in the subjacent lumbar spine, and an 18-degree right-sided curve in the superjacent lower thoracic spine. A vertical line drawn from the center of S1 on a PA view showed minimal coronal imbalance (Fig. 29-1, A). A lateral projection showed 29 degrees of focal kyphosis at the thoracolumbar junction, and the plumb line from C7 was 1.2 cm from the posterosuperior corner of S1, indicating mild positive sagittal balance (Fig. 29-1, B). MRI was performed to rule out concomitant intrathecal abnormalities. CT was performed to ensure that no other abnormalities were present. A tethered cord was noted on MRI, and the L1 level was confirmed to be a fully segmented hemivertebra (Fig. 29-1, C).

The rationale for recommendation of surgical intervention included the patient's young age, significant potential for angular deformities, and positive sagittal balance, which was expected to increase significantly without operative correction. We followed the principles of growth and motion preservation, early intervention, and minimization of construct length and planned an all-posterior approach with complete resection of the anomalous L1 and posterior reconstruction and fusion from T12 to L2. The procedure was performed with a neurosurgeon, who released the tethered cord during the same anesthesia period. No intraoperative or postoperative complications were observed.

Postoperative radiographs showed improved angulation and balance in both planes (Figs. 29-1, D and E). A two-rod construct was used, and the patient was placed in a Risser cast intraoperatively. No interbody graft was used. A posterolateral fusion was accomplished with local autograft from the hemivertebra. The patient underwent uncomplicated removal of instrumentation 2 years later and was followed for the next 5 years. Seven years postoperatively his correction persists (Fig. 29-1, F). Because of his continued growth and strength, his family wanted him to begin to play football at school.

This case is an example of a single thoracolumbar hemivertebra managed with single-level fusion to restore alignment and prevent future deformity at this junction. Because of his young age, short-segment fusion was a viable option. Delayed presentation would likely have necessitated extension of the fusion further into the thoracic and lumbar spines to achieve and maintain correction. This treatment allows these levels to continue longitudinal growth. Stable correction with continued growth is noted several years after implant removal, and patients can grow into adolescence without the effects of spinal instrumentation on adjacent levels.

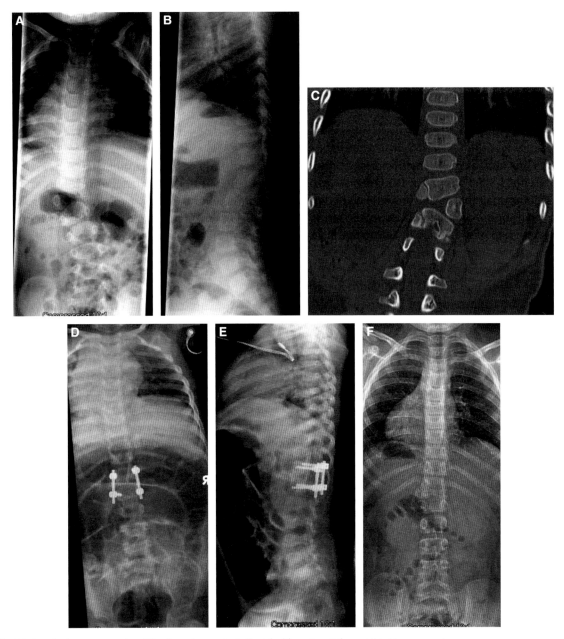

Fig. 29-1 **A,** A preoperative PA view showed a left-sided hemivertebra at L1. Compensatory curves were present at the thoracolumbar junction and within the lumbar spine. **B,** A preoperative lateral projection revealed focal kyphosis from an L1 hemivertebra. **C,** A preoperative coronal CT reconstruction showed disc spaces superior and inferior to the unilateral fully segmented hemivertebra. **D,** A postoperative PA image of the patient in a cast showed two-rod stabilization after resection and short-segment fusion. **E,** A postoperative lateral radiograph demonstrated interval reduction in thoracolumbar kyphosis with near-neutral alignment. **F,** The patient is shown 7 years after hemivertebral excision and short-segment posterior fusion and 5 years after implant removal. Persistent correction and continued growth and maturity of the spine are evident.

Multiple Hemivertebrae in Distinct Locations

This 10-year-old girl had congenital spinal abnormalities noted shortly after birth. This was seen on a chest radiograph obtained for unrelated reasons. Per the mother's report, the patient was referred at 2 years of age to a spine surgeon, who noted 52-degree and 55-degree curves in the thoracic and lumbar spines, respectively. Early operative intervention was recommended; however, the parents did not want their child to have surgery, and because no deformity was obvious, they chose to observe without follow-up across the next 9 years. At a later evaluation, the patient had complaints of truncal asymmetry with thoracic and lumbar spinal deformities that were not painful, occasional shortness of breath, and infrequent urinary retention. Her past medical, surgical, and family histories were unremarkable. On physical examination, she had obvious right thoracic and left lumbar curves with scoliometric readings of 12 degrees and 13 degrees, respectively. She was neurologically intact, and results of her spirometric evaluation were within normal limits.

PA and lateral radiographs showed separate 78-degree right thoracic and 73-degree left lumbar curves. Three-dimensional CT confirmed a diagnosis of congenital scoliosis with right-sided T7-8 and T8-9 fully segmented hemivertebrae and a fully segmented left-sided L2-3 hemivertebra (Fig. 29-2, A through C). Her triradiate cartilages were open and her iliac apophyses were Risser stage 0. Based on interpretations of bone age radiographs of her elbow, she had an 11-year-old immature skeleton.

Because of the separate, severe, and dueling nature of this patient's progressive deformities in a still immature spine, a complex surgical plan was offered to correct both pathologies in a single operative setting. The thoracic hemivertebrae were treated with right-sided subperiosteal exposure, eggshell decancellation, and subtotal excision with instrumentation-assisted collapse with apical fusion of the right side only. The use of pedicle screws in this situation offers three-column fixation to prevent crankshaft later. The lumbar hemivertebra was subject to circumferential excision with anterior interbody fusion using an iliac crest autograft and short-segment three-rod posterior fusion. To harness the remaining growth potential within the rest of her immature spine, the fused areas were left unconnected to allow additional curve correction with continued growth (Fig. 29-2, D and E). Postoperative Cobb measurements showed correction to 48 degrees in the thoracic curve and 41 degrees in the lumbar segment, with 1.0 cm of right-sided coronal and neutral sagittal balances.

This approach treated both areas of pathology in the same surgical setting using separate short-segment fusions, thus minimizing the need to return to the operating room and maximizing growth potential as she aged into maturity. The design of selective, asymmetrical apical fusion allows the unfused opposite concavity to catch up with continued growth, maximizing final spinal column length. Because of her delayed presentation and surgery at 11 years of age, removal of implants is not necessarily recommended.

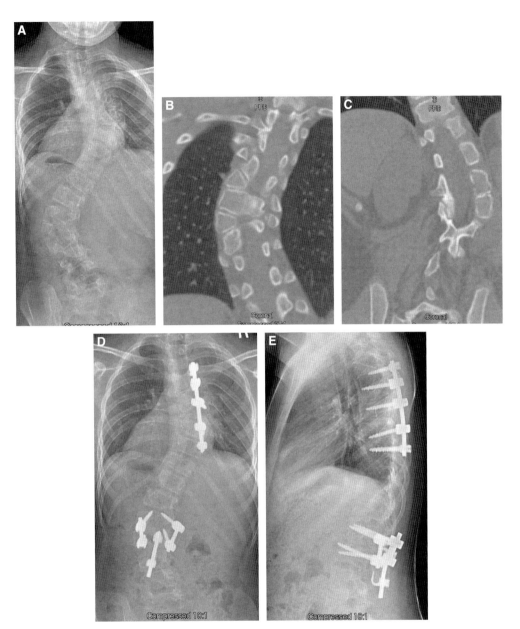

Fig. 29-2   **A,** A preoperative PA view showed significant curves. The overall coronal balance was fairly well maintained because of the opposing structural curves. **B,** A preoperative coronal CT reconstruction of her thoracic spine demonstrated two noncontiguous fully segmented right-sided hemivertebrae. **C,** A preoperative coronal reconstruction of her lumbar spine shows left-sided segmentation of the L2 hemivertebra that was full (not partial) because of the continuous (although diminished) superior disc. **D,** A postoperative PA image reveals the separate instrumentation constructs used for her separate congenital curves. The thoracic curve was treated with decancellation and compression with apical-only fusion to preserve growth on the opposing concavity and to continue her correction with skeletal growth as she nears maturity. The lumbar segment shows a typical three-rod construct after complete hemivertebral excision and fusion. **E,** A postoperative lateral radiograph reveals maintenance of thoracic kyphosis and preservation of lumbar lordosis after instrumentation. Laminar hooks are used with a third rod to improve posterior compression and stabilization after hemivertebral excision.

Thoracic Butterfly Vertebra With Severe Scoliosis

This 10-year-old girl had been seen in a spina bifida clinic for thoracic abnormalities. The effects of her myelomeningocele were very mild. She was neurologically intact to her lower extremities, and she wanted to engage in sports with her friends. Her complaints were related to increasing thoracic deformity with altered coronal and sagittal balance.

An examination revealed obvious midthoracic spinal deviation and rotation; strength and sensation were maintained throughout her lower extremities. Radiographs demonstrated a focal 78-degree left-sided T7-12 coronal curve with compensatory right-sided 37-degree T1-6 and 49-degree L1-5 curves. Her global coronal balance was 3.4 cm to the left, and her global sagittal balance (as determined by the sagittal vertical axis) was −3.9 cm (Fig. 29-3, A and B). A three-dimensional CT scan was obtained to better define the congenital segments. It revealed a butterfly vertebra at T9 with complex abnormalities at T8 and T10 (Fig. 29-3, C and D). A tethered cord was noted on a routine MRI evaluation, which will be released at the time of her deformity correction surgery. Side-bending radiographs showed the congenital curve to be quite rigid. Therefore a vertebral column osteotomy at T10 with posterior spinal fusion from T6 to L3 was believed to be required to allow the degree of deformity correction necessary to restore the patient's coronal and sagittal balance, with reduction of her apex scoliosis. To prevent advancement of kyphosis after the resection, a premachined allograft wedge was ordered to allow both anterior column support for fusion and to create a solid fulcrum for compression through the posterior instrumentation. Additionally, her rib-fusion anomalies were treated with rib harvest at the levels of her resection. The ribs were retained for autograft.

The operation proceeded in an uncomplicated fashion. The patient was admitted to the ICU and was transferred to the floor the next day. Postoperative standing radiographs show neutral balance in the coronal plane and reduction of her SVA to +0.7 cm (Fig. 29-3, E and F). One year postoperatively she has recovered completely and has resumed playing basketball at school.

This case is an example of the powerful correction that is possible with VCR in patients with focal, severe, rigid curves that cannot be managed by soft tissue releases or other osteotomies. The lower thoracic level of this patient's pathology caused significant alterations to her alignment and caused severe scoliosis. This resulted in coronal and sagittal imbalance. All of these problems were corrected with VCR and a nine-level posterior fusion. Although mild residual curvature is seen in the unfused upper thoracic and lower lumbar segments, the neutral overall balance and young age of the patient favored sparing as many levels as possible from the arthrodesis to maximize motion preservation through her adolescence and into parenthood.

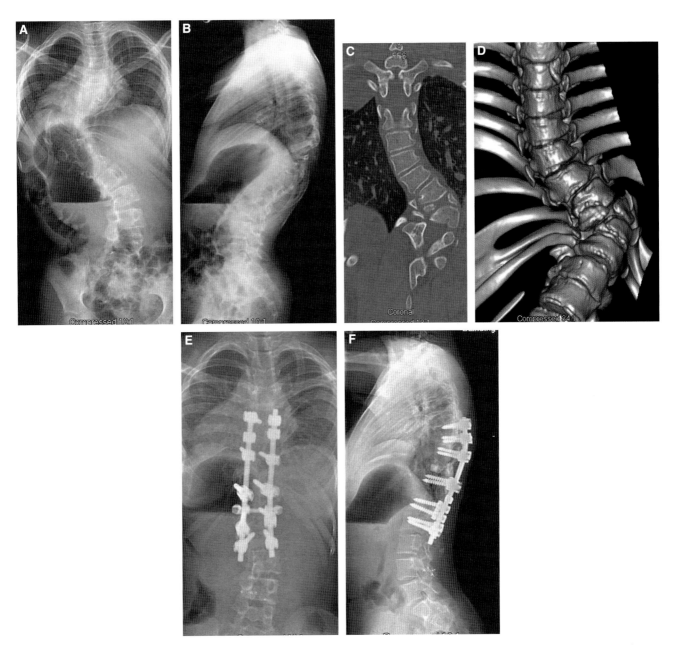

Fig. 29-3 **A,** A preoperative PA view demonstrated significant coronal imbalance and lower thoracic congenital scoliosis, with multiple bilateral rib fusions. **B,** A preoperative standing lateral radiograph showed significant negative sagittal balance. **C** and **D,** Preoperative coronal and three-dimensional CT reconstructions of the lower thoracic congenital abnormality showed a complex T9 butterfly vertebra with adjacent abnormalities in T8 and T10. A significant focal deformity with adjacent compensatory curves had altered her global balance. **E,** A postoperative PA radiograph demonstrates near-neutral coronal alignment with significant reduction in her lower thoracic angulation. **F,** A postoperative lateral view reveals significant reduction of the preoperative negative sagittal balance to +0.7 cm. The allograft interbody graft is evident at the level of resection.

Congenital Hemivertebra at the Lumbosacral Junction

This 14-year-old wheelchair-bound male with spina bifida and a neurologic level of L3 was seen for a known congenital deformity at the lumbosacral junction. He was born with a lipomyelomeningocele, which was closed soon after birth. He had a low-lying conus that was managed nonoperatively by his neurosurgeon. The patient and parents complained of occasional mild low back pain and increasing deformity to his lower back that had progressed clinically as he entered his adolescent growth phase. This was thought to be causing problems with sitting in his chair. Physical examination showed a well-healed midline lumbar scar with an underlying lipoma. His global balance was to the left, causing him to lean against the side of his wheelchair, with a mild amount of pelvic obliquity. He had motor function with hip flexion and weak knee extension with intact sensation throughout his upper thighs, but he had no neurologic function below the knees to either foot.

PA and lateral radiographs (Fig. 29-4, *A* and *B*) demonstrated a fully segmented hemivertebra on the right between L5 and S1, causing a focal scoliosis of 29 degrees and a compensatory left lumbar curve of 49 degrees from L1 to L5. Coronal bending films revealed flexibility within the compensatory curve. Three-dimensional CT reconstruction (Fig. 29-4, *C*) was obtained to develop a three-dimensional printed model (Fig. 29-4, *D*). This highlighted the hemivertebra between L5 and S1, with sacral anomalies, and the expected posterior element deficiency in the lower lumbar spine. Measurements of full-length radiographs showed an overall deviation in coronal balance of 2.5 cm to the left and a sagittal vertical axis of −5.7 cm, with closing triradiate cartilages that suggested modest growth remained.

This patient had coronal and sagittal imbalance, progressive deformity, and sitting problems. He was offered surgical hemivertebrectomy and fusion from L3 to the pelvis with screw and rod instrumentation. After resection, a wedged allograft was inserted to assist in re-creation of lumbar lordosis. Lipoma excision and complex closure were performed by a plastic surgeon. No perioperative complications were observed, and the patient was discharged home on postoperative day 2. Postoperative radiographs show improvements in his coronal balance to 1.2 cm to the left and in his sagittal balance with a sagittal vertical axis of −2.2 cm (Fig. 29-4, *E* and *F*). His compensatory L1-5 lumbar curve is reduced to 6 degrees.

In this patient, global balance was significantly altered because of a single-level hemivertebra, highlighting the large effect attributable to the lumbosacral abnormality that was driving significant focal and compensatory scoliotic curves. Coronal and sagittal balance were restored in a single-level reconstruction and fusion.

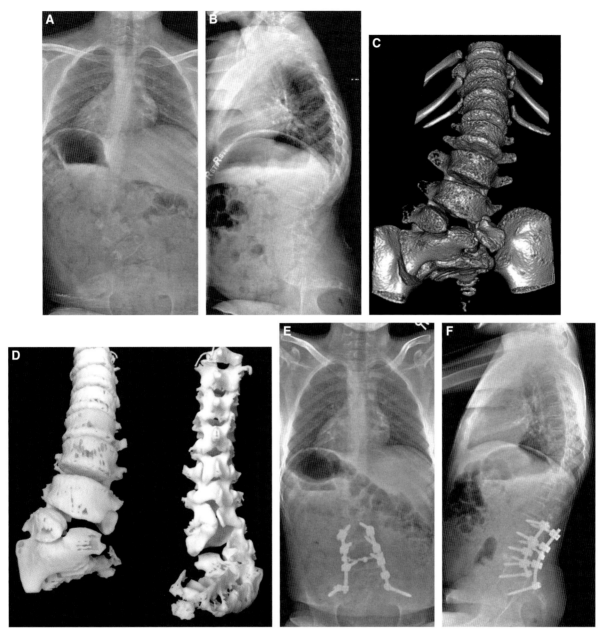

Fig. 29-4 **A,** A preoperative radiograph showed a fully segmented hemivertebra on the right side between L5 and S1, with focal scoliosis and a superjacent compensatory lumbar curve that was flexible on side-bending films. **B,** A preoperative lateral view showed significant negative sagittal balance. **C,** A preoperative three-dimensional CT reconstruction demonstrated the right-sided lumbosacral fully segmented hemivertebra and associated S1 congenital abnormality, causing focal scoliosis and a compensatory lumbar curve. **D,** Anterior and posterior photographs of a three-dimensional printed model of the CT reconstruction. The right-sided lumbosacral hemivertebra is on the *left,* generating a significant focal scoliosis at the junction. Posterior element deficiencies in this patient with spina bifida are seen on the *right.* These models are becoming more useful for preoperative planning. They allow a hands-on appreciation of the deformity, and some can be sterilized for real-time intraoperative use. **E,** A postoperative PA view after hemivertebra resection and fusion from L3 to the pelvis. The patient's coronal balance is significantly improved, and the scoliotic curves are reduced in both the lumbar and lumbosacral areas. **F,** A postoperative lateral radiograph shows improvement in his sagittal balance and re-creation of appropriate lumbar lordosis, with secondary improvement in thoracolumbar kyphosis.

Multiple Upper Thoracic and Cervicothoracic Congenital Abnormalities

This 11-year-old girl had multiple upper thoracic congenital abnormalities and complained of upper back pain. She had been initially seen 7 years previously and was lost to follow-up. Functionally, she had no problems keeping up with other children while at play, and no neurologic deficiencies were noted. She had been diagnosed previously with multiple contiguous congenital bars and formation defects. However, surgical intervention was deferred to allow maximum growth and because her deformity was mild.

Her medical history revealed an associated VATER syndrome without significant current pathologic manifestation. On physical examination she had a 13-degree imbalance in scoliometric testing, restricted motion in her lower cervical spine, and preserved motion throughout the lumbar spine. She was intact neurologically. Current radiographs revealed a rigid 46-degree upper thoracic right-sided curve with a rigid secondary 36-degree left cervicothoracic curve with multiple congenital abnormalities (Fig. 29-5, *A*). MRI showed a fatty filum that, based on a neurologic consultation, was not believed to require release before stabilization surgery. By the time of surgery, her primary curve had increased to 56 degrees, highlighting the potential for rapid progression of congenital curves during peak growth.

This young patient had increasing curve magnitude and was nearing her adolescent growth spurt. She had sufficient cardiopulmonary function. Because of these factors and the complex nature of her deformity, surgical intervention was offered to slow additional progression of her deformity and to limit interference with lung function. Stabilization with a posterior fusion without reduction, with iliac crest autografting from C6 to T8, was offered. Lateral mass screws were placed at C6 and C7, with pedicle screws placed in accessible pedicles to T8. Tapered rods and a cross-link were used (Fig. 29-5, *B*). Her surgery proceeded without complication, and she did well in the postoperative period. She was lost to follow-up.

This case illustrates the principles of the progressive nature of congenital scoliosis and the impact within the cervicothoracic junction, especially within the windows of peak growth. Alternative surgical options might have included complex reconstruction with VCR. However, because the patient's global deformity was acceptable and her curves were rigid, the risk-benefit ratio favored in situ stabilization, without the significant risks of VCR in the cervicothoracic and upper thoracic regions.

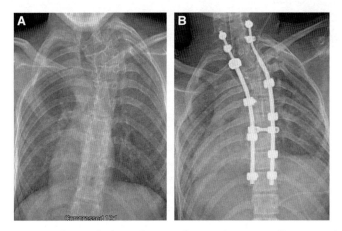

Fig. 29-5   **A,** A preoperative PA radiograph showed a complex combination of hemivertebrae and bar formation in the patient's upper thoracic spine. **B,** A postoperative PA view obtained after in situ fusion across the complex congenital deformity. The tapered rods join the superior lateral mass screws and larger-sized thoracic pedicle screws.

CONCLUSION

Spinal alignment is a critical consideration in the management of patients with congenital scoliosis. The challenges are manyfold and are present throughout the process of patient evaluation and physical examination, radiographic diagnosis, surgical planning, and operative treatment. Patient examination requires careful assessment of the patient's (or parents') concerns regarding pain, deformity, functional status, and neurologic involvement. Physical examination can reveal significant multidimensional and chest wall deformities and other abnormalities such as leg-length discrepancy or other limb anomalies. These can clue the examiner in to important coexisting syndromes or pathologies in addition to scoliosis that may require additional workup or consultation to reduce perioperative complications and improve a patient's overall health.

Imaging evaluation begins with plain radiographs (standing if possible) to assess global coronal and sagittal balance, to measure curves in all planes, and to evaluate for vertebral malformations. Questions about anatomy on plain films warrant CT. Clinicians should make every attempt to minimize the total dose of ionizing radiation. Because of the significant occurrence of coexisting intrathecal abnormalities with congenital deformity, MRI is gaining popularity as a preoperative screening tool that, if positive, merits neurosurgical consultation. This information should allow surgeons to precisely characterize the failures of formation and/or segmentation and to measure the degree of deformity and assess the coronal and sagittal balance.

The principles that shape surgical planning include *early surgical intervention, harnessing of growth potential,* and *patient-specific procedures.* The physician and patient/family should understand the goals of surgery, and the plan should be carefully considered after risks and benefits of intervention are weighed.

For isolated, fully segmented hemivertebrae, the current trend is toward all-posterior complete excision with three-rod posterior instrumentation and circumferential fusion. Adjacent bars portend a lower degree of correction, but can be managed with simultaneous osteotomy. More complex abnormalities may require additional resection or, if reasonably well-balanced, may be amenable to stabilization to halt progression into a more severe curve. Careful design of intended osteotomies and resections allows surgeons to correct alignment in multiple planes and may require additional grafts and instrumentation.

Special attention should be paid to congenital defects affecting the cervicothoracic, thoracolumbar, and lumbosacral junctions, which have a higher rate of malalignment. Whereas longer construct lengths may be necessary for stabilization, early intervention can decrease the length of fused segments and improve alignment while maximizing spinal mobility and remaining growth.

REFERENCES

1. Scoliosis Research Society. Congenital scoliosis and kyphosis. Available at *www.srs.org.*
2. Li W, Sun Z, Guo Z, et al. Analysis of spinopelvic sagittal alignment in patients with thoracic and thoracolumbar angular kyphosis. Spine 38:E813-E818, 2013.
3. Lenke LG, Betz RR, Harms J, et al. Adolescent idiopathic scoliosis: a new classification to determine extent of spinal arthrodesis. J Bone Joint Surg Am 83:1169-1181, 2001.
4. Lin RM, Jou IM, Yu CY. Lumbar lordosis: normal adults. J Formos Med Assoc 91:329-333, 1992.
5. Humbert L, Steffen JS, Vialle R, et al. 3D analysis of congenital scoliosis due to hemivertebra using biplanar radiography. Eur Spine J 22:379-386, 2013.
6. Louis ML, Gennari JM, Loundou AD, et al. Congenital scoliosis: a frontal plane evaluation of 251 operated patients 14 years old or older at follow-up. Orthop Traumatol Surg Res 96:741-747, 2010.
7. Aliabadi H, Grant G. Congenital thoracolumbar spine deformities. Neurosurgery 63(3 Suppl):S78-S85, 2008.
8. Spiro AS, Rupprecht M, Stenger P, et al. Surgical treatment of severe congenital thoracolumbar kyphosis through a single posterior approach. Bone Joint J Br 95:1527-1532, 2013.

9. Aydogan M, Ozturk C, Tezer M, et al. Posterior vertebrectomy in kyphosis, scoliosis and kyphoscoliosis due to hemivertebra. J Pediatr Orthop B 17:33-37, 2008.

10. Li X, Lou Z, Li X, et al. Hemivertebra resection for the treatment of congenital lumbar spinal scoliosis with lateral-posterior approach. Spine 33:2001-2006, 2008.

11. Hedequist DJ. Instrumentation and fusion for congenital spine deformities. Spine 34:1783-1790, 2009.

12. Halm H. Transpedicular hemivertebra resection and instrumented fusion for congenital scoliosis. Eur Spine J 20:993-994, 2011.

13. Obeid I, Bourghli A, Vital JM. Thoracic hemivertebra resection by posterior approach for congenital scoliosis. Eur Spine J 22:678-680, 2013.

14. Wang S, Zhang J, Qiu G, et al. Posterior hemivertebra resection with bisegmental fusion for congenital scoliosis: more than 3 year outcomes and analysis of unanticipated surgeries. Eur Spine J 22:387-393, 2013.

15. McMaster MJ, McMaster ME. Prognosis for congenital scoliosis due to a unilateral failure of vertebral segmentation. J Bone Joint Surg Am 95:972-979, 2013.

16. Ruf M, Jensen R, Letko L, et al. Hemivertebra resection and osteotomies in congenital spine deformity. Spine 34:1791-1799, 2009.

17. Winter RB, Lonstein JE. Scoliosis secondary to a hemivertebra: seven patients with gradual improvement without treatment. Spine 35:E49-E52, 2010.

18. Bollini G, Docquier PL, Viehweger E, et al. Lumbar hemivertebra resection. J Bone Joint Surg Am 88:1043-1052, 2006.

19. Noordeen MH, Garrido E, Tucker SK, et al. The surgical treatment of congenital kyphosis. Spine 34:1808-1814, 2009.

20. Hedequist DJ, Emans J. Congenital scoliosis: a review and update. J Pediatr Orthop 27:106-116, 2007.

21. Hedequist DJ. Surgical treatment of congenital scoliosis. Orthop Clin North Am 38:497-509, 2007.

22. Marks DS, Qaimkhani SA. The natural history of congenital scoliosis and kyphosis. Spine 34:1751-1755, 2009.

23. Yaszay B, O'Brien M, Shufflebarger HL, et al. Efficacy of hemivertebra resection for congenital scoliosis: a multicenter retrospective comparison of three surgical techniques. Spine 36:2052-2060, 2011.

24. Ginsburg G, Mulconrey DS, Browdy J. Transpedicular hemiepiphysiodesis and posterior instrumentation as a treatment for congenital scoliosis. J Pediatr Orthop 27:387-391, 2007.

25. Peng X, Chen L, Zou X. Hemivertebra resection and scoliosis correction by a unilateral posterior approach using single rod and pedicle screw instrumentation in children under 5 years of age. J Pediatr Orthop B 20:397-403, 2011.

26. Campbell RM, Smith MD, Mayes TC, et al. The characteristics of thoracic insufficiency syndrome associated with fused ribs and congenital scoliosis. J Bone Joint Surg Am 85:399-408, 2003.

27. Flynn JM, Emans JB, Smith JT, et al. VEPTR to treat nonsyndromic congenital scoliosis: a multicenter, mid-term follow-up study. J Pediatr Orthop 33:679-684, 2013.

28. Mladenov K, Kunkel P, Stuecker R. Hemivertebra resection in children, results after single posterior approach and after combined anterior and posterior approach: a comparative study. Eur Spine J 21:506-513, 2012.

29. Xu W, Yang S, Wu X, et al. Hemivertebra excision with short-segment spinal fusion through combined anterior and posterior approaches for congenital spinal deformities in children. J Pediatr Orthop B 19:545-550, 2010.

30. Garrido E, Tome-Bermejo F, Tucker SK, et al. Short anterior instrumented fusion and posterior convex non-instrumented fusion of hemivertebra for congenital scoliosis in very young children. Eur Spine J 17:1507-1514, 2008.

31. Bollini G, Docquier PL, Viehweger E, et al. Lumbosacral hemivertebrae resection by a combined approach: medium- and long-term follow-up. Spine 31:1232-1239, 2006.

32. Ding LX, Qiu GX, Wang YP, et al. Simultaneous anterior and posterior hemivertebra resection in the treatment of congenital kyphoscoliosis. Chin Med Sci J 20:252-256, 2005.

33. Hedequist DJ, Hall JE, Emans JB. Hemivertebra excision in children via simultaneous anterior and posterior exposures. J Pediatr Orthop 25:60-63, 2005.

34. Harimaya K, Lenke LG, Son-Hing JP, et al. Safety and accuracy of pedicle screws and constructs placed in infantile and juvenile patients. Spine 36:1645-1651, 2011.

35. Takahashi J, Ebara S, Hashidate H, et al. Computer-assisted hemivertebral resection for congenital spinal deformity. J Orthop Sci 16:503-509, 2011.

36. Sarlak AY, Atmaca H, Tosun B, et al. Isolate pedicle screw instrumented correction for the treatment of thoracic congenital scoliosis. J Spinal Disord Tech 23:525-529, 2010.

37. Atici Y, Sokucu S, Uzumcugil O, et al. The results of closing wedge osteotomy with posterior instrumented fusion for the surgical treatment of congenital kyphosis. Eur Spine J 22:1368-1374, 2013.
38. Li XF, Liu ZD, Hu GY, et al. Posterior unilateral pedicle subtraction osteotomy of hemivertebra for correction of the adolescent congenital spinal deformity. Spine J 11:111-118, 2011.
39. Imrie MN. A "simple" option in the surgical treatment of congenital scoliosis. Spine J 11:119-121, 2011.
40. Halm H. Pedicle subtraction osteotomy for correction of congenital scoliokyphosis. Eur Spine J 20:995-996, 2011.
41. Zeng Y, Chen Z, Qi Q, et al. The posterior surgical correction of congenital kyphosis and kyphoscoliosis: 23 cases with minimum 2 years follow-up. Eur Spine J 22:372-378, 2013.
42. Mirzanli C, Ozturk C, Karatoprak O, et al. Double-segment total vertebrectomy for the surgical treatment of congenital kyphoscoliosis: a case report. Spine J 8:683-686, 2008.
43. Ozturk C, Alanay A, Ganiyusufoglu K, et al. Short-term X-ray results of posterior vertebral column resection in severe congenital kyphosis, scoliosis, and kyphoscoliosis. Spine 37:1054-1057, 2012.

30

Spinal Alignment in the Management of Neuromuscular Scoliosis

Jaysson T. Brooks ▪ *Paul D. Sponseller*

Neuromuscular scoliosis (NMS) is the general term given to a coronal plane deformity caused by aberrant myoneural pathways in the body.[1] A variety of conditions can cause NMS (Table 30-1), but the common end is an inadequate ability to control the muscles surrounding the spine, often resulting in a relentlessly progressive deformity of the spine.

Patients with NMS often have difficulty with ambulation, trunk control, and head control, particularly if their neuromuscular disease is globally involved. Given the varying degree of disability neuromuscular disease causes each patient, it is important for the surgeon, patient, and caregiver to agree on the overall goals for surgical and possibly nonoperative management of the patient's scoliosis. For example, in a patient with global involvement and spastic quadriplegia, restoration of the sagittal and coronal balance that allows the patient to look straight ahead and interact with caregivers can change his or her life. The purpose of this chapter is to explore the recent advances in the knowledge and correction of spinal alignment in patients with NMS.

Table 30-1   Causes of Neuromuscular Scoliosis

Type of Disorder	Cause
Neuropathic	Cerebral palsy
	Friedreich ataxia
	Charcot-Marie-Tooth disease
	Roussy-Lévy disease
	Syringomyelia
	Spinal cord trauma
Myopathic	Poliomyelitis
	Traumatic
	Spinal muscular atrophy
	Dysautonomia
Combined	Myelomeningocele

CORONAL PLANE PARAMETERS

Unlike the various curve combinations described in the classification of Lenke et al,[2] the coronal spinal deformity seen in NMS is usually characterized by a long, continuous, C-shaped curve with an associated pelvic obliquity (PO) (Fig. 30-1, *A*). The development of a coronal plane deformity is closely linked to the global involvement of the patient's neurologic impairment. For example, a patient with spastic hemiplegia will likely not develop the described spinal deformity because of its limited neurologic effect on an isolated limb, whereas a patient with spastic quadriplegia has a near certain chance of developing a classic C-shaped curve.

In the initial evaluation of the patient's coronal plane deformity, it is important to understand the T1 to S1 global alignment. This alignment is evaluated by measuring the offset between a plumb line drawn from T1 and the central sacral vertebral line[3,4] (Fig. 30-1, *B*). Patients with NMS are less likely than patients with idiopathic scoliosis to develop compensatory coronal curves that can restore a relatively normal T1 to S1 alignment.

The degree PO is important when coronal plane deformity is assessed in patients with NMS. PO is determined from a sitting AP radiograph by measuring the angle formed between a line drawn across the upper level of the iliac crests and a line perpendicular to the vertical axis.[3] An angle of more than 10 degrees is abnormal. In patients with NMS, an abnormal PO often develops proximally secondary to muscle imbalance about the spine and pelvis and distally secondary to hip adductor spasticity, resulting in a windswept pelvis appearance on radiographs (Fig. 30-2). In addition, Ko et al[5] recently found intrapelvic asymmetry to be a significant contribution to the PO seen in patients with NMS. They compared the pelvic angles and

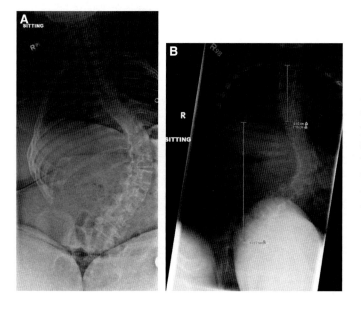

Fig. 30-1   **A,** An AP radiograph shows the characteristic C-shaped spinal curve seen in patients with NMS. **B,** Measuring the T1 to S1 alignment involves drawing a plumb line from the T1 vertebral body and drawing the central sacral vertebral line; the distance between these two points, as denoted by the *red line,* is the result.

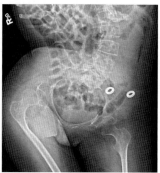

Fig. 30-2   In patients with NMS, an abnormal PO often develops inferiorly secondary to hip adductor spasticity, resulting in a windswept pelvis.

transverse plane symmetry of 27 patients with cerebral palsy (CP) to 20 age-matched controls. They found that patients with CP had asymmetry of at least 10 degrees in multiple pelvic angles, whereas the controls had no asymmetry of more than 10 degrees. In addition, they found that transverse plane asymmetry was much more common in patients with windswept hips. Correction of PO with pelvic fixation in patients with NMS is integral in correcting the coronal and sagittal plane deformities observed in this population and is discussed later in the chapter.

SAGITTAL PLANE PARAMETERS

HYPERKYPHOSIS

Hyperkyphosis, defined as a T2-T12 Cobb angle of at least 50 degrees (Fig. 30-3), has long been known to be a characteristic of patients with NMS; it is part of their battle with gravity.[6] The causes of hyperkyphosis are multifactorial and involve weak extensor muscles of the spine, poor head-trunk balance, spastic trunk musculature, and hamstring contractures.[7] If hamstring contractures are present, it may be helpful to include a proximal hamstring release in the surgical management. Release of the hamstrings also decreases the distal flexion moment, which can sometimes contribute to pullout of pelvic fixation.

Hyperkyphosis can be an important presurgical consideration because recent studies have shown that it increases the risk of developing proximal junctional kyphosis (PJK) after surgery.[8-10] *PJK* is defined as a focal increase in kyphosis of more than 15 degrees that occurs within two levels above and below the upper instrumented vertebra. It has been extensively studied in patients with adolescent idiopathic scoliosis, and risk factors in this population include an associated thoracoplasty, hybrid instrumentation involving proximal hooks and distal pedicle screws, instrumentation involving only pedicle screws proximally, and preoperative kyphosis of more than 40 degrees.[9,11,12] Currently, limited literature is available that characterizes the incidence and risk factors for the development of PJK in patients with NMS.

An ongoing multicenter study examined the risk factors for the development of PJK in patients with CP. (The manuscript has been submitted for publication.) Risk factors shown to be associated with PJK in this population included the absence of mental retardation (resulting in more purposeful and voluntary flexion of the neck), preoperative kyphosis of at least 53 degrees, and a significant operative correction of the patient's kyphosis of at least 29 degrees. Factors not associated with the development of PJK in patients with CP included the upper anchor type, the upper vertebral fusion level, and the patient's hip status, age, Risser sign, lumbar lordosis, and Gross Motor Function Classification System[13] level.

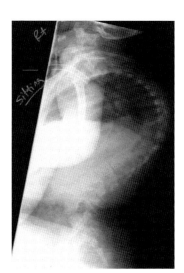

Fig. 30-3   Hyperkyphosis is a common sagittal plane deformity seen in NMS. It is defined as a T2-T12 sagittal Cobb angle of at least 50 degrees.

Hyperlordosis

Hyperlordosis is a rare sagittal plane deformity in patients with NMS; most of the reported studies are case reports[14,15] (Fig. 30-4). Congenital hyperlordosis and lumbar hyperlordosis secondary to lumboperitoneal shunts have been reported; however, this is not common.[15,16] When hyperlordosis is seen, a close evaluation for hip flexion contractures is needed. Vialle et al[17] reported on the presence of hyperlordosis in patients with spastic quadriplegia. They found that all patients in their case series had bilateral hip flexion contractures, an increased sacral slope (SS), and pelvic anteversion. Currently, there is no consensus in the literature as to whether release of hip flexion contractures should take place before correction of the spinal deformity; some cases of hyperlordosis correct with surgery on the spine alone. Lipton et al[7] performed a posterior spinal fusion on eight patients with hyperlordosis with a mean sagittal Cobb angle of 91.8 degrees. After surgery, the mean lumbar lordosis improved to 48.6 degrees. The authors noted the resolution of the patients' preoperative issues of superior mesenteric artery syndrome, bowel and bladder dysfunction, and malnutrition. However, surgery in a spine with lordosis may pose problems with access and wound closure.

Spinopelvic Parameters

Legaye et al[18] first described spinopelvic parameters. Since then, the application of their assessment in patients affected by sagittal plane spinal deformity has become common. They described the following spinopelvic parameters: the pelvic incidence (PI), SS, pelvic tilt (PT), and S1 overhang (OH). The definition of PI is the angle between a line perpendicular to the sacral endplate at its midpoint and a line connecting this point to the axis of the femoral heads. *SS* is defined as the angle between the superior endplate of S1 and a horizontal line. *PT* is defined as the angle between the line connecting the midpoint of the superior sacral endplate to the femoral head's axis and the vertical. The *S1 OH* is defined as the distance between the bicoxofemoral axis and the projection to this level of the midpoint of the sacral plate.

Spinopelvic parameters can be difficult to measure in patients with NMS because of variable posture and associated PO. Few studies in the literature have evaluated the average spinopelvic parameters in patients with NMS. In one such study, Suh et al[19] evaluated the sagittal spinopelvic parameters in 57 patients with

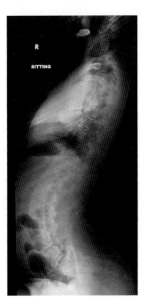

Fig. 30-4 Hyperlordosis is an uncommon sagittal plane deformity in NMS. Patients with this deformity should be evaluated for hip flexion contractures as a cause.

CP (Gross Motor Function Classification System levels I through IV) and compared them to 24 healthy volunteers (controls). They found that across both groups PI values were similar, but patients with CP had higher SS, thoracolumbar kyphosis, lumbar lordosis, and sagittal balance, and lower PT and OH, signifying a much more horizontal sacrum and posterior deviation of the hip joint than in the controls. In addition, correlations were measured between the parameters and symptoms of pain experienced by the patients with CP. PT, OH, and thoracolumbar kyphosis had a positive correlation with the severity of symptoms.

SAGITTAL BALANCE AND CLINICAL OUTCOMES

In the literature on adult patients, interest has increased in the relationship between sagittal and coronal balance and health-related quality of life outcome measures. Glassman et al[20] studied 298 adult patients with degenerative scoliosis who had undergone posterior spinal fusions and correlated their radiographic measurements to their changes in health-related quality of life outcomes. The authors found that a positive sagittal balance was the most reliable predictor of clinical symptoms in patients who had undergone primary and revision posterior spinal arthrodesis.

Literature evaluating the correlation between global sagittal alignment and clinical outcomes in patients with NMS is limited. A recently completed study (manuscript submitted for publication) prospectively evaluated patients with CP who had undergone a posterior spinal fusion for the correction of their sagittal and coronal plane deformities. For a 2-year period, in addition to radiographic parameters, clinical outcomes using the Caregiver Priorities and Child Health Index of Life With Disabilities (CPCHILD) questionnaire were collected.[21] The CPCHILD includes six domains affecting the quality of life of patients with CP. They found that the restoration of global sagittal alignment to a neutral or slightly positive sacral vertebral angle and T1 pelvic angle were associated with better transferring, function, social interaction, and total caregiver satisfaction, whereas a higher pelvic incidence correlated with better sitting tolerance. Although more research is needed on the correlation between clinical and radiographic outcomes in patients with NMS, it is evident that the correction of sagittal and coronal plane deformities has a positive effect on their lives.

NONOPERATIVE MANAGEMENT

It is important to have a discussion with NMS patients and their caregivers about the natural history of the specific neuromuscular disorder, and nonoperative management should be explored as the first treatment option. Nonoperative treatment options include sitting supports, custom seating, and functional sitting programs.[22] Although bracing has been shown to be successful in preventing curve progression in patients with adolescent idiopathic scoliosis, it has not proved effective in preventing progression of curves in patients with NMS.[23] However, for patients with trunk control and flexible curves, a thoracolumbosacral orthosis can help with sitting.

Recent advances have been made in the use of steroids for patients affected by Duchenne muscular dystrophy (DMD). DMD is an X-linked, progressive, degenerative disorder of the muscle secondary to a mutation in the gene dystrophin.[24] In the past, spinal arthrodesis was performed in patients with DMD and scoliosis when the scoliosis curve became larger than 20 degrees because of its rapidly progressive nature, particularly when patients became nonambulatory. However, steroids have now become a viable nonoperative treatment. Lebel et al[25] treated 30 boys with glucocorticoids; the parents of 24 other boys decided against steroid treatment. At the final follow-up, scoliosis developed in only 20% of the boys treated with steroids and in 92% of the boys who were untreated.

PREOPERATIVE PLANNING

Although surgery is often the definitive management for correction of sagittal and coronal plane deformities in patients with NMS, surgeons need to consider whether patients actually benefit from this surgery, given the high complication rate.[26] A preliminary study in patients with totally involved CP showed an improvement in overall comfort noted by their caregivers.[27] In another study, Jones et al[28] surveyed 20 patients with totally involved CP and found an improvement in pain, happiness, frequency of feeling sick and tired, and overall parental satisfaction by 1 year after surgery. Despite the high complication rate, the overall positive impact on the life of patients and their caregivers was thought to be worth the risk.

Because the spinal deformity of most patients with NMS progresses below fusions that do not include the pelvis, it has become the standard of care to extend fusion to the pelvis for the patient with NMS and poor trunk control. Preoperative medical optimization includes adequate nutrition to bring a patient's weight at least to the 10th percentile for the height or arm span, placement of a feeding tube if needed to facilitate nutrition, and assessment by a pulmonologist for evidence of reactive airway disease or restrictive lung disease.[29]

Preoperative evaluation involves obtaining a complete history, performing a thorough physical examination to determine the baseline functional status, and assessment of radiographs. Often, the caregiver will be the only party able to describe a patient's day-to-day activities. Key questions include: Is the patient able to feed himself or herself? Is the patient able to transfer from his or her wheelchair to the bed? These functions are important in planning restoration of spinal alignment. Preoperative radiographs should include an AP view (standing or sitting if nonambulatory), an AP traction view, a lateral view, and an AP pelvis view (to evaluate PO and evidence of any hip dislocation) (Fig. 30-5).

In the past, it was thought that patients with large neuromuscular curves required staged anterior and posterior arthrodesis to fully correct their deformities. However, clinical studies and advances in pedicle screw technology have shown that anterior and posterior arthrodesis performed on the same day and posterior-only arthrodesis have comparable outcomes.[30,31]

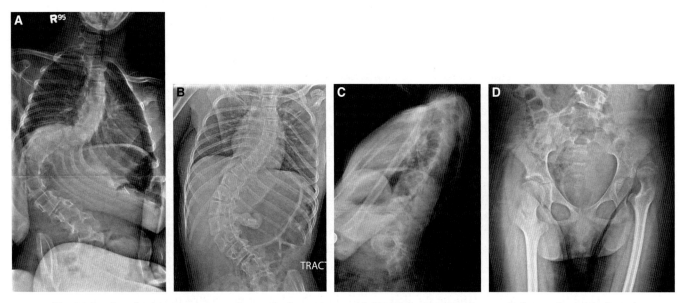

Fig. 30-5   Standard preoperative radiographs for patients with NMS. **A,** An AP radiograph shows classic C-shaped curve and associated PO. **B,** An AP radiograph with traction demonstrates the flexible nature of this coronal plane deformity. **C,** A standard lateral radiograph reveals a patient's global sagittal balance. **D,** A standard AP pelvis radiograph is important for evaluation of a patient's hip status and PO.

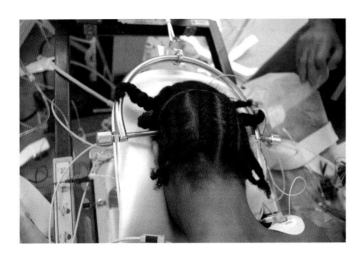

Fig. 30-6   Intraoperative traction can help in the correction of large deformities in patients with NMS.

The decision to use traction should be part of the preoperative plan. Traction may help surgeons to obtain better coronal and sagittal alignment particularly in rigid curve patterns. Halo traction in patients with severe NMS has been shown to decrease the need for vertebral column osteotomies intraoperatively[32] (Fig. 30-6).

OPERATIVE TECHNIQUE

A variety of instrumentation strategies are available for correction of sagittal and coronal plane deformities in patients with NMS, including Luque-Galveston,[33] Cotrel-Duboussett,[34] and the Unit rod,[35] and all have advantages and disadvantages. For example, the Unit rod has been shown to provide excellent correction of PO in patients with NMS.[36] However, the same study also showed that it resulted in higher transfusion requirements, infection rates, and intensive care unit and hospital stays and in more problems at the upper instrumented vertebra.

Patients with NMS usually have substantial abnormalities in spinopelvic parameters. These parameters contribute to the position of the spine over the pelvis and thus to global trunk misalignment. To correctly position the spine over the pelvis in this patient population, it is important to have a rigid fixation as a distal anchor in the form of pelvic fixation. The sacral-alar-iliac (SAI) screw is a versatile anchor that helps to promote global spinal alignment. It provides excellent distal fixation in patients with NMS and allows significant correction of PO.[37]

The advantages of the SAI technique include the following:
- The start point is on the sacrum, which avoids soft tissue dissection needed for the traditional start point of iliac fixation on the posterior superior iliac spine.
- The average length of the SAI pathway is 106 mm, extending far past the lumbosacral pivot point and increasing the stiffness of the fusion construct significantly.[38]
- The narrowest mean width of the ilium is 12 mm; therefore, screws inserted via the SAI pathway can accommodate large diameter screws for increased bone purchase.
- The SAI insertion point on the sacrum is in line with the pedicle screw locations in the rest of the spine.
- The average distance between the skin and the insertion point of the SAI screw is 1.5 cm deeper than the distance between the skin and the posterior superior iliac spine start point, allowing more soft coverage. This coverage is especially important for nonambulatory patients with NMS who are susceptible to pressure sores.

The average start point for the SAI pathway is 25 mm inferior to the S1 endplate and 22 mm lateral from the midpoint of the S2 body (Fig. 30-7, *A*). For pediatric patients, the senior author (P.D.S.) prefers to make the initial pathway with an awl. Others, operating on adults, prefer to use a drill. As the awl is advanced into the sacrum and then the ilium, the trajectory should be angled 40 degrees laterally and 40 degrees caudally[39] (Fig. 30-7, *B* and *C*). As the awl crosses the sacroiliac joint, some resistance is expected. However, if too much resistance is felt, the likely cause is the awl hitting the lateral wall of the ilium. In this case, the awl should be backed out and redirected so that the trajectory is more vertical. The correct position of the awl is routinely just superior to the inferior border of the sacroiliac joint (Fig. 30-7, *D*) and should be confirmed via fluoroscopy.

The length of the screw pathway is measured with a depth gauge (average approximately 90 mm), and a dilator is used to expand the size of the SAI screw pathway. Finally, a guide wire is inserted and impacted into the distal ilium, and the screw is advanced over the guide wire (Fig. 30-7, *E*). This procedure is then performed on the contralateral side.

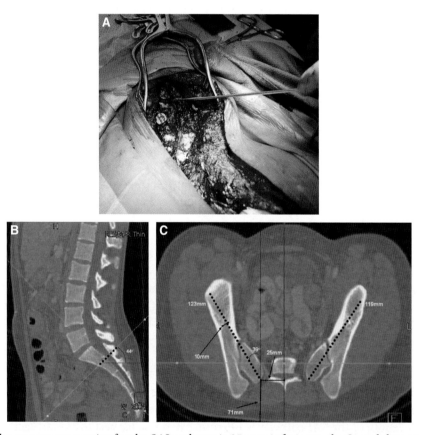

Fig. 30-7   **A,** The average start point for the SAI pathway is 25 mm inferior to the S1 endplate and 22 mm lateral from the midpoint of the S2 body. **B** and **C,** CT imaging shows the SAI screw trajectory. **B,** A sagittal image indicates that the trajectory should be angled 40 degrees caudally when the SAI screw pathway is created with an awl. **C,** The awl should also have a trajectory of 40 degrees laterally. The lateral wall of the ilium should not be penetrated. (**B** and **C,** From Chang TL, Sponseller PD, Kebaish KM, Fishman EK. Low profile pelvic fixation: anatomic parameters for sacral-alar-iliac fixation versus traditional iliac fixation. Spine 34:436-440, 2009.)

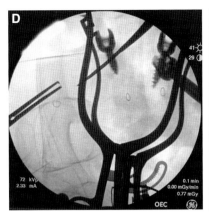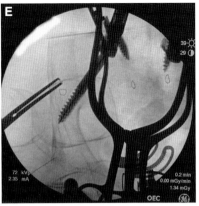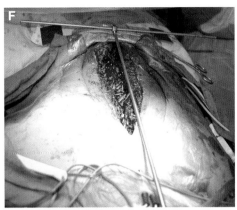

Fig. 30-7, cont'd **D,** Intraoperative fluoroscopic imaging confirms the SAI pathway created with an awl. **E,** The SAI screw should be advanced over the guide wire and its position confirmed with fluoroscopy. **F,** Correction of PO is checked intraoperatively with a T-square instrument. The horizontal limbs are placed parallel to the superior dome of the acetabulum bilaterally. The vertical limb should be in line with the central sacral vertebral line. If PO has been adequately corrected and overall spinal balance achieved, then the top of the T-square instrument will cross the vertebral body of T1.

After both SAI screws are placed, they can easily be connected to the rods superiorly. After the appropriate curves are compressed and distracted to correct the sagittal and coronal deformities, the correction of the patient's PO is assessed with the T-square of Tolo (Fig. 30-7, *F*). The instrument is placed on top of the spine with the horizontal limbs parallel to the superior dome of the acetabulum bilaterally and the vertical limb in line with the central sacral vertebral line. If PO has been adequately corrected and overall spinal alignment achieved, then the top of the T-square instrument will cross the vertebral body of T1.[40]

POTENTIAL COMPLICATIONS AND MANAGEMENT

A variety of complications can arise in the surgical treatment of patients with NMS and spinal instrumentation. Sharma et al[41] performed a random effects analytical meta-analysis of all studies reporting complications in patients with NMS who had spinal surgery. They found an overall pooled estimate rate (PR) of pulmonary complications of 22.71%, an overall PR of neurologic complications of 3.01%, an overall PR of infections of 10.91%, an overall PR of implant-related complications of 12.51%, and an overall PR of pseudarthrosis of 1.88%.

Infection is a particularly difficult complication to prevent in this patient population. At our institution, numerous steps are taken to prevent infection, including pouring povidone-iodine into the incision before closure, soaking all allograft in gentamicin before placement in the body, and sprinkling vancomycin powder onto the hardware and surrounding soft tissues before closure. Zebala et al[42] used a rabbit spine infection model to determine whether local administration of vancomycin eradicated an infection without causing systemic complications. The spines of 20 New Zealand white rabbits were inoculated with methicillin-sensitive *Staphylococcus aureus;* 10 received a local administration of vancomycin at the surgical site, and 10 did not (controls). The bacterial cultures of the surgical site tissues were negative for all 10 vancomycin-treated rabbits and positive for all 10 control rabbits; no systemic effects were seen in either group in this study. Much more needs to be known about the prevention of complications in this patient population, and it is currently the source of active research.

PATIENT EXAMPLE

A 17-year-old patient was admitted to the pediatric medical service for an acute worsening of her baseline decreased respiratory status secondary to pneumonia. During her hospital stay, the pediatric orthopedic service was consulted for possible surgical recommendations for her spinal deformity. She was born by normal vaginal delivery at 42 weeks without complications. Her development appeared normal up until age 6, when her mother noticed that she started to progressively ambulate on the tips of her toes and then along her lateral border of her feet bilaterally. When her daughter started to show signs of clonus, she was

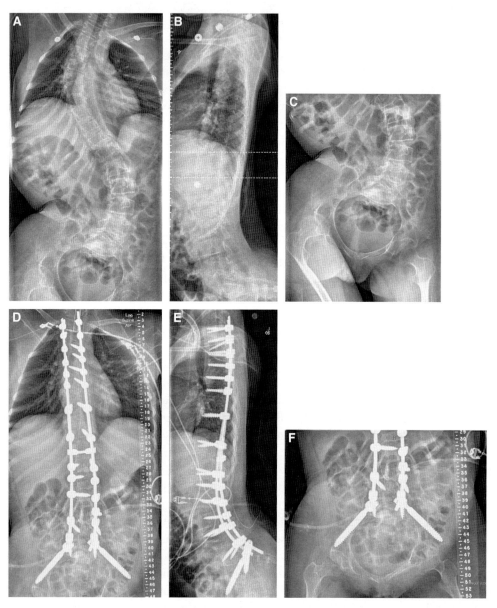

Fig. 30-8   This patient had anterior horn cell degeneration of the spine. **A,** A preoperative AP scoliosis radiograph showed a thoracic curve of 58.5 degrees and a lumbar curve of 61.5 degrees. **B,** A lateral preoperative radiograph showed a neutral to negative sagittal balance. **C,** A preoperative pelvic radiograph showed substantial pelvic obliquity and a dislocated right hip. **D** and **E,** Postoperative AP and lateral radiographs show virtually complete correction of the coronal and sagittal plane deformities. **F,** A postoperative pelvic radiograph reveals substantial correction of the patient's PO and SAI screws in their desired position.

evaluated by a neurologist and found to have a nonspecific form of anterior horn cell degeneration of her spine. By age 18, she was unable to ambulate and was dependent on a wheelchair for mobilization. According to her mother, when the patient became wheelchair-bound, her spinal deformity rapidly progressed to its current state.

On physical examination, the patient was sitting in a motorized wheelchair, with labored breath sounds but in no acute distress. Examination of her back showed no tufts of hair or step-offs. She had gross coronal malalignment of the trunk and was unable to control the muscles of her torso. The patient was tender to palpation throughout her entire spine and had intact sensation in all dermatomes. She was globally weak, with strength testing no higher than 3/5 in any muscle group. She was also tender to palpation in her bilateral hips. Her upper and lower extremity pulses were normal.

Preoperative sitting radiographs of the spine revealed scoliosis composed of a 58.5-degree thoracic curve and a 61.5-degree lumbar curve (Fig 30-8, *A*). A lateral radiograph of the spine revealed a normal to slightly negative global sagittal alignment balance (Fig. 30-8, *B*). A preoperative pelvic radiograph showed a substantial amount of obliquity and a dislocated right hip (Fig. 30-8, *C*). Given the patient's progressively worsening respiratory status secondary to her spinal deformity and her pain, she was taken to the operating room for posterior spinal fusion from T1 to S2. She also underwent a psoas and adductor tendon lengthening on the right hip. Postoperative radiographs show adequate alignment in both the sagittal and coronal planes (Fig. 30-8, *D* through *F*).

CONCLUSION

NMS is a heterogeneous disorder characterized by a loss of normal muscular control involving the spine, often leading to a progressive deformity. In the coronal plane, NMS is characterized by a long, C-shaped curvature and PO. In the sagittal plane, NMS is characterized by hyperkyphosis, hyperlordosis, an increase in SS and global sagittal alignment, with a significantly lower PT and sacral OH correlating to the severity of symptoms. Recently, a nonoperative treatment has shown promising results for patients with DMD: steroids have significantly slowed the progression and development of scoliosis in this population.[25] Posterior spinal fusion with pelvic fixation via the SAI screw technique has provided excellent results in the correction of sagittal and coronal plane deformities and PO.[37] Finally, PJK is a major problem in this patient population, especially because most patients undergo long-segment arthrodesis. Risk factors for the development of PJK in patients with CP include the absence of mental retardation, preoperative kyphosis of at least 53 degrees, and a significant operative correction of the kyphosis by at least 29 degrees. Factors not associated with the development of PJK in patients with CP include the type of upper anchor, the chosen upper instrumented vertebra, the patient's hip status, age, Risser sign, lumbar lordosis, and Gross Motor Function Classification System class.

REFERENCES

1. McCarthy RE. Management of neuromuscular scoliosis. Orthop Clin North Am 30:435-449, 1999.
2. Lenke LG, Betz RR, Harms J, et al. Adolescent idiopathic scoliosis: a new classification to determine extent of spinal arthrodesis. J Bone Joint Surg Am 83:1169-1181, 2001.
3. Auerbach JD, Spiegel DA, Zgonis MH, et al. The correction of pelvic obliquity in patients with cerebral palsy and neuromuscular scoliosis: is there a benefit of anterior release prior to posterior spinal arthrodesis? Spine 34:E766-E774, 2009.
4. Kuklo TR, Potter BK, O'Brien MF, et al; Spinal Deformity Study Group. Reliability analysis for digital adolescent idiopathic scoliosis measurements. J Spinal Disord Tech 18:152-159, 2005.

5. Ko PS, Jameson PG II, Chang TL, et al. Transverse-plane pelvic asymmetry in patients with cerebral palsy and scoliosis. J Pediatr Orthop 31:277-283, 2011.

6. Renshaw TS, Deluca PA. Cerebral palsy. In Morrissy RT, Weinstein SL, eds. Lovell and Winter's Pediatric Orthopaedics. Philadelphia: Lippincott Williams & Wilkins, 2006.

7. Lipton GE, Letonoff EJ, Dabney KW, et al. Correction of sagittal plane spinal deformities with unit rod instrumentation in children with cerebral palsy. J Bone Joint Surg Am 85:2349-2357, 2003.

8. Smith MW, Annis P, Lawrence BD, et al. Early proximal junctional failure in patients with preoperative sagittal imbalance. Evid Based Spine Care J 4:163-164, 2013.

9. Kim YJ, Bridwell KH, Lenke LG, et al. Proximal junctional kyphosis in adolescent idiopathic scoliosis following segmental posterior spinal instrumentation and fusion: minimum 5-year follow-up. Spine 30:2045-2050, 2005.

10. Sink EL, Newton PO, Mubarak SJ, et al. Maintenance of sagittal plane alignment after surgical correction of spinal deformity in patients with cerebral palsy. Spine 28:1396-1403, 2003.

11. Helgeson MD, Shah SA, Newton PO, et al; The Harms Study Group. Evaluation of proximal junctional kyphosis in adolescent idiopathic scoliosis following pedicle screw, hook, or hybrid instrumentation. Spine 35:177-181, 2010.

12. Lee GA, Betz RR, Clements DH III, et al. Proximal kyphosis after posterior spinal fusion in patients with idiopathic scoliosis. Spine 24:795-799, 1999.

13. Palisano R, Rosenbaum P, Walter S, et al. Development and reliability of a system to classify gross motor function in children with cerebral palsy. Dev Med Child Neurol 39:214-223, 1997.

14. Song EW, Lenke LG, Schoenecker PL. Isolated thoracolumbar and lumbar hyperlordosis in a patient with cerebral palsy. J Spinal Disord 13:455-460, 2000.

15. Steel HH, Adams DJ. Hyperlordosis caused by the lumboperitoneal shunt procedure for hydrocephalus. J Bone Joint Surg Am 54:1537-1542, 1972.

16. McIvor J, Krajbich JI, Hoffman H. Orthopaedic complications of lumboperitoneal shunts. J Pediatr Orthop 8:687-689, 1988.

17. Vialle R, Khouri N, Guillaumat M. Lumbar hyperlodosis in cerebral palsy: anatomic analysis and surgical strategy for correction. Childs Nerv Syst 22:704-709, 2006.

18. Legaye J, Duval-Beaupere G, Hecquet J, et al. Pelvic incidence: a fundamental pelvic parameter for three-dimensional regulation of spinal sagittal curves. Eur Spine J 7:99-103, 1998.

19. Suh SW, Suh DH, Kim JW, et al. Analysis of sagittal spinopelvic parameters in cerebral palsy. Spine J 13:882-888, 2013.

20. Glassman SD, Berven S, Bridwell K, et al. Correlation of radiographic parameters and clinical symptoms in adult scoliosis. Spine 30:682-688, 2005.

21. Narayanan UG, Fehlings D, Weir S, et al. Initial development and validation of the Caregiver Priorities and Child Health Index of Life with Disabilities (CPCHILD). Dev Med Child Neurol 48:804-812, 2006.

22. Olafsson Y, Saraste H, Al-Dabbagh Z. Brace treatment in neuromuscular spine deformity. J Pediatr Orthop 19:376-379, 1999.

23. Miller A, Temple T, Miller F. Impact of orthoses on the rate of scoliosis progression in children with cerebral palsy. J Pediatr Orthop 16:332-335, 1996.

24. Wicklund MP. The muscular dystrophies. Continuum 19(6 Muscle Disease):1535-1570, 2013.

25. Lebel DE, Corston JA, McAdam LC, et al. Glucocorticoid treatment for the prevention of scoliosis in children with Duchenne muscular dystrophy: long-term follow-up. J Bone Joint Surg Am 95:1057-1061, 2013.

26. Lonstein JE, Koop SE, Novachek TF, et al. Results and complications after spinal fusion for neuromuscular scoliosis in cerebral palsy and static encephalopathy using Luque Galveston instrumentation: experience in 93 patients. Spine 37:583-591, 2012.

27. Cassidy C, Craig CL, Perry A, et al. A reassessment of spinal stabilization in severe cerebral palsy. J Pediatr Orthop 14:731-739, 1994.

28. Jones KB, Sponseller PD, Shindle MK, et al. Longitudinal parental perceptions of spinal fusion for neuromuscular spine deformity in patients with totally involved cerebral palsy. J Pediatr Orthop 23:143-149, 2003.

29. Jevsevar DS, Karlin LI. The relationship between preoperative nutritional status and complications after an operation for scoliosis in patients who have cerebral palsy. J Bone Joint Surg Am 75:880-884, 1993.

30. Banta JV, Drummond DS, Ferguson RL. The treatment of neuromuscular scoliosis. Instr Course Lect 48:551-562, 1999.

31. Boachie-Adjei O, Lonstein JE, Winter RB, et al. Management of neuromuscular spinal deformities with Luque segmental instrumentation. J Bone Joint Surg Am 71:548-562, 1989.

32. Sponseller PD, Takenaga RK, Newton P, et al. The use of traction in the treatment of severe spinal deformity. Spine 33:2305-2309, 2008.

33. Luque ER. The anatomic basis and development of segmental spinal instrumentation. Spine 7:256-259, 1982.

34. Cotrel Y, Dubousset J. [A new technic for segmental spinal osteosynthesis using the posterior approach] Rev Chir Orthop Reparatrice Appar Mot 70:489-494, 1984.

35. Bell DF, Moseley CF, Koreska J. Unit rod segmental spinal instrumentation in the management of patients with progressive neuromuscular spinal deformity. Spine 14:1301-1307, 1989.

36. Sponseller PD, Shah SA, Abel MF, et al; The Harms Study Group. Scoliosis surgery in cerebral palsy. Differences between unit rod and custom rods. Spine 34:840-844, 2009.

37. Sponseller PD, Zimmerman RM, Ko PS, et al. Low profile pelvic fixation with the sacral alar iliac technique in the pediatric population improves results at two-year minimum follow-up. Spine 35:1887-1892, 2010.

38. McCord DH, Cunningham BW, Shono Y, et al. Biomechanical analysis of lumbosacral fixation. Spine 17:S235-S243, 1992.

39. Chang TL, Sponseller PD, Kebaish KM, et al. Low profile pelvic fixation. Anatomic parameters for sacral alar-iliac fixation versus traditional iliac fixation. Spine 34:436-440, 2009.

40. Andras L, Yamaguchi KT Jr, Skaggs DL, et al. Surgical technique for balancing posterior spinal fusions to the pelvis using the T square of Tolo. J Pediatr Orthop 32:e63-e66, 2012.

41. Sharma S, Wu C, Andersen T, et al. Prevalence of complications in neuromuscular scoliosis surgery: a literature meta-analysis from the past 15 years. Eur Spine J 22:1230-1249, 2013.

42. Zebala LP, Chuntarapas T, Kelly MP, et al. Intrawound vancomycin powder eradicates surgical wound contamination: an in vivo rabbit study. J Bone Joint Surg Am 96:46-51, 2014.

31

Spinal Alignment in the Management of Scheuermann's Kyphosis

Koopong Siribumrungwong ▪ *Munish Chandra Gupta*

Scheuermann's kyphosis was first described in 1920 as a rigid, painful, fixed dorsal kyphosis of the thoracic or thoracolumbar spine that occurs in adolescence.[1] In 1964 Sorensen[2] proposed radiographic criteria defined as a thoracic kyphosis with anterior wedging of 5 degrees or more for at least three consecutive vertebral bodies. Scheuermann's kyphosis can be classified into two different curve patterns. Type I (the typical form), the most common type, has a thoracic curve associated with nonstructural hyperlordosis of the lumbar and cervical spine.[3] Type II, the atypical form, is uncommon, has a thoracolumbar or lumbar curve, and is typically associated with pain that improves with rest and activity modification. Type II is often diagnosed in active athletic adolescents and thought to be likely to progress in adulthood. The incidence of Scheuermann's kyphosis differs depending on the definition. This disease occurs in 1% to 8% of the general population. The true incidence might be underestimated, because the thoracic deformity is attributed to poor posture, or it is a misdiagnosis.[4,5] Previously, Scheuermann's kyphosis was thought to be more common in men than women, but currently the sex ratio is considered to be nearly 1.[5,6]

ETIOLOGIC FACTORS

The cause of Scheuermann's disease is unclear; however, numerous hypotheses have been proposed. Histologic studies show disorganized enchondral ossification similar to Blount's disease, reduced collagen levels, and increased mucopolysaccharide levels in the endplate.[7,8] This was believed to alter enchondral ossification of the endplate and disturb the vertical growth.

MECHANICAL STRESS

Mechanical stress has been proposed as a possible cause of the disease. Van Linthoudt and Revel[9] reported that in identical twins who had similar lesions of localized lumbar Scheuermann's kyphosis, the lesions were worse in the twin who practiced strenuous sports activities. Ravel et al[10] performed a histologic study of vertebral endplates in young rats subjected to intensive passive motion. The results showed that repetitive strain on vertebral endplates can lead to typical Scheuermann's lesions. Bracing can relieve the pain and partially correct the deformity, which possibly supports mechanical stress as a cause of Scheuermann's kyphosis.[11]

Genetic Predisposition

Many investigations showed an increased familial incidence of Scheuermann's kyphosis. Halal et al[12] described five families in which Scheuermann's disease seemed to follow an autosomal dominant pattern of inheritance. Damborg et al[5] reviewed 35,000 twins in the Danish Twin Registry from 1931 to 1982. They found the overall prevalence of Scheuermann's kyphosis to be 2.8%. The pairwise concordance for monozygotic twins was 0.19, compared with 0.07 for dizygotic twins. The probandwise concordance was 0.31 for monozygotic twins and 0.13 for dizygotic twins. The odds ratio was 32.92 and 6.25 in the monozygotic and dizygotic twins, respectively. These differences were significant ($p < 0.01$). Heritability was 74%. Because of the pairwise and probandwise concordance the odds ratios were two to three times higher in monozygotic than in dizygotic twins and the heritability was high, they concluded that genetic makeup is a major etiologic factor in Scheuermann's kyphosis.

Many theories have been proposed to explain the pathogenesis of Scheuermann's kyphosis. These include genetic factors, mechanical stress, and environmental factors. However, further investigation is needed.

NATURAL HISTORY

Murray et al[13] conducted a study of 67 patients with thoracic Scheuermann's kyphosis in North America. They assessed physical examination results, trunk strength measurements, serial radiographs, results of pulmonary function tests, and pain. The mean angle of kyphosis was 71 degrees at presentation (range 37 to 110 degrees), and the average follow-up was 32 years. They found that patients with Scheuermann's kyphosis worked in jobs that were less physically demanding, had higher levels of back pain, and were more concerned about their appearance, compared with the control group.

Ristolainen et al[14] carried out a retrospective study of a Finnish cohort of 49 patients with thoracic Scheuermann's kyphosis. The follow-up period was 37 years. They assessed a questionnaire concerning back pain and disability scores. Compared with the control group, Scheuermann's patients had higher risks for back pain and disabilities during activities of daily living, but the degree of thoracic kyphosis was not related to back pain, quality of life, and general health.

Neither of these studies assessed kyphosis progression, which is the major concern of adolescents seeking medical attention. The natural history of untreated Scheuermann's kyphosis is unknown. Studies in Scheuermann's kyphosis with different curve magnitudes are needed to guide surgeons in conservative and surgical treatment of their patients.

SAGITTAL ALIGNMENT

A radiograph to measure thoracic kyphosis should include the upper thoracic spine. It is very important to have good technique to obtain a measurable radiograph. On a lateral standing view with the arm at the side, the humerus can overlie the upper thoracic spine and prevent good measurement. Lifting the arm forward can induce lumbar hyperlordosis and lead to misinterpretation of the overall alignment. Boseker et al[15] recommended that patients stand in a relaxed posture with the arms forward at a 90-degree angle with the body and resting on a pole in a relaxed posture. Recently, Faro et al[16] and Horton et al[17] described a clavicular position in which patients stand with the arms crossed over the chest, with each fist on the opposite clavicle. Both of these techniques provided an adequate view of the upper thoracic spine and prevented lumbar hyperlordosis.[18]

The method of measuring thoracic kyphosis varies from surgeon to surgeon. Some surgeons routinely measure from T2 to T12 or from T4 to T12, although these might not be the maximally tilted vertebrae. Differences in measurement technique can lead to confusion. Winter et al[18] recommended that thoracic kyphosis be measured from the uppermost tilted vertebra to the lowermost tilted vertebra (true kyphosis technique). Based on this measurement, normal kyphosis in children and adolescents ranges from 33 to 43 degrees with very large ranges of the angle of kyphosis and standard deviations.[15,19]

Spinopelvic balance in the sagittal plane has been referred to as a linear chain that links the spine to the lower extremities.[20] Normal spinal sagittal balance is characterized as kyphosis from T1 to T12 and lordosis from L1 to S1. Not only does the spine play a major role in spinal balance, but the hips, knees, and pelvis are also involved in maintaining sagittal balance. The sagittal vertical axis (SVA) should be balanced by kyphosis and lordosis of the spine, which balance the occiput over the sacropelvic axis in an energy-efficient position.[21] Normally, thoracic kyphosis should be 10 to 40 degrees, and lumbar lordosis should be 40 to 60 degrees.[22] Lumbar lordosis should be 20 degrees more than thoracic kyphosis.

The components of SVA that create overall sagittal balance of the spine are the thoracic spine, the thoracolumbar junction, the lumbar spine, and the pelvis. SVA can be evaluated on a lateral standing radiograph by drawing a plumb line from the C7 vertebral body to the sacral endplate. Patients whose C7 vertical plumb line is anterior to the posterosuperior corner of the sacrum have positive sagittal balance, and those whose C7 vertical plumb line is posterior to the posterosuperior corner of the sacrum have negative sagittal balance. The mean offset of SVA from the posterosuperior corner of the sacrum is 0.5 cm in asymptomatic individuals.[23] An offset of SVA of more than 2.5 cm anterior or posterior is considered abnormal.[23] Mac-Thiong et al[24] described the relation of positive sagittal balance with quality of life in patients with spinal deformity and noted a poor quality of life in patients who had a positive SVA of more than 6 cm. Legaye et al[25] used the pelvic parameters to describe the orientation of the pelvis in relation to the spine. Pelvic parameters have been shown to significantly influence alignment of the spine and pelvis. The spine and pelvis balance around the hip axis to position the gravity line over the femoral heads.[26] Three pelvic parameters have been described: pelvic incidence, sacral slope, and pelvic tilt. Pelvic incidence is the angle formed by a line drawn perpendicular to the midpoint of the sacral endplate and a line drawn to this point from the center of the femoral head. It is a morphometric, fixed parameter after skeletal growth is completed that is different in each person and unaffected by the orientation of the pelvis. Sacral slope is the angle formed by a line drawn along the sacral endplate and a horizontal reference line. Pelvic tilt is the angle formed by a line drawn from the midpoint of the sacral endplate to the center of the femoral head and a vertical reference line. Sacral slope and pelvic tilt are variable parameters that are position dependent and vary with flexion and extension of the pelvis and hip joints. Pelvic incidence is equal to the sum of the sacral slope and pelvic tilt.[25]

Stagnara et al[27] described the relation between lumbar lordosis and sacral slope. When sacral slope increases, the spine adapts with an increased lumbar lordosis. Vaz et al[26] reported on the correlation of pelvic incidence and lumbar lordosis. The greater the pelvic incidence angle the greater the lumbar lordosis. In patients with Scheuermann's kyphosis, thoracic hyperkyphosis is compensated by lumbar hyperlordosis. But lumbar lordosis compensation is limited by facet joint anatomy; therefore additional compensation needs to occur through retroversion of the pelvis on the femoral heads. Pelvic retroversion decreases sacral slope and increases pelvic tilt. Therefore, in Scheuermann's kyphosis, characteristic lumbar hyperlordosis, decreased sacral slope, and increased pelvic tilt occur as a result of pelvic compensation.

Scoliosis correction involves calculating the percentage of correction ([preoperative kyphosis − postoperative kyphosis/preoperative kyphosis] × 100), whereas surgical correction of Scheuermann's kyphosis does not. Kyphosis is not ideally 0 degrees, because this implies a pathologic flat back.[18] Instead, surgeons should report the number of degrees of correction and the final number of degrees of kyphosis.

PRETREATMENT AND PREOPERATIVE PLANNING

CLINICAL PRESENTATION

Most patients with Scheuermann's kyphosis had painful, rigid, dorsal kyphosis in adolescence.[1] A physical examination usually reveals an excessive thoracic kyphosis that is compensated by nonstructural lumbar hyperlordosis, nonstructural cervical hyperlordosis, pelvic anteversion, and rounding of the shoulders. Pain is one of the symptoms for which patients seek medical attention. It might be caused by several factors such as muscle fatigue from decompensated curves of the lumbar or cervical areas, disc inflammation from a Scheuermann's lesion, and disc degeneration.[11] Pain is usually localized at the apex of deformity and the thoracolumbar junction. However, pain at the lumbosacral area should raise suspicion of a spondylolysis lesion. Hyperlordosis in the lumbar area increases stress at the pars interarticularis. Fatigue fractures of the pars can result in spondylolysis.[28] Other clinical findings are tightness of the hamstrings and iliopsoas muscles.[29]

One of the differential diagnoses for Scheuermann's kyphosis is postural kyphosis or round-back deformity. A kyphotic curve secondary to postural kyphosis often disappears after forward bending, whereas forward bending typically accentuates a kyphotic curve with a sharp transition in the thoracolumbar region in Scheuermann's kyphosis.[30] Postural kyphosis can also be differentiated radiographically from Scheuermann's kyphosis by the absence of wedging of the vertebral bodies, irregular endplate, and Schmorl's nodes.

Scheuermann's kyphosis is associated with scoliosis in 15% to 20% of patients.[14,31] Scoliosis probably arises from asymmetrical Scheuermann's lesions. However, it can develop independent of Scheuermann's disease. In this case, the apex of the scoliosis does not correspond with the apex of kyphosis and can cause a more rapid progression.[32]

Neurologic complications are rare in Scheuermann's kyphosis. They are caused by severe kyphosis, thoracic disc herniation, and dural cyst[33,34] triggered by a traumatic event. MRI of the thoracic spine should be performed to evaluate patients with hyperreflexia and motor and sensory abnormalities. Neurologic complications can occur in cases with small, severe angular curves.[34]

Pulmonary complications usually present with restrictive lung disease but are rare. These problems usually present in patients whose kyphosis is more than 100 degrees.[13]

RADIOGRAPHIC STUDIES

Standard standing AP and lateral views of the entire spine should be obtained in patients with Scheuermann's disease. Radiographic criteria are defined as a thoracic kyphosis with anterior wedging of 5 degrees or more for at least three consecutive vertebral bodies. The typical three characteristic findings are anterior vertebral wedging, an irregular endplate, and Schmorl's nodes. Anterior vertebral wedging usually occurs at the primary ossification phase and increases during the secondary ossification phase. Anterior vertebral wedging can occur from excessive pressure on the vertebral endplate. Vertebral wedging will increase from mechanical stress placed on the vertebral endplate (Fig. 31-1).

Schmorl's nodes occur in the secondary ossification phase. They can be isolated without other Scheuermann's lesions. The prevalence of Schmorl's nodes varies from 16% to 48%.[35,36] They can be a central herniation through a weak point of a vertebral endplate or an anterior or posterior herniation through an apophyseal ring fracture. Some studies show an association between Schmorl's nodes and disc degeneration.[35,37] Paajanen et al[38] showed that 55% of the discs in patients with Scheuermann's disease were abnormal on MRI, compared with 10% in patients without Scheuermann's disease. Disc degeneration might be explained by decreased nutrition because of the changes between the disc and vertebral endplate. However, Schmorl's nodes are often asymptomatic in patients younger than 20 years of age.[39]

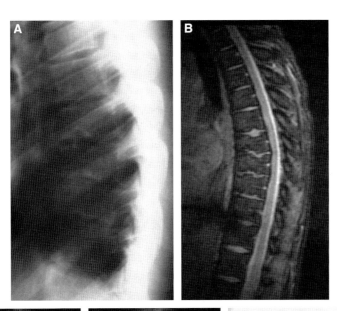

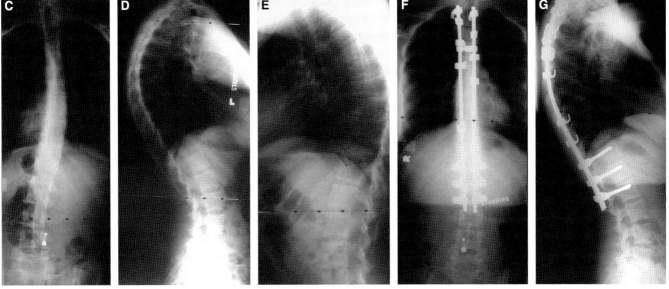

Fig. 31-1   A, This radiograph shows irregular endplates and wedging of the vertebrae, which are commonly seen in patients with Scheuermann's disease. **B,** An MRI demonstrates irregular endplates. **C-E,** The patient is seen preoperatively. Preoperative planning includes hyperextension bolster films to help determine the approach. **F** and **G,** Postoperative radiographs show correction of thoracic kyphosis.

75 degrees   55 degrees   52 degrees

Other causes of abnormal thoracic kyphosis should be differentiated from Scheuermann's kyphosis, such as traumatic compression fracture, postlaminectomy kyphosis, ankylosing spondylitis, tumors, and infection. Overall thoracic kyphosis can be measured with the Cobb angle method on a lateral radiograph.[40] As mentioned previously, two curve types can be identified on lateral radiographs. In type I Scheuermann's kyphosis (typical type), the apex of kyphosis is located between T6 and T8, with curves extending from T1 to T12. In type II Scheuermann's kyphosis (atypical type), the apex of kyphosis is located near the thoracolumbar junction, with curves extending from T4 to L3.

Flexibility of the kyphosis can be evaluated on a hyperextension film by placing a bolster beneath the apex of the kyphosis, with the patient in a supine position. On an AP view, concomitant scoliosis should be evaluated.

INDICATIONS AND CONTRAINDICATIONS

NONOPERATIVE MANAGEMENT

Nonoperative management of patients with Scheuermann's kyphosis includes education, antiinflammatory medication, exercise, physical therapy, and bracing.

Rehabilitation in Scheuermann's kyphosis can relieve pain, enhance general physical conditioning, and improve sagittal balance when the kyphosis can be reduced. Many rehabilitation techniques are advocated, including postural control, strengthening, stretching of the trunk, and musculotendinous stretching especially of the hamstring muscles. Weiss et al[41] reported their results of long-term physical therapy consisting of daily postural education, physiotherapeutic methods with osteopathy, manual therapy, McKenzie and Brügger approaches, and psychological help for pain relief. They reported a 16% to 32% reduction in pain and a decreased frequency of pain that was significant in all cases. However, this study represents Level IV evidence. To our knowledge, no study has been conducted with a high level of evidence of the effectiveness of rehabilitation in patients with Scheuermann's kyphosis.

The goals of bracing are to reduce pressure of the anterior part of the vertebral endplate and relieve pain. It is usually indicated in patients with painful Scheuermann's disease, mild kyphosis with a Cobb angle between 45 and 65 degrees, and ineffective physiotherapy.[42] Many types of braces can be proposed. The main principle consists of posterior support at the apex of kyphosis and two anterior supports above and below the apex of kyphosis. Even in skeletally mature patients, bracing has been reported as a helpful treatment modality.

Sachs et al[43] reported on the long-term results of using a Milwaukee brace in 120 patients with Scheuermann's kyphosis, with a follow-up of at least 5 years. This study showed that a Milwaukee brace is usually an effective method of treatment for these patients; however, 4 of 14 patients who had an initial kyphosis of more than 74 degrees required a spinal fusion.

Riddle et al[44] used a duPont kyphosis brace to treat 22 children with Scheuermann's kyphosis. Nine patients showed improvement, seven were unchanged, and six had progression of kyphosis. Flexible curves were a positive predictor of a successful outcome of bracing with a kyphosis brace. The authors' results were comparable with those previously reported in the literature describing the effectiveness of the modified Milwaukee brace in the treatment of Scheuermann's thoracic kyphosis. The brace provided an additional advantage of concealment under clothing.

SURGICAL INDICATIONS

Operative treatment in patients with Scheuermann's kyphosis is uncommon. The goals of operative treatment are to correct kyphosis, improve sagittal balance, improve cosmetic appearance, prevent progression, and relieve pain. Surgical indications are kyphosis with a Cobb angle of more than 70 degrees, pain that does not response to conservative treatment, an unacceptable cosmetic kyphosis, and rarely a neurologic deficit.[11,30] Restrictive lung disease is a rare indication for surgery that usually occurs in patients with a Cobb angle of more than 100 degrees.[13] MRI should be performed before surgery to rule out other pathologies such as thoracic disc herniation and spinal cord pathology that can result in cord compression after deformity correction. Intraoperative neuromonitoring is recommended in all surgical cases. Surgical management of Scheuermann's kyphosis can be performed with a posterior-only approach, an anterior-only approach, or a combined anterior-posterior approach.

OPERATIVE CONSIDERATIONS

CHOOSING FUSION LEVELS

A general surgical principle is that the whole level of kyphosis should be fused. Lowe and Kasten[45] performed a spinal fusion with Cotrel-Dubousset instrumentation in a patient with severe kyphosis secondary to Scheuermann's disease. The authors recommended fusion of the first lordotic segment distally to prevent distal junctional kyphosis, and not more than 50% of the deformity should be corrected to decrease the risk of proximal junctional kyphosis. Cho et al[46] described the sagittal stable vertebra as the most proximal lumbar vertebral body touched by the vertical line from the posterosuperior corner of the sacrum. They recommended inclusion of this vertebra in the distal end of a fusion for the treatment of thoracic hyperkyphosis. Inclusion of the first lordotic vertebra but not the sagittal stable vertebra is not always appropriate to prevent postoperative distal junctional kyphosis.

POSTERIOR-ONLY APPROACH

The posterior-only approach was the first surgical method used to treat Scheuermann's kyphosis.[47] Many methods have been proposed, but they all consist of three surgical steps: release of the spinal structures, correction of spinal deformity, and fusion with instrumentation (Fig. 31-2). The advantages of a posterior-only approach are a shorter operative time, decreased blood loss, prevention of complications from thoracotomy, and preservation of the anterior blood supply to the spinal cord. Rigid curves that do not correct to less than 50 degrees on a hyperextension film with a bolster might not be suitable for a posterior-only approach.[11] The disadvantage of a posterior-only approach is that the posterior instrument will be under continual tensile stress that can cause pseudarthrosis and implant failure.[48]

Bradford et al[49] showed high rates of correction loss and poor results with a posterior-only approach. In this study, posterior arthrodesis was performed by using Harrington rods, hooks, and wires. However, with the development of new posterior segmental instrumentation systems, pedicle screw fixation from a posterior-only approach has been successfully used as a primary method for fixation in patients with Scheuermann's kyphosis. Pedicular screw fixation and posterior column–shortening techniques such as Ponte osteotomies can successfully correct the deformity with low rates of failure.

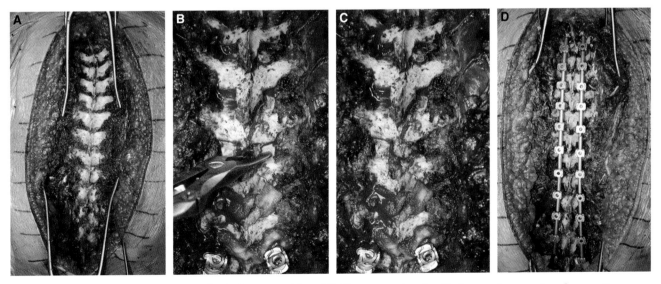

Fig. 31-2   The posterior approach. **A,** Exposure. **B** and **C,** Ponte osteotomies. **D,** Screw placement and correction with a cantilever and compression.

Papagelopoulos et al[50] reported their results in 21 patients with Scheuermann's kyphosis. All patients had posterior spine arthrodesis with segmental compression instrumentation. Seven patients with rigid kyphosis had combined anterior and posterior spine arthrodesis. In the posterior arthrodesis–only group, the mean preoperative thoracic kyphotic curve of 68.5 degrees improved to 40 degrees at the latest review, with an average loss of correction of 5.75 degrees. The combined anterior-posterior arthrodesis group had a mean preoperative thoracic kyphotic curve of 86.3 degrees, which improved to 46.4 degrees at the latest review, with an average loss of correction of 4.4 degrees. The authors concluded that posterior arthrodesis and segmental compression instrumentation seems to be effective for correcting and stabilizing kyphotic deformity in Scheuermann's disease. However, combined anterior and posterior spine arthrodesis was recommended for rigid, more severe kyphotic deformities.

ANTERIOR-ONLY APPROACH

An anterior-only approach includes anterior release of the anterior longitudinal ligament, segmental instrumentation, and anterior arthrodesis (Fig. 31-3). The advantage of this approach is that the fusion between the intervertebral discs is under compression instead of tension, as in a posterior fusion. The disadvantages of an anterior-only approach include complications from an anterior thoracotomy such as pneumothorax, hemothorax, disturbance of the anterior blood supply to the spinal cord, limited access to the number of levels to be instrumented, and the size of the instrumentation, compared with posterior instrumentation.

Kostuik[51] reported results of an anterior-only approach and the use of a Kostuik-Harrington distraction system. The mean kyphosis was reduced from 75 degrees preoperatively to 60 degrees postoperatively.

COMBINED ANTERIOR-POSTERIOR APPROACH

A combined anterior-posterior approach is performed by anterior release and posterior instrumentation with fusion. Anterior release can be performed either through an open thoracotomy or with the assistance of endoscopy. This approach is usually performed in patients with severe kyphosis of more than 80 degrees and rigid deformity that is not corrected on hyperextension films.[30]

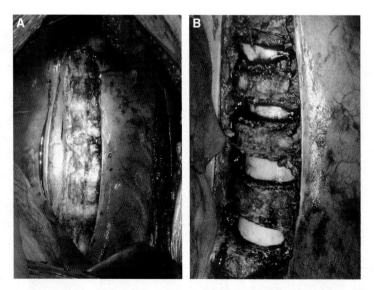

Fig. 31-3 **A** and **B,** An anterior approach involves removal of the disc and placement of structural grafts in the disc space. The grafts are femoral rings cut intraoperatively.

Lee et al[52] compared posterior-only instrumentation with pedicle screw constructs versus a combined anterior-posterior approach in patients with Scheuermann's kyphosis. They showed that a posterior-only approach resulted in less mean residual kyphosis, maintained more correction at the final follow-up, and required shorter surgical times with less blood loss, compared with a combined anterior-posterior approach.

POTENTIAL COMPLICATIONS AND MANAGEMENT

The complication rate after surgical treatment of Scheuermann's kyphosis is significantly higher in adults than in pediatric patients.[53] The overall complication rate is not significantly different between posterior-only and anterior-posterior approaches. The most common complication was wound infection (3.8%). The acute neurologic complication rate was 1.9%, and the mortality rate was 0.6%. Neuromonitoring is very important to alert surgeons during the surgery. Adequate mean artery pressure and oxygenation to the spinal cord should be maintained during surgery.

JUNCTIONAL KYPHOSIS

Junctional degeneration and kyphosis is a pathologic process at the segments caused by accelerated degeneration and instability at the segments proximal or distal to the fusion levels.[54] It has received more attention in the recent literature. Junctional kyphosis can manifest as adjacent disc degeneration, facet joints degeneration, or a combination of both, leading to deformity such as proximal or distal junctional kyphosis. It is characterized by deterioration of sagittal balance at the proximal or distal aspect of the fusion levels that may or may not cause clinical symptoms. Some patients complain of feeling that they are falling forward or of pain at the transitional area. Radiographic features of junctional kyphosis show degenerative changes of the disc or facet joints, disc space narrowing, angulation at the transitional area, and loss of sagittal balance of 10 degrees or more, as measured from the lower endplate of the upper instrumented vertebra to the upper endplate of two levels cephalad to the upper instrumented vertebra. Junctional kyphosis is believed to be the result of kyphogenic forces attempting to return the head to its preoperative position. The change in position can only occur at the spinal segments that have not been instrumented. This is also thought to occur in the upper thoracic segments because of the weakness of the soft tissues at the transitional areas.

Lowe[55] showed treated patients with Scheuermann's kyphosis with double Luque wires and found that the use of sublaminar wires can increase the risk of junctional kyphosis. Lowe and Kasten[45] reported the results of Cotrel-Dubousset instrumentation for severe kyphosis secondary to Scheuermann's disease. The incidence of proximal junctional kyphosis was 31% and that of distal junctional kyphosis was 28%. They recommended that the deformity not be overcorrected by more than 50% to prevent an increased risk of junctional kyphosis.

Denis et al[56] reported that proximal junctional kyphosis in Scheuermann's kyphosis has an incidence as high as 30%. The risk factors of proximal junctional kyphosis were associated with failure to incorporate the proximal-end vertebra, disruption of the junctional ligamentum flavum, and inappropriate vertebral end selection. Distal junctional kyphosis can occur in 12%, most of which is from not including the first lordotic disc in the fusion construct.

Management of junctional kyphosis entails extension of the fusion levels to include the involved segments via a posterior approach.[57] Typically an anterior approach is not necessary unless a patient has significant spondylolisthesis or kyphosis that needs anterior support. However, not all patients with junctional kyphosis need revision surgery. Clinical symptoms are more important than radiographic findings. Proper selection of the fusion levels is very important to minimize the risk of junctional kyphosis.

PATIENT EXAMPLES

This 14-year-old girl had a progressive kyphosis and pain over the thoracic spine (Fig. 31-4, *A* and *B*). She had no extremity numbness, tingling, weakness, bowel symptoms, or bladder symptoms and no other medical problems. Results of a neurologic examination were normal. The patient underwent multiple Ponte osteotomies and a posterior spinal fusion and instrumentation from T2 to L3 (Fig. 31-4, *C* and *D*). She has improvement in her cosmesis and pain at her follow-up.

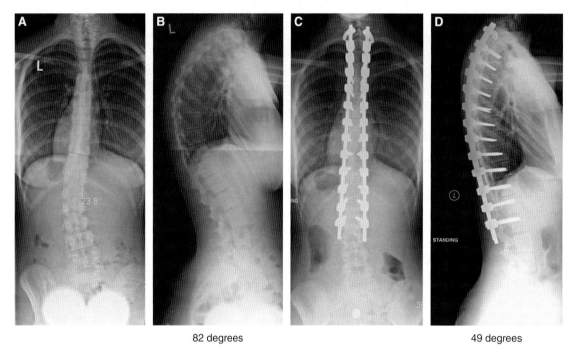

82 degrees   49 degrees

Fig. 31-4   This patient with Scheuermann's kyphosis was treated with posterior instrumentation and fusion. **A** and **B,** Preoperative radiographs. **C** and **D,** Postoperative radiographs.

This 17-year-old patient had Scheuermann's disease with kyphosis and a history of obesity, hypertension, and diabetes (Fig. 31-5, *A* and *B*). He had pain over the apex of the thoracic deformity and at the thoraco-lumbar junction, which is typical of these deformities. The patient had a rigid deformity and was obese. He underwent an anterior release with placement of femoral ring structural grafts in the disc spaces. On the same day, a posterior spinal fusion with instrumentation and multiple Ponte osteotomies were performed (Fig. 31-5, *C* and *D*). He has excellent relief of his pain and cosmetic deformity at his follow-up.

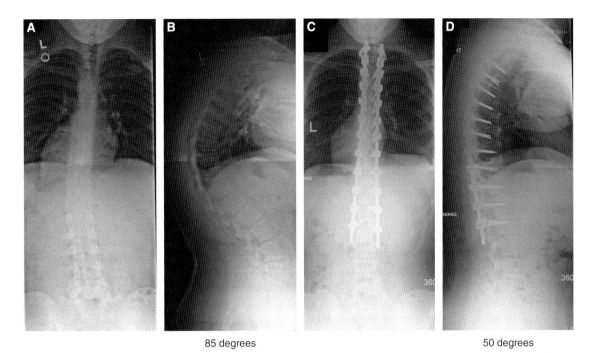

85 degrees   50 degrees

Fig. 31-5 This patient had Scheuermann's disease with kyphosis. He was treated with an anterior release and posterior instrumentation with fusion. **A** and **B,** Preoperative radiographs. **C** and **D,** Postoperative radiographs.

CONCLUSION

Scheuermann's disease with kyphosis is uncommon. A posterior approach with Ponte osteotomies in combination with posterior segmental instrumentation can be successfully used to correct large deformities or those that fail nonoperative treatment.

REFERENCES

1. Scheuermann H. Kyphosis dorsalis juvenilis. Ugesk Leager 82:385-393, 1920.
2. Sorensen K. Scheuermann's Juvenile Kyphosis. Clinical Appearances, Radiography, Aetiology and Prognosis. Copenhagen: Munksgaard, 1964.
3. Jansen RC, van Rhijn LW, van Ooij A. Predictable correction of the unfused lumbar lordosis after thoracic correction and fusion in Scheuermann kyphosis. Spine 31:1227-1231, 2006.
4. Lings S, Mikkelsen L. Scheuermann's disease with low localization. A problem of under-diagnosis. Scand J Rehabil Med 14:77-79, 1982.
5. Damborg F, Engell V, Andersen M, et al. Prevalence, concordance, and heritability of Scheuermann kyphosis based on a study of twins. J Bone Joint Surg Am 88:2133-2136, 2006.
6. Lowe TG, Line BG. Evidence based medicine: analysis of Scheuermann kyphosis. Spine 32:115-119, 2007.
7. Ippolito E, Bellocci M, Montanaro A, et al. Juvenile kyphosis: an ultrastructural study. J Pediatr Orthop 5:315-322, 1985.
8. Scoles PV, Latimer BM, Diglovanni BF, et al. Vertebral alterations in Scheuermann's kyphosis. Spine 16:509-515, 1991.
9. van Linthoudt D, Revel M. Similar radiologic lesions of localized Scheuermann's disease of the lumbar spine in twin sisters. Spine 19:987-989, 1994.
10. Ravel M, Andre-Deshays C, Roudier R, et al. Effects of repetitive strains on vertebral end plates in young rats. Clin Orthop Relat Res 279:303-309, 1992.

11. Tribus CB. Scheuermann's kyphosis in adolescents and adults: diagnosis and management. J Am Acad Orthop Surg 6:36-43, 1998.

12. Halal F, Gledhill RB, Fraser C. Dominant inheritance of Scheuermann's juvenile kyphosis. Am J Dis Child 132:1105-1107, 1978.

13. Murray PM, Weinstein SL, Spratt KF. The natural history and long-term follow-up of Scheuermann kyphosis. J Bone Joint Surg Am 75:236-248, 1993.

14. Ristolainen L, Kettunen JA, Heliovaara M, et al. Untreated Scheuermann's disease: a 37-year follow-up study. Eur Spine J 21:819-824, 2012.

15. Boseker EH, Moe JH, Winter RB, et al. Determination of "normal" thoracic kyphosis: a roentgenographic study of 121 "normal" children. J Pediatr Orthop 20:796-798, 2000.

16. Faro FD, Marks MC, Pawelek J, et al. Evaluation of a functional position for the lateral radiograph acquisition in adolescent idiopathic scoliosis. Spine 29:2284-2289, 2004.

17. Horton WC, Brown CW, Bridwell KH, et al. Is there an optimal patient stance for obtaining a lateral 36″ radiograph? A critical comparison of three techniques. Spine 30:427-433, 2005.

18. Winter RB, Longstein JE, Denis F. Sagittal spinal alignment: the true measurement, norms, and description of correction for thoracic kyphosis. J Spinal Disord Tech 22:311-314, 2009.

19. Mac-Thiong JM, Berthonnaud E, Dimar JR Jr, et al. Sagittal alignment of the spine and pelvis during growth. Spine 29:1642-1647, 2004.

20. Berthonnaud E, Dimnet J, Roussouly P, et al. Analysis of the sagittal balance of the spine and pelvis using shape and orientation parameters. J Spinal Disord Tech 18:40-47, 2005.

21. Schwab F, Lafage V, Patel A, et al. Sagittal plane considerations and the pelvis in the adult patient. Spine 34:1828-1833, 2009.

22. Bernhardt M, Bridwell KH. Segmental analysis of the sagittal plane alignment of the normal thoracic and lumbar spines and thoracolumbar junction. Spine 14:717-721, 1989.

23. Jackson RP, McManus AC. Radiographic analysis of sagittal plane alignment and balance in standing volunteers and patients with low back pain matched for age, sex, and size. A prospective controlled clinical study. Spine 19:1611-1618, 1994.

24. Mac-Thiong JM, Transfeldt EE, Mehbod AA, et al. Can c7 plumbline and gravity line predict health related quality of life in adult scoliosis? Spine 34:E519-E527, 2009.

25. Legaye J, Duval-Beaupere G, Hecquet J, et al. Pelvic incidence: a fundamental pelvic parameter for three-dimensional regulation of spinal sagittal curves. Eur Spine J 7:99-103, 1998.

26. Vaz G, Roussouly P, Berthonnaud E, et al. Sagittal morphology and equilibrium of pelvis and spine. Eur Spine J 11:80-87, 2002.

27. Stagnara P, De Muaroy JC, Dran G, et al. Reciprocal angulation of vertebral bodies in a sagittal plane: approach to references for the evaluation of kyphosis and lordosis. Spine 7:335-342, 1982.

28. Ogilvie JW, Sherman J. Spondylolysis in Scheuermann's disease. Spine 12:251-253, 1987.

29. Lowe TG. Scheuermann's kyphosis. Neurosurg Clin N Am 18:305-315, 2007.

30. Wood KB, Melikian R, Villamil F. Adult Scheuermann kyphosis: evaluation, management, and new developments. J Am Acad Orthop Surg 20:113-121, 2012.

31. Resnick D. Scheuermann's disease. In Resnick D, ed. Diagnosis of Bone and Joint Disorders, ed 3. Philadelphia: WB Saunders, 1995.

32. Beaudreuil J, Marty C, Laredo JD. Maladie de Scheuermann. In Kahn MF, Bardin T, Lioté F, et al, eds. L'Actualité Rheumatologique 2009. Issy-les-Moulineaux: Elsevier Masson, 2009.

33. Chui KY, Luk KD. Cord compression caused by multiple disc herniations and intraspinal cyst in Scheuermann's disease. Spine 20:1075-1079, 1995.

34. Kapetanos GA, Hantzidis PT, Anagnostidis KS, et al. Thoracic cord compression caused by disk herniation in Scheuermann's disease: a case report and review of the literature. Eur Spine J 15:553-558, 2006.

35. Mok FP, Samartzis D, Karppinen J, et al. ISSLS prize winner: prevalence, determinants, and association of Schmorl nodes of the lumbar spine with disc degeneration: a population-based study of 2449 individuals. Spine 35:1944-1952, 2010.

36. Dar G, Peleg S, Masharawi Y, et al. Demographical aspects of Schmorl nodes: a skeletal study. Spine 34:E312-E315, 2009.

37. Williams FM, Manek NJ, Sambrook PN, et al. Schmorl's nodes: common, highly heritable, and related to lumbar disc disease. Arthritis Rheum 57:855-860, 2007.

38. Paajanen H, Alanen A, Erkintalo M, et al. Disc degeneration in Scheuermann disease. Skeletal Radiol 18:523-526, 1989.
39. Takatalo J, Karppinen J, Niinimaki J, et al. Association of modic changes, Schmorl's nodes, spondylolytic defects, high-intensity zone lesions, disc herniations, and radial tears with low back symptom severity among young Finnish adults. Spine 37:1231-1239, 2012.
40. Taylor TC, Wenger DR, Stephen J, et al. Surgical management of thoracic kyphosis in adolescents. J Bone Joint Surg Am 61:496-503, 1979.
41. Weiss HR, Dieckmann J, Gerner HJ. Effect of intensive rehabilitation on pain in patients with Scheuermann's disease. Stud Health Technol Inform 88:254-257, 2002.
42. Bradford DS, Moe JH, Montalvo FJ, et al. Scheuermann's kyphosis and roundback deformity. Results of Milwaukee brace treatment. J Bone Joint Surg Am 56:740-758, 1975.
43. Sachs B, Bradford D, Winter R, et al. Scheuermann kyphosis. Follow-up of Milwaukee-brace treatment. J Bone Joint Surg Am 69:50-57, 1987.
44. Riddle EC, Bowen JR, Shah SA, et al. The duPont kyphosis brace for the treatment of adolescent Scheuermann kyphosis. J South Orthop Assoc 12:135-140, 2003.
45. Lowe TG, Kasten MD. An analysis of sagittal curves and balance after Cotrel-Dubousset instrumentation for kyphosis secondary to Scheuermann's disease. A review of 32 patients. Spine 19:1680-1685, 1994.
46. Cho KJ, Lenke LG, Bridwell KH, et al. Selection of the optimal distal fusion level in posterior instrumentation and fusion for thoracic hyperkyphosis: the sagittal stable vertebra concept. Spine 34:765-770, 2009.
47. Papagelopoulos PJ, Mavrogenis AF, Savvidou OD, et al. Current concepts in Scheuermann's kyphosis. Orthopedics 31:52-58, 2008.
48. de Jonge T, Illes T, Bellvei A. Surgical correction of Scheuermann's kyphosis. Int Orthop 25:70-73, 2001.
49. Bradford DS, Moe JH, Montalvo FJ, et al. Scheuermann's kyphosis. Results of surgical treatment by posterior spine arthrodesis in twenty-two patients. J Bone Joint Surg Am 57:439-448, 1975.
50. Papagelopoulos PJ, Klassen RA, Peterson HA, et al. Surgical treatment of Scheuermann's disease with segmental compression instrumentation. Clin Orthop Relat Res 386:139-149, 2001.
51. Kostuik JP. Anterior Kostuik-Harrington distraction systems. Orthopedics 11:1379-1391, 1988.
52. Lee SS, Lenke LG, Kuklo TR, et al. Comparison of Scheuermann kyphosis correction by posterior-only thoracic pedicle screw fixation versus combined anterior/posterior fusion. Spine 31:2316-2321, 2006.
53. Coe JD, Smith JS, Berven S, et al. Complications of spinal fusion for Scheuermann kyphosis: a report of the scoliosis research society morbidity and mortality committee. Spine 35:99-103, 2010.
54. Lonstein JE. Post-laminectomy kyphosis. Clin Orthop Relat Res 128:93-100, 1977.
55. Lowe TG. Double L-rod instrumentation in the treatment of severe kyphosis secondary to Scheuermann's disease. Spine 12:336-341, 1987.
56. Denis F, Sun EC, Winter RB. Incidence and risk factors for proximal and distal junctional kyphosis following surgical treatment for Scheuermann kyphosis: minimum five-year follow-up. Spine 34:E729-E734, 2009.
57. Cho KJ, Bridwell KH, Lenke LG, et al. Comparison of Smith-Petersen versus pedicle subtraction osteotomy for the correction of fixed sagittal imbalance. Spine 30:2030-2037, 2005.

PART VII

Revision Strategies for Surgical Management of Spinal Deformity

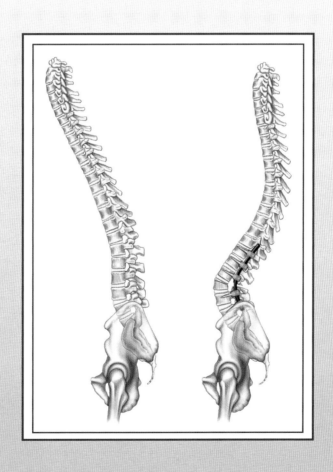

32

Evaluation, Prevention, and Treatment of Proximal Junctional Failure

Satoshi A. Kawaguchi ▪ *Robert A. Hart*

Posterior fusion with segmental pedicle screw instrumentation has been widely used in the treatment of spinal instability and deformity. This procedure is advantageous in creating rigid fixation and correction across multiple spine segments. At the same time, it inherently creates biomechanical vulnerability at proximal and distal mobile segments adjacent to a fused spine, leading in some cases to a biomechanical failure at these segments with various radiographic and clinical manifestations. Adjacent-segment degeneration and adjacent-segment disease are common manifestations of junctional pathology.[1] *Adjacent-segment degeneration,* while adjacent-segment disease is symptomatic, is defined as radiographic changes of intervertebral disc, facet joints, and spinal stenosis at the adjacent segment.[1-3]

Reconstructive strategies for adult spinal deformity comprising long-segment thoracolumbar instrumentation and corrective osteotomies have led to more acute and severe manifestations of adjacent-segment pathology. These deformities include fracture at the top of long-segmental pedicle screw constructs, proximal junctional acute collapse, proximal junctional vertebral fracture, or proximal junctional vertebral fracture–subluxation.[4-7] The term *proximal junctional failure (PJF)* has been proposed to distinguish between patients with mechanical failure and those with proximal junctional kyphosis (PJK).[8-10] PJF is potentially the most severe form of adjacent-segment pathology. It refers to failure of bone (vertebral fracture), of soft tissue (ligament), or at the interface of the implant and bone at the junctional segment as an acute event; in some cases PJF requires urgent surgical reconstruction. The mechanical and clinical features of PJF contrast with degenerative adjacent-segment pathology or junctional deformities such as PJK, which is characterized by increased kyphosis, as seen on radiographs.[9,11-13] In contrast to PJF, most incidents of PJK have limited clinical impact.[9,13]

In this chapter, we describe diagnostic criteria of PJF and PJK and discuss predisposing factors, diagnosis, and prophylactic and therapeutic operative technique for PJF.

DEFINITIONS AND CLINICAL SIGNIFICANCE

PROXIMAL JUNCTIONAL KYPHOSIS

Glattes et al[12] originally described PJK as a postoperative radiographic finding. Diagnostic criteria of PJK are a proximal junctional sagittal Cobb angle between the uppermost instrumented vertebra (UIV) and the two levels above the UIV (UIV + 2) of 10 degrees or more and at least 10 degrees greater than the preoperative measurement[12] (Fig. 32-1). The incidence of PJK above spine deformity fusions is reportedly 17% to 39%.[13] Despite its relative high incidence, most PJK is asymptomatic. To date, only the report by Kim et al[14] has shown a difference in clinical outcomes as a result of PJK.

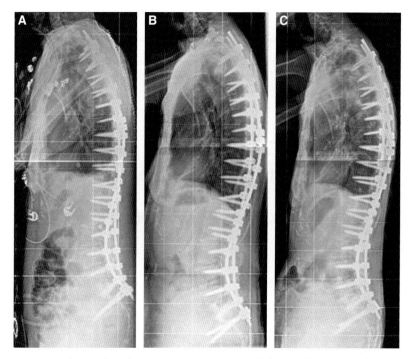

Fig. 32-1 **A,** Postoperative radiographs after posterior instrumented fusion from T4 to the pelvis, L5 laminectomy, and transforaminal lumbar interbody fusion at L5-S1. **B,** A 6-week postoperative lateral radiograph shows that the fracture increased junctional kyphosis from −6 degrees to 5 degrees. **C,** A 2-year postoperative lateral radiograph shows no further increase of proximal junctional kyphosis.

PROXIMAL JUNCTIONAL FAILURE

PJF is distinct from PJK in that it includes features of mechanical failure (see Figs. 32-4 through 32-7). Diagnostic criteria of PJF include the characteristic radiographic finding of PJK, as described previously, along with one or more of the following:

- Fracture of the vertebral body of the UIV or the UIV + 1
- Posterior osseoligamentous disruption
- Failure of instrumentation at the UIV [9]

The incidence of PJF has been reported as 4.7% (57 of 1218 patients) in a multicenter case series.[8] Nearly half (47.4%) of the patients with PJF had revision surgery, indicating the greater clinical significance of PJF, compared with PJK.

RISK FACTORS

Several studies have analyzed predisposing factors for PJK.[12,15-19] A recent systemic review showed the risk factors of PJK to include increased age, fusion to the sacrum, combined anterior-posterior fusion, thoracoplasty, an UIV at T1-3, and nonanatomic restoration of thoracic kyphosis.[13] A comparative analysis of 52 patients who developed PJF after adult spinal deformity surgery and 54 patients who did not have PJF after adult spinal deformity surgery revealed that increased age, greater preoperative sagittal imbalance, and greater sagittal correction were significant predisposing factors for PJF.[20] Older age and larger sagittal correction have also been identified as risk factors for developing PJK that requires revision surgery.[21] Because revision surgery is sometimes required after the development of PJF, these two studies empha-

Table 32-1 Techniques for Proximal Junctional Failure Prevention

Technique	Advantages	Disadvantages
Vertebroplasty of UIV/UIV + 1	Effective Low cost	Added complexity Potential adjacent-disc degeneration
Hook fixation at UIV	Low cost Technically easy	None Does not prevent soft tissue injury
Percutaneous upper screws	Prevents soft tissue injury Added cost	Requires extra implant trays Technically difficult
Undercorrection at upper levels	Zero cost Technically easy	None None
Spinous process tether	Easy Low cost	None Does not prevent soft tissue disruption
Rib fixation of UIV + 1	Technically easy Prevents soft tissue disruption	None Added expense Requires extra implant tray

UIV, Uppermost instrumented vertebra.

sized the importance of considering age and amount of sagittal correction preoperatively.[22] Table 32-1 lists techniques that may help to prevent PJF. An ideal sagittal vertical axis (SVA) and an ideal amount of sagittal correction may differ between older patients with adult spinal deformity and young patients with adolescent idiopathic scoliosis. These issues remain a subject of study.

EVALUATION

Patients with PJF typically present to a clinic or emergency department with acute back pain, although some are asymptomatic. Pain is not always preceded by trauma. PJF needs to be differentiated from PJK, which typically does not need surgical treatment. Improper initial management of PJF can result in devastating neurologic compromise. Typically PJF occurs in patients older than 60 years within 3 months of a long-segment thoracolumbosacral fusion surgery.[8] Patients with acute onset of back pain who meet these criteria should be suspected for PJF.

On examination, kyphotic deformity at the junction of instrumentation and tenderness over the spinal process and interspinal process ligaments should be noted. A thorough neurologic examination should be performed to detect spinal cord injury (thoracic myelopathy) or radiculopathy (intercostal nerve irritation).

Diagnostic imaging includes upright 36-inch long-cassette AP and lateral radiographs of the whole spine. On a lateral film, the proximal junctional Cobb angle is measured between the caudal endplate of the UIV and the cephalad endplate of the UIV + 2. For patients who are unable to stand, thoracic radiographs with the patient in lateral decubitus position can be obtained. In addition to the kyphotic deformity, fracture at the UIV or UIV + 1, subluxation of the UIV + 1, and pullout of instrumentation should be assessed radiographically. Patients whose UIV is in the upper thoracic spine (T2-5) are more likely to have subluxation PFJ (ligament failure) than fracture, whereas those whose UIV is located in the lower thoracic spine (T9-12) are more likely to have a fracture PFJ than subluxation.[23] CT of the thoracic and lumbar spine is useful for further evaluation of vertebral fracture and pullout of instrumentation (Fig. 32-2).

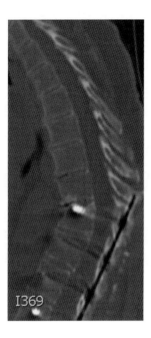

Fig. 32-2   CT performed 6 weeks postoperatively shows a T10 vertebral fracture, which resulted in increased junctional kyphosis from 13 degrees to 37 degrees.

PREOPERATIVE PLANNING

Surgical decompression and stabilization is indicated for virtually all patients with PJF associated with neurologic deficit. Decision criteria for surgical treatment of patients with PFJ with no neurologic deficit vary among surgeons. Hart et al[8] found that the decision for revision surgery was based most strongly on the presence or absence of a trauma episode, severity of PJK angulation, and extent of recurrent sagittal imbalance. Radiographic parameters of sagittal balance thus need to be measured, including SVA, pelvic incidence, pelvic tilt, thoracic kyphosis, and lumbar lordosis. Bone mineral density should be measured if it has not been done in the previous 6 months.

Surgical treatment for PJF typically includes extension of fusion to a more proximal level. Revision posterior instrumented fusion with realignment is most often performed. Extension into the cervical spine may be necessary, depending on the UIV in the primary surgery. Yagi et al[22] recently studied 23 patients who had revision surgery for PJF. Eleven patients (48%) developed additional PJF at the new UIV, and 9 of them had another revision surgery. This suggested the importance of prophylactic procedures to reduce the incidence of PJF after primary and revision reconstructive surgery for adult spinal deformity.

PREVENTION OF PROXIMAL JUNCTIONAL FAILURE: OPERATIVE TECHNIQUE AND CONSIDERATIONS

PREVENTING SOFT TISSUE INJURY AT THE PROXIMAL JUNCTION

Precautions should be taken not to damage supraspinous and interspinous ligaments and the joint capsule at the proximal adjacent segment during exposure and instrumentation. The surgical level should be confirmed fluoroscopically before the UIV is exposed to prevent overexposure and unnecessary soft tissue injury. Special caution is taken when exposing the insertion points of pedicle screws at the UIV, because they are close to the facet joint capsule of the adjacent segment. Some surgeons prefer to use transverse process hooks or pedicle hooks on top of the instrumentation, which may reduce injury to the soft tissues of the UIV.[11] The use of percutaneous screws at the UIV and spinal process fixation, between the UIV and the UIV − 1, have been proposed as alternatives. However, the efficacy of these approaches has not been demonstrated.

Hook Fixation at the Uppermost Instrumented Vertebra

The use of hooks in place of pedicle screws at the UIV has been advocated to decrease stiffness of the instrumentation at the end and to prevent soft tissue injury.[11] This method creates a transition from the rigid instrumentation at the proximal junction. A disadvantage of the use of hooks is a risk of cut-out from the transverse process or lamina, especially in patients with osteoporosis.

Rib Fixation One Level Above the Uppermost Instrumented Vertebra Without Fusion

Hart et al[9] introduced prophylactic rib fixation at the level of UIV + 1. Initially hooks of vertical expandable prosthetic titanium rib (VEPTR) systems were used (see Fig. 32-4, *G* and *H*). They were fixed at the medioposterior section of the ribs at the UIV + 1 and connected with titanium rods bilaterally. More recently, sublaminar tapes have been used in place of VEPTR hooks (Fig. 32-3). Two separate, longitudinal incisions (approximately 3 cm long) are made over the medioposterior portion of the UIV + 1 ribs. The ribs are exposed in a subperiosteal manner circumferentially. Sublaminar tape is then placed in a looped fashion around the indicated rib bilaterally. The tape is tunneled submuscularly to the midline rods and connected with a U clamp, which is then placed under gentle tension and tightened securely using a locking screw.

Vertebral Augmentation

Augmentation with polymethylmethacrylate cement has been proposed to prevent fracture of vertebrae and pullout of the pedicle screw at the UIV.[5,24] A disadvantage of vertebral augmentation is that it can increase the risk of developing vertebral fracture above the level of augmentation; therefore augmentation of vertebrae above the UIV to prevent vertebral body fracture is recommended.[11] However, we have witnessed soft tissue failure with subluxation between the UIV and UIV + 1, causing myelopathy (see Fig. 32-5).

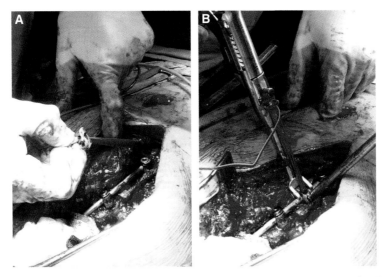

Fig. 32-3 **A,** Sublaminar tape (Universal Clamp Spinal Fixation System, Zimmer Inc.) is fixed to the rib at one level above the uppermost instrumented vertebra (UIV +1) and pulled downward. **B,** With the use of a clamp, the tape is then fixed distally to the rod. Tension is gently applied to the tape and the clamp is immobilized against the rod using a locking screw.

PATIENT EXAMPLES

PROXIMAL JUNCTIONAL FAILURE WITH SEVERE PAIN AND KYPHOSIS BUT WITHOUT NEUROLOGIC DEFICIT AND STENOSIS

This 61-year-old woman presented with progressive symptoms of degenerative lumbar scoliosis (Fig. 32-4, A and B). She underwent posterior instrumented fusion from T10 to her pelvis, laminectomy of L4-5, and transforaminal lumbar interbody fusion at L4-5 and L5-S1 (Fig. 32-4, C and D). Six weeks after the surgery, she began having severe proximal back pain. Radiographs and CT revealed fracture of the T10 vertebra and increased junctional kyphosis from 13 to 37 degrees (Fig. 32-4, E and F). No neurologic deficit was noted. Conservative treatment with a thoracolumbosacral orthosis brace for 6 weeks did not improve her back pain. Revision surgery was performed 3 months after the primary surgery, including extension of posterior instrumented fusion to T4 and prophylactic rib fixation at T3 using VEPTR hooks. Radiographs obtained 10 months postoperatively show a stable spine with junctional kyphosis improved to 13 degrees (Fig. 32-4, G and H).

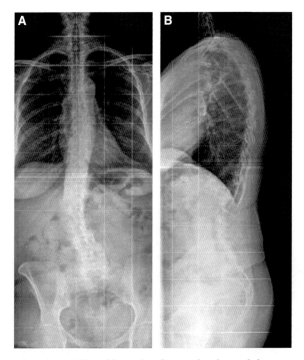

Fig. 32-4   **A** and **B,** Preoperative AP and lateral radiographs showed degenerative lumbar scoliosis.

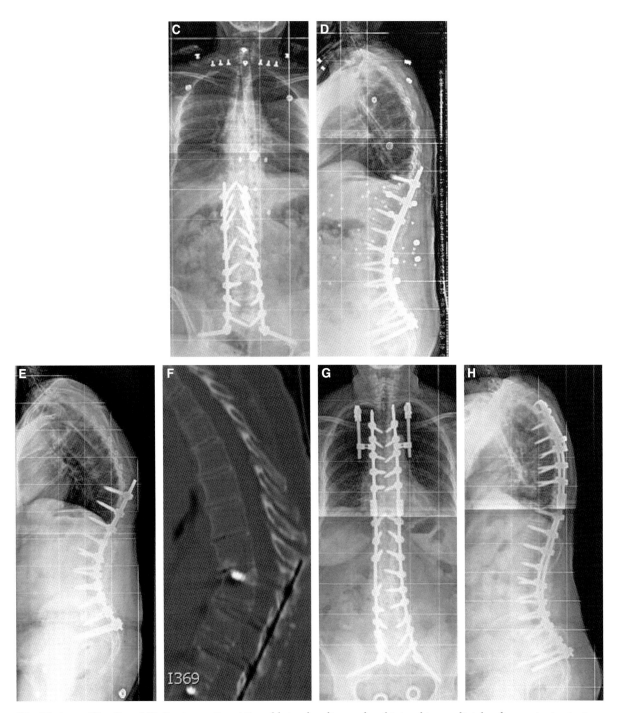

Fig. 32-4, cont'd **C** and **D,** Postoperative AP and lateral radiographs obtained immediately after posterior instrumented fusion from T10 to the pelvis, L4-5 laminectomy, and L4-5 and L5-S1 transforaminal lumbar interbody fusion. **E** and **F,** Six-week postoperative radiographs and CT scan showed fracture of the T10 vertebra and increased junctional kyphosis. **G** and **H,** Ten-month postoperative radiographs after revision surgery that involved extension of the posterior instrumented fusion to T4 and prophylactic rib fixation at T3 using vertical expandable prosthetic titanium rib hooks.

Proximal Junctional Failure With Subluxation Between the Uppermost Instrumented Vertebra and the Uppermost Instrumented Vertebra Plus One and Neurologic Deficit

This 75-year-old woman presented with progressive low back and buttock pain 2 years after having a laminectomy and posterior instrumented fusion at L2-5. Radiographs and CT-myelography showed adjacent-segment spinal stenosis at L1-2 with multilevel nonunion, hardware loosening, and sagittal decompensation (Fig. 32-5, A and B). The patient underwent staged surgery: the first stage consisted of anterior discectomy and fusion at L3-4, L4-5, and L5-S1; the second stage entailed L2 laminectomy, posterior instrumented fusion from T10 to her pelvis, T11 sublaminar wiring, and prophylactic vertebral augmentation with polymethylmethacrylate cement at T9 and T10 (Fig. 32-5, C and D). Five weeks after surgery, she noted pain and weakness in her left thigh following a fall. Radiographs revealed increased junctional kyphosis from 5.5 to 33 degrees with anterior subluxation (Fig. 32-5, E). A CT scan showed a large soft tissue failure between the UIV + 1 and the UIV (Fig. 32-5, F). Revision surgery was performed, including T10 laminectomy, extension of posterior instrumented fusion to T3, and sublaminar wiring at T4. Her pain and weakness have substantially improved, and radiographs 5 years after the revision surgery show a stable spine (Fig. 32-5, G and H).

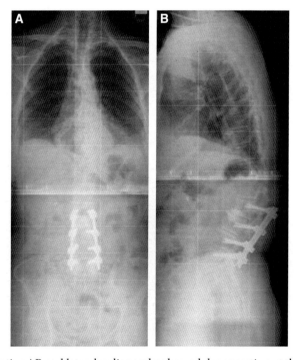

Fig. 32-5   **A** and **B,** Preoperative AP and lateral radiographs showed degeneration at the proximal adjacent segment.

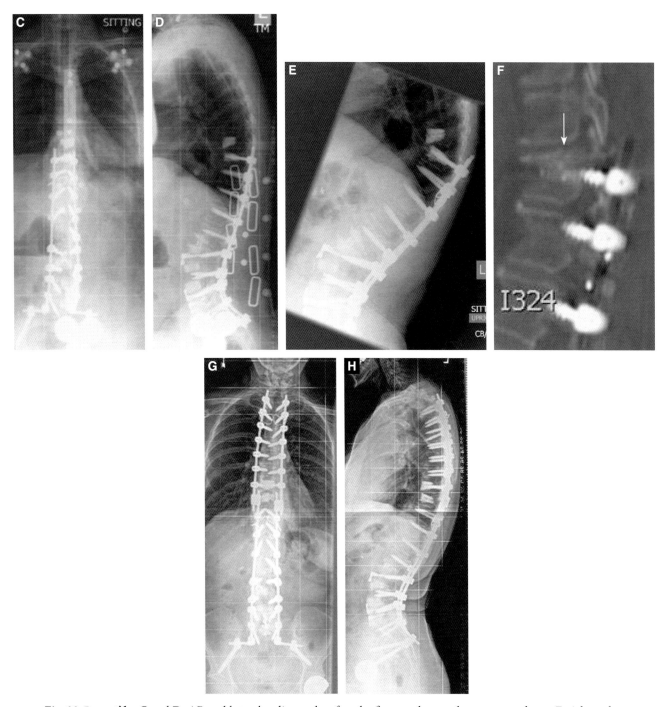

Fig. 32-5, cont'd **C** and **D,** AP and lateral radiographs after the first- and second-stage procedures. **E,** A lateral radiograph obtained 5 weeks postoperatively revealed increased junctional kyphosis to 33 degrees and anterior subluxation. **F,** CT showed a fracture of T10 through the bilateral pedicle. **G** and **H,** Five years after revision surgery, the patient's spine appears stable on AP and lateral radiographs.

LATE PROXIMAL JUNCTIONAL FAILURE WITH DEGENERATIVE CHANGE AND CORD COMPRESSION WITHOUT MYELOPATHY

This 64-year-old woman, who had a laminectomy and posterior instrumented fusion from L4-S1 3 years earlier, presented with progressive low back and leg pain, intermittent claudication, and sagittal imbalance. Radiographs and CT-myelography showed adjacent-segment spinal stenosis at L1-2, L2-3, and L3-4 (Fig. 32-6, *A* and *B*). She underwent staged surgery: the first stage entailed L1-3 laminectomy and posterior instrumented fusion from T10 to her pelvis; the second stage involved anterior discectomy and interbody fusion using eXtreme lateral interbody fusion at L1-2, L2-3, and L3-4 (Fig. 32-6, *C* and *D*). Postoperatively the patient had improved pain and balance for 1 year, until radicular pain developed along her rib cage. Radiographs and CT showed increased junctional kyphosis with significant degeneration of the disc and an endplate fracture at T9-10 (Fig. 32-6, *E* and *F*). Revision surgery was performed, including extension of posterior instrumented fusion to T4, T10 pedicle subtraction osteotomy, interbody fusion at T9-10, prophylactic rib fixation at T3 using the Universal Clamp Spinal Fixation System (Fig. 32-6, *G* and *H*).

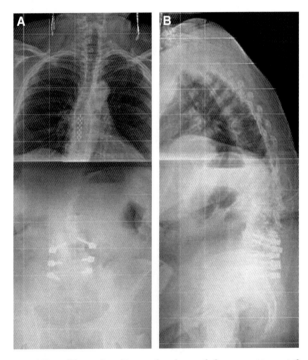

Fig. 32-6   **A** and **B**, Preoperative AP and lateral radiographs showed degeneration at the proximal adjacent segment.

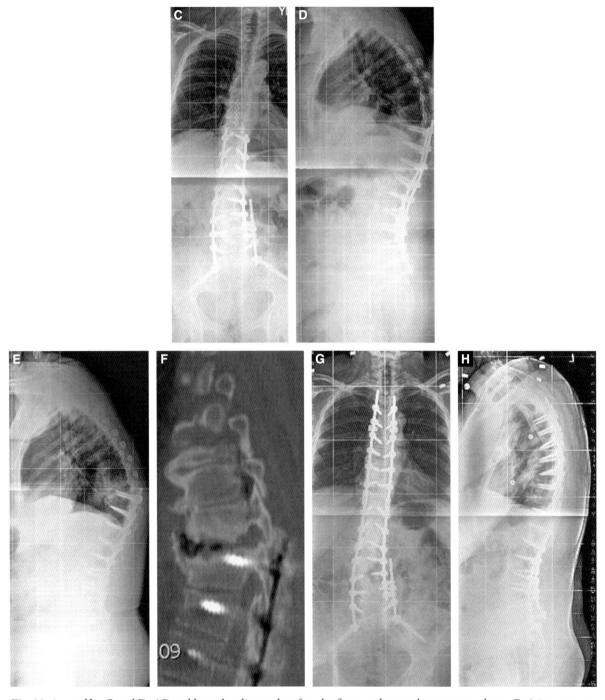

Fig. 32-6, cont'd C and **D,** AP and lateral radiographs after the first- and second-stage procedures. **E,** A 1-year postoperative lateral radiograph showed increased junctional kyphosis. **F,** CT showed degeneration of the intervertebral disc and endplates at T9-10. **G** and **H,** Postoperative AP and lateral radiographs after revision surgery with the Universal Clamp Spinal Fixation System.

PROXIMAL JUNCTIONAL FAILURE WITH SIGNIFICANT KYPHOSIS BUT LIMITED CLINICAL IMPACT

This 62-year-old woman presented with increasing back pain with thoracolumbar scoliosis (Fig. 32-7, *A* and *B*). She had been diagnosed with scoliosis as a child, but was not treated with a brace or surgical correction. Her pain continued despite conservative treatments, including physical therapy and medication. The patient underwent posterior instrumented fusion from T9 to pelvis, L5 laminectomy, transforaminal lumbar interbody fusion at L5-S1, and sublaminar wiring at T11 (Fig. 32-7, *C* and *D*). Radiographs 6 weeks postoperatively revealed increased PJK with a compression fracture of T9 (Fig. 32-7, *E*). The patient tolerated her back pain with a TLSO brace. At 5-year follow-up, she has no back pain despite substantial junctional kyphosis. Radiograph and CT scan show a healed T9 vertebral fracture without further increase of kyphosis (Fig. 32-7, *F* and *G*).

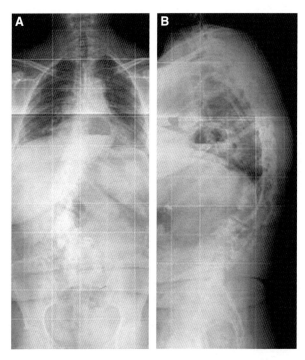

Fig. 32-7   **A** and **B,** AP and lateral radiographs showing thoracolumbar scoliosis.

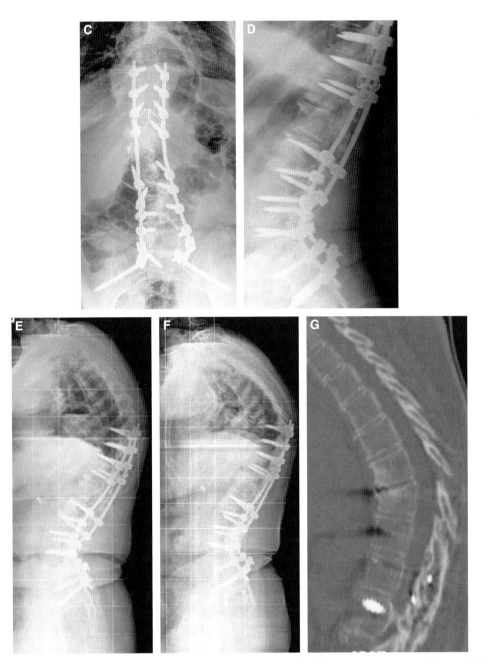

Fig. 32-7, cont'd **C** and **D,** Postoperative AP and lateral radiographs following instrumented fusion, L5 laminectomy, L5-S1 transforaminal lumbar interbody fusion, and T11 sublaminar wiring. **E,** Lateral radiograph 6 weeks postoperatively showing fracture of the T9 vertebra and increased junctional kyphosis. **F** and **G,** Five-year postoperative radiograph and CT scan revealed a healed T9 fracture and no increase of proximal junctional kyphosis.

PROXIMAL JUNCTIONAL KYPHOSIS WITHOUT FAILURE

This 66-year-old woman presented with increasing back pain and imbalance with progressing thoracolumbar kyphoscoliosis (Fig. 32-8, *A* and *B*). She underwent posterior instrumented fusion from T3 to her pelvis, L5 laminectomy, and transforaminal lumbar interbody fusion at L5-S1 (Fig. 32-8, *C* and *D*). Radiographs 6 weeks postoperatively revealed increased PJK without fracture (Fig. 32-8, *E*). The patient denied increased back pain. At her 2-year follow-up, she has no back pain and radiographs show no further increase in PJK (Fig. 32-8, *F*).

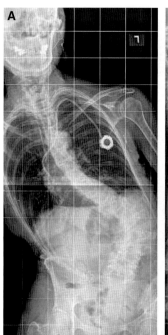
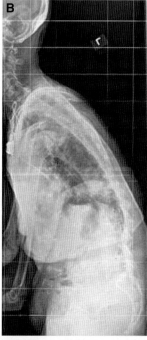

Fig. 32-8　**A** and **B,** Preoperative AP and lateral radiographs showed thoracolumbar kyphoscoliosis. **C** and **D,** Postoperative AP and lateral radiographs after instrumented fusion from T9 to the pelvis, L5 laminectomy, and L5-S1 transforaminal lumbar interbody fusion. **E,** A lateral radiograph 6 weeks postoperatively revealed an increased junctional kyphosis from −6 to 5 degrees. **F,** A 2-year postoperative lateral radiograph shows no further increase of proximal junctional kyphosis.

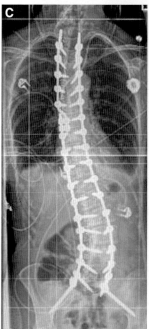
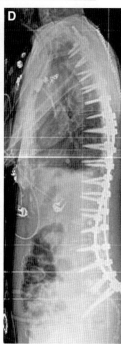
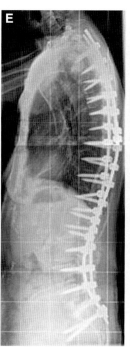
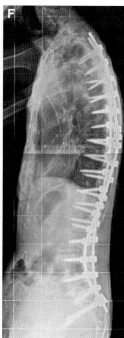

CONCLUSION

With recent advances in surgical technology and technique, aggressive global realignment of the spine is now possible in the treatment of adult spinal deformity. This has led to better surgical outcomes. On the other hand, it has also led to new complications such as PJF. Spine surgeons have begun to reach consensus regarding the definition and cause of PJF, but its treatment and prevention are challenging. Continuous efforts to develop a new prophylactic approach are critical to decrease the incidence of PJF. In addition, continued evaluation of surgery for the primary condition and surgery for resulting junctional complications will help to define ideal final alignment in older patients with adult spinal deformity.

REFERENCES

1. Kraemer P, Fehlings MG, Hashimoto R, et al. A systematic review of definitions and classification systems of adjacent segment pathology. Spine 37(22 Suppl):S31-S39, 2012.
2. Javedan SP, Dickman CA. Cause of adjacent-segment disease after spinal fusion. Lancet 354:530-531, 1999.
3. Kasliwal MK, Shaffrey CI, Lenke LG, et al. Frequency, risk factors, and treatment of distal adjacent segment pathology after long thoracolumbar fusion: a systematic review. Spine 37(22 Suppl):S165-S179, 2012.
4. O'Leary PT, Bridwell KH, Lenke G, et al. Risk factors and outcomes for catastrophic failures at the top of long pedicle screw constructs: a matched cohort analysis performed at a single center. Spine 34:2134-2139, 2009.
5. Hart RA, Prendergast MA, Roberts WG, et al. Proximal junctional acute collapse cranial to multi-level lumbar fusion: a cost analysis of prophylactic vertebral augmentation. Spine J 8:875-881, 2008.
6. Watanabe K, Lenke LG, Bridwell KH, et al. Proximal junctional vertebral fracture in adults after spinal deformity surgery using pedicle screw constructs: analysis of morphological features. Spine 35:138-145, 2010.
7. Fernández-Baillo N, Sánchez Márquez JM, Sánchez Pérez-Grueso FJ, et al. Proximal junctional vertebral fracture-subluxation after adult spine deformity surgery. Does vertebral augmentation avoid this complication? A case report. Scoliosis 7:16, 2012.
8. Hart R, McCarthy I, O'brien M, et al. Identification of decision criteria for revision surgery among patients with proximal junctional failure after surgical treatment of spinal deformity. Spine 38:E1223-E1227, 2013.
9. Hart RA, McCarthy I, Ames CP, et al. Proximal junctional kyphosis and proximal junctional failure. Neurosurg Clin N Am 24:213-218, 2013.
10. Hostin, R, McCarthy I, O'Brien M, et al. Incidence, mode, and location of acute proximal junctional failures following surgical treatment for adult spinal deformity. Spine. 2012 Sep 13. [Epub ahead of print]
11. Arlet V, Aebi M. Junctional spinal disorders in operated adult spinal deformities: present understanding and future perspectives. Eur Spine J 22(Suppl 2):S276-S295, 2013.
12. Glattes RC, Bridwell KH, Lenke LG, et al. Proximal junctional kyphosis in adult spinal deformity following long instrumented posterior spinal fusion: incidence, outcomes, and risk factor analysis. Spine 30:1643-1649, 2005.
13. Kim HJ, Lenke LG, Shaffrey CI, et al. Proximal junctional kyphosis as a distinct form of adjacent segment pathology after spinal deformity surgery: a systematic review. Spine 37(22 Suppl):S144-S164, 2012.
14. Kim HJ, Bridwell KH, Lenke LG, et al. Proximal junctional kyphosis results in inferior SRS pain subscores in adult deformity patients. Spine 38:896-901, 2013.
15. Denis F, Sun EC, Winter RB. Incidence and risk factors for proximal and distal junctional kyphosis following surgical treatment for Scheuermann kyphosis: minimum five-year follow-up. Spine 34:E729-E734, 2009.
16. Kim HJ, Yagi M, Nyugen J, et al. Combined anterior-posterior surgery is the most important risk factor for developing proximal junctional kyphosis in idiopathic scoliosis. Clin Orthop Relat Res 470:1633-1639, 2012.
17. Kim YJ, Bridwell KH, Lenke LG, et al. Proximal junctional kyphosis in adult spinal deformity after segmental posterior spinal instrumentation and fusion: minimum five-year follow-up. Spine 33:2179-2184, 2008.
18. Kim YJ, Lenke LG, Bridwell KH, et al. Proximal junctional kyphosis in adolescent idiopathic scoliosis after 3 different types of posterior segmental spinal instrumentation and fusions: incidence and risk factor analysis of 410 cases. Spine 32:2731-2738, 2007.
19. Wang J, Zhao Y, Shen B, et al. Risk factor analysis of proximal junctional kyphosis after posterior fusion in patients with idiopathic scoliosis. Injury 41:415-420, 2010.

20. Hart RA, Hostin RA, Bess RS, et al. Age, sagittal balance and operative correction are risk factors for proximal junctional failure in adult deformity. In Proceedings of the Annual Meeting of American Academy of Orthopaedic Surgeons, Chicago: The Academy, March 2013.
21. Kim YJ, Bridwell KH, Lenke LG, et al. Patients with proximal junctional kyphosis requiring revision surgery have higher post-op lumbar lordosis and larger sagittal balance corrections. Spine 39:E576-E580, 2014.
22. Yagi M, Rahm M, Gaines R, et al. Characterization and surgical outcomes of proximal junctional failure in surgically treated adult spinal deformity patients. Spine 39:E607-E614, 2014.
23. Ha Y, Maruo K, Racine L, et al. Proximal junctional kyphosis and clinical outcomes in adult spinal deformity surgery with fusion from the thoracic spine to the sacrum: a comparison of proximal and distal upper instrumented vertebrae. J Neurosurg Spine 19:360-369, 2013.
24. Kebaish KM, Martin CT, O'Brien JR, et al. Use of vertebroplasty to prevent proximal junctional fractures in adult deformity surgery: a biomechanical cadaveric study. Spine J 13:1897-1903, 2013.

33

Evaluation and Management of Iatrogenic Sagittal Imbalance

John D. Koerner ▪ *James S. Harrop* ▪ *Todd J. Albert*

Iatrogenic sagittal imbalance has numerous causes and can be defined as failure of the C7 plumb line (the distance from a vertical line drawn from the center of the C7 vertebral body to the posterior superior corner of S1) to fall within 4 cm of the posterior superior aspect of the L5-S1 disc.[1,2] This imbalance leads to high stress on muscles and ligaments and an increasing loss of lumbar lordosis, which decreases the lever arm for the paraspinal muscles.[3] Over time, the dynamic stabilizers gradually fail, followed by failure of the rigid stabilizers (ligaments, capsule).[4] Postsurgical or traumatic disruption of the posterior tension bend will decrease the ability of these muscles to prevent kyphotic deformation. Restoration of sagittal balance is crucial, because this parameter is one of the most reliable indicators of clinical improvement in adult deformity reconstruction.[5]

Classically, iatrogenic loss of lumbar lordosis, also known as *flat-back deformity,* was described after the use of Harrington distraction instrumentation.[6] This deformity creates an inability to stand straight without flexing the hips and knees, which leads to fatigue and pain. A similar clinical picture is seen after other procedures in which sagittal balance is not corrected or over time as a progressive deformity. Other potential causes of sagittal imbalance include proximal junctional kyphosis (PJK), postlaminectomy kyphosis, pseudarthrosis, and posttraumatic kyphosis. The ability of the spine to compensate, however, does not always lead to sagittal imbalance in these conditions.

Revision surgery for adult deformity from all causes is relatively common; one study reported a 10-year survival rate of approximately 61% for primary procedures.[7] The most common reasons for revision in this study were pain from implants, adjacent-segment degeneration, and infection. Sagittal imbalance was not a common reason for revision surgery in this cohort (2/21 patients), although patients having reoperation had a more positive sagittal vertical axis (SVA) and greater thoracic kyphosis. The average age in this cohort was only 42 years, which may explain the low rate of sagittal imbalance. Modern surgical techniques and instrumentation can decrease the rate of revision surgery over time, because the use of pedicle screw constructs instead of hybrid/hook constructs has led to better maintenance of thoracic alignment.[8] A recent study of 643 adult deformity patients reported a revision rate of only 9% (mean follow-up 4.7 years).[9]

Despite the complexity involved in revision cases, patients demonstrate significant improvement, with complication rates similar to those of primary procedures.[10] A thorough understanding of the cause of iatrogenic sagittal imbalance is necessary for appropriate evaluation and treatment of these complex cases. Although we attempt to evaluate our surgical technique and principles to prevent iatrogenic sagittal imbalance, adult deformity is a progressive condition, and many of the findings presented result from natural history or age-related degeneration.

ETIOLOGIC FACTORS

FIXED SAGITTAL IMBALANCE

Fixed sagittal imbalance, or flat-back deformity, was traditionally seen after Harrington distraction instrumentation.[11,12] However, the loss of lumbar lordosis in fixed sagittal imbalance has many causes. In a study of 19 patients undergoing revision surgery for sagittal imbalance, the most common causes were failure to enhance lumbar lordosis at the index procedure and adjacent disc degeneration.[13] After fusion to L4 or L5 without correction of normal lumbar lordosis, the levels below may compensate to correct overall lordosis, with segments above becoming kyphotic.[14] The lower lumbar spine contributes approximately 67% of total lumbar lordosis, and inability to maintain or correct alignment in this region can lead to local kyphosis.[15] Inadequate interbody support or settling can result in decompensation and kyphosis over time.

PROXIMAL JUNCTIONAL KYPHOSIS

PJK in adult deformity is defined as kyphosis of more than 10 degrees at the proximal end of a construct[16] that if not compensated for creates sagittal imbalance. Glattes et al[16] evaluated the outcomes of 81 patients who developed PJK after long posterior fusion and reported an incidence of 26%. Patients with PJK, however, had no significant changes in their SRS-24 scores, nor did they have a more positive sagittal C7 plumb line. It is possible that these patients are able to compensate to prevent sagittal imbalance, and over time clinical symptoms present. Another study reported worse outcomes on the SRS pain subscore in patients who developed PJK.[17]

In a recent systematic review, the incidence of PJK ranged from 17% to 39%, and risk factors for developing PJK included increased age, fusion to the sacrum, combined anterior and posterior spinal fusion, thoracoplasty, upper instrumented vertebra at T1-3, and nonanatomic restoration of thoracic kyphosis.[18] Patients requiring revision surgery for PJK were older and had larger postoperative lumbar lordosis and sagittal balance corrections.[19] SVA correction (average 4.1 cm) did not lead to surgery for PJK, whereas patients with a correction of 8.8 cm were more likely to have revision surgery ($p = 0.02$). The authors postulated that a correction of SVA to zero may not be optimal for all patients. Another study evaluated a cohort of 57 patients who developed proximal junctional failure after adult deformity surgery; patients having revision surgery had a higher SVA, although this was not statistically significant ($p = 0.090$).[20]

POSTLAMINECTOMY KYPHOSIS

Postlaminectomy kyphosis has been reported as a complication that occurs more frequently in the cervical spine and in children and adolescents.[21-23] However, it can lead to sagittal imbalance when it occurs in the thoracic and lumbar spine. One study reported a 100% incidence after multilevel cervical laminectomy in patients younger than 25 years, a 36% incidence in thoracic laminectomy patients, and an incidence of zero after lumbar laminectomy.[24] In adults who had thoracic laminectomy for myelopathy, the increase in kyphosis postoperatively was shown to be relatively small, but females undergoing long-segment laminectomies (at least 3 levels) were at higher risk for developing kyphosis; these patients should be followed closely.[25]

DEVELOPMENT OF PSEUDARTHROSIS

Pseudarthrosis is a common indication for revision deformity surgery, with studies confirming this diagnosis in 41% to 43% of revision cases.[9,10] This is identified most commonly at the L5-S1 level, where it can lead to a local kyphosis and sagittal imbalance. Risk factors for developing pseudarthrosis include preoperative thoracolumbar kyphosis of more than 20 degrees, age older than 55, extent of fusion to S1 compared with a cephalad level, and longer constructs.[26] The prevalence of pseudarthrosis is higher in patients with a positive sagittal balance of at least 5 cm 8 weeks postoperatively.[27]

POSTTRAUMATIC KYPHOSIS

Inadequate treatment of an unstable thoracolumbar injury can lead to progressive deformity, pain, and neurologic deficit. Patients who develop a kyphotic deformity of 30 degrees or more have significant back pain.[28] In an attempt to compensate and maintain sagittal balance, hyperlordosis develops in the lumbar spine, which can place increased stress on facet joints.[29] A similar pattern of muscular fatigue and pain develops over time because of altered biomechanics.

INDICATIONS AND CONTRAINDICATIONS

Indications for revision surgery for iatrogenic sagittal imbalance are similar to those for initial adult deformity surgery and include persistent pain, inability to maintain horizontal gaze, inability to stand for an extended period without the hips and knees flexed, pulmonary compromise, progressive deformity, or neurologic deficit. At least 12 weeks of nonoperative treatment, including physical therapy and medication, should be attempted. In a review of patients with flat back and kyphotic decompensation, Farcy and Schwab[4] found that nonoperative treatment was successful for patients with mild sagittal malalignment (less than 4 cm) who had two intact discs below the fusion, and patients with more severe sagittal imbalance (more than 8 cm) improved with surgical realignment procedures. Patients requiring revision surgery for fusion to the sacropelvis can have good outcomes, compared with primary procedures, with similar complication rates and radiographic alignment.[30]

Most patients with iatrogenic sagittal imbalance are older; therefore they tend to have more medical comorbidities, including osteoporosis. Dual-energy x-ray absorptiometry (DXA) scans will reveal the extent of osteopenia or osteoporosis. The prevalence of osteoporosis has been demonstrated to be higher in patients who develop PJK, compared with those who do not (20.4% versus 9.8%).[17] Physiologic reserve and malnutrition can be assessed by albumin and total protein levels during a preoperative evaluation.

PREOPERATIVE PLANNING

PHYSICAL EXAMINATION

Examination of a patient with iatrogenic sagittal imbalance reveals many important factors that will help to determine treatment. First, previous incisions should be inspected and noted, because they can influence operative planning. If fluctuance, masses, or significant pain is present on palpation, infection should be considered. Infectious markers include complete blood cell count with differential, erythrocyte sedimentation rate, and C-reactive protein.

Patients should be asked to stand straight, and they should be viewed from the side to appreciate overall posture. Flattening of the lower back and forward tilting of the trunk is common, which causes a compensatory hyperextension of the neck and flexion of the knees. Gait analysis can reveal a slow velocity and a short step and stride with a long duration of stance.[31] Patients often demonstrate hip flexion contractures, which are better evaluated with the patient lying down. Attempts should be made to decrease these contractures before surgery by stretching, possibly with a formal physical therapy program. A full neurologic examination should be performed, although a radicular distribution of pain and sensory deficits are not frequently identified.

Radiographic Workup and Preoperative Imaging

Full-length, standing AP and lateral images on 36-inch cassettes that include the femoral heads are required for preoperative evaluation. Flexibility of the deformity should be assessed with flexion/extension radiographs. Supine or prone films are needed to estimate correction. These images, along with clinical evaluation, will help to determine if a deformity is flexible, inflexible or fixed, or partially correctable. CT can be valuable in assessing previous fusions and to help plan osteotomies. MRI is useful to examine the neural elements, and the addition of gadolinium helps to differentiate scar from infection.

Spinopelvic parameters should be evaluated on a standing lateral image. *Pelvic incidence* is a constant spinopelvic parameter that is independent of pelvic positioning. It is the angle formed between the perpendicular from the midpoint of the S1 endplate and a line to the middle of the femoral heads. Sacral slope and pelvic tilt vary based on pelvic position. *Sacral slope* is the angle between the superior endplate of S1 and a horizontal reference line. *Pelvic tilt* is the angle formed between the midpoint of the S1 endplate to the femoral heads and a vertical line.

Gottfried et al[32] evaluated the spinopelvic parameters in normal and flat-back deformity patients (mean sagittal imbalance of 13.1 cm). In asymptomatic adults, the pelvic incidence ranged from 48 to 55 degrees, compared with 66.7 degrees in flat-back deformity patients.[32] Pelvic tilt ranged from 12 to 18 degrees in normal adults, compared with 35.5 degrees in flat-back patients; this was associated with a lower sacral slope and pelvic retroversion to compensate. In normal patients, sacral slope ranged from 36 to 42 degrees. Normal lumbar lordosis, measured by the Cobb angle from the superior endplate of L1 to the caudal endplate of L5, ranged from 43 to 61 degrees. Thoracic kyphosis, measured from T4 to T12, ranged from 41 to 48 degrees. The C7 plumb line was generally less than 4 cm.

OPERATIVE TECHNIQUE

Iatrogenic sagittal imbalance has numerous causes, and a similar treatment strategy can be used for most cases. This involves choosing between anterior, posterior, or a combination of approaches and determining appropriate osteotomies and extension of fusion constructs proximally and distally as needed.

Patient Positioning

Patient positioning and the type of operating room table can significantly affect sagittal alignment. A Jackson OSI (Mizuho OSI, Union City, CA) frame tends to decrease thoracic kyphosis, and it maintains total lumbar lordosis.[33] An Andrews frame (Mizuho OSI) decreases lumbar lordosis especially in the lower levels[34] and should not be used for lumbar fusion procedures if the goal is to increase lumbar lordosis. We prefer patients to be positioned on a Jackson OSI table. The hips are extended if possible, because this positioning may increase lumbar lordosis (Fig. 33-1).

Approaches
Posterior

In primary procedures, posterior only approaches have demonstrated similar correction to combined anterior-posterior procedures, with similar complications rates and radiographic results over a two-year follow-up.[35] With the use of osteotomies, bilateral pedicle screws, and transforaminal lumbar interbody

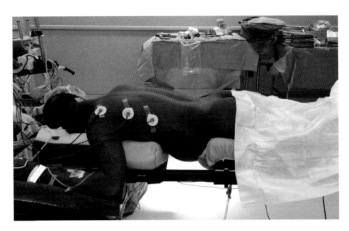

Fig. 33-1 This patient is positioned prone on a Jackson OSI table.

fusion, many procedures can be performed with a posterior-only approach, which limits the morbidity associated with an anterior approach. Comparable sagittal plane radiographic outcomes have been reported for posterior-only and combined anterior-posterior approaches.[36] Posterior osteotomies, which access all three columns of the spine, allows treatment of these cases from an all-posterior approach.

Anterior-Posterior

Alternatively, a single-stage anterior and posterior procedure has been successful in patients with iatrogenic lumbar kyphosis.[37] This technique involves an anterior opening wedge and a posterior closing wedge osteotomy. In a series of 54 patients with iatrogenic flat-back syndrome, this technique was used for patients whose deformity was caused by previous distraction instrumentation, thoracolumbar junctional kyphosis, and degenerative changes above or below the fusion. The authors were able to restore L1-S1 lordosis from 21.5 to 49 degrees.[37] However, anterior-posterior procedures generally have significantly longer surgical times and estimated blood loss,[35] in addition to the added morbidity of an anterior approach. Older patients or those with significant medical comorbidities may not be able to tolerate such a procedure and might benefit from a staged or posterior-only procedure. Kim et al[38] performed combined anterior-posterior fusions on patients considered to be at high risk for pseudarthrosis, including patients with large and stiff deformity or long fusions to the sacrum, and those with pseudarthrosis from previous surgery with kyphosis.

Posterior-Anterior-Posterior

Posterior-anterior-posterior procedures may be necessary for patients with severe fixed deformity. Jang et al[13] described this technique in a series of 19 patients with iatrogenic fixed sagittal imbalance. The first posterior approach included release and removal of instrumentation and the fusion mass followed by closure and turning of the patient to a supine position. From an anterior approach, the disc was removed and structural grafts were placed to create lordosis. The patient was then positioned prone, and a posterior shortening procedure was performed that included removal of ligaments and application of a compressive force with instrumentation. In their series, sagittal imbalance improved from 11.6 to 3.2 cm, and lordosis from 15 to 38 degrees. Excellent or good outcomes were seen in 84.2% of patients. Mean ODI scores improved from 62 ($\pm$ 11) to 36 ($\pm$ 12) ($p <0.0001$).[13]

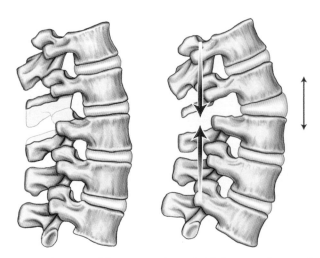

Fig. 33-2   Smith-Petersen osteotomies can achieve approximately 10 degrees of correction per level by closing posteriorly and lengthening anteriorly.

OSTEOTOMIES

Most patients with iatrogenic sagittal imbalance require an osteotomy or multiple osteotomies to correct alignment. These can include anterior osteotomies or posterior osteotomies such as Smith-Petersen osteotomies (SPOs), pedicle subtraction osteotomies (PSOs), posterior wedge resection, or a vertebral column resection (VCR). The degree of correction needed and the rigidity of the deformity will determine the appropriate osteotomy.

Smith-Petersen Osteotomy

An SPO is a posterior closing osteotomy that lengthens the anterior column through the disc space. It was first described in 1945.[39] Because of the anterior lengthening, the disc space needs to be mobile. Bone is resected between the facet joints in the posterior column. With a midline incision, the planned level and one above and one below it are exposed, and the spinous processes are removed (Fig. 33-2). The ligamentum flavum is detached from the inferior lamina and articular process, and an elevator is advanced underneath the lamina until it is visible in the lateral intervertebral notch. The osteotomy is performed at a 45-degree angle with the frontal plane. Approximately 10 degrees of correction per level can be obtained with this technique.[40] Multiple SPOs are appropriate for long curves over multiple segments such as in Scheuermann's kyphosis. For sharp curves, a PSO may be more advantageous.

Pedicle Subtraction Osteotomy

In a PSO, all three columns are incorporated through a V-shaped resection. The posterior column is shortened, but the anterior column is not lengthened as it is in an SPO. This technique is beneficial for acute angular deformities as opposed to curves over multiple segments. Thirty to thirty-five degrees of added lordosis can be expected in the lumbar spine and 25 degrees in the thoracic spine.[38,40] In patients with severe imbalance, SPOs may be necessary at other levels. PSOs can also be performed asymmetrically to correct coronal imbalance. In patients with a prior fusion to L4 and caudal degeneration with sagittal imbalance, Bridwell[40] recommends a PSO if imbalance of 10 to 12 cm or more is present. If the imbalance is less than this, multiple SPOs can be performed with an interbody graft placed at L4-5 and L5-S1.

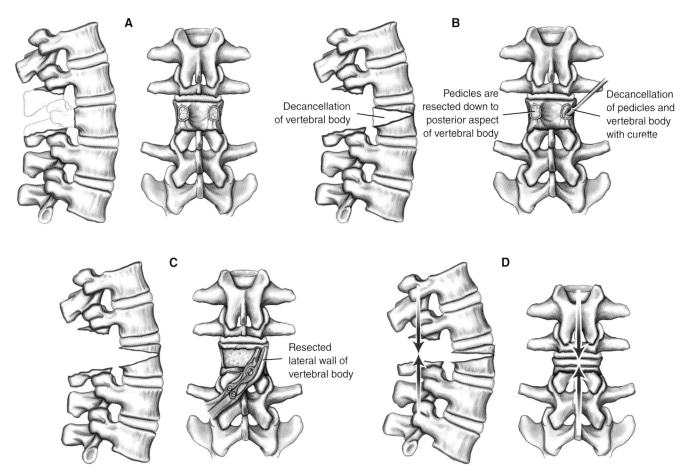

Fig. 33-3   Pedicle subtraction osteotomy. **A,** The posterior elements are resected. **B,** A curette is used to remove bone from the vertebral body. **C,** A part of the lateral body is resected. **D,** The patient's hips can be carefully extended to create lordosis.

This technique involves resection of the posterior elements. After the epidural space is entered, the nerve roots below the pedicle are identified, and all osseous attachments are separated. The dorsal part of the pedicle is removed. A curette is used to remove bone from the vertebral body, including the dorsal margin of the vertebral body (Fig. 33-3). The pedicles are resected, and the posterior vertebral body cortex is fractured medial to the pedicles, pushing the bone into the vertebral body. A part of the lateral vertebral body is resected, and the hips are carefully extended to create lordosis.

Bridwell et al[41] performed this technique in a consecutive series of 27 patients. They demonstrated a 34.1-degree average improvement in lumbar lordosis and sagittal correction of 13.5 cm. Another series with a 5-year follow-up showed no significant decrease in ODI and SRS scores over time, no loss of correction, and overall good satisfaction.[38] van Royen and Slot[42] described a technique similar to a PSO, which involves an L4 posterior closing wedge osteotomy with a partial corpectomy in patients with ankylosing spondylitis, with an average correction of 32 degrees. This V-shaped wedge of bone (comprising spinous processes, lamina, articular processes, and foramen) was resected, followed by the pedicles, the lateral wall of the vertebral bodies, and part of the transverse processes. This technique prevents elongation of the anterior column.

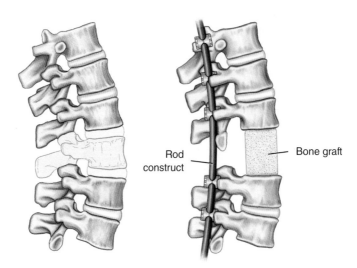

Fig. 33-4 Vertebral column resection. Involves complete resection of a vertebral segment, including the posterior elements, pedicles, and vertebral body.

Posterior Vertebral Resection

Thomasen[43] described a technique similar to a PSO, in which a transpedicular wedge resection osteotomy was performed to correct deformity in patients with ankylosing spondylitis. Berven[44] further modified the procedure as a circumferential wedge excision for the treatment of other conditions leading to sagittal imbalance. Anterior column lengthening is prevented with this technique. In the originally described technique, the articular processes of the osteotomy levels are resected, along with the transverse process and spinous process of the cephalad vertebra. The upper part of the caudal lamina and inferior lamina of the cephalad level is removed. The pedicles of the cephalad level are then removed, and bone is removed from the vertebral bodies through the pedicle roots. Holes are drilled in the spinous processes of the two levels above and below the osteotomy site to place a plate or wire. The reduction is completed, and the plates can be fixed with bolts. Berven et al[44] performed this technique in a series of 13 patients in the lower lumbar spine (L3-5). They improved the C7 sagittal plumb line by 63% and increased lumbar lordosis from 15.5 to 45.4 degrees.

Vertebral Column Resection

VCR involves complete resection of a vertebral segment, including the posterior elements, pedicles, and vertebral body. A VCR may be needed to correct coronal imbalance for which an asymmetrical PSO will not correct the imbalance in the shoulders and pelvis. The benefit of this technique is that it provides access to all three columns of the spine, each from a posterior approach.

After exposure is completed, a minimum of three levels above and below the planned osteotomy level should be instrumented for stabilization. In the thoracic spine, the medial aspect of the rib and transverse process is removed. The lateral vertebral body is exposed until the anterior body is visible. The posterior resection includes a laminectomy and facetectomy at the osteotomy level and partial laminectomies above and below. Temporary rods should be placed to prevent subluxation (Fig. 33-4). The pedicle is entered with a curette, and the corpectomy is completed. The anterior vertebral wall can be left intact, and the adjacent discs are removed. The posterior vertebral wall is then carefully resected after the dura is freed from attachments. The deformity can then be corrected in compression, with placement of an interbody device or graft.

This technique has been used to correct severe rigid deformities.[45-48] Lenke et al[49] demonstrated 45 degrees of correction in 12 patients with global kyphosis and 49 degrees in 10 patients with angular kyphosis. Compared with an anterior-posterior VCR, a posterior-only approach can provide similar outcomes with a shorter operative time and hospital stay.[50]

Anterior Osteotomy

In patients with a prior anterior fusion or ankylosis, an anterior osteotomy through an anterior approach may be necessary for correction. After the disc space or remnant of a disc space is identified, an osteotome can be used to remove bone and the cartilage endplate. The posterior vertebral cortex is then removed with rongeurs. Bone removal is completed with a Kerrison rongeur. An interbody device can be placed, and posterior osteotomies and stabilization are completed. In a series of 34 patients with posttraumatic kyphosis of T11-L2, Zeng et al[29] performed posterior closing wedge osteotomies for angles of 45 degrees or less, and anterior open, posterior closing osteotomiesy if kyphosis was greater than 40 degrees. This technique resulted in improved sagittal alignment.

FUSION LEVEL

If the L5-S1 levels are involved in the symptomatic curve or if spondylolisthesis, obliquity, or stenosis is present at this level, it should be included in the fusion.[30,38] Signs of degeneration of the L5-S1 disc, such as loss of height or signal or a positive discogram, are indications to extend fusion constructs to S1. Extension to the pelvis is likely required in revision cases to obtain adequate fixation in patients with poor bone quality.

The upper instrumented vertebra is generally selected based on the degree and location of thoracic kyphosis. Kim et al[38] recommended a continuation of constructs proximally to the stable and neutral vertebra above the end vertebra in cases of hyperkyphosis or thoracolumar kyphosis (T5-12 greater than 60 degrees or T10-L2 at least 20 degrees, respectively). In primary cases, both proximal and distal thoracic upper instrumented vertebrae have demonstrated similar outcomes[51]; however, in revision cases for sagittal imbalance, longer constructs are likely necessary to obtain adequate stability. Cadaver studies and a small case series have shown the benefits of cement augmentation of the upper instrumented vertebra and first mobile segment to prevent proximal junctional fractures.[52,53]

POTENTIAL COMPLICATIONS AND MANAGEMENT

Although revision surgery is more technically challenging, the rates of complications and outcomes are similar to those of primary deformity surgery, despite the increased frequency of sagittal plane imbalance and use of PSOs.[10] Early complications are often related to osteotomies because of the risk of neurologic injury. In a series of 66 patients having PSOs, 5 had early neurologic deficit.[54] The authors suggested that central canal enlargement and wake-up tests may limit this complication. Early complications after VCR are generally transient neurologic deficits.[46]

Late complications can occur after revision surgery. In a study of 455 patients who underwent revision spinal deformity surgery, 94 (21%) required a second revision surgery, most commonly for pseudarthrosis, pain at the implant site, adjacent-segment disease, and infection.[55] Pain in the low back or buttock after long fusion is rare; however, these patients should be evaluated for sacral fracture.[56] The incidence of clinically significant failure of lumbopelvic fixation is 11.9%, and risk factors included revision procedures and failure to restore lumbar lordosis and sagittal balance.[57] If a second revision procedure is indicated, a similar approach should be used, as previously described.

PATIENT EXAMPLES

POSTLAMINECTOMY KYPHOSIS

This 58-year-old man had a significant forward lean and was unable to stand erect because of a sagittal plane deformity. His lumbar lordosis measured 1.4 degrees, and his pelvic incidence was 52 degrees. He also had a kyphotic deformity of 25 degrees at the thoracolumar junction. His SVA was approximately 20 cm. He had a previous laminectomy from L3 to S1, and at presentation he had severe facet hypertrophy and stenosis at these levels (Fig. 33-5, *A* and *B*).

After exposure from T11-S1, scar tissue was carefully removed from the old laminectomy site. Facetectomies were carried out from the T11-12 levels to the L5-S1 levels. Pedicle fixation was then established from T11-S1, except at L2, the planned osteotomy level. Next, iliac fixation was established bilaterally. A provisional rod was placed to prevent shifting of the spine throughout the osteotomy. A PSO at L2 was then completed. The spine was gently corrected, and rods were contoured and placed. Postoperatively his lumbar lordosis improved to 32 degrees (Fig. 33-5, *C* and *D*).

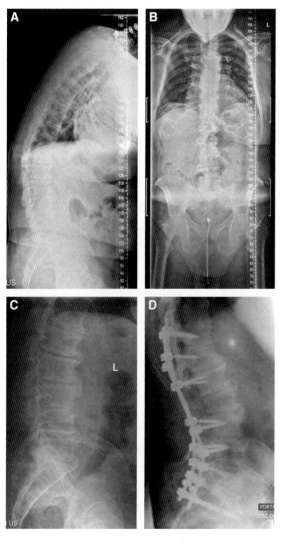

Fig. 33-5 **A** and **B,** Preoperative standing images of a 58-year-old man with postlaminectomy kyphosis. His lumbar lordosis measured 1.4 degrees, and his pelvic incidence was 52 degrees. He had a kyphotic deformity of 25 degrees at the thoracolumar junction, and his SVA was approximately 20 cm. **C** and **D,** Postoperative lateral radiographs of the patient's lumbar spine demonstrate an improvement in lumbar lordosis to 32 degrees.

FLAT-BACK DEFORMITY AFTER PRIOR FUSION

This 74-year-old man was in a motor vehicle accident many years ago and was treated with an L4-5 fusion. His inability to stand upright worsened, and he was wheelchair bound. He had a high pelvic incidence of 82 degrees, a low lumbar lordosis of 6 degrees, and an SVA of approximately 19 cm (Fig. 33-6, *A* and *B*).

A midline incision was made through the previous incision, and instrumentation was identified at L4-5. Exposure was extended from T10 to L5, and the rods were removed. Pedicle screws were placed from T10 to L5, except at L3, the planned osteotomy level. An SPO was performed bilaterally at L3. The transverse processes of L3 were removed, and the L3 pedicle was skeletonized and resected. A pituitary and a Kerrison rongeur were used to remove the vertebral body and a portion of the lateral wall. A temporary rod was then placed, and the contralateral pedicle was resected. The posterior longitudinal ligament was dissected off the body, and an osteotome was used to complete the fracture in the posterior vertebral wall. The nerve roots were inspected throughout their course to confirm that they were not compressed. The patient's legs were then extended, closing the osteotomy, and the rods were locked into place. Postoperatively lumbar lordosis was improved to 35 degrees (Fig. 33-6, *C* and *D*).

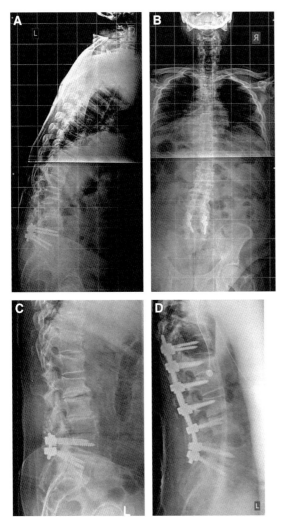

Fig. 33-6 **A** and **B,** Preoperative standing images of a 74-year-old man with flat-back deformity after a prior fusion at L4-5. He had a high pelvic incidence of 82 degrees, a low lumbar lordosis of 6 degrees, and an SVA of approximately 19 cm. **C** and **D,** Postoperative lateral radiographs of the patient's lumbar spine show an improvement in lumbar lordosis to 35 degrees.

CONCLUSION

Iatrogenic sagittal imbalance has many causes, but most patients present in a similar manner. They have difficulty standing upright, fatigue, and pain. A thorough workup and preoperative plan will help to determine the appropriate surgical intervention, which can include multiple approaches, the use of osteotomies, and extension of fusion constructs. The use of a PSO for more acute deformities, with the addition of SPOs at adjacent levels, can drastically improve sagittal alignment, and all can potentially be performed from a posterior approach. Obtaining adequate fixation is crucial in these patients, who may be osteopenic, and proximal and distal extension of constructs is often necessary. Revision cases can be challenging, but complication rates are similar to those of primary procedures, and outcomes are improved with restoration of sagittal alignment.

REFERENCES

1. Schwab F, Farcy JP, Bridwell K, et al. A clinical impact classification of scoliosis in the adult. Spine 31:2109-2114, 2006.

2. Schwab F, Lafage V, Farcy JP, et al. Surgical rates and operative outcome analysis in thoracolumbar and lumbar major adult scoliosis: application of the new adult deformity classification. Spine 32:2723-2730, 2007.

3. Tveit P, Daggfeldt K, Hetland S, et al. Erector spinae lever arm length variations with changes in spinal curvature. Spine 19:199-204, 1994.

4. Farcy JP, Schwab FJ. Management of flatback and related kyphotic decompensation syndromes. Spine 22:2452-2457, 1997.

5. Glassman SD, Berven S, Bridwell K, et al. Correlation of radiographic parameters and clinical symptoms in adult scoliosis. Spine 30:682-688, 2005.

6. Doherty J. Complications of fusion in lumbar scoliosis. Cleveland, OH. Proceedings of the Scoliosis Research Society. J Bone Joint Surg Am 55:438, 1973.

7. Sanchez-Mariscal F, Gomez-Rice A, Izquierdo E, et al. Survivorship analysis after primary fusion for adult scoliosis. Prognostic factors for reoperation. Spine J 14:1629-1634, 2014.

8. Rose PS, Lenke LG, Bridwell KH, et al. Pedicle screw instrumentation for adult idiopathic scoliosis: an improvement over hook/hybrid fixation. Spine 34:852-857; discussion 858, 2009.

9. Pichelmann MA, Lenke LG, Bridwell KH, et al. Revision rates following primary adult spinal deformity surgery: six hundred forty-three consecutive patients followed-up to twenty-two years postoperative. Spine 35:219-226, 2010.

10. Hassanzadeh H, Jain A, El Dafrawy MH, et al. Clinical results and functional outcomes of primary and revision spinal deformity surgery in adults. J Bone Joint Surg Am 95:1413-1419, 2013.

11. Bradford DS, Tribus CB. Current concepts and management of patients with fixed decompensated spinal deformity. Clin Orthop Relat Res 306:64-72, 1994.

12. Lagrone MO, Bradford DS, Moe JH, et al. Treatment of symptomatic flatback after spinal fusion. J Bone Joint Surg Am 70:569-580, 1988.

13. Jang JS, Lee SH, Min JH, et al. Surgical treatment of failed back surgery syndrome due to sagittal imbalance. Spine 32:3081-3087, 2007.

14. Bridwell KH, Lewis SJ, Rinella A, et al. Pedicle subtraction osteotomy for the treatment of fixed sagittal imbalance. Surgical technique. J Bone Joint Surg Am 86(Suppl 1):S44-S50, 2004.

15. Jackson RP, McManus AC. Radiographic analysis of sagittal plane alignment and balance in standing volunteers and patients with low back pain matched for age, sex, and size. A prospective controlled clinical study. Spine 19:1611-1618, 1994.

16. Glattes RC, Bridwell KH, Lenke LG, et al. Proximal junctional kyphosis in adult spinal deformity following long instrumented posterior spinal fusion: incidence, outcomes, and risk factor analysis. Spine 30:1643-1649, 2005.

17. Kim HJ, Bridwell KH, Lenke LG, et al. Proximal junctional kyphosis results in inferior SRS pain subscores in adult deformity patients. Spine 38:896-901, 2013.

18. Kim HJ, Lenke LG, Shaffrey CI, et al. Proximal junctional kyphosis as a distinct form of adjacent segment pathology after spinal deformity surgery: a systematic review. Spine 37(22 Suppl):S144-S164, 2012.

19. Kim HJ, Bridwell KH, Lenke LG, et al. Patients with proximal junctional kyphosis requiring revision surgery have higher postoperative lumbar lordosis and larger sagittal balance corrections. Spine 39:E576-E580, 2014.

20. Hart R, McCarthy I, O'Brien M, et al; International Spine Study Group. Identification of decision criteria for revision surgery among patients with proximal junctional failure following surgical treatment for spinal deformity. Spine 38:E1223-E1227, 2013.

21. Wiggins GC, Shaffrey CI. Dorsal surgery for myelopathy and myeloradiculopathy. Neurosurgery 60(1 Suppl 1):S71-S81, 2007.

22. Papagelopoulos PJ, Peterson HA, Ebersold MJ, et al. Spinal column deformity and instability after lumbar or thoracolumbar laminectomy for intraspinal tumors in children and young adults. Spine 22:442-451, 1997.

23. Otsuka NY, Hey L, Hall JE. Postlaminectomy and postirradiation kyphosis in children and adolescents. Clin Orthop Relat Res 354:189-194, 1998.

24. Yasuoka S, Peterson HA, MacCarty CS. Incidence of spinal column deformity after multilevel laminectomy in children and adults. J Neurosurg 57:441-445, 1982.

25. Aizawa T, Sato T, Ozawa H, et al. Sagittal alignment changes after thoracic laminectomy in adults. J Neurosurg Spine 8:510-516, 2008.

26. Kim YJ, Bridwell KH, Lenke LG, et al. Pseudarthrosis in adult spinal deformity following multisegmental instrumentation and arthrodesis. J Bone Joint Surg Am 88:721-728, 2006.

27. Kim YJ, Bridwell KH, Lenke LG, et al. Pseudarthrosis in long adult spinal deformity instrumentation and fusion to the sacrum: prevalence and risk factor analysis of 144 cases. Spine 31:2329-2336, 2006.

28. Gertzbein SD. Scoliosis Research Society. Multicenter spine fracture study. Spine 17:528-540, 1992.

29. Zeng Y, Chen Z, Sun C, et al. Posterior surgical correction of posttraumatic kyphosis of the thoracolumbar segment. J Spinal Disord Tech 26:37-41, 2013.

30. Fu KM, Smith JS, Burton DC, et al; International Spine Study Group. Revision extension to the pelvis versus primary spinopelvic instrumentation in adult deformity: comparison of clinical outcomes and complications. World Neurosurg. 2013 Feb 21. [Epub ahead of print]

31. Sarwahi V, Boachie-Adjei O, Backus SI, et al. Characterization of gait function in patients with postsurgical sagittal (flatback) deformity: a prospective study of 21 patients. Spine 27:2328-2337, 2002.

32. Gottfried ON, Daubs MD, Patel AA, et al. Spinopelvic parameters in postfusion flatback deformity patients. Spine J 9:639-647, 2009.

33. Marsicano JG, Lenke LG, Bridwell KH, et al. The lordotic effect of the OSI frame on operative adolescent idiopathic scoliosis patients. Spine 23:1341-1348, 1998.

34. Stephens GC, Yoo JU, Wilbur G. Comparison of lumbar sagittal alignment produced by different operative positions. Spine 21:1802-1806; discussion 1807, 1996.

35. Good CR, Lenke LG, Bridwell KH, et al. Can posterior-only surgery provide similar radiographic and clinical results as combined anterior (thoracotomy/thoracoabdominal)/posterior approaches for adult scoliosis? Spine 35:210-218, 2010.

36. Burkett B, Ricart-Hoffiz PA, Schwab F, et al. Comparative analysis of surgical approaches and osteotomies for the correction of sagittal plane spinal deformity in adults. Spine 38:188-194, 2013.

37. Kostuik JP, Maurais GR, Richardson WJ, et al. Combined single stage anterior and posterior osteotomy for correction of iatrogenic lumbar kyphosis. Spine 13:257-266, 1988.

38. Kim YJ, Bridwell KH, Lenke LG, et al. Results of lumbar pedicle subtraction osteotomies for fixed sagittal imbalance: a minimum 5-year follow-up study. Spine 32:2189-2197, 2007.

39. Smith-Petersen ML, Larson CB, Aufranc OE. Osteotomy of the spine for the correction of deformity in rheumatoid arthritis. J Bone Joint Surg Am 27:1-11, 1945.

40. Bridwell KH. Decision making regarding Smith-Petersen vs. pedicle subtraction osteotomy vs. vertebral column resection for spinal deformity. Spine 31(19 Suppl):S171-S178, 2006.

41. Bridwell KH, Lewis SJ, Lenke LG, et al. Pedicle subtraction osteotomy for the treatment of fixed sagittal imbalance. J Bone Joint Surg Am 85:454-463, 2003.

42. van Royen BJ, Slot GH. Closing-wedge posterior osteotomy for ankylosing spondylitis. Partial corporectomy and transpedicular fixation in 22 cases. J Bone Joint Surg Br 77:117-121, 1995.

43. Thomasen E. Vertebral osteotomy for correction of kyphosis in ankylosing spondylitis. Clin Orthop Relat Res 194:142-152, 1985.

44. Berven SH, Deviren V, Smith JA, et al. Management of fixed sagittal plane deformity: results of the transpedicular wedge resection osteotomy. Spine 26:2036-2043, 2001.

45. Suk SI, Chung ER, Kim JH, et al. Posterior vertebral column resection for severe rigid scoliosis. Spine 30:1682-1687, 2005.
46. Suk SI, Chung ER, Lee SM, et al. Posterior vertebral column resection in fixed lumbosacral deformity. Spine 30:E703-E710, 2005.
47. Suk SI, Kim JH, Kim WJ, et al. Posterior vertebral column resection for severe spinal deformities. Spine 27:2374-2382, 2002.
48. Bradford DS, Tribus CB. Vertebral column resection for the treatment of rigid coronal decompensation. Spine 22:1590-1599, 1997.
49. Lenke LG, Sides BA, Koester LA, et al. Vertebral column resection for the treatment of severe spinal deformity. Clin Orthop Relat Res 468:687-699, 2010.
50. Pahys JL, Lenke LG, Bridwell KH, et al. Matched cohort analysis of posterior-only vertebral column resection versus combined anterior/posterior vertebrectomy for severe spinal deformity. Spine Deformity 1:439-446, 2013.
51. Ha Y, Maruo K, Racine L, et al. Proximal junctional kyphosis and clinical outcomes in adult spinal deformity surgery with fusion from the thoracic spine to the sacrum: a comparison of proximal and distal upper instrumented vertebrae. J Neurosurg Spine 19:360-369, 2013.
52. Kebaish KM, Martin CT, O'Brien JR, et al. Use of vertebroplasty to prevent proximal junctional fractures in adult deformity surgery: a biomechanical cadaveric study. Spine J 13:1897-1903, 2013.
53. Lattig F. Bone cement augmentation in the prevention of adjacent segment failure after multilevel adult deformity fusion. J Spinal Disord Tech 22:439-443, 2009.
54. Bridwell KH, Lewis SJ, Edwards C, et al. Complications and outcomes of pedicle subtraction osteotomies for fixed sagittal imbalance. Spine 28:2093-2101, 2003.
55. Kelly MP, Lenke LG, Bridwell KH, et al. The fate of the adult revision spinal deformity patient: a single institution experience. Spine 38:E1196-E1200, 2013.
56. Papadopoulos EC, Cammisa FP Jr, Girardi FP. Sacral fractures complicating thoracolumbar fusion to the sacrum. Spine 33:E699-E707, 2008.
57. Cho W, Mason JR, Smith JS, et al. Failure of lumbopelvic fixation after long construct fusions in patients with adult spinal deformity: clinical and radiographic risk factors: clinical article. J Neurosurg Spine 19:445-453, 2013.

34

Evaluation and Management of Traumatic and Infectious Kyphosis

Matthew McDonnell ▪ *Alice Jane Hughes* ▪ *Alexander R. Vaccaro*

Injury to the spinal column or spinal cord after trauma can be devastating. Despite improved methods for evaluating and managing spinal fractures, many chronic or late complications can develop in this patient population. Posttraumatic spinal deformity is a potential complication that can result in pain and neurologic compromise and poses one of the greatest challenges for spinal surgeons.

The most common posttraumatic spinal deformity is kyphosis. It most commonly occurs at the thoracolumbar region followed by the thoracic and lumbar regions of the spine and is progressive. Kyphosis can develop after compression fractures and subsequent adjacent-level degeneration because of altered spinal biomechanics. It can also occur after a more severe burst or flexion-distraction type of injury in which the anterior and posterior spinal elements are disrupted.[1-3] Posttraumatic kyphosis can develop in patients initially treated nonoperatively with or without bracing. However, patients treated surgically at the time of injury can develop late deformity from pseudarthrosis, implant failure, or prior laminectomy. Additionally, progressive posttraumatic kyphosis is seen in patients treated with short-segment fixation or fusions.[4,5] Finally, posttraumatic kyphosis and instability are observed in patients with a neuropathic spinal arthropathy. Also known as *Charcot spine,* it is reported in patients with paralysis and lack of sensation from spinal cord injury. The lack of sensory feedback is thought to lead to abnormal movement between spinal segments and destruction of joint surfaces, and fractures and vertebral collapse lead to pseudarthrosis and deformity.[6-8]

Similarly, spinal deformity can be a late or chronic complication after spinal infections. Spinal infections are typically pyogenic and are further categorized as osteomyelitis, discitis, or epidural abscess. Atypical spinal infections are fungal or granulomatous processes often caused by tuberculous. Patients generally have an indistinct clinical presentation and most commonly present with vague back pain. A diagnosis is often delayed until clinical deterioration occurs, causing sepsis, pathologic fracture, or a neurologic deficit. Spinal deformity can result from pathologic fracture or progressive destruction of the vertebral body later in the process.

INDICATIONS AND CONTRAINDICATIONS

Posttraumatic Kyphosis

Clinical manifestations of posttraumatic kyphosis are generally described as mechanical or neurologic. Patients with mechanical sequelae can present with pain, fatigue, progression of deformity, and instability or imbalance in either the sitting or standing position. Neurologic sequelae include either a new or progressive deficit in the setting of a previously stable neurologic examination.

Pain is the most common presenting symptom of patients with posttraumatic deformity. It is thought to result from abnormal spinal biomechanics caused by trauma and subsequent deformity, which places altered forces on the bony and soft tissue structures.[1,9] Additionally, vertebral levels above and below the deformity may degenerate prematurely because of the altered biomechanics. Surgical correction of posttraumatic deformity has demonstrated modest improvement in pain in a number of studies assessing clinical outcomes after surgery.[10-12] Surgery improves pain in some patients, but this result is not entirely predictable.

Patients often present with a new or increasing neurologic deficit after previously presenting with a "late" posttraumatic deformity. Disruption of the spinal column and supporting ligamentous structures may result in instability, stenosis, kyphosis, and scoliosis. The development or progression of deformity and the resultant stenosis can cause direct compression or tenting of the neural elements, which worsens an existing neurologic deficit or creates a new one. Such a deficit can result from a posttraumatic syringomyelia.

Posttraumatic syringomyelia accounts for approximately 25% of all cases of syringomyelia. A syrinx develops in 21% to 28% of patients with a spinal cord injury, and 1% to 9% become clinically symptomatic.[13] Posttraumatic syringomyelia can develop years after injury. Patients usually present with pain in a segmental distribution, sensory loss, and progressive weakness. The cause of this condition is poorly understood, but it is thought to be related to initial cord injury, persistent cord compression, altered blood supply, and arachnoiditis.[13,14] Treatment for this condition should first involve correction of the deformity, decompression of compressive pathology, untethering of the cord, arachnolysis, and duraplasty.[13,15,16]

In the setting of posttraumatic kyphosis, surgery is considered for increasing pain, progression of neurologic deficit, pseudarthrosis or malunion, and breakdown of levels above or below the deformity. The goals of surgery include appropriate decompression of neural elements, restoration of sagittal balance, adequate structural support, and stabilization to obtain a solid bony fusion.

INFECTIOUS KYPHOSIS

Nonoperative treatment for spinal infections such as osteomyelitis and discitis is often appropriate initially. The offending organism can be diagnosed from blood cultures or image-guided biopsy to determine an appropriate antibiotic regimen. Parenteral antibiotics should be selected based on an organism's sensitivity profile and can usually be switched to an oral regimen. Involvement of an infectious disease specialist can be helpful to determine the most appropriate antibiotic regimen and duration. Rigid bracing is useful for spinal immobilization to allow patient mobilization, ambulation, and pain control. Indications for surgical intervention for spinal infections include failure of nonoperative treatment, the need for an open biopsy, the presence of a spinal abscess, sepsis, instability, progressive deformity, neurologic compromise, or refractory pain.

PREOPERATIVE PLANNING

POSTTRAUMATIC KYPHOSIS

Surgical planning requires consideration of both the focal deformity and the overall sagittal alignment. Plain radiographs are critical for evaluation of the overall balance of a patient with posttraumatic kyphosis. Standard full-length AP and lateral radiographs should be obtained initially to assess the C7 plumb line (which should fall through the posterosuperior corner of S1) and the cervical and lumbar lordosis and thoracic kyphosis. The magnitude of a focal kyphotic deformity is measured and should be further characterized as either sharp or smooth and flexible or stiff, because these can affect the choice of treatment.[17] Based on overall sagittal balance, the deformity can be characterized as type I or type II[18] (Fig. 34-1). Patients with a type I deformity present with a focal deformity or kyphosis but have normal overall sagittal

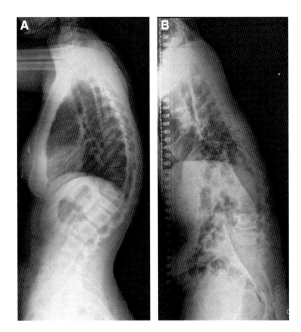

Fig. 34-1 **A,** A full-length lateral radiograph of a patient with a type I focal kyphosis secondary to T10 and T11 compression fractures but normal overall sagittal balance. The patient's lumbar spine is hyperlordotic to compensate for the kyphotic deformity. **B,** A full-length lateral radiograph of a patient with a type II deformity shows a focal kyphotic deformity and a positive sagittal imbalance.

balance. The segments above and below the focal deformity can compensate and thus maintain normal global sagittal alignment. For example, a patient with a posttraumatic kyphosis at the thoracolumbar junction might compensate with hyperlordosis of the lumbar spine. A patient with a type II deformity has a global, nonphysiologic sagittal imbalance and cannot compensate for the focal deformity. These patients may require more extensive surgery. Flexion, extension, and lateral-bending radiographs allow further assessment of the flexibility of the deformity and the potential extent of correction that can be anticipated at the time of surgery.

Fine-cut CT scans with sagittal and coronal reconstructions are excellent for visualizing the bony anatomy and are useful for surgical planning or assessment of pseudarthrosis. In patients with a neurologic deficit, a preoperative MRI needs to be evaluated to identify sites of compressive pathology.

A pseudarthrosis can occur after an unsuccessful surgical intervention. If suspected, dynamic flexion-extension radiographs and a scan should be evaluated. If a pseudarthrosis is diagnosed, a combined anterior-posterior approach or a posterior approach with an interbody fusion should be considered to increase the chance of a successful fusion.

INFECTIOUS KYPHOSIS

Preoperative planning for the treatment of infectious kyphosis is similar to that described for posttraumatic kyphosis, with a few important, unique considerations. Imaging of the entire spinal axis to evaluate for noncontiguous sites of infection is of paramount importance. Additionally, surgeons should be prepared to obtain samples for culture and biopsy analysis, because tumors can mimic infection. If the offending organisms have not yet been identified by image-guided biopsy, preoperative antibiotics should be withheld until intraoperative cultures are obtained. However, in the setting of bacteremia or sepsis, intravenous administration of antibiotics should not be delayed. In either setting, blood cultures are recommended. Surgeons should also be prepared to perform a decompression if an epidural abscess is identified.

Anterior infections such as osteomyelitis and discitis with or without an epidural abscess should be debrided and decompressed from an anterior approach, followed by structural bone grafting and posterior stabilization. In the setting of infection, structural autograft is preferred over allograft or anterior instrumentation. For deformity management, the necessary imaging studies are similar to those performed for posttraumatic kyphosis. Standard full-length AP and lateral radiographs allow assessment of the focal deformity and overall sagittal alignment.

OPERATIVE TECHNIQUE

POSTTRAUMATIC KYPHOSIS

The operative technique can be performed from an all-posterior approach, an all-anterior approach, or a combined anterior-posterior approach. Surgeons need to consider the surgical goals to select the best approach.

A thorough decompression is performed at the time of surgery (before deformity correction) when stenosis is present. This ensures adequate correction of the deformity in a safe manner. In the presence of a kyphotic deformity, anterior compression of the neural elements is common, and an anterior approach is often required. In addition to providing direct access to the site of compression, an anterior approach facilitates placement of anterior structural support.[19,20]

A patient with a flexible deformity that appears corrected on extension radiographs generally does not require an osteotomy. Such a deformity is often corrected after the patient is positioned on the operating table and properly instrumented. A stiff or inflexible deformity usually requires an osteotomy from either a posterior-only approach (Smith-Petersen or pedicle subtraction osteotomies) or a combined anterior-posterior approach. A Smith-Petersen osteotomy or chevron osteotomy involves resection of the posterior elements (facets) and posterior compression to shorten the posterior column. It lengthens the anterior column, with the posterior margin of the vertebral body serving as the axis of correction or pivot point. The average correction obtained with a single-level Smith-Petersen osteotomy is about 10 to 15 degrees (1 degree for each millimeter of bone resected).[21,22] Pedicle subtraction osteotomies have proved very effective for obtaining significant sagittal deformity correction. In this procedure, all posterior elements are removed, the pedicles are taken down, and the vertebral body is decancellated. The posterior and lateral body walls can be removed in the shape of a closing wedge to extend the spine, with hinging on the anterior margin of the vertebral body. Posterior compression across instrumentation in the posterior column allows maximal deformity correction. A single-level pedicle subtraction osteotomy provides 30 to 35 degrees of correction. An advantage is that kyphosis can be corrected without lengthening the anterior column. The technique, however, is technically demanding and can be associated with a large amount of epidural and cancellous bleeding.[10,23]

The most important principle and goal of correction is to restore sagittal balance. Ahn et al[11] reported on radiographic parameters and functional outcomes in patients having an osteotomy. They wanted to identify radiographic parameters associated with improved functional outcomes. The authors found a significant association between improved outcomes and radiographic correction if the postoperative lumbar lordosis was larger than 25 degrees and if the postoperative coronal C7 plumb line was correct to within 2.5 cm of midsacrum.

INFECTIOUS KYPHOSIS

The key surgical principles for the treatment of spinal infections are adequate debridement, decompression of neural elements, and rigid stabilization. Anterior infections such as osteomyelitis and discitis with or without epidural abscess should be debrided and decompressed from an anterior approach. Generally, structural bone grafting is required, followed by either immediate or staged posterior instrumentation/fusion. Structural autograft (for example, iliac crest) is generally preferred over anterior cages, rods, or plates because of the concern for potential pathogen incubation on the surface of the implants and difficulty eradicating the infection. Posterior instrumentation in the form of pedicle screws and rods provides rigid stabilization, allowing early mobilization and diminishing pain. Posterior-only approaches are generally only indicated in the setting of posterior epidural abscess without anterior spinal involvement. Decompression of anterior elements and placement of structural graft through a posterior approach is possible, but it is technically demanding and risks iatrogenic neurologic injury. The principles of deformity management are the same as those for posttraumatic deformity.

Postoperative broad-spectrum, empirical parenteral antibiotics are discontinued, and pathogen-specific antibiotics are given based on microbiology results and organism sensitivity. Sequential laboratory markers such as erythrocyte sedimentation rate and C-reactive protein should be followed to confirm eradication of the infection.

OUTCOMES AND POTENTIAL COMPLICATIONS

Although the procedures can be challenging and complications may occur, surgery for posttraumatic deformity generally has favorable results. Early surgery showed better results in a study of 16 patients with posttraumatic instability of thoracolumbar fractures.[24] Patients who had surgery more than 13 months after injury had inferior results, compared with those who had earlier surgery. Suk et al[25] compared surgical results of a combined anterior-posterior procedure with a posterior closing wedge osteotomy in patients with posttraumatic kyphosis. In the anterior-posterior surgery group, the authors reported 11.2 degrees of correction at the final follow-up, but they noted a 27% loss of correction, compared with measurements on immediate postoperative radiographs. In the posterior closing wedge osteotomy group, the mean correction at the final follow-up was 25.7 degrees, and loss of correction was 11%, compared with results on initial postoperative radiographs. The authors concluded that a posterior wedge osteotomy was more reliable at restoring sagittal alignment, despite being technically demanding. Wu et al[26] reported their results in 13 patients treated with a posterior decancellation osteotomy procedure for rigid posttraumatic kyphosis.[26] They achieved fusion in all 13 patients and reported an average correction of 38 degrees with no neurologic injuries. Other studies have reported successful correction of posttraumatic kyphotic deformity using posterior closing wedge osteotomies, with the average correction ranging from 34 to 51 degrees.[27-29] These results indicated that a greater degree of mean correction was obtained with a posterior closing wedge or pedicle subtraction osteotomy, compared with anterior-only procedures.[30,31]

Complications associated with deformity correction surgery include neurologic injury and infection. Surgical management of posttraumatic kyphosis has an increased potential for neurologic injury. Factors that predispose patients to this complication include the presence of a preexisting spinal cord injury, draping of the neural elements over the anterior vertebral body, the presence of scar tissue, or a tethered cord.

Neurologic injury ranges from mild neuropathy to paraplegia. As previously discussed, adequate decompression of neural elements before deformity correction can help to minimize this risk. Additionally, intraoperative monitoring with motor-evoked potentials and somatosensory-evoked potentials can be an early warning system for potential neurologic injury. If results of neuromonitoring raise concerns intraoperatively, a wake-up test can potentially allow alteration of instrumentation or curve correction while a patient is anesthetized.

PATIENT EXAMPLES

This 46-year-old man was injured at the gym while attempting to lift 250 pounds. He was originally diagnosed with a T12 compression fracture and was neurologically intact. The patient presented to our institution 2 years later with severe back pain and a sharp angular kyphosis measuring 45 degrees (Fig. 34-2, A through D). Results of a neurologic examination were normal. A T12 pedicle subtraction osteotomy, a T12-L1 laminectomy, and a T10-L1 posterior spinal fusion were performed, all through a posterior-only approach, to restore normal sagittal alignment. He is shown postoperatively (Fig. 34-2, E and F).

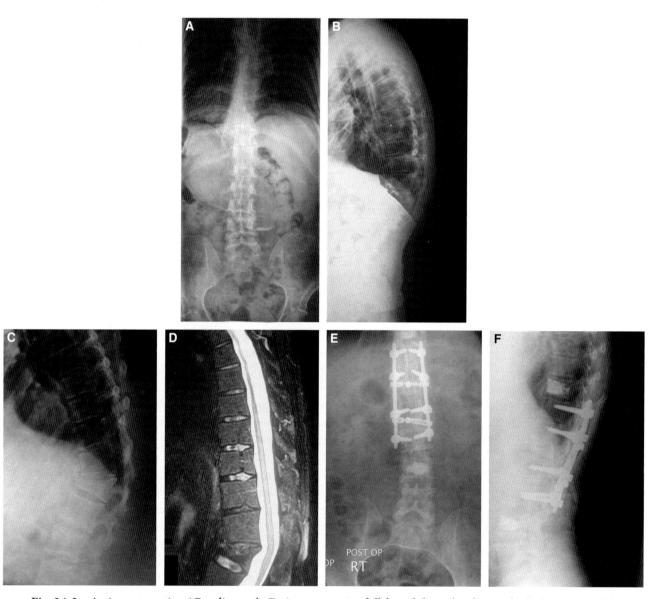

Fig. 34-2   **A,** A preoperative AP radiograph. **B,** A preoperative full-length lateral radiograph. **C,** A preoperative lateral radiograph of fracture and deformity. **D,** Preoperative sagittal T2-weighted MRI. **E,** A postoperative AP radiograph. **F,** A postoperative lateral radiograph.

This 69-year-old man presented 4 months after sustaining an L1 burst fracture in an automobile accident. He was initially neurologically intact and treated with a thoracolumbosacral brace. On presentation to our institution, the patient had severe back pain, neurogenic claudication, progressive lower extremity weakness, and a focal hyperkyphosis of 45 degrees (Fig. 34-3, *A* and *B*). He required a walker to ambulate. He was treated with a combined anterior-posterior approach. The general surgeons performed an anterior approach along the course of the twelfth rib, requiring resection of the rib, with a patient in the lateral decubitus position. An L1 corpectomy was then performed, decompressing the neural elements. An expandable cage and local autologous bone graft were placed, along with anterior Moss-Miami instrumentation (DePuy Spine, Raynham, MA) with a longitudinal rod. The patient was then placed in a prone position, and posterior stabilization was performed with posterior T11-L3 fusion. Immediate postoperative radiographs are shown (Fig. 34-3, *C* and *D*).

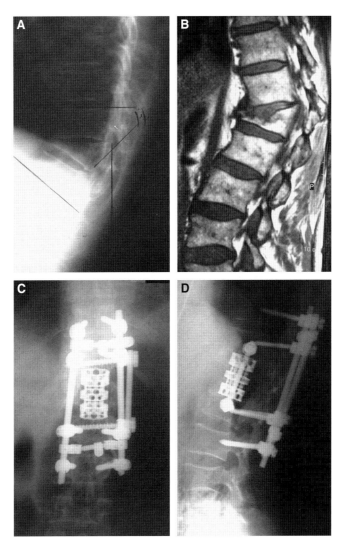

Fig. 34-3 **A,** A preoperative lateral radiograph. **B,** Preoperative sagittal MRI. **C,** A postoperative AP radiograph. **D,** A postoperative lateral radiograph.

This 44-year-old woman was transferred from an outside hospital with L2-3 discitis/osteomyelitis. Her history was notable for right lower extremity necrotizing fasciitis, diagnosed 1 year previously. The patient presented with mild, symmetrical, bilateral lower extremity weakness (grade 4/5). Blood cultures were positive for *Klebsiella* organisms. A CT-guided biopsy of her spine was negative. Radiographs and CT revealed destruction of the L2-3 disc space with focal kyphosis and lateral listhesis of L2 on L3 (Fig. 34-4, *A* through *D*). An MRI with contrast demonstrated an anterior epidural abscess from L2 to L4 and significant central and foraminal narrowing (Fig. 34-4, *E* and *F*). A posterior bilateral extracavitary approach was chosen to drain the epidural abscess and to perform a posterior laminectomy and L3 pedicle subtraction osteotomy and T10- L5 posterior fusion using local bone graft. Immediate postoperative radiographs are shown (Fig. 34-4, *G* and *H*).

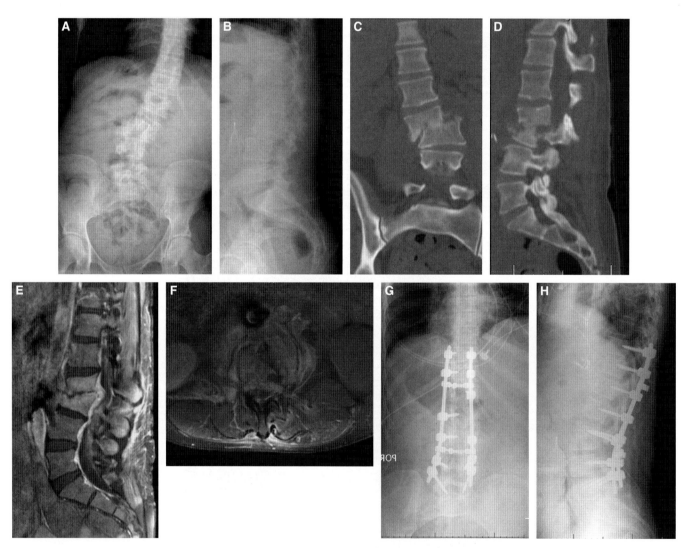

Fig. 34-4   **A,** A preoperative AP radiograph. **B,** A preoperative lateral radiograph. **C,** Preoperative coronal CT. **D,** Preoperative sagittal CT. **E,** Preoperative sagittal MRI with contrast. **F,** Preoperative axial MRI with contrast. **G,** A postoperative AP radiograph. **H,** A postoperative lateral radiograph.

CONCLUSION

Posttraumatic kyphotic deformity can develop as a complication in patients with spinal trauma. Pain is the most common presenting clinical symptom. Indications for surgery include severe pain, progressive deformity, neurologic compromise, or pseudarthrosis. The principle goals of surgery include decompression of neural elements if neurologic deficit or claudication is present, re-creation of normal sagittal alignment and balance, and stabilization and successful fusion. These can be achieved with various surgical approaches, with or without osteotomy depending on patient and curve characteristics. Similar surgical principles apply to deformity in the setting of infection, along with appropriate medical management. In either case, a careful preoperative assessment with appropriate imaging is necessary to fully understand characteristics of the deformity and overall alignment before a surgical approach and technique are selected.

REFERENCES

1. Vaccaro AR, Silber JS. Post traumatic spinal deformity. Spine 26(24 Suppl):S111-S118, 2001.
2. Polly DW Jr, Klemme WR, Shawen S. Management options for the treatment of posttraumatic thoracic kyphosis. Semin Spine Surg 12:110-116, 2000.
3. Vaccaro AR, Jacoby SM. Thoracolumbar fractures and dislocations. In Fardon DF, Garfin SR, Abitbol JJ, et al, eds. Orthopaedic Knowledge Update: Spine 2. Rosemont, IL: American Academy of Orthopaedic Surgeons, 2002.
4. McLain RF, Burkus JK, Benson DR. Segmental instrumentation for thoracic and thoracolumbar fractures: prospective analysis of construct survival and five-year follow-up. Spine J 1:310-313, 2001.
5. Knop C, Fabian HF, Bastian L, et al. Late results of thoracolumbar fractures after posterior instrumentation and transpedicular bone grafting. Spine 26:88-99, 2001.
6. McBride GG, Greenberg D. Treatment of Charcot spinal arthropathy following traumatic paraplegia. J Spinal Disord 4:212-420, 1991.
7. Harrison MJ, Sacher M, Rosenblum BR, et al. Spinal Charcot arthropathy. Neurosurgery 28:273-277, 1991.
8. Schwartz HS. Traumatic Charcot spine. J Spinal Disord 3:269-275, 1990.
9. Malcolm BW, Bradford DS, Winter RB, et al. Posttraumatic kyphosis: a review of forty-eight surgically treated patients. J Bone Joint Surg Am 63:891-899, 1981.
10. Bridwell KH, Lewis SJ, Edwards C, et al. Complications and outcomes of pedicle subtraction osteotomies for fixed sagittal imbalance. Spine 28:2093-2101, 2003.
11. Ahn UM, Ahn NU, Buchowski JM, et al. Functional outcome and radiographic correction after spinal osteotomy. Spine 27:1308-1311, 2002.
12. Bohlman HH, Kirkpatrick JS, Delamarter RB, et al. Anterior decompression for late paralysis after fractures of the thoracolumbar spine. Clin Orthop Relat Res 300:24-29, 1994.
13. Bordbelt AR, Stoodley MA. Post-traumatic syringomyelia: a review. J Clin Neurosci 10:401-408, 2003.
14. Edgar R, Quail P. Progressive post-traumatic cystic and non-cystic myelopathy. Br J Neurosurg 8:7-22, 1994.
15. Batzdorf U, Lekamp J, Johnson JP. A critical appraisal of syrinx cavity shunting procedures. J Neurosurg 89:382-388, 1998.
16. Lee TT, Alameda GJ, Gromelsk EB, et al. Outcome after surgical treatment of progressive posttraumatic cystic myelopathy. J Neurosurg 92:149-154, 2000.
17. Buchowski JM, Kuhns CA, Bridwell KH, et al. Surgical management of posttraumatic thoracolumbar kyphosis. Spine J 8:666-677, 2008.
18. Booth KC, Bridwell KH, Lenke LG, et al. Complications and predictive factors for the successful treatment of flatback deformity (fixed sagittal imbalance). Spine 24:1712-1720, 1999.
19. Roberson JR, Whitesides TE Jr. Surgical reconstruction of late posttraumatic thoracolumbar kyphosis. Spine 10:307-312, 1985.
20. Kostuik JP, Matsusaki H. Anterior stabilization, instrumentation, and decompression for post-traumatic kyphosis. Spine 14:379-386, 1989.

21. Smith-Petersen MN, Larson CB, Aufranc OE. Osteotomy of the spine for correction of flexion deformity in rheumatoid arthritis. Clin Orthop Relat Res 66:6-9, 1969.

22. Yang C, Wood KB. Surgical management of posttraumatic kyphosis. In Vaccaro AR, Fehlings MG, Dvorak MF, eds. Spine and Spinal Cord Trauma: Evidence-Based Management. New York: Thieme, 2011.

23. Bridwell KH, Lewis SJ, Lenke LG, et al. Pedicle subtraction osteotomy for the treatment of fixed sagittal imbalance. J Bone Joint Surg Am 85:454-463, 2003.

24. Keene JS, Lash EG, Kling TF Jr. Undetected posttraumatic instability of "stable" thoracolumbar fractures. J Orthop Trauma 2:201-211, 1998.

25. Suk SI, Kim JH, Lee SM, et al. Anterior-posterior surgery versus posterior closing wedge osteotomy in posttraumatic kyphosis with neurologic compromised osteoporotic fracture. Spine 28:2170-2175, 2003.

26. Wu SS, Hwa SY, Lin LC, et al. Management of rigid posttraumatic kyphosis. Spine 21:2260-2266, 1996.

27. Lehmer SM, Keppler L, Biscup RS, et al. Posterior transvertebral osteotomy for adult thoracolumbar kyphosis. Spine 19:2060-2067, 1994.

28. Gertzbein SD, Harris MB. Wedge osteotomy for the correction of posttraumatic kyphosis: a new technique and a report of three cases. Spine 17:374-379, 1992.

29. Heary RF, Bono CM. Pedicle subtraction osteotomy in the treatment of chronic, posttraumatic kyphotic deformity. J Neurosurg Spine 5:1-8, 2006.

30. Been HD, Poolman RW, Ubags LH. Clinical outcome and radiographic results after surgical treatment of posttraumatic thoracolumbar kyphosis following simple type A fractures. Eur Spine J 13:101-107, 2004.

31. Atici T, Aydinli U, Akesen B, et al. Results of surgical treatment for kyphotic deformity of the spine secondary to trauma or Scheuermann's disease. Acta Orthop Belg 70:344-348, 2004.

35

Transpsoas Techniques for Restoration of Spinal Alignment

Michael S. Park ▪ Luiz Pimenta ▪ Juan S. Uribe

Sagittal spinopelvic harmony is increasingly targeted as a primary goal during the surgical management of adult spinal deformity. The cause of adult spinal deformity is usually iatrogenic or related to progressive degenerative changes, and patients most commonly present with pain. Scoliosis can be present with a component in the sagittal plane, although coronal deformity correction is outside the scope of this chapter. Spinopelvic harmony, as demonstrated by a sagittal vertical axis (SVA) of less than 50 mm, a pelvic incidence (PI) within 9 degrees of lumbar lordosis (LL), and a pelvic tilt (PT) of less than 25 degrees, has been shown to correlate with improvements in health-related quality of life scores.[1-4] Conversely, a high postoperative SVA increases the risk of pseudarthrosis, adjacent-segment disease, and proximal junctional kyphosis.[5-7]

Surgical correction of sagittal imbalance can be accomplished with techniques that lengthen the anterior column, shorten the posterior column, or both (Table 35-1). The effects, complication rates, technical challenges, complications, and radiographic outcomes vary with these techniques. Those that lengthen the anterior column include placement of an interbody cage with or without release of the anterior longitudinal ligament (ALL).

Posterior shortening techniques include Smith-Petersen osteotomy, pedicle subtraction osteotomy, and vertebral column resection. A Smith-Petersen osteotomy is generally considered a safe technique with low morbidity. It is confined to resection of the laminae and articular facets and hinges on the middle column in an attempt to stretch an intact ALL. Each millimeter of bone resected provides approximately 1 degree of correction, with a maximum correction of 10 to 15 degrees.[8-12] In contrast, a pedicle subtraction

Table 35-1 Surgical Options for Treating Sagittal Imbalance

Techniques That Lengthen the Anterior Column	Techniques That Shorten the Posterior Column	Techniques That Affect Both the Anterior and Posterior Columns
Minimally invasive-lumbar interbody fusion Anterior column release/anterior longitudinal ligament release	Facetectomy Smith-Petersen osteotomy Pedicle subtraction osteotomy	Anterior longitudinal ligament–total column release Vertebral column resection

osteotomy is a challenging procedure involving all three spinal columns and is associated with significant blood loss. After the posterior elements are resected, the anterior vertebral body is fractured while the osteotomy is closed to achieve lordosis. Pedicle subtraction osteotomy procedures have reportedly achieved LL correction of approximately 30 to 40 degrees and SVA improvement of 5.5 to 13.5 cm.[5,8,13] In a vertebral column resection, the entire vertebral segment is resected in an attempt to correct significant rigid spinal deformities. This procedure generally requires prolonged operative times and has a significantly higher complication rate.[14]

Most of these techniques can now be performed through minimally invasive approaches, either lateral or posterior or both. Minimally invasive surgical techniques have the potential for muscle mass preservation and decreased physiologic stress, operative times, blood loss, narcotic use, and length of hospitalization, but they have challenges and limitations, including a steep learning curve.[15-19] Patient selection is an important factor, because patients with severe deformity may not be appropriate candidates for a minimally invasive approach. We describe the range of options that can be performed from a minimally invasive lateral approach for the correction of spinal deformity.

TREATMENT OPTIONS

Sagittal imbalance can be corrected surgically by shortening the posterior column, lengthening the anterior column, or a combination of both. Numerous techniques are available to spine surgeons to achieve this goal. In increasing order of achievable correction, these combinations include:

- Interbody cage placement
- Interbody cage placement with a facetectomy
- ALL release or anterior column release without posterior column manipulation
- ALL release with a facetectomy
- ALL release with a Smith-Petersen osteotomy
- ALL release with a total column release (that is, ALL release with complete resection of the posterior elements)
- Pedicle subtraction osteotomy
- Vertebral column resection

A pedicle subtraction osteotomy can be performed in a hybrid fashion, which has been previously described.[20,21] It requires a staged approach, as do all procedures involving manipulation of the posterior column (for example, a facetectomy). The development of lateral transpsoas techniques has allowed these procedures or portions of them to be performed in a minimally invasive fashion.

INDICATIONS AND CONTRAINDICATIONS

Indications for surgical application of these techniques include sagittal and coronal deformity. The selection of techniques that are appropriate for a patient depends on the degree of sagittal imbalance, the desired amount of lordotic correction, and the presence of prior fusion.[22] Relative contraindications to transpsoas approaches are generally limited to prior abdominal or especially retroperitoneal surgery and aberrant vascular anatomy on the side of the planned approach, although the procedure may possibly be safely performed from the other side. We do not recommend that ALL release be performed in the presence of significant vascular pathology or prior surgical reconstruction, given that the aorta, inferior vena cava, and/or iliac vessels are retracted during this portion of the procedure.

PREOPERATIVE EVALUATION AND PLANNING

The diagnosis of adult spinal deformity and sagittal imbalance begins with the history and physical examination. In particular, it is important to obtain a patient's history of prior surgical intervention, especially laminectomy, facetectomy, or instrumentation and fusion, and all prior abdominal or retroperitoneal procedures. This information may dictate the side for a chosen approach or preclude a lateral approach altogether.

Standing 36-inch scoliosis films form the cornerstone of spinal deformity evaluation, because they allow measurement of the SVA, the coronal sagittal vertical line (CSVL) with the C7 plumb line, and all other spinopelvic parameters. The femoral heads should be visualized for accurate measurement of the PI and PT. Often the femoral heads are not truly superimposed on a lateral film, in which case the midpoint of the line connecting the centers of the femoral heads can be used for parameter measurement. Some patients are not able to stand erect without flexing the hips and knees to compensate for positive sagittal balance and pelvic retroversion and to achieve horizontal gaze.[23] This can preclude the ability to obtain optimal films. Coronal and rotational spinal deformities, which are not discussed in this chapter, can preclude truly accurate measurement of spinopelvic parameters. The presence of pelvic obliquity should be noted if lower lumbar levels (L3-4 or L4-5) are involved. This is determined with a horizontal line drawn across the tops of the iliac crests. During patient assessment for correction of sagittal deformity, lateral hyperextension bolster films can help to determine whether the deformity is fixed or flexible.

CT is useful for additional surgical planning especially in the setting of prior lumbar surgery to determine the presence of laminectomy, instrumentation, and the status of the facet joints. More often, MRI or CT-myelography is obtained as part of the evaluation. It is important to identify the configuration of the psoas musculature and the major vascular anatomy, including the aorta, inferior vena cava, and iliac vessels, for a planned lateral approach. If possible, the relative location of the segmental vessels is noted in relation to the disc space, because these vessels can be injured during contralateral annulus release.

OPERATIVE TECHNIQUE: MINIMALLY INVASIVE LATERAL TRANSPSOAS APPROACH

In 2006 Ozgur et al[24] described the anterolateral (or direct lateral) transpsoas approach for placement of a large interbody cage. The patient is given general endotracheal anesthesia and positioned in a true lateral decubitus position. Proper orthogonal visualization is confirmed on cross-table AP and lateral films. The skin is marked with the use of fluoroscopic guidance and then incised. The abdominal wall muscles and transversalis fascia are gently split, and the retroperitoneal space is entered in a blunt fashion. In the retroperitoneal space, a finger is used to sweep the peritoneum anteriorly and palpate down to the psoas muscle (Fig. 35-1, A). The anteroposterior midpoint of the psoas muscle is approximated by locating the greatest bulk of the psoas muscle with palpation. It serves as a suitable initial entry point for the first dilator, which is safely guided to the surface of the psoas muscle with an index finger. The location is confirmed with lateral fluoroscopy.

The fibers of the psoas muscle are gently dissected using a dilator with directional EMG monitoring to assess the proximity of the lumbar plexus nerve roots. If EMG readings are appropriate, serial dilators are passed over the initial dilator, and an expandable tubular retractor (for example, MaXcess, NuVasive, San Diego, CA) is passed over the largest dilator and attached to a table-mounted system (Fig. 35-1, B).

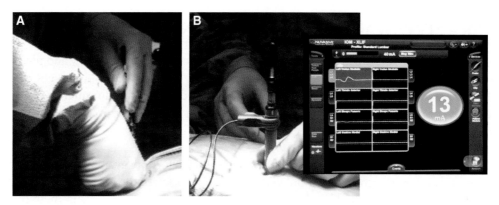

Fig. 35-1 A minimally invasive lateral approach. **A,** The retroperitoneal space is entered, and blunt finger dissection is performed. **B,** Placement of serial directional EMG dilators. Sample directional EMG monitoring is shown in the inset.

ANTEROLATERAL LUMBAR INTERBODY FUSION

With the retractor in place, the discectomy can be performed with a combination of curettes, rongeurs, rasps, and broaches. The contralateral annulus is released with a Cobb elevator to accommodate a long (wide) implant that can rest on both lateral margins of the epiphyseal ring, maximizing endplate support. Interbody distraction and implant placement in an anterior and bilateral epiphyseal location restores disc height and corrects sagittal and coronal plane imbalance. Le et al[25] have shown that placement of a 10-degree cage corrects segmental lordosis by approximately 1.5 degrees.

ANTERIOR LONGITUDINAL LIGAMENT RELEASE

ALL release can be accomplished safely from a lateral approach, with placement of a hyperlordotic cage fixed to the vertebral body. The positioning and approach are the same as those used for an interbody fusion. After a retractor is placed, an annulotomy and discectomy are performed, with care to prepare and preserve the endplate. A custom-curved retractor is then gently passed along the anterior edge of the ALL and positioned between the large vessels and sympathetic plexus and the ventral disc. The great vessels are not visualized, because the extent of dissection required would likely place a patient at greater risk than placement of a 2 to 4 mm wide retractor. A custom disc blade and intradiscal retractor are used to section the ALL in a sequential fashion, easing the curved retractor to the contralateral side of the disc space. Complete ALL release is confirmed when the adjacent vertebral body endplates are mobilized with minimal resistance and a *fish-mouth* opening of the ventral disc space is evident.

After the endplates are prepared, an appropriately sized polyetheretherketone cage is selected. These cages range from 8 to 18 mm in height and from 50 to 60 mm in length, and they have 20 to 30 degrees of lordosis. The cages are packed with allograft, placed into the disc space, and anchored to the adjacent vertebral body with one or two screws to prevent ventral migration into the peritoneal cavity and loss of indirect decompression.

OUTCOMES

Initial cadaveric studies suggested approximately 10 degrees of segmental lordosis and 10 to 20 degrees of regional LL correction per level of ALL release.[26] Deukmedjian et al[27,28] performed 11 ALL releases in 7 patients. They described a gain of segmental lordosis ranging from 9 to 20 degrees, with an average of 17 degrees per level. Regional lumbar lordosis improved by an average of 24 degrees, and mean SVA improved by 4.9 cm, from a mean preoperative sagittal balance of 9 cm to a postoperative value of 4.1 cm. PT decreased by a mean value of 7 degrees, from 32 to 25 degrees. The only complication noted in this series was a superficial wound infection.

Akbarnia et al[29] described their results in a series of 17 patients. Two patients had ALL release with placement of 10-degree lordotic cages. (The other 15 patients underwent different procedures, which are described later in the chapter.) Segmental lordosis (motion segment angle) improved from 13 to 42 degrees and from 9 to 32 degrees for an increase of 29 degrees and 23 degrees, respectively. Regional lumbar lordosis changed from 26 to 33 degrees and from 34 to 44 degrees for an increase of 7 degrees and 10 degrees, respectively. Sagittal balance, as measured by the T1 spinopelvic inclination (another measure of global sagittal balance), was unchanged and improved by 4 degrees in each patient. Pelvic tilt worsened in one case by 2 degrees and improved by 7 degrees in the other.

In a more recent series, Manwaring et al[30] reviewed results of 15 anterior column releases in 9 patients. Per level released, the segmental lordotic correction was 12 degrees, and SVA correction was 3.1 cm. Per patient, the (regional) LL was corrected by 16.5 degrees, and SVA was corrected by 4.8 cm. All patients in this series had multilevel minimally invasive lumbar interbody fusions (MI-LIFs). The mean though nonsignificant improvement in sacral slope and PT were 7.5 degrees and 5.2 degrees, respectively. In a comparison group of 27 patients who had MI-LIF without anterior column release, no significant difference was noted in preoperative and postoperative SVA, regional LL, or segmental LL, although the study was underpowered to detect such differences. The authors reported that the use of posterior segmental instrumentation did not alter the degree of lordotic or sagittal balance correction.[30]

Anterior longitudinal ligament total column release can be achieved by performing an ALL release in addition to a facetectomy and removal of the inferior vertebral pedicles. This provides an *accordion* effect by simultaneously shortening the middle and posterior columns, while allowing additional length gain in the anterior column. This procedure increases lordosis more than an anterior column release only. Initial results from a single case (unpublished data) demonstrated improvement of lumbar lordosis from 27 degrees kyphosis to 27 degrees lordosis, which was a 54-degree change. PT decreased from 32 degrees preoperatively to 8 degrees postoperatively. Overall, the sagittal balance corrected from 23 to 10 cm.

In the series of Akbarnia et al,[29] two other patients underwent pedicle subtraction osteotomies at the released level; the motion segment angle improved from 14 degrees and 9 degrees of kyphosis preoperatively to 21 degrees and 18 degrees of lordosis, for a gain of 35 degrees and 36 degrees of segmental lordosis, respectively. The regional LL improved from 15 degrees of kyphosis and 20 degrees of lordosis to 34 degrees and 51 degrees of lordosis postoperatively, for an increase of 49 degrees and 31 degrees, respectively. The T1 spinopelvic inclination changed from 8 degrees and 1 degree preoperatively to −5 degrees and 0 degrees postoperatively, for a change of −13 degrees and −1 degree, respectively. Pelvic tilt improved from 37 to 26 degrees in one case and from 41 to 32 degrees in the other.

The other possible variation of an anterior column release is a straightforward ALL release, followed by facetectomies or Smith-Petersen osteotomies. The remaining 13 patients described by Akbarnia et al[29] underwent this procedure (2 of them had Smith-Petersen osteotomies at additional levels). The motion segmental angle improved from a mean value for all patients from 11 degrees of kyphosis to 21 degrees of lordosis for an average lordotic correction of 32 degrees. Regional LL improved from a mean value of 16 degrees to 53 degrees for an average improvement of almost 37 degrees. The mean improvement in T1 spinopelvic inclination was approximately −4 degrees, and the average improvement in PT was nearly 12 degrees. Compared with the previously described variations of ALL release, we believe that the lordotic correction effected by ALL release and facetectomy is between the value achieved with ALL release alone and an ALL release with total column release.

ALL release has the potential for catastrophic aortic or inferior vena cava injury. These vessels are manipulated without adequate proximal and distal control.[28] As mentioned previously, severe aortic, caval, or iliac vessel calcification or other pathology or prior surgical reconstruction, in conjunction with fixed kyphotic deformity, is an absolute contraindication to ALL release. Significant vascular calcification or pathology alone and the inability to define the appropriate plane of retraction are relative contraindications. In the latter situation, ALL release is aborted at that level. Fixed sagittal deformity is another relative contraindication; anterior fixed deformities necessitate more extensive surgery, whereas posteriorly fixed deformities require osteotomy before anterior column release.[31] Based on results of cadaveric studies, it is possible to inadvertently damage the sympathetic plexus by passing a retractor ventral to it (while passing the retractor dorsal to the vessels and ventral to the ALL), although the clinical manifestations of such injury are unknown.[27]

A systematic review of minimally invasive techniques for adult degenerative spinal deformity revealed scant literature. Of thirteen papers meeting inclusion criteria for review, two were considered high quality, two demonstrated improvement in SVA of four that documented SVA, three demonstrated improvement in PT, and seven demonstrated increased LL. Complication rates ranged from 14.3% to 87.5%, with an overall rate of 45% in the pooled data. Thirty-seven neurologic complications were identified in the meta-analysis for a rate of 14%, although the authors noted that these were largely transient.[32]

OPERATIVE TECHNIQUE: HYBRID PEDICLE SUBTRACTION PEDICLE OSTEOTOMY

The technique for a hybrid pedicle subtraction osteotomy has been previously described.[20,21] The positioning and approach are the same as those performed for an interbody fusion. Rostral to L1 a retrodiaphragmatic-pleural approach is possible, which includes release of the diaphragmatic attachments from the costal insertions, vertebral body, and posterior spinal elements. The approach is retroperitoneal for levels caudal to L1. During placement of the retractor at the vertebral body and dissection for the osteotomy, one of the principal difficulties involves manipulation and coagulation of the segmental vessels, which run along the inferolateral border of the vertebral body from anterior to posterior.

The bony resection is the same as that of a lateral corpectomy, which is described later. It involves the use of curettes, osteotomes, rongeurs, and a high-speed drill (see Fig. 35-4). In our experience, a lateral osteotomy can be performed in one of at least two ways. If a patient is fused above and below the target level (for example, with Harrington rods in a previous interbody fusion), then a retractor is placed at the level of the vertebral body, and a wedge osteotomy is performed with resection of the ipsilateral pedicle and posterior longitudinal ligament (PLL). If the desired level is not fused, then the retractor is placed at the immediately adjacent disc spaces, and discectomies are performed followed by cage/graft placement, as described previously. A retractor is then placed at the level of the vertebral body and the wedge osteotomy (including the ipsilateral pedicle and PLL resection) is completed. The retractor must be placed three times to prevent unnecessary retraction of the psoas muscle and the lumbar plexus.

After bony resection is performed in the lateral position, the PLL is fully resected and the dura exposed to prevent buckling of the dura during closure of the osteotomy from a posterior direction. Closure should include multiple layers, and a drain is placed in the surgical bed or intrapleural space as needed. Between the lateral and posterior stages, we believe that patients should be restricted to bed rest until completion of the second stage because of the potential instability after wedge osteotomy and unilateral pedicle resection.

We recommend that the second stage be completed shortly after the initial stage. A laminectomy, bilateral facetectomy, and removal of the contralateral pedicle are performed with the patient in the prone position. If pedicle screws were not previously present, we instrument at least two levels above and below the osteotomized level. A temporary rod is placed on the contralateral side of the pedicle being resected. The osteotomy is closed in a standard fashion, with care to prevent thecal sac buckling and entrapment or impingement of the two nerve roots exiting on each side. Electrophysiologic monitoring should be performed during closure.

With this hybrid approach, a pedicle subtraction osteotomy can be completed with minimal manipulation of the neural elements, particularly during posterior longitudinal ligament resection and wedge osteotomy. This is especially important at more rostral levels (for example, T12-L2) because of the relative inflexibility of the neural structures at these levels. This approach allows interbody fusion at the corresponding rostral and caudal levels, reducing the risk of pseudarthrosis and hardware failure, which can occur with a posterior-only approach. Additional advantages include the potential for decreased blood loss and direct visualization of vascular structures and the anterior thecal sac. However, the hybrid approach requires two procedures (or a staged procedure) and involves a steep learning curve, as with all minimally invasive surgical techniques.

Outcomes

In two cases of hybrid pedicle subtraction osteotomy, we were able to improve segmental lordosis from 20 degrees of kyphosis to 3 degrees of lordosis and from 4 degrees of lordosis to 18 degrees of lordosis, a lordotic correction of 23 degrees and 14 degrees, respectively. Regionally, LL was improved in the first case from 10 to 35 degrees; in the other case, regional LL remained unchanged at 31 degrees. PT improved from 40 degrees preoperatively in each case to 30 degrees and 31 degrees postoperatively. The SVA was decreased by 1.6 cm and 1.0 cm, respectively.

OPERATIVE TECHNIQUE: MINIMALLY INVASIVE LATERAL CORPECTOMY

Vertebral corpectomy via a minimally invasive lateral approach has been previously described.[33-35] The positioning and approach are performed as for an interbody fusion. The approach is modified with regard to the ribs and diaphragm depending on the vertebral level, as described earlier for a hybrid pedicle subtraction osteotomy procedure. For a thoracic or upper lumbar level, in the lateral position, the borders of the vertebral body of interest are outlined using fluoroscopy, and the ribs above are palpated. The rib directly overlying the vertebral body is outlined, and this is the incision mark. A 7 cm incision is made over the rib line, with a slight posterior offset from the vertebral body outline. Dissection using electrocautery is carried down directly on top of the rib, without entering the neurovascular bundle below each rib segment.

Subperiosteal dissection is performed to clear the tissue off of the rib and to maintain the pleura intact. Once the rib is freed, a rib cutter is used to remove as much rib ventrally and dorsally as possible. For a retropleural approach, the endothoracic fascia is dissected along the medial border of the rib. This dissection is carried bluntly down to the vertebral body, and segmental vessels coming from anterior are ligated as proximally as possible. After adequate exposure is obtained with the retractor in place, a vertebral corpectomy is performed using standard surgical techniques with a combination of rongeurs, curettes, osteotomes, and high-speed drills (Fig. 35-2, *A*). Ventral reconstruction is then performed using expandable titanium

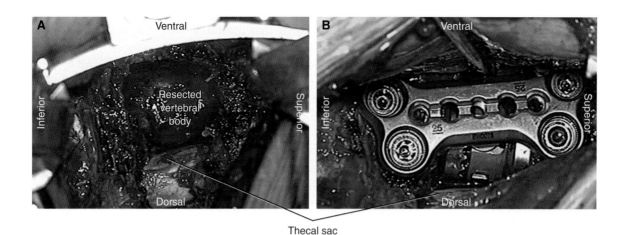

Thecal sac

Fig. 35-2   Minimally invasive lateral corpectomy. **A,** Exposure after a corpectomy proper. **B,** Placement of an expandable cage and lateral plate.

cages, biologic allograft, and any autograft obtained during the approach. Spinal instrumentation with ventrolateral plate-screw fixation through the expandable retractor (Fig. 35-2, *B*) and/or percutaneous posterior pedicle screw–rod fixation is necessary. The intended correction and anterior column lengthening need to be considered during selection and expansion of the cage and application of the anterolateral plating.

When combined with posterior osteotomies, a vertebral corpectomy provides the greatest amount of deformity correction of the lateral retroperitoneal techniques. It approaches the degree of correction achievable by circumferential or anteroposterior vertebral column resection, which is limited only by the degree of neural element manipulation. A vertebral column resection, performed either in a circumferential or posterior-only fashion, involves a significant amount of risk of neurologic compromise.

PATIENT EXAMPLES

ANTERIOR LONGITUDINAL LIGAMENT RELEASE

This 57-year-old woman presented with axial back pain, limited mobility of her left leg, and tingling and burning paresthesias to her knee. She had a left L3-4 microdiscectomy 2 years earlier. Her preoperative films revealed lumbar dextroscoliosis with stable grade I retrolistheses at L2-3 and L3-4. Standing 36-inch films showed an SVA of 3 cm, an LL of 40 degrees, a PI of 59 degrees, and a PT of 29 degrees (Fig. 35-3, *A;* Table 35-2). In a staged fashion, we performed anterior column release at L2-3 and L4-5, with L3-4 interbody fusion, followed by L5-S1 facetectomy and transforaminal lumbar interbody fusion with L2-S1 percutaneous pedicle screw instrumentation. Her pain was improved after the procedure. On postoperative lateral standing scoliosis films, her SVA is 4 cm, LL is 56 degrees, PI is 59 degrees, and PT is 20 degrees (Fig. 35-3, *B;* Table 35-2). She has remained neurologically intact.

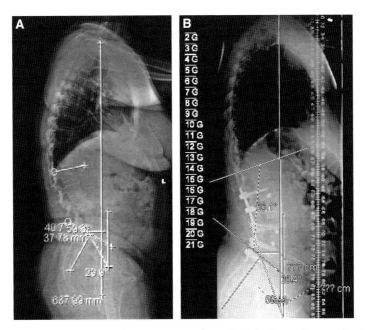

Fig. 35-3 **A** and **B,** Preoperative and postoperative lateral 36-inch standing scoliosis radiographs.

Table 35-2 Preoperative and Postoperative Spinopelvic Parameters

	Preoperative Values	**Postoperative Values**
Sagittal vertical axis (cm)	3	4
Lumbar lordosis (degrees)	40	56
Pelvic incidence (degrees)	59	59
Pelvic tilt (degrees)	29	20

Hybrid Pedicle Subtraction Osteotomy

This 69-year-old man had multiple previous thoracolumbar operations. The most recent was a T10-S1 instrumentation and fusion (Fig. 35-4, *A*). He presented with gluteal and thigh pain, limiting his ambulation and other activities of daily living. Preoperatively he had 8 cm of positive sagittal imbalance and 10 degrees of LL, with anterior wedging of his L1 vertebral body. In a staged procedure, an anterior wedge resection of the L1 vertebral body was performed using a minimally invasive retroperitoneal lateral approach (Fig. 35-4, *C* through *E*). The patient was then placed in a prone position for completion of the pediculectomies, closure of the pedicle subtraction osteotomy, and definitive posterior rod instrumentation. Blood loss was minimal. On postoperative lateral standing scoliosis films, his LL was 35 degrees, a gain of 25 degrees (Fig. 35-4, *B*; Table 35-3). He was discharged home 4 days after the procedure. Six months postoperatively, the patient is neurologically intact.

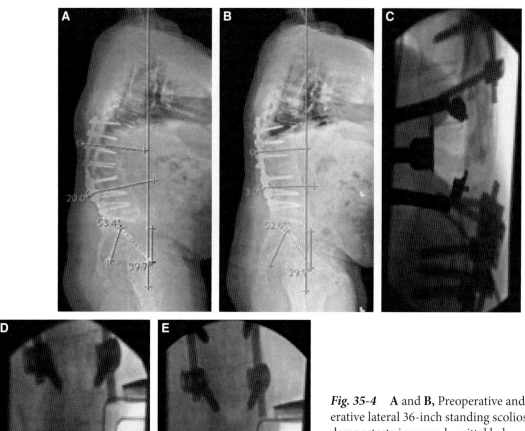

Fig. 35-4 **A** and **B,** Preoperative and postoperative lateral 36-inch standing scoliosis films demonstrate improved sagittal balance and lumbar lordosis. **C,** Intraoperative fluoroscopy of the lateral pedicle subtraction osteotomy. A lateral projection confirmed retractor placement at the posterior L1 vertebral body. **D** and **E,** AP projections showed the use of an osteotome and drill, respectively, during a pedicle subtraction osteotomy.

Table 35-3   Preoperative and Postoperative Spinopelvic Parameters

	Preoperative Values	Postoperative Values
Sagittal vertical axis (cm)	8	6.4
Lumbar lordosis (degrees)	10	35
Segmental (T12-L1) lordosis (degrees)	−20	3
Pelvic incidence (degrees)	53	53

CONCLUSION

Global sagittal balance is gaining recognition for its patient outcomes. Goals of sagittal imbalance correction surgery include an SVA of less than 50 mm, a PI within 9 degrees of lumbar LL, and a PT of less than 25 degrees. Patients in whom these goals are met, with good postoperative sagittal balance and spinopelvic harmony, have superior outcomes. Multiple techniques have been described for sagittal imbalance correction; several of these can be performed through a minimally invasive lateral approach, including interbody cage placement solely or with ALL release and a minimally invasive lateral corpectomy. A minimally invasive lateral approach can also be performed as a part of staged or hybrid techniques combining traditional osteotomies, including facetectomies, Smith-Petersen osteotomies, and pedicle subtraction osteotomies.

REFERENCES

1. Schwab F, Patel A, Ungar B, et al. Adult spinal deformity–postoperative standing imbalance: how much can you tolerate? An overview of key parameters in assessing alignment and planning corrective surgery. Spine 35:2224-2231, 2010.
2. Blondel B, Schwab F, Ungar B, et al. Impact of magnitude and percentage of correction on health-related quality of life at 2-years follow-up. Neurosurgery 71:341-348; discussion 348, 2012.
3. Glassman SD, Bridwell K, Dimar JR, et al. The impact of positive sagittal balance in adult spinal deformity. Spine 30:2024-2029, 2005.
4. Lafage V, Schwab F, Patel A, et al. Pelvic tilt and truncal inclination: two key radiographic parameters in the setting of adults with spinal deformity. Spine 34:E599-E606, 2009.
5. Schwab FJ, Patel A, Shaffrey CI, et al. Sagittal realignment failures following pedicle subtraction osteotomy surgery: are we doing enough? Clinical article. J Neurosurg Spine 16:539-546, 2012.
6. Kim YJ, Bridwell KH, Lenke LG, et al. Pseudarthrosis in long adult spinal deformity instrumentation and fusion to the sacrum: prevalence and risk factor analysis of 144 cases. Spine 31:2329-2336, 2006.
7. Jackson RP, Hales C. Congruent spinopelvic alignment on standing lateral radiographs of adult volunteers. Spine 25:2808-2815, 2000.
8. Bridwell KH. Decision making regarding Smith-Petersen vs. pedicle subtraction osteotomy vs. vertebral column resection for spinal deformity. Spine 34:E766-E774, 2009.
9. Bridwell KH, Lewis SJ, Lenke LG, et al. Pedicle subtraction osteotomy for the treatment of fixed sagittal imbalance. J Bone Joint Surg Am 85:454-463, 2009.
10. Buchowski JM, Bridwell KH, Lenke LG, et al. Neurologic complications of lumbar pedicle subtraction osteotomy: a 10-year assessment. Spine 32:2245-2252, 2007.
11. Cho KJ, Bridwell KH, Lenke LG, et al. Comparison of Smith-Petersen versus pedicle subtraction osteotomy for the correction of fixed sagittal imbalance. Spine 30:2030-2038, 2005.
12. Gill JB, Levin A, Burd T, et al. Corrective osteotomies in spine surgery. J Bone Joint Surg Am 90:2509-2520, 2008.
13. Lafage V, Schwab F, Vira S, et al. Does vertebral level of pedicle subtraction osteotomy correlate with degree of spinopelvic parameter correction? J Neurosurg Spine 14:184-191, 2011.
14. Lenke LG, Sides BA, Koester LA, et al. Vertebral column resection for the treatment of severe spinal deformity. Clin Orthop Relat Res 468:687-699, 2010.
15. Fessler RG, Khoo LT. Minimally invasive cervical microendoscopic foraminotomy: an initial clinical experience. Neurosurgery 51:S37-S45, 2002.
16. Oppenheimer JH, DeCastro I, McDonnell DE. Minimally invasive spine technology and minimally invasive spine surgery: a historical review. Neurosurg Focus 27:E9, 2009.
17. Guiot BH, Khoo LT, Fessler RG. A minimally invasive technique for decompression of the lumbar spine. Spine 27:432-438, 2002.
18. Khoo LT, Palmer S, Laich DT, et al. Minimally invasive percutaneous posterior lumbar interbody fusion. Neurosurgery 51(5 Suppl):S166-S171, 2002.
19. Mummaneni PV, Rodts GE Jr. The mini-open transforaminal lumbar interbody fusion. Neurosurgery 57:256-261, 2005.

20. Park MS, Deukmedjian AR, Ahmadian AA, et al. Global sagittal balance: experience with the lateral retroperitoneal approach. Contemp Neurosurg 35:1-6, 2013.

21. Deukmedjian A, Uribe JS. Minimally invasive anterior column reconstruction for sagittal plane deformities. In Wang MY, Lu Y, Anderson DG, et al, eds. Minimally Invasive Spinal Deformity Surgery: An Evolution of Modern Techniques. Wien: Springer-Verlag, 2014.

22. Deukmedjian AR, Ahmadian A, Bach K, et al. Minimally invasive lateral approach for adult degenerative scoliosis: lessons learned. Neurosurg Focus 35:E4, 2013.

23. Bridwell KH, Lewis SJ, Edwards C, et al. Complications and outcomes of pedicle subtraction osteotomies for fixed sagittal imbalance. Spine 28:2093-2101, 2003.

24. Ozgur BM, Aryan HE, Pimena L, et al. Extreme Lateral Interbody Fusion (XLIF): a novel surgical technique for anterior lumbar interbody fusion. Spine J 6:435-443, 2006.

25. Le TV, Vivas AC, Dakwar E, et al. The effect of the retroperitoneal transpsoas minimally invasive lateral interbody fusion on segmental and regional lumbar lordosis. ScientificWorldJournal 2012:516706, 2012.

26. Uribe JS, Smith DA, Dakwar E, et al. Lordosis restoration after anterior longitudinal release and placement of lateral hyperlodrotic cages during the minimally invasive lateral transpsoas approach: a radiographic study in cadavers. J Neurosurg Spine 17:476-485, 2012.

27. Deukmedjian AR, Le TV, Baaj AA, et al. Anterior longitudinal ligament release using the minimally invasive lateral retroperitoneal approach: a cadaveric feasibility study and report of 4 clinical cases. J Neurosurg Spine 17:530-539, 2012.

28. Deukmedjian AR, Dakwar E, Ahmadian A, et al. Early outcomes of minimally invasive anterior longitudinal ligament release for correction of sagittal imbalance in patients with adult spinal deformity. ScientificWorldJournal 2012:789698, 2012.

29. Akbarnia BA, Mundis GM Jr, Moazzaz P, et al. Anterior column realignment (ACR) for focal kyphotic spinal deformity using a lateral transpsoas approach and ALL release. J Spinal Disord Tech 27:29-39, 2013.

30. Manwaring JC, Bach K, Ahmadian AA, et al. Management of sagittal balance in adult spinal deformity with minimally invasive anterolateral lumbar interbody fusion: a preliminary radiographic study. J Neurosurg Spine 20:515-522, 2014.

31. Nomoto EK, Kabirian N, Akbarnia BA, et al. XLIF® for anterior column realignment. In Goodrich JA, Volcan IJ, eds. eXtreme Lateral Interbody Fusion, ed 2. St Louis: Quality Medical Publishing, 2013.

32. Bach K, Ahmadian A, Deukmedjian A, et al. Minimally invasive surgical techniques in adult degenerative spinal deformity: a systematic review. Clin Orthop Relat Res 472:1749-1761, 2014.

33. Uribe JS, Dakwar E, Le TV, et al. Minimally invasive surgery for thoracic spine tumor removal. Spine 35(26 Suppl):S347-S354, 2010.

34. Uribe JS, Dakwar E, Cardona RF, et al. Minimally invasive lateral retropleural thoracolumbar approach: cadaveric feasibility study and report of 4 clinical cases. Neurosurgery 68 [ONS Suppl 1]:ons32-ons39, 2011.

35. Park MS, Deukmedjian AR, Uribe JS. Minimally invasive anterolateral corpectomy for spinal tumors. Neurosurg Clin North Am 25:317-325, 2014.

36

Transforaminal Interbody Fusion Techniques for Restoration of Spinal Alignment

Cyrus C. Wong ▪ *Clifford M. Houseman*
John C. Barr ▪ *Joseph S. Cheng*

Restoration of coronal and sagittal balance in spinal surgery requires knowledge of the biomechanical parameters for proper alignment and the appropriate surgical techniques. Proper alignment is crucial whether fusion is performed at one level or thirteen levels. Restoration of normal physiologic energy requirements for upright posture is a surgical endpoint that may include re-creation of lumbar lordosis (improving sagittal balance), neural decompression (directly or indirectly), restoration of the height of disc spaces, and increased surface area for arthrodesis. Providing long-standing clinical benefit is an important goal in surgical management that extends beyond ensuring surgical and radiographic balance. The effects of transforaminal lumbar interbody fusion (TLIF) correlate with fusion and restitution of pelvic and spinal parameters.[1] The use of TLIF techniques has demonstrated increased segmental lordosis in patients with isthmic spondylolisthesis.[2] The goal of this chapter is to review the literature for TLIF, profiles of patients who have undergone this procedure, and TLIF techniques that provide radiographic and clinical success.

Scoliosis and loss of lordosis can result from degenerative changes of the lumbar spine and from surgical techniques that hasten spinal imbalance. Patient symptoms associated with these changes include back pain, lower extremity pain, and weakness.[2] Radiographic findings include loss of lordosis with either straightening of the spine, resulting in a flat-back deformity, or reversal of lordosis secondary to kyphotic motion segments receiving eccentric loading.[2] These changes can be translated through the transition segment into the thoracic spine, leading to extensive deformity.

Current techniques for the restoration of global spinal balance include extensive decompression and mobilization of the spine with various osteotomy techniques such as a Smith-Petersen, Ponte, pedicle subtraction, and/or vertebral column shortening. The choice of technique depends on the degree of correction needed and the instrumented fusion planned to maintain the proper alignment. In addition to the vertebral resection techniques, vertebral augmentation techniques can be used such as TLIF to modify the spinal alignment and augment the fusion bed. TLIF techniques allow a significant degree of rotational correction and the preservation of more mobile segments. TLIF also affects arthrodesis. Jagannathan et al[3] reported a pseudarthrosis rate of 2.5% in a study of 80 patients who had TLIF procedures for deformity correction. The minimum follow-up was 2 years. In a study of 40 patients with Cobb angles of 20 to 60 degrees, each patient was randomized to have posterolateral fusion or TLIF treatment.[4] TLIF patients had significant recovery, compared with posterolateral fusion patients, of lumbar lordosis (62.5% versus 36%, respectively) and spinal sagittal balance (64.1% versus 44.8%, respectively).[4] In the same study, clinical outcome was determined by the SRS-22 questionnaire. The scores for pain control and satisfaction with the treatment were higher for the TLIF group.

Current evidence indicates that interbody grafting has positive outcomes radiographically and clinically. The TLIF maneuver has been compared with posterior lumbar interbody fusion (PLIF) and anterior lumbar interbody fusion (ALIF). Advantages of TLIF over PLIF include the requirement for less dural retraction, less risk of traversing a nerve root injury, and the option to apply a larger interbody graft that contacts more surface area. Fusion rates of these two techniques do not differ significantly. ALIF techniques have a significant advantage in that the anterior column is directly released, thereby benefiting patients with fixed deformities and revision surgery candidates.[5] Release of the anterior longitudinal ligament before a posterior corrective procedure results in a more pliable lumbar spine, a concept that is also demonstrated with the Smith-Peterson osteotomy technique. Additionally, ALIF allows placement of a graft that is both much larger with increased surface area contact and more lordotic, because the anterior interspace can be distracted. Hsieh et al[6] reported that the ALIF procedure increased foraminal height by 18.5%, the local disc angle by 8.3 degrees, and lumbar lordosis by 6.2 degrees. In the same study, TLIF decreased the local disc angle by 0.1 degrees and lumbar lordosis by 2.1 degrees. These radiographic findings of improvement, however, did not correlate with clinical improvement, and radiographic improvement of severe preoperative imbalance was not statistically different.[7] Additionally, clinical outcome measures in patients who had TLIF for thoracolumbar deformity correction were not higher than those in patients who had ALIF. The difference in complication rates between the two procedures was not statistically significant in patients with worst outcomes. Disadvantages of the ALIF procedure are that it typically requires an access surgeon, and it carries an increased risk of vascular and/or peritoneal/visceral organ injury. TLIF procedures provide direct visualization and decompression of the exiting and traversing nerve roots. ALIF provides indirect decompression by restoring disc space height. In men the superior hypogastric plexus with an anterior approach can be injured, which can result in retrograde ejaculation. The literature states that the risk is approximately 0.42%[8] to 5.9%[9] and is higher at the L5-S1 level, compared with more rostral levels.

Surgical techniques have evolved. Direct lateral (or extreme lateral) interbody grafting is an alternative method that allows the placement of a large interbody graft and anterior column release. These techniques carry the risk of immediate postoperative problems such as psoas weakness. However, long-term disability significantly diminishes over time, and modifications with neuromonitoring, proper docking, and working channels have mitigated the once-profound effect on the psoas muscle. As with ALIF, this technique does not provide direct nerve root visualization and decompression. Both techniques require a staged procedure, compared with TLIF, which is completed in the same setting as the primary posterior deformity correction and fixation.

INDICATIONS AND CONTRAINDICATIONS

Surgical indications for degenerative adult scoliosis continue to be debated. More studies such as a prospective controlled clinical trials are needed to compare nonsurgical with surgical treatments. These patients are typically older with multiple comorbidities, which can make major operations and rehabilitation more complicated.[10] Therefore careful patient selection and knowledge of indications are paramount. TLIF techniques should be indicated in patients with a high risk of nonfusion. This includes elderly patients, those with a known pseudarthrosis who are having revision surgery, and patients with the following characteristics: tobacco abuse, chronic steroid therapy, immunosuppression, osteoporosis, postmenopausal status, suspected noncompliance with external orthoses, a history of thyroid/parathyroid disorders, renal osteodystrophy, or osteopenia on bone density imaging. Patients with any of these conditions merit strong consideration for TLIF during preoperative planning. TLIF is warranted in patients with an obvious radiculopathy that can be directly correlated to MRI results, because the exiting and traversing nerve root can be decompressed with minimal retraction and detraction of the disc space. A TLIF technique should be strongly considered for patients with radiographic evidence of a grade I or II spondylolisthesis, because this is one of the strongest qualifiers for known patient improvement with radiculopathy and axial back pain.

Preoperatively the presence of a fixed or nonfixed deformity requires consideration. In a patient with a fixed deformity and a native abdomen, an ALIF is favored to provide anterior column release before a posterior reduction, facilitating the degree of correction. Contraindications based on preoperative imaging include the presence of sclerotic or chronic Modic changes. Either of these postinflammatory conditions will prevent osteoinduction and conduction necessary for fusion to occur. MRI scans should be carefully reviewed for the presence of a conjoined nerve root within the foramen. Although this is a rare condition, it is a strong contraindication for TLIF. In these patients, the conjoined root overlies the typical graft entry site and cannot be significantly retracted, increasing the incidence of nerve root injury. Another contraindication is placement of an interbody graft adjacent to fracture fragments. This can worsen the fracture and inadvertently lead to the development of a kyphotic deformity.

PREOPERATIVE PLANNING

Physical Examination

A thorough history-taking and physical examination are essential for all patients who are considered for surgical correction of a spinal deformity. Understanding a patient's chief complaints is imperative for appropriate surgical decision-making and planning. For instance, a patient with axial mechanical back pain alone is treated differently from a patient who has axial back pain in combination with radicular or claudication symptoms. Factors that aggravate and ameliorate symptoms should be documented, along with all signs or symptoms of focal weakness.

A detailed neurologic examination should be performed in all patients with spinal deformity. This should include assessment for focal weakness, hyperreflexia, clonus, a Babinski sign, decreased rectal tone, and saddle anesthesia. Evidence of myelopathy should prompt surgeons to evaluate the cervical and thoracic area for significant neural compression that may need to be treated at the time of surgery.

A detailed musculoskeletal examination is imperative in this patient population. Other causes of spinal deformity need to be identified such as intrinsic muscular disease (that is, muscular dystrophy), poor posture, and leg-length discrepancy; these need to be treated before surgical intervention is considered.[11] If a leg-length discrepancy is noted, a shoe lift should be used and scoliosis films repeated for accurate measurements of the patient's deformity. The presence of a rib hump deformity and elevated clavicles are noted and considered when planning surgical intervention. Cosmetic appearance has been documented and evaluated in pediatric deformity patients, but its impact on adult degenerative scoliotic patients is less evident.[11]

Osteoporosis or osteopenia is assessed in the preoperative examination. Results may prompt a bone metabolic workup that includes laboratory evaluation of parathyroid hormone, calcium, and vitamin D levels. A formal endocrinology consult may be prudent before any surgical intervention. Medical optimization by the primary care physician is essential specifically in the adult degenerative population, because many of these patients have significant comorbidities that can lead to increased perioperative complications.

Radiographic Evaluation

Radiographic evaluation of spinal deformity patients typically involves a multimodal approach. Most patients have a combination of MRI and CT. A CT-myelogram is performed in patients who cannot tolerate MRI or if MRI is contraindicated. These imaging modalities provide information about neural compression either in the central canal or lateral gutter/foramen that may need to be decompressed during the surgical procedure. They also reveal anterior or lateral osteophytes that need to be treated during coronal or sagittal plane correction. In patients with osteopenia or osteoporosis, a DXA scan can help to evaluate bone mineral density and the risk for osteoporotic fractures. These results are reported in T-scores and Z-scores. T-scores represent a patient's results compared with those of a 30-year-old sex-matched patient.[11] A T-score of less than −2.5 is diagnostic for osteoporosis. A T-score between −1.0 and −2.5 indicates osteopenia. A Z-score is a patient's bone density compared with an age-matched and sex-matched average and is typically not used to diagnose osteoporosis.[11]

In complex patients who have a history of previous surgical intervention and difficulty pinpointing their back pain, nuclear bone scanning can sometimes be a helpful diagnostic tool. Increased uptake shows active bone metabolism/inflammation and is typically seen in scoliotic patients at the apex of the curve. This information can be useful when following patients who have no significant progression on their scoliosis radiographs but who have increased complaints of back pain.

Arguably the most important radiographic evaluations for global spinal alignment are 36-inch side-bending and flexion/extension scoliosis films. These images are obtained with the patient standing, with knees and hips extended, arms flexed, and hands on the clavicles. This allows an accurate evaluation of sagittal and coronal alignment, eliminating potential compensatory mechanisms in the knees or pelvis to maintain alignment. The importance of sagittal alignment cannot be underestimated when planning surgical intervention for these patients. These films are used to measure thoracic, lumbar, and thoracolumbar curves with the Cobb method on neutral and side-bending films. The results help to diagnosis curves that may need to be included in surgical constructs (that is, major and minor curves) and compensatory curves that can be excluded from surgical fusions. Flexion/extension films assist in diagnosing areas of focal instability and in determining reducibility of global sagittal imbalance. Other maneuvers that help to evaluate flexibility of curves include non-weight-bearing views such as supine side-bending films. Radiographs can be obtained with the patient in push or traction views or with the patient positioned over a bolster.[11] These images can be useful in identifying the amount of closed correction to expect from positioning and general anesthesia.

The main parameters measured on these films are the sacral slope, pelvic tilt, pelvic incidence, lumbar lordosis, thoracic kyphosis, C7 plumb line, sagittal vertical axis, and the central sacral vertical line.[11] Pelvic incidence, sacral slope, and pelvic tilt are geometrically related, as indicated in the following equation: Pelvic incidence = Sacral slope + Pelvic tilt (Fig. 36-1). Coronal curves are measured using the Cobb method. These curves are classified by size and their ability to reduce to less than 20 degrees. The largest curve is the main curve. Of the other curves, those that measure more than 20 degrees are minor curves, and curves that are flexible to less than 20 degrees are compensatory.[11]

These measurements provide an overall evaluation of a patient's global spinal alignment and help surgeons determine the amount of correction, the location of the correction, and levels that need to be instrumented. Many patients retrovert the pelvis in an attempt to maintain sagittal alignment. Understanding these parameters and their relationships allows surgeons to estimate the amount of pelvic compensation a patient is using. This is important during planning to prevent underestimation of the amount of correction needed. A detailed discussion of these parameters is beyond the scope of this chapter; however, several surgical goals involving these values are as follows: Lumbar lordosis = Pelvic incidence ± 9 degrees; pelvic tilt is less than 14 degrees; and the sagittal vertical axis is within 4 cm of the posterior superior aspect of the S1 vertebral body.[12]

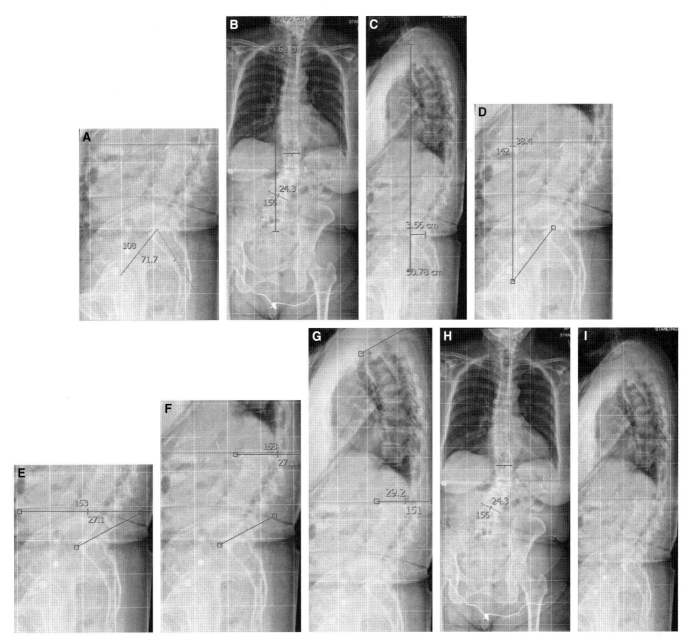

Fig. 36-1 **A,** Pelvic incidence is the angle between a line perpendicular to the endplate of S1 and a line running to the center of the femoral head. **B,** The central sacral vertical line is a line measured from the midline of the sacrum. The distance between this line and another vertical line drawn downward from the spinous process of C7 is the amount of coronal shift of a patient's head off the midline. **C,** The sagittal vertical axis is the horizontal distance between the C7 plumb line and a vertical line from the posterosuperior corner of the sacral endplate. This provides a measure of sagittal balance. **D,** Pelvic tilt is the angle formed by a line that extends from the middle of the femoral head to the midpoint of the S1 endplate and a horizontal reference line. **E,** Sacral slope is the angle between a line parallel to the S1 endplate and a horizontal reference line. **F,** Lumbar lordosis is the angle between a line parallel to the superior endplate of L1 and a line parallel to the superior endplate of S1. **G,** Thoracic kyphosis is the angle between a line parallel to the superior endplate of T2 (or the highest measurable thoracic vertebral body) and a line parallel to the inferior endplate of T12. **H,** A 36-inch scoliosis film is an AP film of a patient standing with knees extended to show overall global coronal balance. The Cobb angle of the main coronal nerve is measured. **I,** A 36-inch scoliosis film is a lateral film of a patient standing with knees extended and hands on the clavicles to show overall global sagittal balance.

OPERATIVE TECHNIQUE

In this section, we describe our procedure for placement of a transforaminal interbody graft. Careful preoperative planning helps to delineate the levels at which to perform this procedure and the optimal position of the interbody device to correct sagittal or coronal deformity.

The patient is brought to the operating room and placed under general anesthesia. Appropriate IV access is obtained with either two large-bore IV catheters or placement of central line. An arterial line is then placed for appropriate blood pressure monitoring during the case. At the discretion of the surgeon, neuromonitoring personnel place leads in preparation for a baseline measurement after the patient is placed in a prone position. At our institution, typically somatosensory evoked potentials and EMG are monitored.

We use a Jackson rail-top bed (Mizuho OSI, Union City, CA) with a hard footboard for extension of the hips for lordosis. We believe that this bed allows adequate thoracic kyphosis and lumbar lordosis using the chest and hip pads. The hip pads are placed slightly more caudally than usual for increased lumbar lordosis. Numerous pillows are placed on the footboard, and the knees are bent and placed on gel pads to exaggerate lumbar lordosis. If the patient has a coronal imbalance, a sheet is placed before prone positioning and is used for closed reduction of the deformity before an incision is made. After the patient is positioned, AP and lateral baseline fluoroscopic images are obtained. These will be compared with images obtained after completion of the osteotomies and correction. The patient's heels and shoulders are aligned to prevent introduction of an obliquity. The patient's skin is prepared and draped in the normal sterile fashion.

An incision is made to encompass the levels needed for osteotomies and stabilization. We generously infiltrate the skin with local anesthetic, and sharp dissection is then carried down to the fascia. Monopolar cautery is used to release the muscle attachments to the spinous processes, and subperiosteal dissection is carried down to the lamina and facet joints (Fig. 36-2, *A*). Levels are confirmed to be correct with the use of fluoroscopy or by identification of the sacrum. Lateral dissection is carried to the transverse processes of the levels to be fused.

The decompression or osteotomies are performed. Depending on the patient's preoperative symptoms, a full laminectomy or Ponte (chevron) osteotomies are required. These begin by removal of the inferior articular process. A strip laminectomy is then performed bilaterally, and the superior aspect of the superior articular process is removed to provide adequate room for the nerve root when the osteotomy is closed (Fig. 36-2, *B*). The inferior articular process can be removed with a high-speed drill and Kerrison rongeurs or with osteotomes, depending on the surgeon's preference (Fig. 36-2, *C*). The tip of the superior articular process is typically removed with Kerrison rongeurs (Fig. 36-2, *D*). This is done at multiple levels to allow mobilization of the spinal segments needed for correction. Conversely, if the spine is deemed fixed, then a pedicle subtraction osteotomy may be appropriate. This procedure begins with a partial laminectomy above and below the level of interest and a full laminectomy at the level of interest. The inferior and superior articular processes are removed, creating a superforamen once the pedicle is removed. Removal of these processes and identification of the nerve roots facilitates skeletonization of the pedicle. We typically disarticulate the transverse process and dissect the lateral body/pedicle with a No. 1 Penfield dissector. Once full exposure is obtained a pediculectomy is performed, taking the pedicle down flush with the posterior aspect of the vertebral body. A progressive wedge-shaped defect is made into the body down to the anterior cortical edge. When an appropriate amount of bone has been removed, downward-angled curettes are used to dissect the posterior aspect of the vertebral body away from the thecal sac. The posterior cortical wall of the vertebral body is then fractured into the pedicle subtraction osteotomy defect. Last, the lateral edge of the pedicle is drilled away or removed with an Adson or Lempert rongeur. The defect is then closed with back and forth compression with temporary rods. A permanent rod can be placed and final tightening performed to maintain the correction.

The TLIF graft can be placed before or after full osteotomies are completed. The levels of placement and location in the disc space affect spinal alignment. Generally, the more anterior the graft placement, the more lordosis is obtained with compression, and unilateral placement at multiple levels may help to correct a coronal imbalance. We typically plan the insertion side to be on the concavity of the coronal deformity to maximize coronal correction, as reported in several recent papers.[7,11,13] The inferior articular process and the tip of the superior articular process are removed at the level of placement, and the exiting and traversing nerve root are identified to protect them during discectomy and graft placement (Fig 36-2, E). Once the disc space is identified, the traversing nerve root is dissected and retracted gently to allow access to the annulus. This is cauterized with bipolar cautery. The annulus is opened with a No. 11 blade, and a discectomy is performed (Fig. 36-2, F). The disc is removed using straight and upward-angled pituitary rongeurs. Once room is made, we typically use paddle shavers to scrape the endplate to facilitate removal of the remaining disc. The shavers provide an estimate of the graft size. If entering the disc space is difficult because of disc space collapse, then distraction on this side may be helpful. This is performed in one of several ways. Screws are placed and the tulip heads are distracted (with the use of a laminar spreader if the lamina is intact); temporary rods are placed, and the contralateral screws are distracted; or the segment is sequentially distracted from inside the disc space with shavers or distractors.[13]

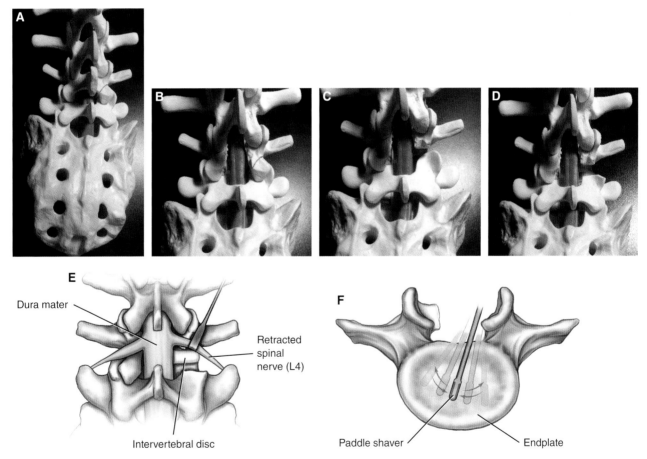

Fig. 36-2 Sequential steps of bony removal for a right-sided L4-5 TLIF. **A,** A subperiosteal exposure is performed. **B,** A full laminectomy is completed. The bony resection is carried laterally to transect the pars at the level of the *blue line*. **C,** The inferior articular process is removed en bloc to reveal the superior articular process and pedicle. **D,** The superior articular process is removed flush to the pedicle laterally with a Kerrison rongeur to allow maximal access to the disc space. **E,** The nerve root is protected during discectomy and graft placement. **F,** A discectomy is performed.
Continued

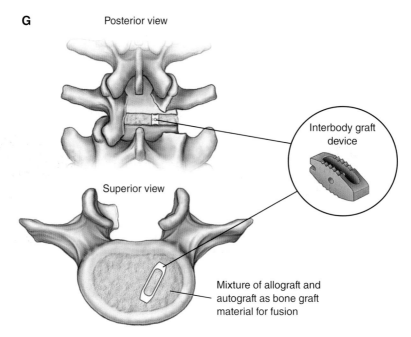

Fig. 36-2, cont'd   **G,** The vertebral body has fusion material and a cage in place.

After the endplates are appropriately shaved, angled curettes are used to scrape the upper and lower endplates to remove remaining disc and to detect potential violations of the endplates. An appropriately sized implant is selected. We place a mixture of allograft, autograft, and demineralized bone matrix into the disc space. This fusion material is tamped anteriorly to allow room for the cage. Once the disc space is adequately packed with fusion material, the interbody cage is placed. The cage is packed with the same combination of fusion material. We place the cage just below the posterior aspect of the vertebral body and use a downward-angled curette (no depth stopper) to turn the cage into its final position (Fig 36-2, *G*). Many graft options are available. We use polyetheretherketone interbodies, though the choice of interbody is the surgeon's preference. Recent literature shows that wedge-shaped interbodies tend to provide more lordosis than rectangular-shaped counterparts.[13] We use fluoroscopy to confirm appropriate disc space, depth of placement, and side of placement if attempting a more unilateral placement for correction of coronal deformity. Once the graft is placed in the final position, hemostasis is achieved using a combination of bipolar cautery, Gelfoam, and Surgiflow with gentle cottonoid compression. This procedure can be carried out at multiple levels to help with overall coronal and sagittal spinal correction.

POTENTIAL COMPLICATIONS AND MANAGEMENT

Complications from TLIF procedures can be categorized as vascular, neural, or bony.

VASCULAR

Though exceedingly rare, injury to the anterior retroperitoneal vessels is possible during discectomy and graft placement. The inferior vena cava branches at the level of L4-5 into the common iliac veins. These venous structures are at particular risk of injury given their weaker vessel walls, compared with arterial vasculature. To minimize this risk, the integrity of the anterior longitudinal ligament and annulus should be assessed on a preoperative MRI scan particularly if the disc has herniated at the level of interest. Intraoperatively during discectomy the integrity can be evaluated through gentle probing with a blunt-tip instrument such as the tip of a closed pituitary rongeur. By performing this assessment before biting with a rongeur, surgeons can prevent inadvertent violation through a defect in the annulus and injury to a vessel.

During graft placement for a TLIF, the graft should be turned once it is in the disc space before it is advanced too far anteriorly. The broad surface of the graft is less likely to breach the annulus than the narrow portion. A mallet is used to hammer the graft deeper into the space to an anterior position for optimal lordosis. During this process, sequential fluoroscopic imaging should be performed to minimize the chance of breaching the annulus.

If a vascular injury is suspected or if the graft is dislodged into the retroperitoneal space, the patient's hemodynamic stability is immediately assessed and the anesthesia team is notified. The patient may need to be emergently closed and turned over, with emergent consultation with vascular surgery personnel for a laparotomy. Overall, the risk of bowel or vascular injury from a posterior TLIF approach is less than with direct anterior retroperitoneal approaches such as ALIF or XLIF procedures.

Neural

Both the traversing nerve root and exiting nerve root are at risk during trial or graft placement, either because of excessive retraction or irritation/injury to the nerve root by the actual graft as it is inserted. Severe cases have a risk of endoneural fibrotic changes, resulting in chronic radiculopathy.[14]

Postoperatively patients can have new or worsening radicular dysesthesia or weakness. Reversible causes such as misplaced instrumentation should first be ruled out. Radiographic assessment can be performed. CT may be required to rule out breach by a pedicle screw, causing nerve root impingement. If imaging is negative and suspicion of nerve irritation was high during graft placement (that is, radiculopathy corresponding to the side and level of graft placement), patients can be given low-dose steroids or neuropathic medications such as gabapentin or trileptal.

The rate of postoperative neuralgia after PLIF has been reported to be as high as 7.1%.[15] TLIF offers the advantage of a more lateral approach to the disc space through complete resection of the superior articular process, thereby minimizing retraction on the traversing nerve root and thecal sac.

Bony/Structural

The endplates require thorough preparation to ensure that cartilaginous and disc material are removed to prevent soft tissue impedance of fusion. However, endplates should not be violated, because this can increase the risk of subsidence, pseudarthrosis, and graft migration. Shavers should be used carefully and overdistraction avoided during graft placement. The advent of polymer cage materials such as polyetheretherketone has decreased the risk of endplate violation and subsidence.[14] Unlike early titanium cages, these have a modulus of elasticity comparable to that of bone.

The overall rate of pseudarthrosis in deformity surgery involving combined TLIF and posterior instrumentation was 17% in one series.[10] Failure of fusion at the TLIF level may require extension of the posterior construct (that is, extension of a failed L5-S1 TLIF to the ilium). Revision arthrodesis of the actual disc space can be difficult to perform from a posterior approach. In these cases an anterior retroperitoneal approach may be needed to remove the failed graft and to place a new, larger ALIF graft. This can allow greater arthrodesis and lordotic correction given the larger ALIF graft footprint and the ability to ensure anterior placement.

PATIENT EXAMPLES

This 61-year-old woman presented with chronic, severe low back pain and radiating right leg pain. Conservative management was unsuccessful. She had a history of a lumbar laminectomy (Fig. 36-3, *A* through *C*). She underwent lumbar laminectomies and Ponte osteotomies from L2-S1. We also performed L2-iliac posterior spinal fixation with L5-S1 TLIF. Anterior placement of graft enhanced the lordosis. Her preoperative lumbar lordosis was 18 degrees. Postoperatively her lumbar lordosis is 53 degrees, and her coronal deformity is corrected (Fig. 36-3, *D* through *F*).

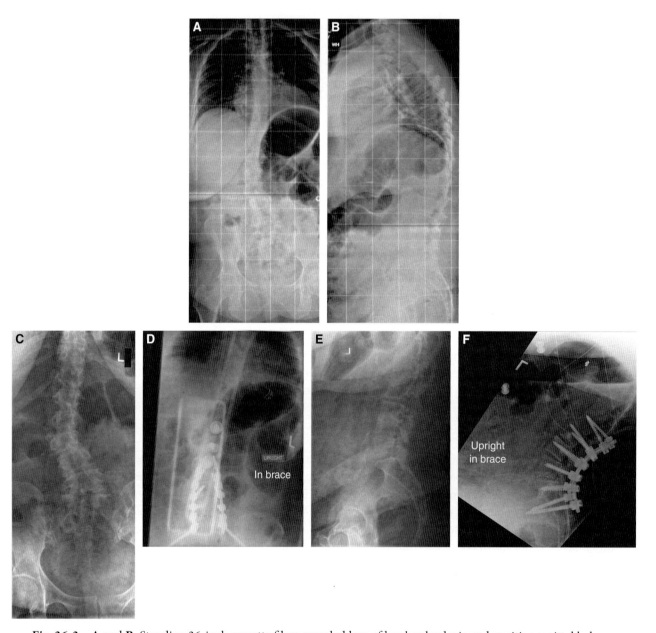

Fig. 36-3   **A** and **B,** Standing 36-inch cassette films revealed loss of lumbar lordosis and positive sagittal balance (sagittal vertical axis 9 cm). The patient had dextroscoliosis, a pelvic incidence of 59 degrees, thoracic kyposis of 31 degrees, and lumbar lordosis of 18 degrees. Inadequate lumbar lordosis results in a mismatch with the other parameters. Ideal lumbar lordosis should be approximately 45 degrees. **C-F,** Preoperative and postoperative lumbar upright radiographs.

This 65-year-old woman presented with severe low back pain and radiating lower extremity pain that was greater on the left side (Fig. 36-4, *A* and *B*). Conservative therapy, including epidural steroid injections and physical therapy, was unsuccessful. She reported that foot dragging caused falls. She underwent L1-5 Ponte osteotomies with laminectomies and foraminotomies, followed by left-sided L4-5 TLIF and T11-iliac posterior spinal fixation. She is shown preoperatively and postoperatively on lumbar upright radiographs (Fig. 36-4, *C* through *F*). The left-sided placement of a TLIF graft at L4-5 assisted in reducing the coronal deformity.

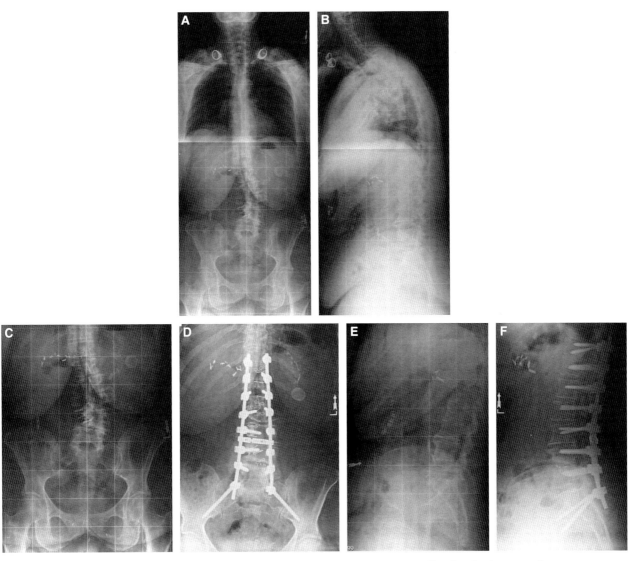

Fig. 36-4 **A** and **B,** Preoperative standing 36-inch films demonstrated loss of lumbar lordosis, resulting in a significant sagittal vertical axis of 8 cm. An AP film revealed a levoscoliotic curve with a Cobb angle of 28 degrees. **C-F,** Preoperative and postoperative lumbar upright radiographs.

This 40-year-old man presented with a remote history of a motor vehicle collision with chronic, worsening mechanical axial back pain. Preoperative lumbar CT (Fig. 36-5, *A*) demonstrated grade II spondylolisthesis at L3-4 with bilateral, chronic corticated pars fractures. He had an L3-4 TLIF with decompression and reduction of the listhesis (Fig. 36-5, *B*).

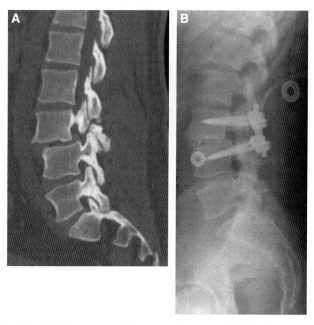

Fig. 36-5 **A,** Preoperative lumbar CT demonstrated L3-4 grade II spondylolisthesis with bilateral chronic pars fractures. **B,** Postoperative upright lumbar radiograph.

REFERENCES

1. Ould-Slimane M, Lenoir T, Dauzac C, et al. Influence of transforaminal lumbar interbody fusion procedures on spinal and pelvic parameters of sagittal balance. Eur Spine J 21:1200-1206, 2012.
2. Recnik G, Kosak R, Vengust R. Influencing segmental balance in isthmic spondylolisthesis using transforaminal lumbar interbody fusion. J Spinal Disord Tech 26:246-251, 2013.
3. Jagannathan J, Sansur CA, Oskouian RJ Jr, et al. Radiographic restoration of lumbar alignment after transforaminal lumbar interbody fusion. Neurosurgery 64:955-963; discussion 963-954, 2009.
4. Barami K, Lincoln T, Bains R. Experience with transforaminal interbody fusion in corrective surgery for adolescent idiopathic scoliosis. J Clin Neurosci 20:1256-1258, 2013.
5. Li FC, Chen QX, Chen WS, et al. Posterolateral lumbar fusion versus transforaminal lumbar interbody fusion for the treatment of degenerative lumbar scoliosis. J Clin Neurosci 20:1241-1245, 2013.
6. Hsieh PC, Koski TR, O'Shaughnessy BA, et al. Anterior lumbar interbody fusion in comparison with transforaminal lumbar interbody fusion: implications for the restoration of foraminal height, local disc angle, lumbar lordosis, and sagittal balance. J Neurosurg Spine 7:379-386, 2007.
7. Crandall DG, Revella J. Transforaminal lumbar interbody fusion versus anterior lumbar interbody fusion as an adjunct to posterior instrumented correction of degenerative lumbar scoliosis: three year clinical and radiographic outcomes. Spine 34:2126-2133, 2009.
8. Flynn JC, Price CT. Sexual complications of anterior fusion of the lumbar spine. Spine 9:489-492, 1984.
9. Tiusanen H, Seitsalo S, Osterman K, et al. Retrograde ejaculation after anterior interbody lumbar fusion. Eur Spine 4:339-342, 1995.

10. Burneikiene S, Nelson EL, Mason A, et al. Complications in patients undergoing combined transforaminal lumbar interbody fusion and posterior instrumentation with deformity correction for degenerative scoliosis and spinal stenosis. Surg Neurol Int 3:25, 2012.

11. Heller JE, Kai-Ming GF, Smith JS, et al. Adult thoracic and lumbar deformity. In Benzel EC, ed. Spine Surgery: Techniques, Complication Avoidance and Management, ed 3. Philadelphia: Elsevier, 2012.

12. Dorward IG, Lenke LG, Bridwell KH, et al. Transforaminal versus anterior lumbar interbody fusion in long deformity constructs: a matched cohort analysis. Spine. 2013 Feb 25. [Epub ahead of print]

13. Godde S, Fritsch E, Dienst M, et al. Influence of cage geometry on sagittal alignment in instrumented posterior lumbar interbody fusion. Spine 28:1693-1699, 2003.

14. Cole CD, McCall TD, Schmidt MH, et al. Comparison of low back fusion techniques: transforaminal lumbar interbody fusion (TLIF) or posterior lumbar interbody fusion (PLIF) approaches. Curr Rev Musculoskelet Med 2:118-126, 2009.

15. Krishna M, Pollock RD, Bhatia C. Incidence, etiology, classification, and management of neuralgia after posterior lumbar interbody fusion surgery in 226 patients. Spine J 8:374-379, 2008.

37

Anterior Access to the Thoracic and Lumbar Spine

Michael F. O'Brien ▪ *Randall P. Kirby*
R. Mark Hoyle ▪ *Richard Hostin*

In 1934 Ito et al[1] reported a paramedian retroperitoneal approach for treatment of Pott's disease. In 1956 Hodgson and Stock[2] were first to report drainage of a tuberculosis abscess through a transpleural approach. Hodgson and colleagues[3-5] described thoracotomy and retroperitoneal approaches for treatment of the same disease. Since then, anterior approaches to the thoracic and lumbar spine have been performed to treat spinal deformity, trauma, tumor, and infection, with good results. The proliferation and popularization of posterior and lateral approaches to the spine, with their attendant tools and specialized instrumentation, has resulted in a movement away from open anterior spinal surgery. Although posterior approaches provide powerful techniques for spinal reconstruction, posterior-only techniques cannot solve all spinal reconstruction challenges and can only poorly treat others. Anterior approaches for releasing rigid spinal deformities and achieving maximal lordotic reconstruction of the lumbar spine are unparalleled for difficult sagittal and coronal reconstruction problems encountered in spinal deformity surgery. Most anterior lumbar exposures are quick and straightforward. However, most general and vascular surgeons have not been trained in these procedures because of the shift away from open anterior spinal surgery and consequently find them challenging. When properly performed, typical one- to three-level anterior lumbar exposures are completed in approximately 30 to 60 minutes. They are typically accomplished with little blood loss and performed through a relatively small incision with low morbidity. However, this is not an operation to be taken lightly, because major complications can occur. Injury to the inferior vena cava or iliac veins can be a life-threatening event in an elective procedure.[6] Even the best access surgeons injure these vessels. An access surgeon should be comfortable treating these problems and able to quickly perform iliac arterial thrombectomy, arterial bypass, and repair of venous injuries. The most talented orthopedic, neurosurgical, general, or vascular surgeon without experience with this procedure can suddenly find themselves confronted with a life-threatening situation. Aspiring access surgeons should at least observe several exposures by an experienced access surgeon. Texts and videos are available and can be helpful in educating surgeons, but these are not substitutes for actual participation and mentoring by an experienced access surgeon. The technique that we use is efficient, straightforward, easy to teach and learn, safe to perform on a regular basis, and requires few special tools.

OPERATIVE TECHNIQUE

Numerous skin incisions have been described in the surgical approach for anterior lumbar exposures: oblique, paramedian, midline, and transverse. We prefer to make a midline skin, fascial, and muscle incision followed by a left retroperitoneal dissection to expose the spine (Fig. 37-1, A). In a thin patient who needs only one- or two-level exposure, we may use a transverse skin incision with a midline fascial and muscle incision to approach the retroperitoneal space. We do not approach the retroperitoneal space lateral to the rectus by pulling the muscle across the midline. The spine is a midline structure and can be approached from the midline, preventing considerable morbidity associated with more lateral approaches. The access surgeon starts a left retroperitoneal approach (preferred) on the right side of the patient, adjacent to the abdomen. This position is satisfactory for the access surgeon for the entire surgery, unless the deep anatomy becomes problematic. The spinal surgeon will typically be positioned on the left (ipsilateral) side of the retroperitoneal approach. If a right retroperitoneal approach is required the access surgeon will start the case standing on the left side of the patient. The steps for the deep exposure are the same as for a left retroperitoneal, only directed towards the right side. A right-sided approach would be appropriate if a left-sided approach is not possible. This position is satisfactory for the entire surgery, unless the deep anatomy becomes problematic. Rostrocaudal placement of the incision depends on the levels being exposed and the appearance of the anatomy on fluoroscopic imaging before the patient is prepared and draped. The lateral fluoroscopic radiograph can be performed to visualize the disc levels which require access. The skin incision can then be marked on the patient precisely. The vertebral level and the trajectory for approach to the spine and discs can be clearly identified with these fluoroscopic images. In general, the L5-S1 level is distal to the umbilicus and about two thirds of the way to the pubic symphysis. The interspace at L4-5 is 2 cm below the umbilicus, and the interspace at L3-4 is 2 cm above the umbilicus. The L2-3 interspace is usually 5 to 8 cm above the umbilicus. The placement and length of the incision also depend on the size and girth of the patient. In a thin patient undergoing a one-level anterior lumbar interbody fusion, exposure through a 5 cm incision is often adequate.

After the skin is incised, the anterior fascia is cut vertically in the midline with Bovie electrocautery and held up on the left side with either a Kocher or preferably a Richardson retractor (Fig. 37-1, B). A retro-rectus dissection plane is then developed, with dissection of the endoabdominal fascia off of the posterior rectus muscle. This is accomplished first with Bovie electrocautery and then with blunt hand or sponge stick dissection, proceeding as far laterally and to the left as possible. We attempt to stay in front of the inferior epigastric vessels that run vertically under the left rectus muscle. These vessels sometimes need to be mobilized bluntly laterally and/or anteriorly with the muscle. If they are injured during dissection, they can be ligated with clips. The endoabdominal fascia is then cut vertically with a scissors, in a lateral position near the anterior axillary line (Fig. 37-1, C). Blunt sponge-stick dissection achieves entry into the left retroperitoneal space. Once the space is entered, blunt hand dissection is used to further develop the space and identify the sacral promontory, ureter, and the iliac vessels (Fig. 37-1, D).

The authors prefer a Bookwalter retractor, which is then fixed to the operating table. Other retractor systems have been used successfully, including the Omni, Baulfour, and others. The Bookwalter retractor set has right-angled, nonflexible-type blades. Appropriate-length retractor blades from a Bookwalter set are positioned to hold the peritoneal sac to the right and cephalad. The retractor blades are carefully placed to protect the ureter from direct pressure. Generally they are placed anterior or superficial to the ureter to prevent a direct stretch or compression of the ureter by the retractor blades. In this position the left ureter can be visualized throughout the procedure on the right side of the surgical field, anterior to the spine and attached to the peritoneal sac. A rostral blade is placed to retract the peritoneal sac superiorly, and the ureter is protected as it traverses from the right side of the surgical field toward the left kidney. Another blade is placed on the left lateral abdominal wall. The regional anatomy is then reviewed to identify and verify the position and integrity of the major vessels, ureter, peritoneal sac, psoas, and spine. The vasculature is evaluated and dissected. The veins are bluntly dissected. This is in contrast to the sharp dissection tech-

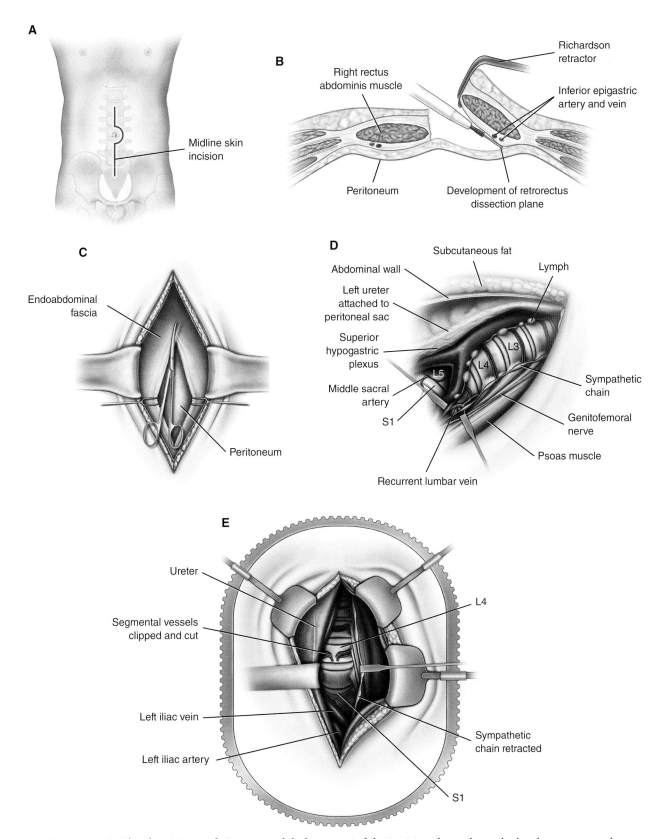

Fig. 37-1 A, The skin is incised. Rostrocaudal placement of the incision depends on the level exposure and appearance of anatomy on fluoroscopic imaging. **B,** The anterior fascia is dissected. The access surgeon begins the left retroperitoneal approach while standing on the right side of the table to facilitate the initial stages of the retroperitoneal exposure. **C,** The endoabdominal fascia is cut vertically with scissors. **D,** The retroperitoneal space is entered. **E,** The sympathetic chain is retracted.

nique advocated for mobilizing arterial structures in vascular surgery. The veins are thin-walled, tenuous structures and do not tolerate sharp dissection well.

At L5-S1, the left common iliac artery and vein are mobilized to the left of the spine, and the peritoneal sac and ureter are mobilized bluntly to the right of the spine using long Kitner sponge blunt dissectors. They are held in place with Wiley vein retractors. Standard Wiley vein retractors are usually sufficient, but occasionally specially made bayoneted, long Wiley retractors are necessary in very obese patients. The middle sacral vessels over the L5-S1 disc are identified and encircled with a right-angle clamp and doubly clipped with medium, automatically dispensed clips.

The vessels are then divided with scissors or coagulated with an Aquamantys System (Medtronic Sofamor Danek, Minneapolis, MN) and bipolar cautery. Usually, only one middle sacral artery and two veins are present, with one venous branch off of the common iliac vein coursing toward the left lateral border of the spine. If this branch is not identified and divided, it can be avulsed and cause significant blood loss. The areolar tissue over the anterior disc space is then cleaned with a Kitner sponge blunt dissector on a long clamp to expose the lateral, superior, and inferior borders of the disc.

At the L4-5 interspace, the aorta, inferior vena cava, and left iliac artery and vein are swept to the right of the spine using blunt dissection with a Kitner sponge blunt dissector and held in place with Wiley vein retractors. The sympathetic chain is held out of harm's way if possible to the left of the spine (Fig. 37-1, E).

If the sympathetic chain is injured accidently or needs to be divided to provide access to the spine, there is typically no clinical sequela. A sympathectomy typically requires at least three sympathetic ganglia to be removed from the ipsilateral chain. If a partial or complete sympathectomy results from an anterior approach to the spine, the patient may perceive that the lower extremity on the side contralateral to the side of the approach is cold, as the resultant sympathectomy vasodilation of the ipsilateral leg makes it feel warmer. This increased warmth of the ipsilateral lower extremity is often misinterpreted as a "cold right leg" and sometimes interpreted as an arterial occlusion on the contralateral side of the sympathectomy. The segmental lumbar vessels, artery and vein, traverse L4 at the midvertebral body above the L4-5 disc space. Once identified, they are encircled with a right-angle clamp and doubly clipped and cut (see Fig. 37-1, E). Ligation of the segmental vessels facilitates mobilization of the great vessels toward the right side so that they can be retracted across the midline to allow visualization of the anterior aspect of the spine.

Before retraction of the great vessels, the large iliolumbar vein is identified. This vessel arises from the left lateral side of the common iliac vein and dives deep between the psoas muscle and the lateral aspect of the spine adjacent to L5 or L4. It usually is a significant, tethering structure that resists rightward mobilization of the left common iliac vein toward the midline. Premature attempts to achieve rightward mobilization of the vessels during exposure of the L4-5 disc can avulse the iliolumbar vein. When this vessel is avulsed, it usually retracts under the psoas muscle, making access to it difficult. This side of the injury can be controlled by packing the iliolumbar vein beneath the psoas muscle. It also results in a significant posterior wall tear of the common iliac vein. The use of Floseal and Surgicel and maintaining pressure with a sponge stick for at least 3 minutes are effective in achieving at least temporary control. Definitive ligation, however, is preferred. Repair of the common iliac vein injury is required.

At L3-4 and L2-3 the aorta and inferior vena cava need to be bluntly mobilized to the right of the spine. The transverse segmental lumbar vessels, above and below the disc space, need to be double clipped and cut to facilitate mobilization of the great vessels. These vessels can be tied with suture, but this is often difficult and time consuming in this deep dissection. Once mobilized, the great vessels can be held in the appropriate position with Wiley vein retractors.

Prolonged retraction with any retractor can lead to thrombosis of the common iliac artery, necessitating thrombectomy and/or iliac artery bypass. This is of most concern at L4-5. Here, we intermittently remove the Wiley vein retractors to allow frequent flow to the vessels. This ensures blood flow to the left lower extremity and prevents arterial thrombosis. The L4-5 level is the most treacherous level with regard to potential vasculature injury. There are more venous injuries and more arterial thromboses at this level than at all the others combined.[6] Judgment and experience are essential to know how much the inferior vena cava and iliac vein can be stretched or mobilized at this level without being torn. However, even in the best of hands this occasionally occurs. If the vein is tight during the exposure, tethering structures should be suspected and located, including segmental lumbar vessels or a missed iliolumbar vessel arising from the left lateral side of the iliac vein. More than one such vessel can be present. We have seen patients with two or three iliolumbar veins in close proximity to each other at the L4-5 level. If visualization and release of the vessels are difficult while standing on the right side of the table, surgeons can move to the left side of the table. Deep exposure and mobilization of the vessels at L4-5 and superiorly can occasionally be easier from the left side of the table. The spine surgeon will typically assist the access surgeon and perform the spine surgery standing on the patient's left side. If the sympathetic chain is encroaching on the left side of the spine, where the discectomy needs to be performed, it can be mobilized by making a vertical longitudinal incision anterior (toward the midline) to the sympathetic chain in the aerolar tissue to which it is attached. The sympathetic chain then can be bluntly mobilized with a Kitner, Wiley, or nerve root retractor. At L2-3 and sometimes L3-4 the diaphragmatic crura (muscle-tendon) overlies the disc. These can be mobilized sharply with either a Bovie device or a knife or bluntly with a Cobb elevator or a cloverleaf-shaped Walley Cobb elevator. If iliac arteries at L4-5 are severely diseased, we leave the artery to the left of the spine and mobilize the vein to the right of the spine to help prevent iliac artery injuries. If an atherosclerotic vessel is retracted too far to the right, a plaque can crack, resulting in thrombosis of the vessel with partial or complete occlusion of blood supply to the left (ipsilateral) leg. In this instance we mobilize the artery sharply but not the vein. We now only do this when the artery is palpably diseased with atherosclerosis, and extensive arterial mobilization seems unwise.

When working around atherosclerotic vessels, it is important to check for a distal pulse in the left iliac artery within the surgical field. A pulse oximeter on both lower extremities is helpful to monitor right-to-left differential oxygen saturation. Surgeons should be mindful of the electrophysiologic somatosensory evoked potential signals in the lower extremity. The SSEPs are very sensitive to decreased arterial blood flow. L2-3 occasionally can be exposed through a retroperitoneal approach, but this is usually difficult because of the vascular anatomy in this area. This level can be accessed through a transperitoneal approach, with the small bowel retracted into the right upper quadrant and the left colon mobilized to the left of the spine. The ligament of Treitz is taken down, as it is for an aortic aneurysm or bypass procedure. Dissection between the aorta and vena cava is performed with ligation of the segmental lumbar vessels with double clips as they cross the spine. The mesentery is closed, as it is with placement of an aortic graft, to prevent small bowel obstruction. Exposures of the L1-2 disc space are performed by an intraperitoneal approach, with dissection and mobilization of the ligament of Treitz. The aorta is bluntly mobilized to the left and the vena cava to the right. The renal artery and vein may need sharp and blunt dissection and superior mobilization to expose the L1-2 level. Alternatively, L1-2 can be exposed through a lateral decubitus position in the retroperitoneal plane. L1 approaches are best performed with the patient placed in a lateral decubitus position. We have performed them transperitoneally with a midline abdominal incision; it is necessary to approach more distal lumbar levels during the same procedure.

Once the discs have been identified, they are quickly and efficiently removed to prepare for a lordotic reconstruction at each level. The process is simple but relies on efficient tools. A generous annulotomy is performed with a knife on a long handle. It is important to release the disc to the right and left anterolateral corners so that the disc can be lordotically distracted in preparation for the lordotic sagittal plane reconstruction. This thorough release will also facilitate realignment of the stiff fractional lumbosacral coronal deformities that often accompany adult spinal deformity. A large, double-action rongeur is used to remove the anterior annulus (Fig. 37-2, *A*). The cartilaginous endplates are then separated from the vertebral bodies with up- and down-angled cloverleaf-shaped Walley Cobb elevators. A large, double-action rongeur and long-handled straight and angled curettes are used to clean the disc space and remove the cartilaginous endplates in preparation for fusion (Fig. 37-2, *B*). It is essential to completely mobilize the disc annulus to allow correction of sagittal and coronal plane malalignment. Occasionally it is even necessary to release the right and left lateral sides of the annulus to achieve maximum mobilization. This can be done sharply under direct visualization on the ipsilateral side of the retroperitoneal approach and bluntly through the disc space on the contralateral side. The endplates are prepared for fusion. This requires disruption of the endplate centrally to create a bleeding osseous surface that is amenable to fusion. It is important to preserve the structural subchondral bone to support the intradiscal device and prevent settling of the cage. The interspace is then reconstructed with a structural lordotic cage filled with the chosen bone graft material (Fig. 37-2, *C*). Segmental instrumentation is placed to stabilize the anterior construct and prevent graft dislodgement.

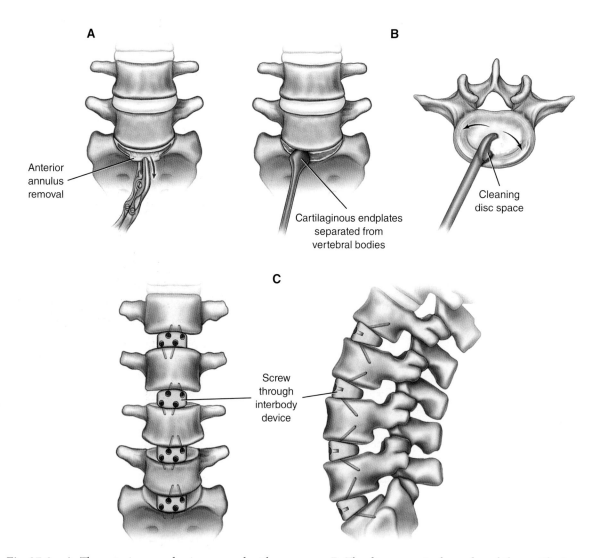

Fig. 37-2   **A,** The anterior annulus is removed with a rongeur. **B,** The disc space is cleaned, and the cartilaginous endplates are removed in preparation for fusion. **C,** The final reconstruction with the graft in place. The cage should be stabilized with instrumentation to prevent dislodgement while performing the posterior procedure with the screws as shown above or with some other instrumentation.

Box 37-1 outlines pearls to consider when performing anterior access surgery.

BOX 37-1 Surgical Pearls

- With experience, every access surgeon develops unique strategies. With a steep L5-S1 angle, often seen in hyperlordosis, the anesthesiologist should place the patient in Trendelenburg (head down) position as tolerable to facilitate access to the disc. This technique can be helpful in patients with grade II or III spondylolisthesis with excessive lordosis. This positioning trick, in conjunction with incising the fascia to the pubic symphysis, can be helpful in achieving the angulation necessary to gain access to the L5-S1 disc. Conversely, at L3-4 and more so at L2-3, reverse Trendelenburg (head up) positioning may be useful, because the angle into the disc is opposite that at L5-S1. For typical anterior lumbar procedures, the patient is placed on the operating table in a supine position over a large, 8- to 9-inch gel roll to induce lumbar lordosis. The gel roll should be positioned rostrocaudally so that the middle of the intended operative segment is pointing straight up or perpendicular to the table, as visualized on cross-table lateral fluoroscopy.
- We use a standard supine midline anterior retroperitoneal approach for vertebrectomies of L3, L4, and L5. A lateral decubitus approach is used for vertebrectomies of L1 and above. L2 vertebrectomies are best performed through either a lateral decubitus or transperitoneally from an anterior approach.
- Small holes in the peritoneum are closed with 3-0 Vicryl suture on an SH needle if they are easily accessible. If they are hard to repair or if multiple rents occur, we usually make the rents bigger, connect them, and leave them open. After intraperitoneal exposures, small bowel obstructions may occur if the mesentary is not repaired or if the closure dehisces postoperatively.
- A postoperative pain pump such as an On-Q (I-Flow, Irvine, CA) is useful. We place the catheter or catheters directly on top of the closed fascia and give 0.5% Marcaine for pain control at a rate of 4 to 5 ml per hour.
- If a vein is injured during the case but can be controlled with Wiley or Kitner retractors, the spine surgery should be completed before definitive repair is attempted. Any attempt to repair it first can disrupt the repair, worsening the injury and causing excessive bleeding. This may require that the spinal procedure be aborted. If bleeding cannot be controlled, repair takes precedence. If there is any doubt about ongoing hemorrhage, a transperitoneal approach may be necessary to expose the vena cava and iliac vessels proximally and distally to control bleeding. For uncontrolled hemorrhage, ligation of the left common iliac vein may be necessary.
- At L5-S1, fat from below the sacral promontory will obstruct the spine surgeon's view. A Ray-Tec sponge placed in front of and deep to the promontory usually prevents this problem. Alternatively, placement of a medium malleable retractor anterior and distal to the sacral promontory can be useful.
- For a standard L3-S1 anterior intradiscal fusion, the L3-4 cage is placed first, because it will be difficult to place last, after distraction of the L5-S1 and L4-5 interspaces. The L3-4 disc space should not be overfilled. Re-creation of angular lordosis is more important than distraction of the disc space. The L5-S1 cage is placed second. This disc is most important in reestablishing lumbar lordosis. Access to this disc can be difficult, and maximum mobilization of this interspace is required to re-create the lordotic angulation necessary to reconstruct the sagittal plane. The L4-5 cage is placed last, because this location is easiest to visualize for access and manipulation in the surgical field
- Minor venous bleeding from the iliac vein or inferior vena cava may be controlled with Floseal and surgical packing held in place for 3 to 4 minutes. Many of the venous injuries that we previously tried to repair with suture or vascular clips can now be stopped with this method. Floseal packing is very effective, especially for smaller injuries which are the majority and which are often deep in the retroperitoneum or pelvis where it is difficult to sew or even apply clips.

POTENTIAL COMPLICATIONS AND MANAGEMENT OF ANTERIOR SPINAL EXPOSURES

During anterior approaches to the lumbar spine, most complications are vascular injuries such as holes or tears in the vena cava or iliac veins or thrombosis of the iliac arteries. It is extremely difficult to obtain circumferential proximal and distal control of these major vessels with such exposures. Small incisions, deep operative sites, and complex anatomy sometimes make repairs challenging. Partial control can be achieved with the use of a Kitner dissection sponge on a clamp, sponge sticks, and Wiley vein retractors. We prefer to clip injured veins with a medium, automatic clip device, with the clips placed as tangential to the vein as possible to prevent narrowing. It is difficult to sew these injuries in a deep operative site with restricted access for tool manipulation, especially in an obese patient. The clips usually work well, and we try not to narrow the vein by more than 5% or 10%; however, we accept up to 30% narrowing. Attempting to perform a primary suture repair or oversewing an injury may be dangerous, where the slightest torque with a needle driver can worsen the injury. Longer tears may need to be sewed. We typically use 5-0 Prolene on a C-1 needle. For venous injuries the use of Floseal and Surgicel/Gelfoam with gentle sponge-stick pressure for 3 minutes controls bleeding. We have not had to reoperate for postoperative hemorrhage when we have used this technique. Most small venous injuries should probably be treated this way, unless the vessel is easily clipped with no venous narrowing. An Aquamantys bipolar device is of great assistance in controlling nuisance hemorrhage. A small injury can become a significant injury with a slight misstep. Rarely, we have had to pack a major venous injury and convert to a transperitoneal approach to obtain proximal and distal control of the inferior vena cava. Conversion to a transperitoneal approach may be necessary to visualize and control large tears or for suture repair.

The left common iliac artery can clot, despite a surgeon's best efforts. When this occurs, 5000 units of heparin is given immediately, and circumferential control is obtained proximal and distal to the probable area of thrombosis. This typically requires proximal control on the common iliac vessel down to the external iliac artery takeoff. We use a Rommel tourniquet or latex vessel loops proximally and a doubly passed vessel loop distally. We open the common iliac artery transversely with a No. 11 blade and pass a 4 Fr Fogarty catheter proximally and distally and retrieve all clots. The transverse arteriotomy is closed with a 5-0 Prolene suture. This usually solves the problem, and an angiogram is seldom required. Within a few minutes, the patient should have a palpable pulse, if they had pulses preoperatively. It is important to verify pulses preoperatively. Spasm of lower extremity arteries can last several minutes. However, if inflow is good and no resistance to the Fogarty catheter is noted distally to the knee, arterial flow should return. If flow is questionable, an angiogram is performed through the external iliac artery. Occasionally, a Fogarty catheter cannot be passed beyond the groin, and a femoral cutdown is necessary to remove a clot and pass the catheter distally. If a cracked plaque is the cause of thrombosis, it may be necessary to perform an endarterectomy or a short ilioiliac or iliofemoral bypass with 6 mm, ringed, polytetrafluoroethylene graft with standard vascular techniques.

The chance of venous injury is 3% to 5%, with a 1% transfusion rate and a 1% incident of deep venous thrombosis (DVT) postoperatively. Most DVTs manifest clinically as unilateral left leg swelling. Patients with significant venous injuries can benefit from postoperative DVT prophylaxis with Lovenox (30 mg every 12 hours) for the length of hospitalization. In 2013 over 500 spinal exposures were performed, and five patients (1%) developed a postoperative DVT. All of these patients sustained a venous injury during the anterior approach. If a patient develops leg swelling postoperatively, an ultrasound is warranted to rule out DVT. If the ultrasound results are negative, a CT-venogram or MRA of the iliac veins should be performed, because ultrasonography cannot be used to evaluate the vasculature above the inguinal ligament and a thrombus could be present and undetected in the iliac vein or vena cava.

Some patients develop small hematomas (2 to 4 cm) around the spine postoperatively. These are typically not symptomatic and should not be treated. Large postoperative hematomas (9 cm or larger on CT) that are palpable and symptomatic, causing pain, may require evacuation. Generally, the cause of hemorrhage that resulted in the hematoma has stopped bleeding and is not identifiable by the time the hematoma is evacuated. Some large hematomas that are asymptomatic and not tender but are palpable can be observed and treated nonoperatively. This is typically successful. Occasionally, with multilevel exposures that are "wet," we place a 19 Fr round Blake drain. This is rarely needed.

Hemostatic agents such as Surgicel or Gelfoam that are placed in the operative site or bone graft that is placed in front of the cages will look like an abscess on postoperative CT. We have never seen an abscess in the early postoperative period (up to 3 months) after an anterior lumbar exposure. We have argued this point with many radiologists who have made this diagnosis based on CT results in the early postoperative period. To our knowledge, none of our patients has developed a postoperative abscess after this procedure.

Ureteral injuries are a rare complication.[6] Injuries can occur intraoperatively from lacerations with a knife, a Bovie device, or from instruments used in the discectomy. These result in the immediate appearance of urine in the wound. We have never encountered a primary ureteral injury in our patients during an anterior approach to the spine. Alternatively, ischemic injuries may result from traction on a tethered ureter or from extended periods of direct pressure. This may result in delayed necrosis and an incompetent ureter. This will likely manifest as a urinoma 1 to 2 weeks postoperatively. A ureteral stricture can manifest as hydronephrosis from restricted drainage of the kidney on the ipsilateral side of the approach. If a particularly difficult anterior spinal approach is anticipated, ureteral stents can be placed preoperatively to help identify the ureter in the surgical field, however no data exists to substantiate that this will prevent ureteral injuries during anterior spinal approaches. Alternatively, a contralateral retroperitoneal approach or a transperitoneal approach may also be performed, avoiding the laterally placed ureters if stents are not used. Injuries to the ureter require the assistance of a surgical urologist for repair. Delayed ureteral injuries require urological consult with an attempt to stent the ureter with a retrograde cystourethrogram or through a nephrostomy tube with ureteral stenting. Long-term stenting and repairs over a stent typically result in good outcomes. If stenting cannot be accomplished because of technical reasons, the ureter should be explored and repaired if possible before retroperitoneal scarring has occurred.

Retrograde ejaculation can result in sterility. *Sterility* is a lack of delivery of sufficient sperm to impregnate the female. This needs to be differentiated from *impotence,* which is failure to achieve an erection. Retrograde ejaculation is reported to occur in up to 0.42% of patients. It results from disruption or irritation of the superior hypogastric plexus, which is located on the left side of the spine and courses over the sacral promontory. These nerves regulate the internal vesicular sphincters. Failure to work synergistically results in ejaculation of sperm into the bladder rather than out of the penis, hence sterility. Within 3 to 6 months, most cases resolve. Permanent cases of retrograde ejaculation are rare. This injury results less commonly from mechanical disruption of the superior hypogastric plexus with surgical dissection than from thermal injury caused by the use of a monopolar cautery, that is, Bovie electrocautery. Blunt dissection or bipolar cautery should only be used for this part of the dissection, especially in reproductive-age males. Impotence can result from injury to the inferior hypogastric plexus. These nerves, however, are found well below the sacral promontory and are not usually in the surgical field for anterior lumbar approaches. Impotence after anterior spinal surgery is reported but is probably not a direct result of the surgical procedure. Impotence is reported in approximately 0.44% of cases and is typically short lived. It generally resolves with time and therapy.[6,7]

Small bowel injuries are rare and can result from difficult intraperitoneal exposures, revision exposures, or small unrecognized injuries to the peritoneal sac during a retroperitoneal dissection. These can be serious injuries, because the diagnosis is usually only made definitively at reoperation, at which time patients may be very sick.

Several days of postoperative ileus is common. Most patients are given clear liquid diets in the immediate postoperative period in anticipation of this problem. Prolonged ileus is treated with Reglan, MiraLax, and mineral oil or milk of magnesia by mouth. Nasogastric tube suction is reserved for patients in whom unresolved ileus causes vomiting.

ALTERNATIVE EXPOSURE CONSIDERATIONS

EXPOSURE FOR REVISION SURGERY

Revision anterior access procedures can be very challenging. We always attempt a retroperitoneal approach. However, many revision anterior lumbar spine exposures will require conversion to a transperitoneal approach. The retroperitoneum is usually scarred and vessels can more easily be controlled proximally and distally with a transperitoneal approach. We typically do not perform transperitoneal approaches for primary procedures, because the incidence of small bowel obstruction and postoperative ileus is higher. An exception might be isolated approaches to L5-S1. If a revision approach is performed, we may attempt a right retroperitoneal exposure and convert to transperitoneal exposure as necessary. With revision access at the same level as the primary procedure, the vessels are adhered to the adjacent anatomy and usually have to be mobilized with sharp dissection using a No. 15 blade. Once we enter the plane below the vessels, we find that a down-cutting Epstein curette is helpful to push the vessels off the disc space. The curette cuts downward against the disc but is blunt against the vessels. Surgeons should anticipate injuries to the veins with revision exposures. We do not hesitate to gain proximal and distal control of the vessels if necessary before final exposure of the spine. We sometimes approach a revision surgery at L2-3, L3-4, or L4-5 laterally with the patient in a lateral decubitus position with the left side up. This allows a retroperitoneal approach to the spine, which is accessed laterally under or posterior to the great vessels and obviates the need to manipulate or move the great vessels. To approach the disc, the psoas muscle needs to be mobilized off the lateral aspect of the spine. We prefer this approach for patients who have infected cages and/ or infected vertebral bodies. Revision surgery at L5-S1 is anterior through a transperitoneal approach. This is very straightforward and a very useful approach for this level. Placement of temporary ureteral stents before revision access procedures can help to identify the ureter in the surgical field.

THORACIC EXPOSURE

An anterior approach to the thoracolumbar junction and the thoracic spine up to approximately T5 involves a standard left-side-up lateral decubitus thoracotomy.[8-10] Fluoroscopy should be used to determine the exact location of the skin incision. The incision follows the rib that is immediately lateral to the area of surgical interest, as projected on a standing AP radiograph. If the ability to access the surgical site from this level is questionable, the incision is made one or perhaps two ribs more proximally. It is always easier to work more distally in a thoracotomy than more proximally through the same incision. If bone graft is necessary, a rib can be removed as part of the approach. Alternatively, the chest wall can be entered between the ribs, thus preventing some of the postoperative morbidity and pain often associated with standard thoracotomy. These approaches are much easier than anterior lumbar approaches in that minimal if any vascular mobilization is required. In addition, little soft tissue is retracted or mobilized other than the lung. If a double-lumen endotracheal tube is placed, the ipsilateral lung can be deflated during the procedure. This provides excellent visualization of the lateral aspect of the thoracic spine. The segmental vessels can either be preserved and worked around or sacrificed as needed. Much discussion has taken place in the last two decades regarding preservation of the segmental vessels to protect the occasionally tenuous blood supply to the spinal cord. Simple discectomies do not require that the vessels be sacrificed. Vertebrectomies and procedures requiring anterior thoracic instrumentation will likely require ligation of the segmental vessels. The aorta requires minimal mobilization from a lateral approach.

Discectomies usually do not require rib resection. However, removal of the rib head allows maximal access to the lateral disc and annulus and increases mobilization of the segment through removal of the tethering fibers of the costovertebral joint.[11] Vertebrectomies are facilitated by medial rib and rib head removal.

Rarely, thoracotomy incisions need to proceed past the anterior axillary line. The incision is more lateral and posterior. T4 to T11-12 exposures are fairly straightforward from a left-sided approach. We typically do not take the diaphragm down unless we have to go below the T11-12 disc. In this case, the diaphragm can be elevated but not completely detached, leaving little to suture back in place. Typically, if the twelfth rib is removed, the pleural space does not need to be entered. However, if the eleventh rib is removed, the pleural space will be entered.

CONCLUSION

Anterior spinal exposures are, in general, poorly understood and poorly performed by most surgeons who have no exposure experience. The spine can be exposed safely and quickly through small incisions and with acceptable morbidity when regional anatomy is defined in a stepwise fashion and when the techniques required to identify and mobilize the important anatomy are acquired.

REFERENCES

1. Ito H, Tsuchiya J, Asami G. A new radical operation for Pott's disease. J Bone Joint Surg 16:499-515, 1934.
2. Hodgson AR, Stock FE. Anterior spinal fusion: a preliminary communication on the radical treatment of Pott's disease and Pott's paraplegia. Br J Surg 44:266-275, 1956.
3. Hodgson A, Stock F. Anterior spinal fusion for the treatment of tuberculosis of the spine, the operative findings and results of treatment in the first one hundred cases. J Bone Joint Surg Am 42:295-310, 1960.
4. Hodgson AR. Correction of fixed spinal curves. J Bone Joint Surg Am 47:1221-1227, 1965.
5. Hodgson AR, Wong SK. A description of a technique and evaluation of results in anterior spinal fusion for deranged intervertebral disk and spondylolisthesis. Clin Orthop Relat Res 56:133-161, 1968.
6. O'Brien M, Jones A. Complications of anterior spine surgery. In Lenke L, Betz R, Harms J, eds. Modern Anterior Scoliosis Surgery. St Louis: Quality Medical Publishing, 2004.
7. O'Brien M. Nervous system. In DeWald RL, Arlet V, Carl AL, et al, eds. Spinal Deformities: The Comprehensive Text. New York: Thieme Medical Publishing, 2003.
8. O'Brien M. Cervical spine and cervicothoracic junction. In Bauer R, Kerschbaumer F, Poisel S, eds. Operative Approaches in Orthopedic Surgery and Traumatology. New York: Thieme Medical Publishing, 1987.
9. Bauer R, Kerschbaumer F, Poisel S, et al. Approaches. In Bauer R, Kerschbaumer B, Poisel S, eds. Atlas of Spinal Operations. New York: Thieme Medical Publishing, 1993.
10. Bauer R. Kyphosis. In Bauer R, Kerschbaumer F, Poisel S, eds. Atlas of Spinal Operations. New York: Thieme Medical Publishing, 1993.
11. O'Brien M. Surgical anatomy of the thoracic spine. In DeWald RL, Arlet V, Carl AL, et al, eds. Spinal Deformities: The Comprehensive Text. New York: Thieme Medical Publishing, 2003.

38

Anterior Interbody Techniques
for Restoration of Spinal Alignment

David M. Benglis, Jr. ▪ *Laura Ellen Prado* ▪ *Regis W. Haid, Jr.*

Anterior lumbar interbody fusion (ALIF) is an important tool in a spine surgeon's armamentarium for the treatment of degenerative joint disease, multiplanar deformity such as spondylolisthesis, postsurgical spinal instability, failed posterior fusion, infection, tumor, and trauma. Advantages of this approach are numerous. They include access to the anterior and middle columns of the lumbar spine for realignment of spinal balance, reestablishment of lordosis, restoration of disc space height, and indirect foraminal decompression. This approach can help to prevent direct nerve retraction and muscle dissection from posterior procedures. ALIF provides an ideal environment for placement of a large lordotic graft, with higher rates of fusion.[1] After sectioning of the anterior longitudinal ligament, lateral annular release, and sequential distraction, ALIF is superior for correction and improvement of lumbar lordosis and restoration of sagittal balance.

HISTORY

Muller[2] was first to describe traditional open anterior abdominal approaches to the spine for the treatment of Pott's disease. Over the course of the twentieth century, open, stand-alone ALIF was established as treatment for a wide variety of spinal degenerative disorders.[3] Early reports of success and morbidity were widely variable, and ALIF was not yet established as a safe and effective supplement or alternative to posterior approaches. Low fusion rates were reported with stand-alone femoral ring allografts.[4] Barnes et al[5] reported significantly lower fusion rates in patients receiving stand-alone ALIF with threaded cortical bone dowels versus PLIF with instrumentation. Some groups began to advocate front-back procedures to support the ventral constructs, notably with allograft as the fusion matrix.[6] Other materials and biologics were eventually developed such as the Ray (Stryker, Kalamazoo, MI), BAK (Bagby and Kuslich; Spine-Tech, Inc., Minneapolis, MN), Inter Fix (Medtronic Sofamor Danek, Minneapolis, MN), and SR (Synthes, West Chester, PA) threaded titanium cages, polyetheretherketone (PEEK) interbody devices and PEEK devices with stand-alone screws, and hyperlordotic implants.

LAPAROSCOPIC VERSUS MINI-OPEN ANTERIOR LUMBAR INTERBODY FUSION

Laparoscopic ALIF became popular, along with minimally invasive posterior spine techniques, in the mid to late 1990s.[7,8] Surgeons learned to work in smaller corridors, and technological advancements in the surgical instruments, retractor systems, lighting, and spinal implants employed in these confined spaces opened a new field. Laparoscopic ALIF resulted in a reduction in morbidity, compared with early traditional open approaches. Mayer[9] described the mini-open ALIF approach as an alternative to the laparoscopic technique (Fig. 38-1).

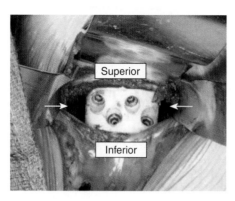

Fig. 38-1 A hyperlordotic (30 degrees, 10 by 28 by 38 mm) ALIF polyetheretherketone graft (NuVasive, San Diego, CA) is placed at L5-S1 through a mini-open incision, demonstrating lateral annulus release *(white arrows)*.

Kaiser et al[7] reported on a study of patients who had laparoscopic ALIF versus those who had a mini-open procedure. Patients in the mini-open group had lower incidences of retrograde ejaculation, less need for technically demanding instruments, and reduced operative times. Patients with laparoscopic ALIF, however, had a slightly reduced hospital stay and morbidity. (Most extended stays were for transient ileus.) Chung et al[10] found no statistical difference in perioperative or postoperative parameters up to 2 years postoperatively between laparoscopic ALIF and mini-open procedures. The introduction of laparoscopic instrumentation led to the development of the mini-open approach through the modification of retractors, implants, and biologics.

SAGITTAL BALANCE AND ASSESSMENT OF SPINOPELVIC ALIGNMENT

Schwab et al,[11] Lafage et al,[12,13] Dubousset,[14] and others have stressed the importance of spinal balance in obtaining good outcomes. Spinopelvic malalignment has been reported to increase pain and disability as the plumb line shifts anteriorly.[15] The threshold values for severe disability include an ODI higher than 40, pelvic tilt of 22 degrees or more, sagittal vertical axis of 47 mm or more, and pelvic incidence–lumbar lordosis mismatch of at least 11 degrees.[15] These measurements should be considered in both short- and long-segment spinal constructs. Sagittal vertical axis or sagittal balance is measured as the distance from the posterosuperior corner of the sacrum to a vertical line dropped from the center of C7 (Fig. 38-2).

The sagittal vertical axis can be assessed on standing lateral 36-inch vertical plain films. Balance is negative when the plumb line falls behind the sacrum, and it is positive when the line is in front of the sacrum. *Radiographic sagittal imbalance* is defined as a value larger than 5 cm. As a person ages, however, a positive sagittal balance is normal. For example, a normal sagittal vertical axis in an 80-year-old might be +6 to 8 cm. In patients with severe kyphosis, it may be important not to overcorrect, notably in elderly patients.

Lumbar lordosis and pelvic alignment contribute to the sagittal vertical axis. The average lumbar lordosis angle in normal adults, measured from L1 to L5, ranged from 40 to 60 degrees.[16] The greatest amount occurred at L4-S1 (approximately 50 degrees, 80% of lordosis in the lumbar spine), 60% of which was present at L5-S1[16] (Fig. 38-3; Box 38-1).

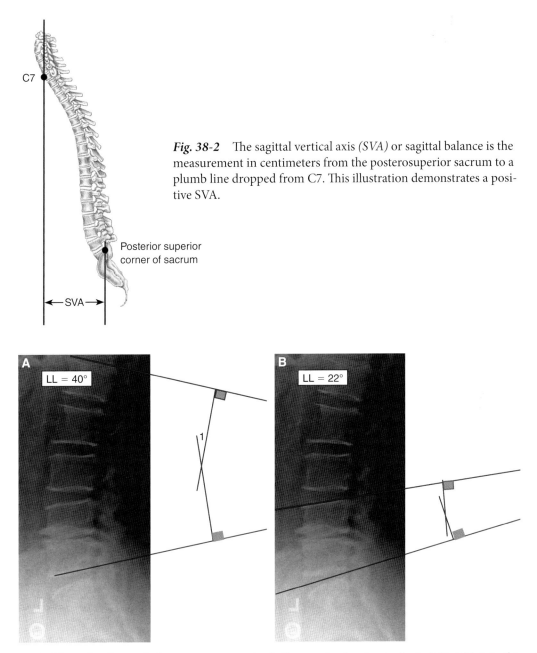

Fig. 38-2 The sagittal vertical axis *(SVA)* or sagittal balance is the measurement in centimeters from the posterosuperior sacrum to a plumb line dropped from C7. This illustration demonstrates a positive SVA.

Fig. 38-3 **A,** A lateral radiograph demonstrates a method of measuring lumbar lordosis *(LL)* at L1-5. In this patient, LL or *(1)* is 40 degrees. A normal, average LL is 40 to 60 degrees. **B,** A lateral radiograph shows a method of measuring LL at L4-S1. LL = 22 degrees. A normal, average LL is approximately 50 degrees at L4-S1.

BOX 38-1 Average Lumbar Lordosis

- Average, normal lumbar lordosis is 61 degrees.
- Average, normal L4-5 lordosis is 16.8 degrees.
- Average, normal L5-S1 lordosis is 32.4 degrees.

From Troyanovich SJ, Cailliet R, Janik TJ, et al. Radiographic mensuration characteristics of the sagittal lumbar spine from a normal population with a method to synthesize prior studies of lordosis. J Spinal Disord 10:380-386, 1997.
Eighty percent of lordosis occurs at L4-5 and L5-S1.

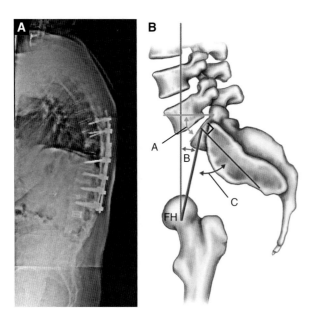

Fig. 38-4 **A,** A lateral radiograph of a patient in whom foundational lordosis was not achieved and subsequent surgeries resulted in further spinal sagittal imbalance. **B,** Measurements of pelvic alignment include sacral slope *(A)*, pelvic tilt *(B)*, and pelvic incidence *(C)*. *(FH,* Femoral head.)

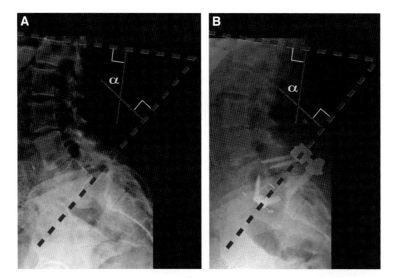

Fig. 38-5 **A,** This preoperative standing lateral lumbar radiograph revealed spondylolisthesis at L5-S1. Pelvic tilt was 25 degrees, pelvic incidence was 64 degrees, and lumbar lordosis *(α)* was 48 degrees. **B,** Anterior lumbar interbody fusion with posterior instrumentation was performed. A postoperative standing lateral lumbar radiograph demonstrates a pelvic tilt of 19 degrees, pelvic incidence of 67 degrees, and lumbar lordosis of 63 degrees. In both images, the patient's sagittal vertical axis is less than 5 cm.

Foundational lordosis should be established in the lower lumbar spine. Fig. 38-4, *A,* is an example of a patient with prior lower lumbar operations that did not achieve foundational lordosis. Worsening spinal sagittal balance developed after subsequent operations in the thoracic region. Common measurements of pelvic alignment include sacral slope, pelvic tilt, and pelvic incidence[17] (Fig. 38-4, *B*).

Pelvic incidence is defined as the angle formed by a perpendicular line extending downward from the center of the S1 endplate and a line from the center of the sacral endplate to the center of the femoral head. This value is generally fixed after puberty.[17] Lumbar lordosis should be matched to pelvic incidence. **The most common error in surgical correction is too little lumbar lordosis.** *Pelvic tilt* is a compensatory parameter. It is defined by the angle subtended from a line drawn to the center of the femoral head from the midpoint of the sacral endplate and a plumb line drawn upward from the center of the femoral head. *Sacral slope* is an angle derived from a horizontal line parallel to the endplate of S1 and a horizontal reference line drawn from the anterior corner of the S1 endplate. Pelvic incidence is the sum of pelvic tilt and sacral slope.

A patient can compensate for decreased lumbar lordosis and maintain the sagittal vertical axis by retroverting the pelvis or increasing pelvic tilt. This action requires high energy during walking and forces the hips into external rotation, while the knees internally rotate as a compensatory mechanism.[16]

In our practice, we obtain postoperative scoliosis standing 36-inch films, which we compare with preoperative standing 36-inch films. After a fusion procedure, we tend to strive for a sagittal vertical axis of less than 5 cm and a pelvic tilt smaller than 20 degrees. *Lumbar lordosis and pelvic incidence should be within 10 degrees of each other on postoperative standing scoliosis films.* The pelvic incidence calculated preoperatively can help to predict what a patient's lordosis should be postoperatively and plays a role in the planning[17] (Fig. 38-5). Lumbar lordosis can be reestablished with patient positioning (on a Jackson table [Mizuho OSI, Union City, CA] with hips extended), interbody grafts, and facetectomy/osteotomies with posterior compression.

ADVANTAGES AND DISADVANTAGES

One of the greatest advantages of ALIF is the restoration of sagittal alignment through correction of lordosis (Box 38-2). To achieve spinal balance, L5-S1 lordosis is essential. It is literally the foundation of all the spine levels located above it. Eighty percent of a patient's lumbar lordosis is at the L4-5 and L5-S1 segments, with most at L5-S1. Lordotic correction is achieved by sectioning and release of the anterior longitudinal ligament, direct distraction, placement of lordotic/hyperlordotic cages, and the application of large-surface-area implants, which have greater load-sharing capabilities than transforaminal lumbar interbody fusion (TLIF) and posterior lumbar interbody fusion (PLIF). Bone morphogenic protein (BMP) can be employed in an on-label fashion for an increased fusion rate. Another advantage of ALIF is that it can reduce spondylolisthesis. L5-S1 is the foundation of the spine.

BOX 38-2   Advantages and Disadvantages of Anterior Lumbar Interbody Fusion

---

Advantages
- Better restoration of lordosis
  - Release of the anterior longitudinal ligament
  - Direct distraction
  - The placement of lordotic/hyperlordotic cages
  - The placement of larger implants
- A larger surface area for fusion
- Compression of the graft
- An increased rate of fusion (compared with posterior lateral fusion with pedicle screws, with or without interbody graft)
- Less risk of neurologic injury, cerebrospinal leakage
- A lower deep infection rate

Disadvantages
- Possible requirement of an access surgeon
- Retrograde ejaculation is 2% to 10%
- The potential for vascular and visceral complications
- Difficulty in patients with prior intraperitoneal surgery

Disadvantages of the approach include the potential requirement of a vascular surgeon, retrograde ejaculation (2% to 10%), the development of ileus or vascular and visceral complications, and the technical difficulty in patients with prior intraperitoneal surgery.[1]

ANTERIOR LUMBAR INTERBODY FUSION VERSUS OTHER FUSION METHODS

Multiple studies have compared ALIF and its ability to restore lordosis with other fusion techniques. Watkins et al[19] reported a significant average increase in lordosis per level after ALIF (4.5 degrees) versus TLIF (0.8 degrees). Hsieh et al[20] conducted a retrospective study on 32 patients having ALIF and 25 having TLIF (a ventrally placed cage with a unilateral facetectomy and compression); most of the levels treated were at L4-S1. ALIF resulted in a 6.2-degree increase in lordosis and an 18.5% increase in foraminal height, whereas TLIF led to a 2.1-degree decrease in lordosis and a −0.4% change in foraminal height. Later correspondence (2014) revealed an average increase in lordosis and local correction of 5.7 degrees when bilateral Smith-Petersen osteotomies were performed. Kim et al[21] compared 48 patients having mini-open ALIF with 46 patients having mini-TLIF with tubular retractors. They noted that segmental lordosis increased by an average of 8.6 degrees in the ALIF group versus 2.5 degrees in the TLIF group. Dorward et al[22] observed similar findings in a comparison of ALIF and TLIF for establishing additional lordosis in long-segment scoliosis constructs (L4-5 lordosis was increased by 5.6 degrees after ALIF and by −1.7 degrees after TLIF; L5-S1 lordosis increased by 2.5 degrees with ALIF versus −1.4 degrees with TLIF).

Dimar et al[23] conducted a retrospective review of 88 patients (n = 22 in each group) and evaluated four techniques for spinal fusion: instrumented posterolateral fusion, transforaminal lumbar interbody fusion, anterior posterior fusion with posterior instrumentation, and anterior interbody fusion with lumbar tapered (LT) cages (Medtronic Sofamor Danek, Minneapolis, MN). All preoperative radiographic parameters were similar. Following are some of the authors' comments. The LT cage was best for lordosis. The PEEK spacer blocked the ability to compress and increase lordosis posteriorly. No osteotomies were performed with TLIF. They noted no placement of TLIF spacers. The technique, size, and placement of an interbody graft have a major impact on the ability to restore lordosis. The authors found that instrumented posterolateral fusion produced an actual loss of lordosis. The maintenance of lordosis and disc space height was significantly better with stand-alone ALIF with LT cages, compared with all other fusion methods. Despite the placement of 8-degree or 12-degree ramped PEEK cages, anterior-posterior fusion did not result in superior lordotic measurements, compared with TLIF. The authors proposed that the position and size of the cages blocked compression in the posterior part of the disc once the pedicle screws were placed. Lateral approaches provided good coronal correction but less satisfactory sagittal correction than ALIF.

Fusion rates are high for ALIF and subsidence is low because of the large area for fusion available after decortication and osteotome use centrally and because of the structural support provided by a rigid apophyseal ring (that is, a structural foundation at the periphery of the interspace) (Fig. 38-6). Grafts should be

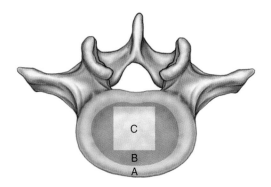

Fig. 38-6   Three critically important regional areas to know for an ALIF: the zone of periphery/apophyseal ring for structural support *(A)*, the decortication zone for fusion *(B)*, and the central zone also known for fusion, where cancellous bone is exposed with an osteotome *(C)*. The central portion of the disc space is the portion for fusion.

sized to cover these three critically important areas. Zdeblick[24] demonstrated higher fusion rates and shorter return to work times in a prospective randomized series comparing ALIF with posterolateral fusion with pedicle screws with and without interbody graft. Reported rates of fusion with ALIF are variable. Burkus et al[25] reported on the impact of BMP on fusion rates in ALIF with bone dowels. They noted no pseudarthroses in the ALIF group with BMP, whereas 20% of patients in whom an autograft was used did not fuse. Fusion rates vary with the type of interbody used (titanium, PEEK, and allograft; see Cage Morphology and Assessment of Fusion). ALIF has a decreased risk of neurologic injury (because the nerves are not directly retracted, lower incidences of CSF leakage, and a trend toward lower incidences of deep infections (for anterior stand-alone procedures) requiring revision operations.[1,26-29]

PREOPERATIVE PLANNING

IMAGING

Preoperatively we obtain standing scoliosis 36-inch upright films, dynamic flexion-extension views, MRI, and sometimes CT of the lumbar region. Surgical planning is influenced by the desired spinopelvic alignment measurements described previously. DXA scans reveal osteoporosis or osteopenia. We usually refer these patients to an osteoporosis specialist before we proceed (see The Link Between Biologics and Fusion).

VASCULAR CONSULTATION

A vascular surgeon is consulted on the feasibility of this approach in patients with comorbid conditions such as severe peripheral vascular disease, prior abdominal surgery, or anatomy inhibiting appropriate access to the L5-S1 interspace, for example, the angle of the pubic ischium. Preoperative imaging of vascular structures may be indicated for surgical planning in some high-risk patients. This includes MRI of the vessels and radiographs in patients with calcification. Relative contraindications include multiple prior intraabdominal surgeries. Patients are strongly advised to quit smoking before the procedure. NSAIDs should not be taken beginning 4 weeks before to at least 6 weeks after the procedure, because they can affect fusion.

OPERATIVE TECHNIQUE

The key steps of an ALIF technique are the following:
- Cleaning of the endplate; preservation of the endplate integrity
- Release of the lateral annulus
- Sequential dilation of the disc space with distractors
- Optimization of lordosis

The patient is placed in a supine position on the operating table. A small bolster is placed under the patient to accentuate lordosis. The arms are placed to the side at right angles. The table is reversed to facilitate intraoperative lateral and AP fluoroscopy. Bowel preparation the night before is not necessary. However, a nasogastric tube may be placed and removed intraoperatively, and postoperative metoclopramide (Reglan, Schwarz Pharma, Germany) given to promote gastric emptying. Blood salvage and recycling with a Cell Saver device (Haemonetics Corporation, Braintree, MA) is useful if vascular injury occurs.

In our practice we perform a mini-open ALIF procedure with the assistance of a vascular surgeon. The incision depends on the patient's anatomy, the surgical history and the presence of scars (for example, from a caesarean section), and the surgeons' preferences.

Typically, from L4-S1, the incision is below the umbilicus in a vertical or slightly oblique orientation in the midline for a transperitoneal approach, or a left paramedian incision is made for a left retroperitoneal

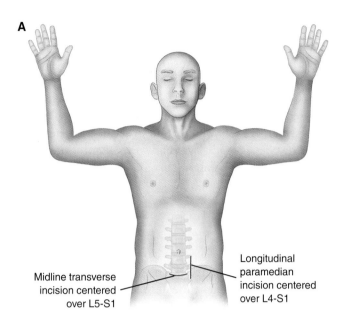

A

Midline transverse
incision centered
over L5-S1

Longitudinal
paramedian
incision centered
over L4-S1

Fig. 38-7   **A,** The patient is positioned with the arms to the side at right angles to the chest. A longitudinal paramedian left-sided incision is made below the umbilicus for a left retroperitoneal approach to include L4-S1. A midline transverse incision can be used for L5-S1.

approach (Fig. 38-7, *A*). Transperitoneal approaches are often performed for revision operations, because they introduce virgin surgical planes.

The superior hypogastric plexus is usually adherent to the peritoneum and is mobilized from left to right in a left retroperitoneal approach with blunt dissection. The surgeon should not use Bovie electrocautery (high energies) at the disc space to lower the risk of thermal injury to the plexus. During mobilization of the vascular and visceral structures at L4-5, the left iliolumbar vein is ligated. Dissection is typically more challenging at L4-5 versus L5-S1 because of the bifurcation of the great vessels. Right-sided retroperitoneal approaches are more difficult because of the location of the vena cava and should be performed only in specific cases.

The surgeon deploys a retractor that is attached to a device fixed to the operating table (Fig. 38-7, *B*). Some retractor designs are radiolucent and lighted. We prefer a rigid blade that optimizes vessel mobilization. The disc is then incised, and a Cobb instrument is moved under the superior and over the inferior endplates. Most of the disc is delivered en bloc with straight and angled pituitary instruments or a large rongeur. Disc is further cleaned off the endplates with curettes (Fig. 38-7, *C*). For collapsed discs, distractors or bullet-shaped trial instruments are placed in the lateral edges on alternating sides for further disc work and posterior osteophyte removal.

A complete anterior discectomy is critical, because it creates a large surface area for fusion, eliminates movement of distracters when they are countersunk in the depths of the disc space, provides anterior release for optimizing distraction and lordosis, prevents retropulsion of posterior disc fragments, and serves as a visualization tool to orient the surgeon to midline to facilitate optimal graft placement.[1] After visualizing the posterior longitudinal ligament, a surgeon may choose to open it for a herniated nucleus pulposus if indicated.

The central portion of the disc space is the portion for fusion (see Fig. 38-6, *B* and *C*). Decortication with curettes, osteotomes, or a drill is essential until bleeding bone is noted, because it facilitates a robust fusion (Fig. 38-7, *D*). I (senior author R.W.H.) prefer a curved osteotome at this step in the non–load-bearing central portion of the implant. After a trial deployment, an interbody device of the same size is chosen. A 2- to 3-minute waiting period is needed for the disc space to adjust to the new increase in axial length (that is, tissue hysteresis).

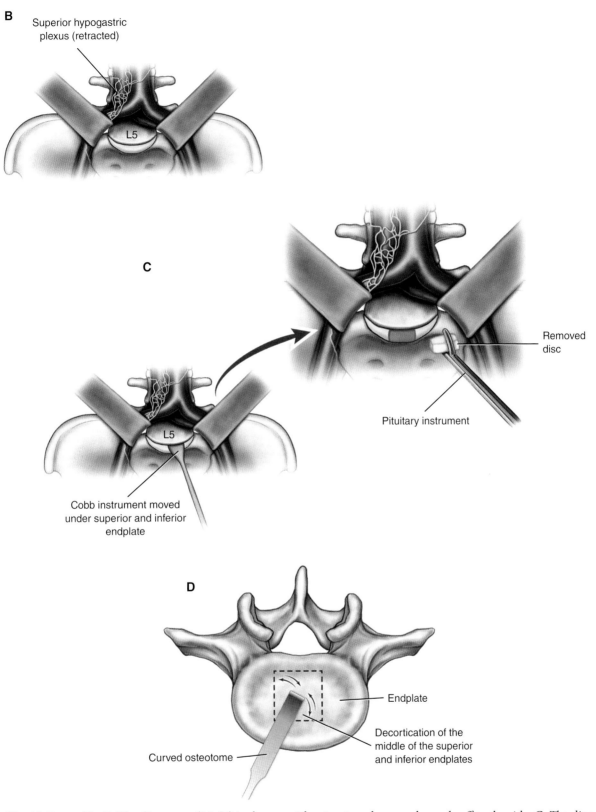

Fig. 38-7, cont'd **B,** The disc space (L5-S1) is shown, with retractors down and vessels off to the side. **C,** The disc and endplates are cleaned. The annulus is released laterally. **D,** The middle of the superior and inferior endplate is decorticated. The senior author (R.W.H.) prefers to perform this step with a curved osteotome.

Continued

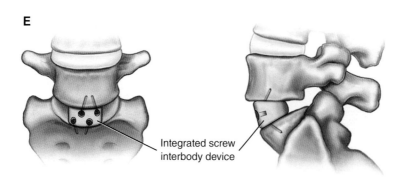

Fig. 38-7, cont'd   **E,** A screw is placed through the interbody device to secure it.

An approximate interbody height is determined preoperatively by measuring normal, nonsurgical levels on a lateral lumbar radiograph. The center of the interbody graft is filled with cancellous bone chips, demineralized bone matrix, or BMP. I (R.W.H.) prefer BMP with allograft bone chips and dust. The graft is countersunk a few millimeters. With an integrated screw interbody device, starter holes are made with an awl, and two to three screws are placed (Fig. 38-7, *E*). Lateral and AP radiographs are obtained to confirm correct positioning. The retractors are removed, and a lateral radiograph is obtained to optimize visualization. The muscle and fascia are closed in a meticulous fashion to prevent abdominal hernia development.

POSTOPERATIVE CARE

Postoperatively patients are given a liquid diet overnight. The diet is advanced in the morning as tolerated. Metoclopramide is continued for approximately 24 to 48 hours. Ileus is treated by continuing fluids and maintaining an NPO status. Rarely a nasogastric tube may be required. Postoperative deep venous thrombosis management includes heparin 5000 units subcutaneously on induction and 5000 mg subcutaneously twice daily until the patient is ambulatory, sequential compression devices, and early ambulation. Early deep venous thromboses are treated with inferior vena cava filters. Peripheral pedal pulses are monitored every 2 hours for the first 8 hours postoperatively.

POTENTIAL COMPLICATIONS AND MANAGEMENT

The incidence of retrograde ejaculation (RE) reported in the literature ranges from 2% to 10%. Sasso et al[30] demonstrated a higher incidence of RE after transperitoneal ALIF versus retroperitoneal ALIF. Kaiser et al[7] noted a 4% incidence of RE with laparoscopic ALIF. Two recent studies (one with statistical significance) revealed a higher incidence of RE in patients in whom BMP was used: 3.4% versus 1.7% without BMP (Burkus et al[31]) and 6.3% versus 0.9% without BMP (Comer et al[32]). Mobilization of the hypogastric plexus requires care, as described previously, to prevent this adverse event. BMP as a direct cause of RE has not been confirmed but only suggested in the literature. Lubelski et al[33] examined 59 patients who received BMP after ALIF and 51 who did not. They noted no difference in RE occurrence between the two groups (8% versus 8%).

A patient who has postoperative radicular pain with or without motor weakness might have a retroperitoneal hematoma, posteriorly displaced graft, or a disc fragment. An imaging study should be ordered to rule out these complications. Patients with radiculopathy from interbody distraction and nerve stretch are treated with an oral steroid taper and neuroleptic medication. This pain typically resolves over the course of weeks to months. Continued back pain in the postoperative course warrants laboratory evaluation and imaging to rule out infection or nonunion.

THE LINK BETWEEN BIOLOGICS AND FUSION

Bone healing and fusion are influenced by a variety of factors. A basic understanding of the physiology of bone repair is critical for spine surgeons, because an unsuccessful fusion results in construct failure and return of symptoms.

Bone-healing phases include early inflammation, repair, and late remodeling. Bone consists of osteogenic progenitor cells, osteoblasts (bone-creating cells), osteoclasts (bone-resorbing cells), and osteocytes (osteoblasts within bone matrix). Osteocytes secrete osteoid, which is a demineralized organic matrix of protein and collagen (30% of the weight) that combines with inorganic substances, including calcium phosphate (70% of the weight), providing strength and leading to bone formation.[34]

Bone metabolism is influenced externally by hormonal factors that include parathyroid hormone, testosterone, vitamin D, and calcitonin. Osteoblasts have parathyroid hormone receptors. This hormone keeps extracellular calcium concentrations at constant levels, whereas vitamin D stimulates absorption of calcium into the body through the gastrointestinal tract. Calcitonin acts in an opposite manner by limiting absorption of calcium in the body.[35] Low levels of testosterone have been found in 20% to 40% of older men. Patients with low-T syndrome can be considered for replacement therapy. Restoration of testosterone to normal, age-matched levels improves muscle mass, increases bone mineral density, reduces body fat, and improves libido and mood.[36]

In our practice we work closely with an osteoporosis specialist. All patients are placed on high-protein diets and protein supplements. At-risk patients can be placed on hormonal bone-stimulating medications such as teriparatide (parathyroid hormone) (Forteo, Eli Lilly, Indianapolis, IN), ideally for 2 to 6 months in the perioperative period. Ohtori et al[37] compared results in 57 patients given bisphosphonates or teriparatide after lumbar fusion. Rates of bone fusion and time to fusion were improved in the group who received teriparatide. In another study, this group of authors reported a reduction in screw loosening after fusion in patients who were given teriparatide.[38]

CAGE MORPHOLOGY AND ASSESSMENT OF FUSION

Structural grafts and cages and the substances that are placed in them for arthrodesis have physiologic properties. Osteogenesis (the ability of a graft or substance to produce new bone) is a property of iliac crest. Osteoconductivity (the ability to act as a scaffold for bone formation and vascular ingrowth) is a property of allograft and DBM. Osteoinduction (the ability to induce stem cells to change into mature bone cells) is a characteristic of BMPs.[39] Three factors to consider when choosing a specific interbody device for ALIF are the following:
- The modulus of elasticity or stiffness (The higher the modulus of elasticity, the more stiff the device.)
- The ability of a device to incorporate bony ingrowth (conductivity)
- The degree of radiolucence of a device, which allows fusion for assessment

Ideally a graft should have a high modulus of elasticity, high conductivity, and low radiolucency (Table 38-1). Burkus et al[40] described the fusion criteria for anterior lumbar interbody devices. They assessed fusion with dynamic plain radiographs and thin-cut CT scans and described different zones of bone growth (Fig. 38-8).

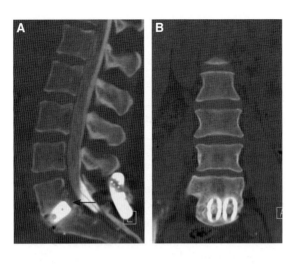

Fig. 38-8   **A** and **B,** These CT myelogram images were obtained 5 years after placement of a stand-alone LT cage and BMP at L5-S1. Relative to the position of the cage, bony ingrowth *(red arrow)* is evident laterally, posteriorly, and anteriorly.

Table 38-1   Comparison of Properties of Cage and Graft Materials

Materials	Titanium	Polyetheretherketone	Allograft
Modulus of elasticity	+++	++	+
Bony ingrowth	+++	+	++
Radiolucency	+	+++	++

Bagby and Kuslich and Lumbar Tapered Titanium Cages

The BAK design was a cylindrical cage that was first implanted in 1992. It consisted of two symmetrical titanium devices that were threaded into the endplates, with open spaces for bone graft placement.[41] Other titanium-based ALIF devices were also developed, including the Ray, Inter Fix, and Synthes SR titanium cage (Fig. 38-9). This device had a high modulus of elasticity and the ability to withstand stress forces. In a prospective study, Sasso et al[42] revealed superior fusion rates with titanium-based ALIF devices, compared with femoral ring allografts. The use of BMPs enhanced fusion rates for all devices. It also eliminated the need for iliac crest bone harvest and the associated morbidity.[43]

Older titanium cylindrical cages required significant reaming of the disc endplates (mainly posterior), which resulted in limited distraction/neuroforaminal height restoration and significant subsidence.[44] Lumbar tapered titanium cages (LT) cages allowed more physiologic distraction and symmetrical reaming for fusion; that is, they were better for correction and maintenance of lordosis. These are currently the only FDA-approved interbody devices for concurrent use with rhBMP-2 (Infuse bone graft, Medtronic Sofamor Danek, Minneapolis, MN) in spinal surgery[45] (Fig. 38-10).

Allograft

Machined allograft structural bone grafts had the advantages over older-design titanium cages of better osteoconductivity and incorporation over time, and they were easier to revise and assess for fusion.[46] Early studies were promising for their use as an alternative to lumbar tapered titanium cages, along with BMP.[47] Disadvantages of allograft devices included increased graft-host resorption, loosening, and nonunion when used with BMP, presumably during the remodeling phase of bone healing.[48,49]

Polyetheretherketone/Titanium

Radiolucent PEEK grafts have a lower modulus of elasticity than titanium and do not remodel when BMP is present, as in some femoral ring allograft implants. They can, however, form a biofilm at the PEEK-bone interface, inhibiting conductivity compared with allograft and newer, rough titanium designs[50,51] (Fig. 38-11). These biofilms can also increase rates of infection and pseudarthrosis.

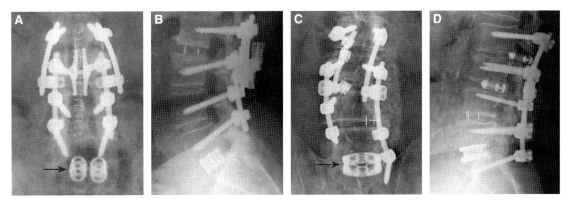

Fig. 38-9 **A** and **B,** Postoperative AP and lateral radiographs of a patient who had revision surgery with lateral L2-3 interbody and posterior instrumentation. The patient had two previous lumbar fusion procedures. The *red arrow* points to the original BAK cages at L5-S1. **C** and **D,** Postoperative AP and lateral radiographs of a patient who had revision surgery, with extension of fusion to treat adjacent-level segment degeneration through lateral interbody fusions with pedicle screws. The patient had a previous ALIF with placement of a Synthes SR titanium cage *(red arrow).*

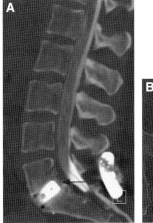

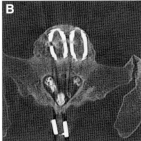

Fig. 38-10 **A** and **B,** A 5-year postoperative sagittal radiograph and an axial lumbar myelogram show an ALIF LT titanium cage with a spinous process clamp. Bony growth *(red arrow)* is present posterior to the cage.

Fig. 38-11 A lordotic, 15-degree integrated screw interbody device, titanium (NuVasive).

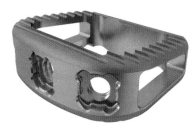

As mentioned previously, the need to optimize lordosis during surgery is critical to long-term success. Lordotic implants (15-degree devices) and hyperlordotic implants (20-, 25-, and 30-degree devices) are currently available for use in ALIF procedures (Fig. 38-12). Theoretically these implants achieve greater restoration of lordosis and potentially reduce adjacent-segment disease.

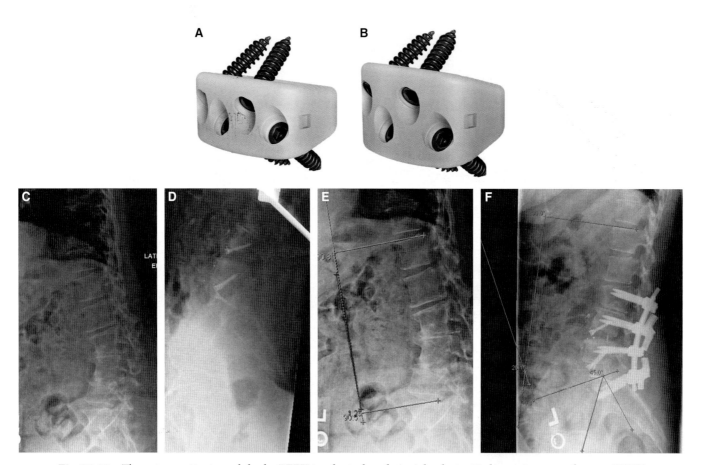

Fig. 38-12   These two patients each had a PEEK implant placed. **A,** A lordotic, 15-degree integrated screw PEEK interbody implant (NuVasive). **B,** A hyperlordotic, 30-degree integrated screw PEEK interbody implant (NuVasive). **C** and **D,** Patient example 1. A preoperative standing radiograph and a postoperative supine radiograph, before posterior supplementation with an integrated screw interbody lumbar hyperlordotic implants at L4-5 and L5-S1. **E** and **F,** Patient example 1. Preoperative and postoperative standing radiographs. The postoperative view shows posterior supplementation with an integrated screw interbody lumbar hyperlordotic implant at L4-S1. Preoperatively the pelvic incidence was not measured and the lumbar lordosis was 1.2 degrees. Postoperatively the pelvic incidence is 45 degrees and the LL is 25 degrees. An attempt was made at L3-4, but the patient was fused anteriorly at this level and an interbody graft was not placed.

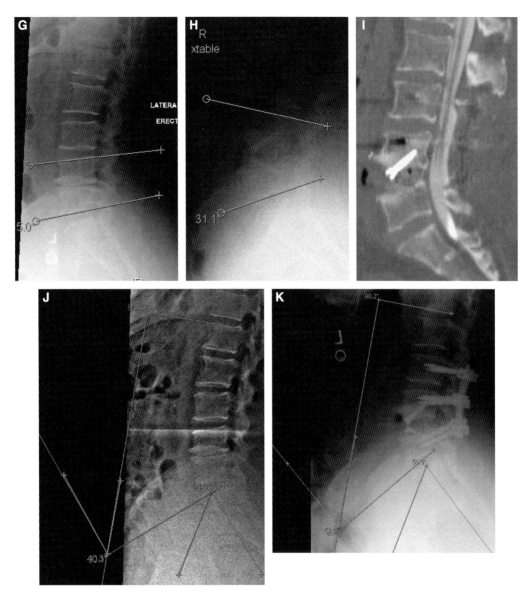

Fig. 38-12, cont'd **G,** Patient example 2. A preoperative standing radiograph. **H,** Postoperative supine radiograph obtained before posterior supplementation demonstrating an integrated screw interbody lumbar hyperlordotic implant at L4-5. **I,** A postoperative CT image of the hyperlordotic graft at L4-5. The preoperative focal lordosis at L4-5 was 5 degrees. This is improved to 31 degrees postoperatively. **J** and **K,** Preoperative and postoperative standing films with measurements. Preoperatively the patient's pelvic incidence was 54 degrees, and lumbar lordosis was 40 degrees. Postoperatively the pelvic incidence is 59 degrees, and lumbar lordosis is 54 degrees.

GRAFT EXTRUSION AND DEVICE INSTABILITY

Various fixation options exist for anterior interbody devices. Anterior longitudinal ligament sectioning has a caveat: the graft, unless fixated, is more prone to extrusion.[1] Risk of graft extrusion can be reduced by the addition of a cancellous screw with a washer in the lower vertebral body. Another option is a buttress plate with screws that restores the anterior tension band and has a locking mechanism to inhibit screw backout. Newer, integrated screw interbody devices (see Fig. 38-13) reduce the anterior profile of a construct, compared with plating systems.

Table 38-2   Biomechanical Stability of Devices

Construct	Flexion-extension	Lateral Bending	Axial Rotation
Stand-alone/no anterior screws	+	+	Increased instabilty
Stand-alone/three to four anterior screws	+ +	+ +	+ +
Stand-alone/no screws anterior plate	+ + +	+ +	+ +
Stand-alone/no anterior screws with bilateral pedicle screws	+ + + +	+ + +	+ + +
Stand-alone/three anterior screws with spinous process plate	+ + + +	+ +	+ +

Adapted from Kornblum MB, Turner AW, Cornwall GB, et al. Biomechanical evaluation of stand-alone lumbar polyether-etherketone interbody cage with integrated screws. Spine J 13:77-84, 2013.
+, Rigidity.

Kornblum et al[52] reported on the biomechanical stability of stand-alone devices versus three- and four-screw integrated devices with or without posterior supplementation in an L4-5 cadaver model (Table 38-2). A stand-alone device without supplementation limited the motion in flexion, extension, and lateral bending, compared with motion in intact spines, but it increased motion by 8% in axial rotation. They reported that placement of a fourth screw in an anterior device added no significant benefit. A posterior spinal fixation plate with an interbody screw device provided more rigidity in flexion and extension than an interbody screw device alone. Results with the spinous process model were similar to those with bilateral pedicle screws.

Biomechanical Considerations for Anterior Lumbar Interbody Fusion Constructs

Knowledge of spine biomechanics and sagittal balance/pelvic parameters is critical in understanding why some constructs work and others fail. A patient might be a candidate for a stand-alone ALIF device if he or she has primarily axial instability, foraminal and lateral recess stenosis without critical central stenosis, and a flat endplate angle at the disc space (that is, a small sacral slope angle). The patient shown in Fig. 38-13 benefited from anterior-only surgery, which does not require posterior muscle disruption and potentially shortens postoperative recovery time.

Alternatively, a stand-alone device is not an ideal option for patients with translational instability or marked global sagittal plane malalignment. In these cases posterior supplementation is often required. Spinous process clamping, with or without unilateral pedicle screws, is an alternative posterior supplemental option when a laminectomy is not required. Bone surface is available for a laminar, facet, or transverse process fusion/arthrodesis (Fig. 38-14).

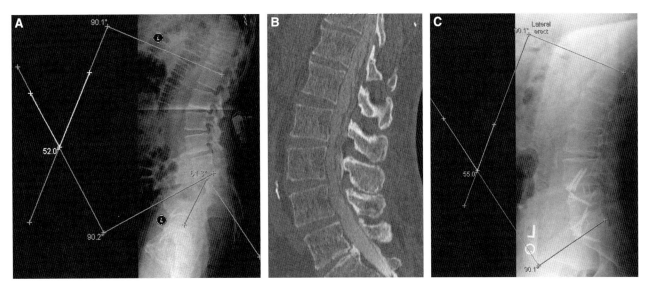

Fig. 38-13 **A-C,** A preoperative standing scoliosis radiograph, a lumbar CT image, and a postoperative standing scoliosis radiograph, respectively, of a 40-year-old man. He had no central canal stenosis, but he had significant foraminal stenosis and intractable back and leg pain. Preoperatively his lumbar lordosis was 52 degrees and pelvic incidence was 61 degrees. Anterior-only surgery was performed. Postoperatively his lumbar lordosis was 55 degrees. Postoperative pelvic incidence was not measured.

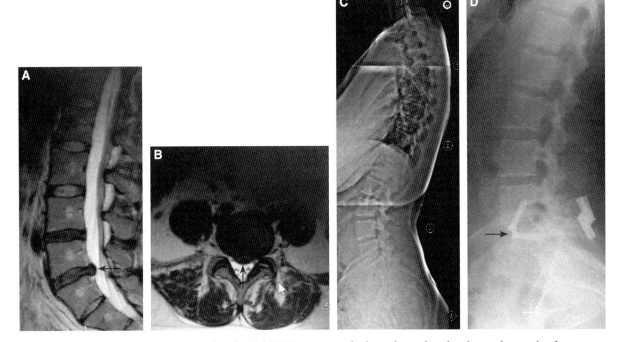

Fig. 38-14 **A-C,** Preoperative sagittal and axial MRI images and a lateral standing lumbar radiograph of a woman with axial back pain and central disc herniation at L5-S1 *(red arrows).* Conservative therapy was unsuccessful. She had a positive discogram with concordant pain at L5-S1. **D,** A postoperative lateral standing radiograph shows an implanted hyperlordotic ALIF device at L5-S1 *(red arrow)* with supplemental spinous process fixation. Central disc herniation was removed through an anterior approach.

In a biomechanical study, Wang et al[53] compared the following posterior fusion constructs in a cadaveric ALIF model: spinous process plating (SPP), bilateral/unilateral pedicle screws, and facet screws. ALIF with SPP provided the greatest stability in flexion-extension, compared with other fixation methods, followed by bilateral pedicle screws and facet fusion. Unilateral pedicle screws and SPP showed increased motion in lateral bending, compared with bilateral pedicle screws. In an operative study of SPP after ALIF, Wang et al[54] found that spinous process clamping versus bilateral open pedicle screw constructs had shorter operative times and reduced blood loss with similar results in fusion percentage. Burton et al[55] reported similar findings in a cadaver model when they compared the stability of various constructs supporting an anterior titanium ALIF cage. They noted that a unilateral pedicle screw construct was inferior in stability, compared with bilateral pedicle screws or transfacet screws in all planes except axial loading, where it showed equivalence. Biomechanically, ALIF–bilateral pedicle screw fixation provides the greatest strength and stability in all planes (see Fig. 38-12).

Open, traditional pedicle screws allow direct decompression in patients with central stenosis and provide an area available for posterolateral fusion on the transverse processes. Opponents of open posterior fixation techniques argue that retractor pressures and muscle denervation cause atrophy and potentially lead to higher incidences of adjacent-level degeneration, compared with minimal access or muscle-splitting approaches. Surgeons who place percutaneous pedicle screws can decorticate the facet complex for arthrodesis or rely only on the interbody for fusion.

Ferrera et al[56] found similar biomechanical stability of facet screws versus bilateral pedicle screws when posterior support was provided for an ALIF construct. Best and Sasso[57] listed certain advantages of facet screws over open pedicle screw placement, including decreased operative time, smaller incision, less muscle stripping, lower prominence of instrumentation, and clearance from manipulating the adjacent facet complex.

Anterior Lumbar Interbody Fusion Long-Segment Constructs

Interbody fusions are performed at the end of long-segment deformity constructs. Dorward et al[22] compared TLIF and ALIF for long-deformity constructs (13.6 segments). They found that ALIF improved lordosis better than TLIF (8.1 degrees versus −3.1 degrees at L4 S1) and had lower blood loss. TLIF, however, reduced operative time and improved scoliotic curvature (through facetectomy and distraction) better than ALIF. Differences in fusion rates were not significant.

CONCLUSION

The ability of ALIF to restore sagittal alignment through disc distraction and correction of lordosis is one of its greatest advantages over posterior approaches. Surgeons have direct access to the anterior and middle columns of the lumbar spine through sectioning of the anterior longitudinal ligament. The fusion rates are superior and subsidence low because of the large area for fusion available after decortication and the structural support that a rigid apophyseal ring provides. The rate of deep infections may be reduced with stand-alone ALIFs, compared with open posterior fusions. Additional key considerations for ALIF are presented in Box 38-3.

BOX 38-3 Key Considerations

- ALIF establishes lordosis better than TLIF.
- The *left* iliac vein is at greater risk at L5-S1.
- Fifty-three percent of lumbar lordosis is obtained at L5-S1.
- Eighty percent of lumbar lordosis is obtained at L4-S1.
- Spinopelvic parameters are critical to obtaining long-term clinical success.
- The goal is to match pelvic incidence and lumbar lordosis within 10 degrees.
- rhBMP-2 increases the fusion rate but can slightly increase retrograde ejaculation.
- The need for posterior supplemental fixation depends on bone quality, degree of translational instability, presence of a pars defect, the need for concomitant posterior decompression, and the sacral slope.
- ALIFs do not always require posterior fixation.
- PEEK has optimal postoperative fusion, as assessed with CT scan, but titanium might promote better bone ingrowth.

REFERENCES

1. McLaughlin MR, Haid R, Rodts GE, et al. Current role of anterior lumbar interbody fusion in lumbar spine disorders. Semin Neurosurg 11:221-229, 2000.
2. Muller W. Transperitoneale freilegung der wirbelsaule bei tuberkuloser spondylitis. Dtsch Z Chir 85:128-135, 1906.
3. Harmon PH. Anterior disc excision and fusion of the lumbar vertebral bodies. A review of diagnostic level testing, with operative results in more than seven hundred cases. J Int Coll Surg 40:572-586, 1963.
4. Kumar A, Kozak JA, Doherty BJ, et al. Interspace distraction and graft subsidence after anterior lumbar fusion with femoral strut allograft. Spine 18:2393-2400, 1993.
5. Barnes B, Rodts GE, McLaughlin MR, et al. Threaded cortical bone dowels for lumbar interbody fusion: over 1-year mean follow up in 28 patients. J Neurosurg 95(1 Suppl):S1-S4, 2001.
6. Kozak JA, O'Brien JP. Simultaneous combined anterior and posterior fusion. An independent analysis of a treatment for the disabled low-back pain patient. Spine 15:322-328, 1990.
7. Kaiser MG, Haid RW Jr, Subach BR, et al. Comparison of the mini-open versus laparoscopic approach for anterior lumbar interbody fusion: a retrospective review. Neurosurgery 51:97-103; discussion 103-105, 2002.
8. Rodts GE Jr, McLaughlin MR, Zhang J, et al. Laparoscopic anterior lumbar interbody fusion. Clin Neurosurg 47:541-556, 2000.
9. Mayer HM. A new microsurgical technique for minimally invasive anterior lumbar interbody fusion. Spine 22:691-699; discussion 700, 1997.
10. Chung SK, Lee SH, Lim SR, et al. Comparative study of laparoscopic L5-S1 fusion versus open mini-ALIF, with a minimum 2-year follow-up. Eur Spine J 12:613-617, 2003.
11. Schwab F, Lafage V, Boyce R, et al. Gravity line analysis in adult volunteers: age-related correlation with spinal parameters, pelvic parameters, and foot position. Spine 31:E959-E967, 2006.
12. Lafage V, Schwab F, Skalli W, et al. Standing balance and sagittal plane spinal deformity: analysis of spinopelvic and gravity line parameters. Spine 33:1572-1578, 2008.
13. Lafage V, Schwab F, Patel A, et al. Pelvic tilt and truncal inclination: two key radiographic parameters in the setting of adults with spinal deformity. Spine 34:E599-E606, 2009.
14. de Jonge T, Debousset JF, Illés T. Sagittal plane correction in idiopathic scoliosis. Spine 27:754-760, 2002.
15. Schwab FJ, Blondel B, Bess S, et al. Radiographical spinopelvic parameters and disability in the setting of adult spinal deformity: a prospective multicenter analysis. Spine 38:E803-E812, 2013.
16. Troyanovich SJ, Cailliet R, Janik TJ, et al. Radiographic mensuration characteristics of the sagittal lumbar spine from a normal population with a method to synthesize prior studies of lordosis. J Spinal Disord 10:380-386, 1997.
17. Ames CP, Smith JS, Scheer JK, et al. Impact of spinopelvic alignment on decision making in deformity surgery in adults: a review. J Neurosurg Spine 16:547-564, 2012.

18. Schwab F, Patel A, Ungar B, et al. Adult spinal deformity-postoperative standing imbalance: how much can you tolerate? An overview of key parameters in assessing alignment and planning corrective surgery. Spine 35:2224-2231, 2010.

19. Watkins RG IV, Hanna R, Chang D, et al. Sagittal alignment after lumbar interbody fusion: comparing anterior, lateral, and transforaminal approaches. J Spinal Disord Tech 27:253-256, 2014.

20. Hsieh PC, Koski TR, O'Shaughnessy BA, et al. Anterior lumbar interbody fusion in comparison with transforaminal lumbar interbody fusion: implications for the restoration of foraminal height, local disc angle, lumbar lordosis, and sagittal balance. J Neurosurg Spine 7:379-386, 2007.

21. Kim JS, Kang BU, Lee SH, et al. Mini-transforaminal lumbar interbody fusion versus anterior lumbar interbody fusion augmented by percutaneous pedicle screw fixation: a comparison of surgical outcomes in adult low-grade isthmic spondylolisthesis. J Spinal Disord Tech 22:114-121, 2009.

22. Dorward IG, Lenke LG, Bridwell KH, et al. Transforaminal versus anterior lumbar interbody fusion in long deformity constructs: a matched cohort analysis. Spine. 2013 Feb 25. [Epub ahead of print]

23. Dimar JR II, Glassman SD, Vemuri VM, et al. Lumbar lordosis restoration following single-level instrumented fusion comparing 4 commonly used techniques. Orthopedics 34:e760-e764, 2011.

24. Zdeblick TA. Laparoscopic spinal fusion. Orthop Clin North Am 29:635-645, 1998.

25. Burkus JK, Sandhu HS, Gornet MF. Influence of rhBMP-2 on the healing patterns associated with allograft interbody constructs in comparison with autograft. Spine 31:775-781, 2006.

26. Rihn JA, Patel R, Makda J, et al. Complications associated with single-level transforaminal lumbar interbody fusion. Spine J 9:623-629, 2009.

27. Hackenberg L, Halm H, Bullmann V, et al. Transforaminal lumbar interbody fusion: a safe technique with satisfactory three to five year results. Eur Spine J 14:551-558, 2005.

28. Rajaraman V, Vingan R, Roth P, et al. Visceral and vascular complications resulting from anterior lumbar interbody fusion. J Neurosurg 91(1 Suppl):60-64, 1999.

29. Brau SA. Mini-open approach to the spine for anterior lumbar interbody fusion: description of the procedure, results and complications. Spine J 2:216-223, 2002.

30. Sasso RC, Burkus KJ, LeHuec JC. Retrograde ejaculation after anterior lumbar interbody fusion: transperitoneal versus retroperitoneal exposure. Spine 28:1023-1026, 2003.

31. Burkus JK, Dryer RF, Peloza JH. Retrograde ejaculation following single-level anterior lumbar surgery with or without recombinant human bone morphogenetic protein-2 in 5 randomized controlled trials: clinical article. J Neurosurg Spine 18:112-121, 2013.

32. Comer GC, Smith MW, Hurwitz EL, et al. Retrograde ejaculation after anterior lumbar interbody fusion with and without bone morphogenetic protein-2 augmentation: a 10-year cohort controlled study. Spine J 12:881-890, 2012.

33. Lubelski D, Abdullah KG, Nowacki AS, et al. Urological complications following use of recombinant human bone morphogenetic protein-2 in anterior lumbar interbody fusion: presented at the 2012 Joint Spine Section Meeting: clinical article. J Neurosurg Spine 18:126-131, 2013.

34. Muschler GF, Lane JM, Dawson EG, eds. The Biology of Spinal Fusion. New York: Springer-Verlag, 1990.

35. Kalfas IH. Principles of bone healing. Neurosurg Focus 10:E1, 2001.

36. Dandona P, Rosenberg MT. A practical guide to male hypogonadism in the primary care setting. Int J Clin Pract 64:682-696, 2010.

37. Ohtori S, Inoue G, Orita S, et al. Teriparatide accelerates lumbar posterolateral fusion in women with postmenopausal osteoporosis: prospective study. Spine 37:E1464-E1468, 2012.

38. Ohtori S, Inoue G, Orita S, et al. Comparison of teriparatide and bisphosphonate treatment to reduce pedicle screw loosening after lumbar spinal fusion surgery in postmenopausal women with osteoporosis from a bone quality perspective. Spine 38:E487-E492, 2013.

39. Benglis DM, Boden SD, Wang MY. Biology of Spine Fusion, ed 3. Philadelphia: Elsevier, 2012.

40. Burkus JK, Foley K, Haid RW, et al. Surgical Interbody Research Group–radiographic assessment of interbody fusion devices: fusion criteria for anterior lumbar interbody surgery. Neurosurg Focus 10:E11, 2001.

41. Kuslich SD, Ulstrom CL, Griffith SL, et al. The Bagby and Kuslich method of lumbar interbody fusion. History, techniques, and 2-year follow-up results of a United States prospective, multicenter trial. Spine 23:1267-1278; discussion 1279, 1998.

42. Sasso RC, Kitchel SH, Dawson EG. A prospective, randomized controlled clinical trial of anterior lumbar interbody fusion using a titanium cylindrical threaded fusion device. Spine 29:113-122; discussion 121-122, 2004.

43. Sasso RC, LeHuec JC, Shaffrey C; Spine Interbody Research Group. Iliac crest bone graft donor site pain after anterior lumbar interbody fusion: a prospective patient satisfaction outcome assessment. J Spinal Disord Tech 18 Suppl:S77-S81, 2005.
44. Burkus JK, Schuler TC, Gornet MF, et al. Anterior lumbar interbody fusion for the management of chronic lower back pain: current strategies and concepts. Orthop Clin North Am 35:25-32, 2004.
45. Burkus JK, Gornet MF, Dickman CA, et al. Anterior lumbar interbody fusion using rhBMP-2 with tapered interbody cages. J Spinal Disord Tech 15:337-349, 2002.
46. Sasso RC, Reichard AK, Shah S. Anterior Lumbar Interbody Fusion, ed 2. New York: Thieme, 2008.
47. Burkus JK, Gornet MF, Schuler TC, et al. Six-year outcomes of anterior lumbar interbody arthrodesis with use of interbody fusion cages and recombinant human bone morphogenetic protein-2. J Bone Joint Surg Am 91:1181-1189, 2009.
48. Pradhan BB, Bae HW, Dawson EG, et al. Graft resorption with the use of bone morphogenetic protein: lessons from anterior lumbar interbody fusion using femoral ring allografts and recombinant human bone morphogenetic protein-2. Spine 31:E277-E284, 2006.
49. Hansen SM, Sasso RC. Resorptive response of rhBMP2 simulating infection in an anterior lumbar interbody fusion with a femoral ring. J Spinal Disord Tech 19:130-134, 2006.
50. Olivares-Navarrete R, Gittens RA, Schneider JM, et al. Osteoblasts exhibit a more differentiated phenotype and increased bone morphogenetic protein production on titanium alloy substrates than on poly-ether-ether-ketone. Spine J 12:265-272, 2012.
51. Olivares-Navarrete R, Hyzy SL, Gittens RA, et al. Rough titanium alloys regulate osteoblast production of angiogenic factors. Spine J 13:1563-1570, 2013.
52. Kornblum MB, Turner AW, Cornwall GB, et al. Biomechanical evaluation of stand-alone lumbar polyether-ether-ketone interbody cage with integrated screws. Spine J 13:77-84, 2013.
53. Wang JC, Spenciner D, Robinson JC. SPIRE spinous process stabilization plate: biomechanical evaluation of a novel technology. Invited submission from the Joint Section Meeting on Disorders of the Spine and Peripheral Nerves, March 2005. J Neurosurg Spine 4:160-164, 2006.
54. Wang JC, Haid RW Jr, Miller JS, et al. Comparison of CD HORIZON SPIRE spinous process plate stabilization and pedicle screw fixation after anterior lumbar interbody fusion. Invited submission from the Joint Section Meeting On Disorders of the Spine and Peripheral Nerves, March 2005. J Neurosurg Spine 4:132-136, 2006.
55. Burton D, McIff T, Fox T, et al. Biomechanical analysis of posterior fixation techniques in a 360 degrees arthrodesis model. Spine 30:2765-2771, 2005.
56. Ferrara LA, Secor JL, Jin BH, et al. A biomechanical comparison of facet screw fixation and pedicle screw fixation: effects of short-term and long-term repetitive cycling. Spine 28:1226-1234, 2003.
57. Best NM, Sasso RC. Efficacy of translaminar facet screw fixation in circumferential interbody fusions as compared to pedicle screw fixation. J Spinal Disord Tech 19:98-103, 2006.

39

Osteotomies for Restoration of Spinal Alignment

John Paul Kelleher ▪ *Justin S. Smith* ▪ *Paul J. Schmitt*
Christopher P. Ames ▪ *Christopher I. Shaffrey*

As the population's life expectancy lengthens and the desire for maintaining an active lifestyle increases, more and more patients are seeking medical and surgical evaluation for fixed sagittal deformity. These deformities may have degenerative, posttraumatic, neoplastic, infectious, metabolic, or congenital causes.[1,2] The four most common presentations are (1) previous fusion for idiopathic scoliosis to L3 or L4 with resulting hypolordosis and caudal disc level degeneration, (2) flat-back syndrome secondary to loss of lumbar lordosis (LL) caused by a previous surgery, (3) sharp-angular posttraumatic kyphosis, often with a component of pseudarthrosis, and (4) in the setting of ankylosing spondylitis.[1] These patients often have associated functional disability and can have limited ability to walk a significant distance without intractable pain or fatigue.

With the widespread use of polysegmental three-column fixation with pedicle screws and advances in spinal instrumentation, posterior-only approaches for correcting kyphotic or kyphoscoliotic deformities have become feasible and more common in recent years, obviating the need for and the morbidity of anterior release and corpectomy approaches.[3] The use of posterior-only osteotomies with pedicle screw instrumentation can provide significant equivalent alignment correction in all three dimensions, and greater pedicle screw pullout strength and stiffness limit the number of levels fused, preserving more mobile spinal segments.[3,4]

Surgeons who treat patients with kyphotic deformities should have experience with the various osteotomy techniques and understand their appropriate uses. Determining whether a spinal deformity is fixed or flexible helps significantly with the surgical decision-making process. Assessment of curve flexibility and the compensatory ability of adjacent segments of the spine helps to determine the surgical approach, the number of spinal levels to be fused, and the need for corrective osteotomies. This can be determined radiographically based on supine, bending, or bolster films and by evaluating the magnitude of deformity correction. Deformities that demonstrate more than 30% correction on bending radiographs are generally considered flexible and are less likely to require osteotomies, whereas curves that correct less than 30% with bending are generally considered fixed or rigid deformities and are more likely to require osteotomies.[5] Another important feature to consider is whether the kyphosis is more rounded, long, and sweeping or short and angular.[6] Many adult patients with spinal deformity have had previous fusion surgery, which may contribute to rigidity of the deformity and increase the need for an osteotomy for sufficient alignment. Flexibility should be evaluated in all curves considered for surgical correction.

Fixed sagittal deformity makes erect posture difficult without flexion of the knees, hyperextension of the hips, and/or pelvic retroversion. The sagittal vertical axis (SVA), which is the horizontal offset between the C7 plumb line and the posterosuperior corner of the S1 vertebra, is often significantly positive in patients with fixed sagittal spinopelvic deformity. No clear consensus exists regarding normal SVA, but in the recent Scoliosis Research Society (SRS)–Schwab adult spine deformity classification, Schwab et al[7] considered an SVA of less than 4 cm to be normal, an SVA of 4 to 9.5 cm to be moderately increased, and an SVA greater than 9.5 cm to be severely increased. The T1 spinopelvic inclination (SPI) and T9 SPI are alternative measures of global sagittal alignment that rely on angular measurements rather than distances. T1 SPI has been shown to have a slightly greater correlation with health-related quality of life (HRQOL) scores than the SVA, perhaps because SPI accounts for the relationship of the pelvis and lower extremities to the spine by measurement of the offset of T1 from the pelvis in relation to the femoral heads and not the sacrum.[8] Lafage et al[8] found that T1 SPI had the strongest correlation with HRQOL, followed by SVA and pelvic tilt (PT).

Recent studies have demonstrated the importance of pelvic parameters, including pelvic incidence (PI), PT, and sacral slope (SS), in assessing sagittal spinal alignment.[9,10] Positive sagittal malalignment can lead to increased pelvic retroversion (increased PT) as a means of compensation. Although increased PT may help to mitigate positive sagittal malalignment, abnormal pelvic retroversion can adversely affect ambulation and increase energy expenditure, resulting in a negative impact on HRQOL.[1-13] Regardless of the cause of adult spinal deformity, a strong correlation exists between sagittal malalignment and pain and disability based on standardized measures of HRQOL.[14] Correction of both SVA and PT has been reported to result in better outcome scores than correction of SVA alone.[8-10] Schwab et al[15] recommended that the goal of surgical correction for sagittal spinopelvic malalignment, based on normative data and HRQOL-based postoperative outcomes, should be an SVA of less than 50 mm, T1 SPI of less than 0 degrees, PT of less than 20 degrees, and LL within 9 degrees of PI. The results of a study from Blondel et al[16] that assessed the amount of sagittal correction needed for patients to perceive improvement in HRQOL scores were consistent with the correction goals proposed by Schwab et al for realignment surgery. The best HRQOL outcomes for adult patients with severe sagittal plane deformity were achieved with an SVA correction of more than 120 mm or at least 66%. Furthermore, they found that the greater the magnitude of correction of SVA, the better the improvement in SRS pain and ODI scores. The goal of surgery should be a complete or near-complete correction of sagittal malalignment if feasible; partial correction may in some cases increase the risks of instrumentation failure, proximal junctional kyphosis, and suboptimal improvement of HRQOL.[15,16] Corrective surgery for fixed sagittal imbalance or kyphoscoliosis often involves osteotomies such as a Smith-Petersen osteotomy (SPO), pedicle subtraction osteotomy (PSO), or vertebral column resection (VCR) with transpedicular segmental instrumentation. The use of osteotomies to restore sagittal spinopelvic alignment in adults depends on the pathology, patient age, medical comorbidities, and experience of the surgeon. To determine which osteotomy or combination of osteotomies to employ for deformity correction, a working appreciation for the applications and limitations of all three key posterior osteotomies (SPO, PSO, and VCR) is important. In this chapter we will focus on the indications, surgical technique, complications, and outcomes of SPO and PSO for the correction of kyphoscoliotic deformities; VCR is discussed in Chapter 40.

Smith-Petersen Osteotomy

Smith-Petersen et al[17] first described SPO in 1945 for correction of fixed sagittal deformity in patients with a kyphotic deformity and an ankylosed spine caused by rheumatic conditions such as anklyosing spondylitis. Also referred to as *Chevron osteotomy, extension osteotomy,* or *Ponte osteotomy,* SPO involves removal of the posterior bony elements, including the bilateral facet joints, inferior portion of the lamina, and inferior portion of the spinous process, and removal of the posterior ligaments at the osteotomy level.[3,18,19] The osteotomy is closed with the axis of rotation at the posterior aspect of the disc space, which results in widening of the anterior disc space and disruption of the anterior longitudinal ligament and hence requires a mobile disc space. SPO produces shortening of the posterior column and lengthening of the anterior column. One modification of the SPO procedure is to use an interbody graft or spacer in the middle or anterior third of the disk space and then compress posteriorly using the graft as a fulcrum; this can provide a greater degree of lordosis, with less risk of compromising the neural foramina.[18] The amount of correction typically achieved with SPO is approximately 10 degrees per level or 1 degree of correction for each millimeter of bone removed.[3,17-19]

INDICATIONS AND PREOPERATIVE PLANNING

SPO is typically indicated for patients with long, gradual sweeping deformity, with mobile intervertebral disc spaces, who have no more than moderate elevation of SVA (6 to 8 cm), features typically not associated with rigid deformities.[6] The classic indication for SPO is Scheuermann's kyphosis, but it can be used in the treatment of mild iatrogenic fixed sagittal imbalance.[6,18] The role of SPO is limited in fixed sagittal deformity, because these osteotomies have limited effectiveness in sharp, angular kyphosis and are not effective in the presence of anterior bridging osteophytes or across previously fused segments because of the lack of disc mobility.

Standing 36-inch scoliosis radiographs in AP and lateral views are necessary to assess the global and regional spinopelvic alignment. Both global and regional parameters should be measured. Radiographs taken over a bolster can provide valuable information about the flexibility (or rigidity) of the deformity. The severity and character (foraminal versus central) of a patient's stenosis can be assessed with MRI or CT-myelography. Myelography has the added benefits of allowing an assessment of fusion masses and providing a clearer picture of pathology in the setting of previous instrumentation, whereas MRI is more susceptible to metallic artifact. Opening-wedge osteotomies are not advisable across levels with significant foraminal stenosis, because the foramina are compressed when the osteotomy is closed unless more extensive facetectomies and pars resections are performed to ensure sufficient decompression.

OPERATIVE TECHNIQUE

The patient is positioned prone on a Jackson frame (Mizuho OSI, Union City, CA), with pads across the chest and at each of the iliac crests. The Jackson frame encourages the spine to reduce into a more anatomic curvature as the posterior elements are released. The posterior elements are exposed at all levels planned for surgery. Care is taken to preserve the facet capsules and the supraspinous ligament at the upper instrumented level to prevent adjacent-level disease. Otherwise, soft tissue is meticulously dissected from all of the bony structures to facilitate arthrodesis. Pedicle screws can be placed before or after the osteotomies depending on surgeon preference. Opening-wedge osteotomies will not typically destabilize the spine enough to necessitate fixation across the levels of interest before these osteotomies are performed.

The SPO technique is illustrated in Fig. 39-1. The interspinous ligament at the level of the osteotomy is removed, and the spinous process shortened. A drill is used to create a trough laterally through the inferior articular process, extending from the border of the interlaminar space to the foramen. Once the ligamentum flavum is identified, the facet complex is separated from the superior articular process by a single cut with an osteotome. A Capener gouge can then be used to remove the inferior facet, angling it to remain above the level of the exposed ligamentum flavum (see Fig. 39-1, A and B). By using rongeurs and osteotomes, and by minimizing the use of the drill, bone can be collected and morselized for use in the arthrodesis. Alternatively, the lamina, ligament, and superior and inferior facet can be removed in a chevron fashion with rongeurs and Kerrison punch.

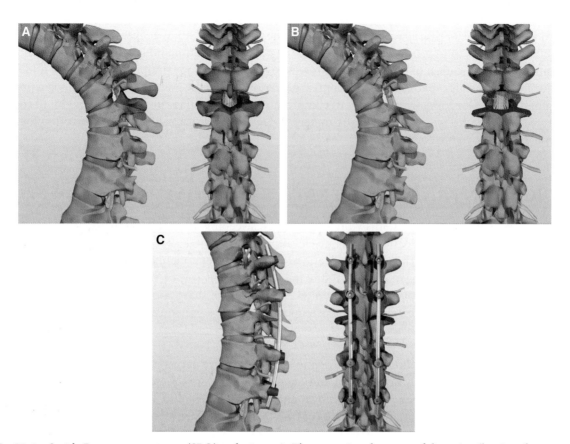

Fig. 39-1 Smith-Petersen osteotomy (SPO) technique. **A,** The posterior elements of the spine (lamina, facets, and pars) to be removed for the SPO are highlighted in orange. **B,** The bony defect following the SPO. Note that pedicle screws are shown at two vertebral levels above and below the SPO. **C,** The SPO following closure via compression across the pedicle screw-rod construct spanning the osteotomy level. The posterior column is shortened and the anterior column is lengthened. (Illustrations copyright© Kenneth X. Probst. Published with permission from Xavier Studio.)

Rods are cut and contoured appropriately before being placed across the pedicle screw heads. Locking caps are tightened to an appropriate torque and sequentially compressed across the levels at which opening wedge osteotomies have been performed (see Fig. 39-1, *C*). The arthrodesis is completed using a combination of autograft with allograft and/or osteobiologic materials, which can be laid across the posterior elements in the thoracic spine and in the lateral gutters of the lumbar spine. Subfascial drains are placed, followed by a multilayered closure.

POTENTIAL COMPLICATIONS AND OUTCOMES

SPO is not free of risks, because anterior column lengthening places vascular structures at risk, particularly in older patients and in patients with ankylosing spondylitis, who may have calcified major vessels.[3,18] Gastrointestinal complication can occur secondary to superior mesenteric artery syndrome. Neurologic complications have been reported, mainly radiculopathy secondary to compression of nerve roots in the foramen from closure of the SPO.[3] Other complications include but are not limited to pseudarthrosis, bleeding, durotomy, and pedicle fracture. Compared with three-column osteotomies, SPOs are usually associated with shortened operative time, decreased blood loss (1392 ml for three-column SPO compared with 2617 ml for single PSO for a similar degree of correction), and decreased rates of neurologic complication.[20]

PATIENT EXAMPLE

MULTILEVEL SMITH-PETERSEN OSTEOTOMIES

This 22-year-old woman with a known history of Scheuermann's kyphosis was involved in a motor vehicle collision and sustained an unstable C5 flexion fracture that was treated with corpectomy and fusion. She also had a T8 compression fracture, which was treated with bracing. The combination of her preexisting Scheuermann's kyphosis and T8 traumatic compression fracture resulted in progressive kyphosis over the 3 years after her injury. She presented with grossly apparent kyphotic deformity and intractable back pain. Preoperative full-length standing AP and lateral radiographs showed no coronal deformity, but they revealed significant thoracic hyperkyphosis (T3-L2 Cobb angle of 82 degrees) and global positive sagittal malalignment (SVA of +11 cm; Fig. 39-2, *A* and *B*). A preoperative full-length lateral supine radiograph obtained with the patient over a bolster revealed thoracic curve flexibility, with correction of the kyphosis from 82 to 39 degrees (Fig. 39-2, *C*). Surgical treatment included T3-L2 instrumented arthrodesis with T7-8 to T11-12 SPOs. On postoperative full-length standing AP and lateral radiographs she has no coronal deformity and significant improvement of her thoracic kyphosis (from 82 to 36 degrees) and of her global sagittal alignment (SVA of −1 cm; Fig. 39-2, *D* and *E*).

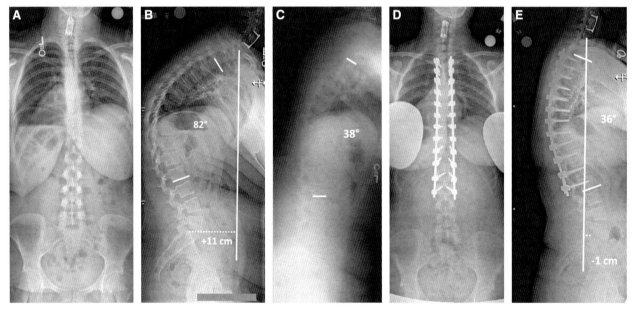

Fig. 39-2   **A** and **B,** Preoperative full-length standing AP and lateral radiographs showed no coronal deformity, but they revealed significant thoracic hyperkyphosis (a T3-L2 Cobb angle of 82 degrees) and global positive sagittal malalignment (a sagittal vertical axis of 11 cm). **C,** A preoperative full-length supine lateral radiograph with the patient over a bolster revealed thoracic curve flexibility, with correction of the kyphosis to 38 degrees. **D** and **E,** Postoperative full-length standing AP and lateral radiographs after T3-L2 instrumented arthrodesis with multilevel Smith-Petersen osteotomies. The thoracic kyphosis (T3-L2 Cobb angle) has been corrected to 36 degrees, and the global positive sagittal malalignment has been corrected (sagittal vertical axis of −1 cm). *Vertical white lines* represent C7 plumb lines, and *horizontal dashed lines* represent the C7 offset from the posterosuperior corner of S1 (a sagittal vertical axis).

Pedicle Subtraction Osteotomy

Since Thomasen[21] first described the PSO procedure in 1985, it has been performed increasingly for the surgical correction of fixed sagittal plane deformity. PSO can be used to restore alignment in the thoracic, lumbar, and more recently the cervical spine.[22,23] In the lumbar spine, it can typically provide approximately 30 degrees of lordosis, although the magnitude of correction varies based on technique. Li et al[24] obtained a mean 36.4-degree correction with standard PSO and a mean 48.5-degree correction with a modified, extended PSO in a cadaveric study. Multiple clinical studies have shown deformity correction from 26.2 to 40.1 degrees, with an average correction of 32 degrees with PSO.[1,25,26] In a study from Bridwell et al,[1] the average improvement in SVA was 13.5 cm. Expected correction for PSO in the thoracic spine is less than in the lumbar spine, likely because of the shorter heights of thoracic vertebral bodies compared with lumbar vertebral bodies.

PSO comprises a three-column osteotomy with a transpedicular vertebral wedge resection, extending from the posterior elements through the pedicles bilaterally and into the vertebral body (Fig. 39-3).[1,2,4,23] The extended PSO technique involves resection of the cephalad endplate and disc at the osteotomy level, with closure of the inferior endplate of the supradjacent vertebral body directly onto the inferior aspect of the osteotomy wedge. The anterior cortex is left intact and acts as a hinge for the closure of the wedge defect.

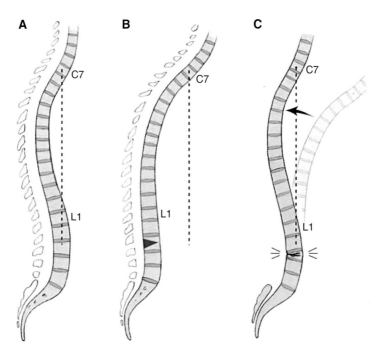

Fig. 39-3   Sagittal alignment correction with pedicle subtraction osteotomy (PSO). **A,** Normal sagittal spinal curvature, with the C7 plumb line *(dashed vertical line)* aligned with S1. **B,** A kyphotic spine, with the C7 plumb line substantially offset in front of S1. The *triangular wedge* overlying the L3 vertebral body represents the planned bone removal for alignment correction with PSO. **C,** Closure of the L3 PSO and sagittal realignment of the spine, with the C7 plumb line now aligned over S1.

Closing the wedge provides a substantial surface area for osseous union from closure of the bony surfaces of the anterior, middle, and posterior columns. It shortens the posterior column without lengthening the anterior column, thus providing maximal healing potential with less risk of stretching the major abdominal vessels and viscera anterior to the spine.[1,23] After the posterior wedge has been closed, two nerve roots exit on each side at the vertebral level of the osteotomy through the newly formed neural foramina.

INDICATIONS AND PREOPERATIVE PLANNING

PSO is typically used to correct fixed sagittal deformity with sharp or angular kyphosis in patients with an SVA of more than 8 cm or fixed positive sagittal spinopelvic malalignment requiring more than a 30-degree correction of lumbar lordosis. PSO is often performed to treat acquired or iatrogenic flat-back syndrome, ankylosing spondylitis, and rigid deformities that lack the anterior flexibility needed for an effective SPO.[18] In addition to patients with fixed positive sagittal malalignment, patients with a PI-LL mismatch who remain globally sagittally aligned can benefit from PSO. In a recent study, Smith et al and the International Spine Study Group[27] found this form of compensated flat-back syndrome to be a significant source of pain and disability. They demonstrated magnitudes of improvement in HRQOL measures after surgical correction similar to those for surgical correction of positive sagittal malalignment.

In patients with focal fixed-angle sagittal deformity, PSO is typically performed at the level of kyphosis; however, in the absence of focal thoracolumbar kyphosis, lumbar PSO is preferable. PSO can be performed in patients with circumferential fusion across multiple segments, previous laminectomy, and an area of rotation, although these features potentially increase the technical difficulty and the risk of complications.[6] The extensive cancellous bony contact associated with the wedge osteotomy increases stability and reduces the risk of pseudarthrosis. Furthermore, both sagittal and coronal plane deformity can be corrected with an asymmetrical wedge resection osteotomy. PSO tends not to be performed in distal lumbar vertebrae, because fewer fixation points are available distally.[6] PSO is most commonly performed at L2 or L3, because these levels are generally below the conus and have a sufficient number of fixation points distally. Nevertheless, the vertebral level of the PSO should be guided by the type and location of pathology.

Preoperative assessment should include standing 36-inch AP and lateral spine radiographs to measure global and regional spinopelvic parameters. In addition, a supine 36-inch lateral radiograph and films obtained with the patient over a bolster can help to assess the flexibility of the deformity. Less rigid deformities may demonstrate considerable correction on these alternative views, which is useful to determine whether osteotomies are needed for correction and whether multiple SPOs will suffice instead of a more aggressive PSO.

OPERATIVE TECHNIQUE

The PSO technique is illustrated in Fig. 39-4. After the exposure, instrumentation is placed. This typically includes pedicle screws but can include hooks. We prefer to place all fixation points, including pedicle and iliac screws, before starting the osteotomy. Generally, at least two levels of fixation above and below the planned level of the PSO are needed, but in most patients with deformity, multilevel posterior segmental fixation points are used for correction.

Laminectomies and posterior decompression are performed next. A partial laminectomy that extends through the pars interarticularis bilaterally at the level superior to the level of the PSO and a complete laminectomy that extends through the pars interarticularis bilaterally at the level of the PSO, with bilateral facetectomies, are performed. Central decompression is achieved with excision of the ligamentum flavum. If a laminectomy has been performed at the level of the planned PSO, scar tissue overlying the thecal sac should be removed, because this tissue can buckle during osteotomy closure and compromise neural structures. The initial stages of a PSO include an SPO both cephalad and caudal to the pedicle for the PSO level. The bone surrounding the pedicle is then completely removed, including the transverse process, exposing the cephalad and caudal nerve roots. The pedicles are isolated and separated from all osseous attachments other than the vertebral body. The medial wall of each pedicle is carefully delineated, and the thecal sac and exiting nerve roots are protected with a nerve root retractor.

The pedicle is then decancellated using curettes or a drill. The nerve root superior to the pedicle is usually sufficiently far from the pedicle to limit the risk of injury during pedicle resection, but the inferior nerve root and the thecal sac should be carefully retracted and protected. With the use of a Leksell rongeur, the cortical walls of the pedicles are resected flush with the vertebral bodies, because osseous remnants can impinge on the nerve roots when the wedge osteotomy is closed (see Fig. 39-4, A). Hemostatic agents and cottonoids can help to control epidural bleeding during isolation and resection of the pedicle.

The plane between the lateral aspects of the vertebral body and the adjacent soft tissues is developed. This can be achieved by carefully passing a small Cobb elevator into the subperiosteal plane along the lateral vertebral body wall, sweeping from cephalad to caudal and reflecting the soft tissue away from the lateral vertebral wall. Care is needed to prevent injury to the segmental vessel, the exiting nerve roots, and the sympathetic chain. If a segmental artery is compromised, hemostasis can be achieved with bipolar coagulation or a hemostatic agent. Defining the lateral aspects of the vertebral body helps to visualize the bony anatomy, including the anterior depth and lateral aspects of the vertebral body, and to protect adjacent structures. The plane along the lateral aspects of the vertebral body is maintained during the osteotomy with the use of a sponge or one of many specially designed retractors.

Vertebral body decancellation is performed in a preplanned, wedge-shaped fashion using an osteotome primarily or with a combination of a high-speed drill, curettes, and pituitary rongeurs (see Fig. 39-4, B). Proper orientation is critical during the decancellation and osteotomy, with a wider resection posteriorly that leads to a focal point anteriorly. Fluoroscopic guidance can be helpful. Both the decancellation and osteotomy are typically completed on one side before performing the same procedure on the opposite side. We use an L-shaped osteotome to make a cut at the inferior and medial margin of the pedicle, followed by a straight osteotome to cut the lateral cortex of the vertebral body. The initial bone wedge is removed, and further medial decancellation of the vertebral body is performed in a symmetrical fashion using a curette, drill, and/or pituitary rongeur from lateral to medial and ventral to the posterior vertebral wall. A wedge shape with an anterior apex needs to be maintained, or closure of the defect may only shorten the column, rather than correct the sagittal alignment. The osteotomy wedge should extend laterally to include the lateral cortical walls of the vertebral body, because residual cortical wall can prevent closure of the osteotomy (see Fig. 39-4, C).

To maximize the potential osteotomy angle, vertebral body removal begins below the pedicle stump inferiorly and extends to just below the cephalad endplate superiorly. The anterior cortex is preserved, including at the apex of the wedge to act as a hinge and to prevent translation at the time of closure of the osteotomy. In addition, preservation of the anterior cortex helps to minimize risk to the great vessels and potentially other structures. During an osteotomy, the thecal sac and nerve roots are protected with nerve root retractors. Gentle traction may be applied with the retractor on the thecal sac if the level of osteotomy is below the level of the conus. Heavy bleeding is usually controlled with surface hemostatic agents, by packing with cottonoids or sponges and by an organized and efficient osteotomy. After completion of the osteotomy on one side, it is packed to control bleeding and a temporary rod is placed across the osteotomy prevent premature, uncontrolled closure. Temporary rods also help to prevent translation of the spine in patients with long fusion above or below the osteotomy. The osteotomy is then completed on the opposite side in a similar fashion, and decancellation continues until the sides connect. Underneath the posterior vertebral cortex, the cortex is thinned as much as possible by thoroughly removing the cancellous bone behind the posterior vertebral cortical wall. The epidural space between the posterior vertebral wall and the anterior dura is then carefully developed using a Woodson elevator to free adhesions between the dura and bone and to prevent an anterior dural tear. The risk of durotomy and spinal fluid leak is high, because many patients have had one or more previous surgeries and therefore have scar tissue that can disrupt normal tissue planes. Epidural bleeding is controlled with judicious use of bipolar electrocautery and hemostatic agents.

Next, the posterior cortical wall of the vertebral body is carefully pushed into the cavity created from the wedge resection with the use of a Woodson elevator, reverse-angled curette, or one of many specially designed posterior vertebral wall impactors (see Fig. 39-4, *D*). The fractured posterior cortex is removed with pituitary rongeurs. Careful attention and orientation will create a symmetrical wedge osteotomy, which is necessary to achieve symmetrical closure and the desired sagittal correction. However, in the presence of kyphoscoliotic deformity, an asymmetrical osteotomy can be performed and should be well planned preoperatively. Resection of a larger wedge on the convex side rather than the concave side of the vertebral body, allows correction of the coronal plane during wedge closure. All bone removed during the osteotomy is preserved for use as graft for posterolateral arthrodesis.

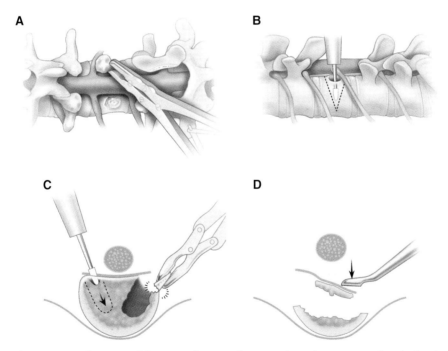

Fig. 39-4 **A,** The posterior elements of the spine (lamina, facets, and pars) are removed at the level planned for pedicle subtraction osteotomy (PSO). The pedicles are exposed and can be removed with a rongeur or drill. The adjacent exiting nerve root should be protected. The posterior elements, including pedicles, are removed, allowing access to the vertebral body. **B,** An osteotome or high-speed drill can be used to decancellate a triangular wedge. **C,** A rongeur or osteotome is used to remove portions of the lateral walls of the vertebral body based on a similar wedge pattern. **D,** After the PSO wedge is created, including decancellation and removal of the corresponding lateral cortical walls, the remaining anterior cortical wall adjacent to the dura is removed by collapsing this bone into the decancellated cavity with a down-pushing curette.

Continued

E

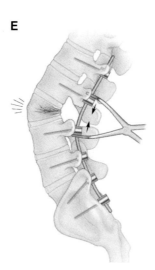

Fig. 39-4, cont'd   **E,** The PSO wedge is closed with compression across pedicle screws spanning the osteotomy level. This may be achieved by spanning the level with short, temporary rods, with subsequent placement of permanent rods, or by cantilevering prebent lordotic rods.

The wedge is closed by compression with manual pressure or by cantilevering the spine (see Fig. 39-4, *E*). Before the osteotomy is closed, a Kerrison rongeur can be used to enlarge the central canal and remove all bone fragments or residual elements of the pedicles that might impinge on the exiting nerves, because the two adjacent foramina are now combined into one foramen with two exiting nerve roots on each side.

The temporary rod-screw construct is loosened but not removed, because it can provide a guide during closure of the wedge resection. The neural elements are carefully observed for compression from bony or ligamentous structures during the closure. If the osteotomy closes adequately with no changes in neurophysiologic monitoring information, a permanent, contoured rod spanning the entire segment is placed, with caps applied loosely over the screws on the side contralateral to the temporary rod. A compressor is placed along the heads of the pedicle across the osteotomy on each side and gently compressed, thereby further closing the osteotomy defect. The temporary rod on the opposite side is then replaced with a contoured, permanent rod and compression is applied across the osteotomy level before final tightening of the screw caps. The thecal sac and nerve root are inspected again for bony compression or excessive buckling of the thecal sac, in which case additional bony resection should be performed.

If the osteotomy does not completely close, intervening residual bone fragments, inadequate rod contouring, or subluxation should be considered as a possible cause. Residual bony fragments can be removed with a curette or rongeur. The rod can be further contoured with in situ benders. Some surgeons routinely place a satellite rod on one or both sides across the PSO level using side connectors.[28,29] Subluxation can occur during closure, most commonly posterior subluxation of the proximal elements over the distal elements. This should be corrected for proper closure and anatomic alignment and to prevent spinal cord or cauda equina compromise. Reduction screws can be placed at the caudal adjacent level to reduce subluxation with rod reduction into the screw head. If neurophysiologic monitoring indicates concerning changes during closure, it should be stopped and reversed. Further decompression posteriorly or laterally may be necessary, depending on whether the changes are in the motor evoked potentials or EMGs, respectively, before attempting to reclose the osteotomy wedge. Neurophysiologic monitoring changes can also result from subluxation that causes impingement of the thecal sac. Monitoring should be continued until the end of surgery to assess for delayed neurologic compromise, even if no monitoring changes occurred during the closure.

The procedure is completed with posterolateral decortication using a high-speed drill, followed by placement of harvested bone graft from the osteotomy and iliac crest for posterolateral fusion. The use of osteobiologic agents may enhance the fusion. We typically place two subfascial drains and close the wound in a standard, multilayer fashion.

Modification of the PSO technique may increase the amount of deformity correction. An extended PSO involves including the rostral disc space in the osteotomy and closing the wedge onto the endplate of the adjacent vertebral body. For an extended PSO, an interbody device can be placed anteriorly into the osteotomy defect to serve as a fulcrum and to prevent compromise of the neural foramina.

POTENTIAL COMPLICATIONS AND OUTCOMES

Patients treated with PSO have shown improvement in sagittal balance, thoracic kyphosis, lumbar lordosis, height, pain scale score, and ODI score. However, PSO is also associated with relatively high rates of complications. Careful planning and understanding of the risks and benefits by both the patient and surgeon are necessary.[30] More common complications include durotomy, wound infection, neurologic deficit, implant failure, wound hematoma, epidural hematoma, and pulmonary embolism. According to Smith et al,[20] the overall complication rates associated with procedures that include any type of osteotomy were significantly higher than those not requiring an osteotomy (34.8% compared with 17%, respectively). This difference remained significant after adjusting for patient age, surgeon experience, and history of previous surgery. The study reported a progressive increase in complication rates with more aggressive osteotomy, with PSO having a complication rate of 39.1%. In addition, a higher rate of complications was found in patients who underwent revision procedures than in those who did not (24.5% compared with 18.2%, respectively). The spine should be carefully observed for subluxation when closing a PSO osteotomy. PSO has been associated with an 8% incidence of new neurologic deficit.[6] These tend to be related to a single root, with somewhat higher incidence at L4 and L5 compared with L2 or L3.[31] These new deficits can be related to either a mild subluxation of the spine, dural buckling, dorsal compression of nerve roots, or traction on distal roots, particularly with previous surgery. These risks should be carefully considered during patient counseling and surgical planning. Evaluation of this risk-benefit balance should be personalized and carefully discussed with the patient. Consideration for surgical treatment should include the patient's age and overall health, severity of the symptoms, the impact on the patient's quality of life, and willingness of the patient to accept the risks of surgery. A recent multicenter study assessed risk factors for major perioperative complications in adult spinal deformity surgery and found that significantly higher rates of complications were associated with staged and combined anterior-posterior surgeries.[32] Osteoporosis places a patient at increased risk of proximal junctional kyphosis. Preoperative DXA and treatment, if indicated, can be of benefit. Smith et al[28] recently documented high rates of rod fracture across PSO sites; as a result, some surgeons routinely use side connectors to place a satellite rod on one or both sides across the PSO level.[29] Although these complex surgical procedures have been shown on average to be significantly beneficial in treating these patients, surgery is not necessarily indicated for every patient with sagittal deformity, and nonoperative methods should generally be attempted first.

PATIENT EXAMPLE

Pedicle Subtraction Osteotomy

This 63-year-old woman with a history of multiple previous thoracolumbar surgeries presented with intractable back pain and very early fatigue with standing or walking. She was found to have significant kyphoscoliosis and positive sagittal malalignment. Preoperative full-length standing AP and lateral radiographs revealed thoracolumbar scoliosis, a +5.5 cm coronal imbalance, LL of 31 degrees, PI of 68 degrees, PT of 30 degrees, PI-LL mismatch of 37 degrees, and SVA of +13 cm (Fig. 39-5, *A* and *B*). Surgical treatment included T3-ilium instrumented arthrodesis with an extended PSO at L3. Postoperative full-length standing AP and lateral radiographs show significant correction of her thoracolumbar scoliosis and coronal imbalance (+1.2 cm) and significant improvement of her SVA (+2.5 cm), PT (22 degrees), LL (61 degrees), and PI-LL mismatch (7 degrees) (Fig. 39-5, *C* and *D*).

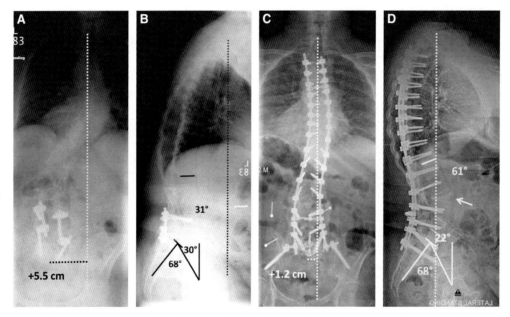

Fig. 39-5 **A** and **B,** Preoperative standing full-length AP and lateral radiographs revealed thoracolumbar scoliosis, a +5.5 cm coronal imbalance, LL of 31 degrees, PI of 68 degrees, PT of 30 degrees, PI-LL mismatch of 37 degrees, and SVA of +13 cm. She underwent T3-ilium instrumented arthrodesis with an extended L3 PSO. **C** and **D,** Postoperative AP and lateral radiographs show significant correction of her thoracolumbar scoliosis and coronal imbalance (+1.2 cm) and significant improvement of SVA (+2.5 cm), PT (22 degrees), LL (61 degrees), and PI-LL mismatch (7 degrees). *Vertical dashed lines* represent C7 plumb lines, and *horizontal dashed lines* represent the coronal C7 offset from the central sacral vertical line. Lumbar lordosis is indicated (preoperative and postoperative), measured from the inferior endplate of T12 and the sacral endplate.

ACKNOWLEDGMENT

The authors wish to acknowledge the talents of Ms. Chris Gralapp, who provided the pedicle subtraction osteotomy technique illustrations for this chapter.

REFERENCES

1. Bridwell KH, Lewis SJ, Lenke LG, et al. Pedicle subtraction osteotomy for the treatment of fixed sagittal imbalance. J Bone Joint Surg Am 85:454-463, 2003.
2. Wang MY, Berven SH. Lumbar pedicle subtraction osteotomy. Neurosurgery 60(Suppl 1):ONS140-ONS146; discussion ONS146, 2007.
3. Dorward IG, Lenke LG. Osteotomies in the posterior-only treatment of complex adult spinal deformity: a comparative review. Neurosurg Focus 28:E4, 2010.
4. Steinmetz MP, Rajpal S, Trost G. Segmental spinal instrumentation in the management of scoliosis. Neurosurgery 63:131-138, 2008.
5. Silva FE, Lenke LG. Adult degenerative scoliosis: evaluation and management. Neurosurg Focus 28:E1, 2010.
6. Bridwell KH. Decision making regarding Smith-Petersen vs. pedicle subtraction osteotomy vs. vertebral column resection for spinal deformity. Spine 31(19 Suppl):S171-S178, 2006
7. Schwab F, Ungar B, Blondel B, et al. Scoliosis Research Society–Schwab adult spinal deformity classification: a validation study. Spine 37:1077-1082, 2012.
8. Lafage V, Schwab F, Patel A, et al. Pelvic tilt and truncal inclination: two key radiographic parameters in the setting of adults with spinal deformity. Spine 34:E599-E606, 2009.
9. Ames CP, Smith JS, Scheer JK, et al. Impact of spinopelvic alignment on decision making in deformity surgery in adults: a review. J Neurosurg Spine 16:547-564, 2012.
10. Schwab FJ, Blondel B, Bess S, et al; International Spine Study Group. Radiographical spinopelvic parameters and disability in the setting of adult spinal deformity: a prospective multicenter analysis. Spine 38:E803-E812, 2013.
11. Lazennec JY, Ramare S, Arafati N, et al. Sagittal alignment in lumbosacral fusion: relations between radiological parameters and pain. Eur Spine J 9:47-55, 2000.
12. Sarwahi V, Boachie-Adjei O, Backus SI, et al. Characterization of gait function in patients with postsurgical sagittal (flatback) deformity: a prospective study of 21 patients. Spine 27:2328-2337, 2002.
13. Yoshimoto H, Sato S, Masuda T, et al. Spinopelvic alignment in patients with osteoarthrosis of the hip: a radiographic comparison to patients with low back pain. Spine 30:1650-1657, 2005.
14. Glassman SD, Bridwell K, Dimar JR, et al. The impact of positive sagittal balance in adult spinal deformity. Spine 30:2024-2029, 2005.
15. Schwab F, Patel A, Ungar B, et al. Adult spinal deformity-postoperative standing imbalance: how much can you tolerate? An overview of key parameters in assessing alignment and planning corrective surgery. Spine 35:2224-2231, 2010.
16. Blondel B, Schwab F, Ungar B, et al. Impact of magnitude and percentage of global sagittal plane correction on health-related quality of life at 2-years follow-up. Neurosurgery 71:341-348; discussion 348, 2012.
17. Smith-Petersen MN, Larson CB, Aufranc OE. Osteotomy of the spine for correction of flexion deformity in rheumatoid arthritis. Clin Orthop Relat Res 66:6-9, 1969.
18. La Marca F, Brumblay H. Smith-Petersen osteotomy in thoracolumbar deformity surgery. Neurosurgery 63(3 Suppl):163-170, 2008.
19. Sansur CA, Fu KM, Oskouian RJ Jr, et al. Surgical management of global sagittal deformity in ankylosing spondylitis. Neurosurg Focus 24:E8, 2008.
20. Smith JS, Sansur CA, Donaldson WF III, et al. Short-term morbidity and mortality associated with correction of thoracolumbar fixed sagittal plane deformity: a report from the Scoliosis Research Society Morbidity and Mortality Committee. Spine 36:958-964, 2011.
21. Thomasen E. Vertebral osteotomy for correction of kyphosis in ankylosing spondylitis. Clin Orthop Relat Res 194:142-152, 1985.
22. Deviren V, Scheer JK, Ames CP. Technique of cervicothoracic junction pedicle subtraction osteotomy for cervical sagittal imbalance: report of 11 cases. J Neurosurg Spine 15:174-181, 2011.
23. Gill JB, Levin A, Burd T, et al. Corrective osteotomies in spine surgery. J Bone Joint Surg Am 90:2509-2520, 2008.

24. Li F, Sagi HC, Liu B, et al. Comparative evaluation of single-level closing-wedge vertebral osteotomies for the correction of fixed kyphotic deformity of the lumbar spine: a cadaveric study. Spine 26:2385-2391, 2001.

25. Gupta MC, Kebaish K, Blondel B, et al. Spinal osteotomies for rigid deformities. Neurosurg Clin N Am 24:203-211, 2013.

26. Kim YJ, Bridwell KH, Lenke LG, et al. Results of lumbar pedicle subtraction osteotomies for fixed sagittal imbalance: a minimum 5-year follow-up study. Spine 32:2189-2197, 2007.

27. Smith JS, Singh M, Klineberg E, et al; International Spine Study Group. Surgical treatment of pathological loss of lumbar lordosis (flatback) in patients with normal sagittal vertical axis achieves similar clinical improvement as surgical treatment of elevated sagittal vertical axis. J Neurosurg Spine 21:160-170, 2014.

28. Smith JS, Shaffrey CI, Ames CP, et al. Assessment of symptomatic rod fracture after posterior instrumented fusion for adult spinal deformity. Neurosurgery 71:862-867, 2012.

29. Tang JA, Leasure JM, Smith JS, et al. Effect of severity of rod contour on posterior rod failure in the setting of lumbar pedicle subtraction osteotomy (PSO): a biomechanical study. Neurosurgery 72:276-282; discussion 283, 2013.

30. Smith JS, Shaffrey CI, Glassman SD, et al. Risk-benefit assessment of surgery for adult scoliosis: an analysis based on patient age. Spine 36:817-824, 2011.

31. Cho KJ, Bridwell KH, Lenke LG, et al. Comparison of Smith-Petersen versus pedicle subtraction osteotomy for the correction of fixed sagittal imbalance. Spine 30:2030-2037; discussion 2038, 2005.

32. Schwab FJ, Hawkinson N, Lafage V, et al; International Spine Study Group. Risk factors for major peri-operative complications in adult spinal deformity surgery: a multi-center review of 953 consecutive patients. Eur Spine J 21:2603-2610, 2012.

40

Vertebral Column Resection for Restoration of Spinal Alignment

Isaac O. Karikari ▪ *Lawrence G. Lenke*

Rigid spinal malalignment can present in the coronal plane, the sagittal plane, or a combination of both. The treatment of any type of spinal malalignment depends on whether the deformity is fixed or flexible. With stiff or flexible deformities, posterior column osteotomies (Ponte or Smith-Petersen) can be useful for the restoration of normal alignment.[1] Deformities that are fixed or fused often require three-column osteotomies to restore normal alignment. These osteotomies consist of pedicle subtraction osteotomies or vertebral column resections (VCRs).[1] The VCR technique involves the complete resection of one or more vertebral segments in their entirety, including the posterior elements (spinous process, laminae, and pedicles), the vertebral body, and the adjacent discs; this allows circumferential access to the vertebral column and the spinal cord. VCRs can be used to treat a diverse spectrum of pathologies that affect the thoracic and lumbar spine, including spinal column tumors, hemivertebrae, infection, trauma, and complex structural deformities. During the late 1980s Bradford[2] was the first to describe the use of VCR for the correction of severe and rigid spinal deformities. Boachie-Adjei and Bradford[3] later published a case series of 16 patients who underwent circumferential VCR. In 2005 Suk et al[4] were the first to describe an all-posterior VCR technique for rigid spinal deformity. A VCR facilitates powerful correction of severe spinal deformities. During the past decade it has become a major component in the armamentarium of many spinal deformity surgeons who treat severe and rigid deformities.[5]

INDICATIONS AND CONTRAINDICATIONS

The VCR technique is indicated for cases in which less aggressive surgical options would be inadequate for the correction of a given spinal deformity. Severe fixed coronal and sagittal malalignment, global kyphosis, angular kyphosis, and kyphoscoliosis are common indications for a VCR. Revision deformity surgery in which the presence of a fusion mass creates spinal rigidity may also necessitate a VCR to allow optimal correction. Any disease process with vertebral body involvement and ventral or ventrolateral spinal cord compression can be treated with a VCR.[5-7] A case example is illustrated in Fig. 40-1.

The VCR procedure is technically demanding and often performed in patients with severe deformities, therefore it should be executed by spine surgeons with adequate experience and avoided by novices. A neurologically intact patient with unobtainable neuromonitoring data is a relative contraindication to the procedure unless multiple wake-up tests are planned and can be reliably executed. Any deformity that can be treated with less complex osteotomies (for example, posterior column osteotomies) should not be treated with VCR. An example of a case in which VCR would not be the best option is shown in Fig. 40-2.

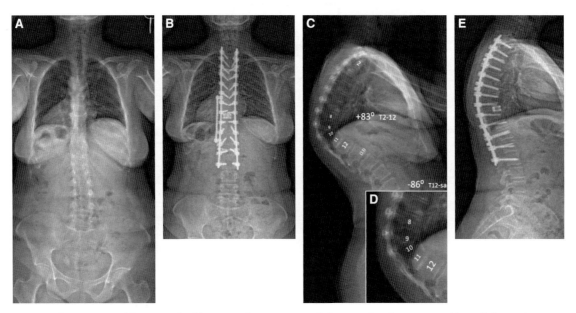

Fig. 40-1 This 51-year-old woman had longstanding congenital thoracic kyphosis caused by a failure of segmentation and lumbar hyperlordosis. She had increasing back pain but no leg pain. She underwent a T10 vertebral column resection with partial T9 and T11 corpectomies and an instrumented posterior spinal fusion from T2-L2.

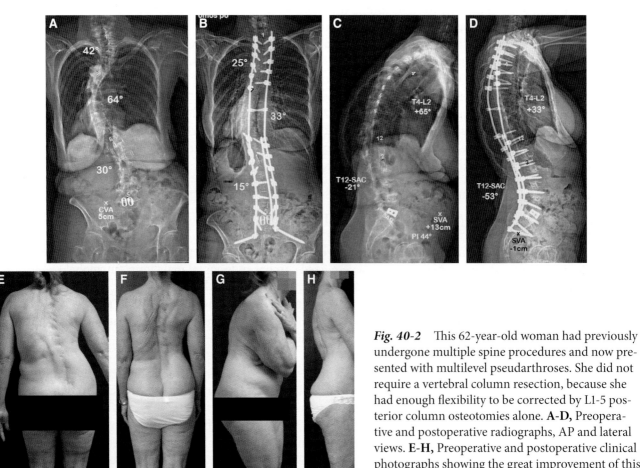

Fig. 40-2 This 62-year-old woman had previously undergone multiple spine procedures and now presented with multilevel pseudarthroses. She did not require a vertebral column resection, because she had enough flexibility to be corrected by L1-5 posterior column osteotomies alone. **A-D,** Preoperative and postoperative radiographs, AP and lateral views. **E-H,** Preoperative and postoperative clinical photographs showing the great improvement of this patient's deformity.

PREOPERATIVE PLANNING

PHYSICAL EXAMINATION

A thorough history, physical examination, and neurologic examination are imperative to the preoperative evaluation. It is not uncommon for some patients—especially those with angular kyphosis—to present with thoracic myelopathy. All attempts should be made to assess the relative flexibility of the deformity. This is accomplished by examining the patient in the supine, prone, suspended, and stretched positions. Attention should be paid to overall sagittal/coronal balance, shoulder height, rib prominences, abdominal creases, pelvic obliquity, hamstring contractures, and leg-length discrepancies. Because many patients—especially in the pediatric population—carry concomitant diagnoses or undiagnosed conditions, genetic, cardiopulmonary, hematologic, and neurologic consultations may be needed for optimization prior to surgery. The effects of spinal deformity on overall pulmonary function necessitate pulmonary function testing before surgery.

RADIOGRAPHIC EXAMINATION

In addition to the routine erect, side-bending, and recumbent diagnostic radiographs, further radiographic evaluation is useful when planning a VCR for severe deformity. This includes a three-dimensional CT scan of the spine that accurately depicts the anterior and posterior vertebral bony landmarks, some of which are not well visualized on plain radiographs. Anatomic three-dimensional models of severe deformities can be quite helpful for delineating the patient's precise anatomy. An MRI of the entire neural axis is required to gain a better appreciation of any craniocervical junctional abnormalities (for example, Chiari malformations, syringomyelia, or intrinsic spinal cord lesions) and to assess the overall caliber and position of the spinal cord.

A complete laboratory evaluation that includes a complete blood count, chemistry panel, nutritional values, and platelet function assessment should be performed. Blood products must be available intraoperatively as a result of the extensive nature and length of the surgical procedure.

OPERATIVE TECHNIQUE

ANESTHETIC CONSIDERATIONS

One of the most critical components of a safe VCR is the presence of anesthesia personnel with vast experience providing intraoperative care for complex spine cases. All patients require central venous access and arterial lines for strict blood pressure monitoring. For cases that involve severe proximal thoracic or cervicothoracic deformities, fiberoptic intubation may be required. Because VCR procedures are often associated with significant blood loss, the use of antifibrinolytic agents is highly recommended.[8] At our institution, we prefer tranexamic acid given as a 50 mg/kg loading dose and a 5 mg/kg maintenance dose for pediatric patients and a 10 mg/kg loading dose and a 1 mg/kg maintenance dose for adults during the entire procedure. Strict blood pressure control with the maintenance of a mean arterial pressure between 75 and 80 mm Hg is required throughout the case. The anesthesiology team should make all attempts to prevent sudden hypotension.

SPINAL CORD MONITORING

Intraoperative monitoring of the sensory and motor spinal tracts is critical for the safe execution of a VCR.[9] This can be accomplished in the form of somatosensory evoked potentials and either transcranial motor evoked potentials or descending neurogenic evoked potentials continuously throughout the procedure. Spontaneous EMGs can be useful when working in the lumbar spine. EMGs can also be used in a triggered fashion to test the integrity of pedicle screws from T6-S1. In unique situations (for example, patients with prior intraspinal lesions, tethered cord release, or Charcot-Marie-Tooth disease), spinal cord monitoring may not be obtainable. Such cases carry a high risk of neurologic deficit and will therefore require multiple intraoperative wake-up tests for the confirmation of normal or stable neurologic function.

INTRAOPERATIVE POSITIONING

Cases that require VCR tend to be inherently lengthy, so proper patient positioning is essential. The face and eyes should be free from any pressure. This is best achieved with the application of 5 to 15 pounds of traction via Gardner-Wells tongs or a halo; care must be taken to prevent overdistraction, as the tenuous spinal cord may not tolerate any further lengthening. The arms should be placed in a 90-degree position with the elbows resting on soft pads and the axillae free of any compression to prevent brachial plexopathy. The chest and pelvic pads should be positioned so that the abdomen hangs free, and the ankles and feet should be placed on pillows and free from any compression.

SETUP/EXPOSURE

The planned incision begins at the spinous process one level above the upper instrumented vertebra and ends at the spinous process of the planned lower instrumented vertebra. A subperiosteal dissection is then performed to expose the posterior elements out to the tips of the transverse processes (Fig. 40-3, A). At the level of the planned resection, the dissection should be continued laterally to expose at least 4 to 5 cm of rib (see Fig. 40-3, B). For patients with severe deformities with prominent rib humps, convex medial rib thoracoplasties may need to be performed to gain access to the transverse processes at the apex. The entire exposure should be performed expeditiously and thoroughly, with the aim of minimizing blood loss to prevent early coagulopathy.

POSTERIOR COLUMN OSTEOTOMIES AND SCREW PLACEMENT

After the exposure and accurate identification of the operating levels and anatomy, an inferior facetectomy is performed by removing 3 to 4 mm of the inferior facet at all levels that will be fused. This serves as a great source for autograft, creates a good surface area for fusion, and delineates the anatomy for pedicle screw placement. Multilevel posterior column osteotomies are then performed, typically around the apex of the deformity. This allows increased flexibility in the periapical segments and palpation of the medial pedicle on the concavity of the curve, which permits safe and efficient free-hand pedicle screw placement (Fig. 40-3, C). During the treatment of patients with angular kyphosis, it is important to obtain pedicle screw fixation before posterior column osteotomies are performed. This avoids the risks of a sagging of the spinal column and subsequent ventral compression of the spinal cord, which can cause loss of spinal cord monitoring data. After the screws are placed, AP and lateral radiographs or intraoperative CT scans are obtained to verify the position of the screws. Every screw placed from T6 to the sacrum is tested with triggered EMG-based screw stimulation.

VERTEBRAL COLUMN RESECTION

If the VCR is to be performed in the thoracic spine, a costotransversectomy is first performed bilaterally at the level of the planned resection by removing 4 to 5 cm of the medial rib (see Fig. 40-3, B). A wide laminectomy that spans from the inferior aspect of the pedicle above the planned resection to the superior pole of the pedicle below the planned resection is performed (Fig. 40-3, D). A temporary rod is then placed on the contralateral side to prevent inadvertent subluxation of the spine (Fig. 40-3, E). The dura should be freed of all scar tissue and epidural fat. In the thoracic spine the corresponding nerve roots are first cross-clamped for approximately 5 minutes to ensure that blood flow to the spinal cord is not compromised. If there are no changes in neurophysiologic monitoring data, the clamp is removed, and the nerve is double ligated with a 2-0 silk suture medial to the dorsal root ganglion. This is most commonly performed unilaterally, but it can be bilateral if absolutely required.

The pedicles are then isolated with a combination of Bovie electrocautery and a No. 1 Penfield dissector. The lateral vertebral wall is carefully dissected free of soft tissue, making sure not to violate of the parietal pleura (Fig. 40-3, *F*). A spoon retractor or a malleable retractor is placed to protect the ventral and lateral vasculature and viscera. Removal of the vertebral segment begins with removal of the pedicle using a combination of cutting burrs, curettes, and Leksell rongeurs. The concavity of the deformity is often quite sclerotic, which necessitates its removal with the use of a high-speed burr. The concave pedicle should be removed first to prevent the pooling of blood in the concavity that is created if the convex pedicle is removed first. The cancellous bone in the vertebral body is then removed with a curette and saved for later use as bone graft. The entire vertebral body is removed except for the ventral cortical shell, which should be thin enough to allow easy closure of the remaining spinal column. Next, the discs above and below are removed with the use of a combination of curettes, pituitary rongeurs, and a high-speed burr, with care taken to not violate the endplates (Fig. 40-3, *G* through *I*). The remaining posterior vertebral wall should be thinned down and removed with a combination of Kerrison rongeurs and a customized posterior wall impactor. To prevent inadvertent injury to the spinal cord, all force should be directed ventrally into the created defect at all times (Fig. 40-3, *J* and *K*). It is not uncommon to encounter significant bleeding from the epidural venous plexus during this stage. Such bleeding can be controlled effectively with a combination of Floseal, Gelfoam, cottonoids, and careful use of bipolar electrocautery. After the removal of all bone (aside from the ventral cortical rim), the defect is closed. This is a critical part of the case, and it requires keen attention from the neuromonitoring team and the anesthesiologist.

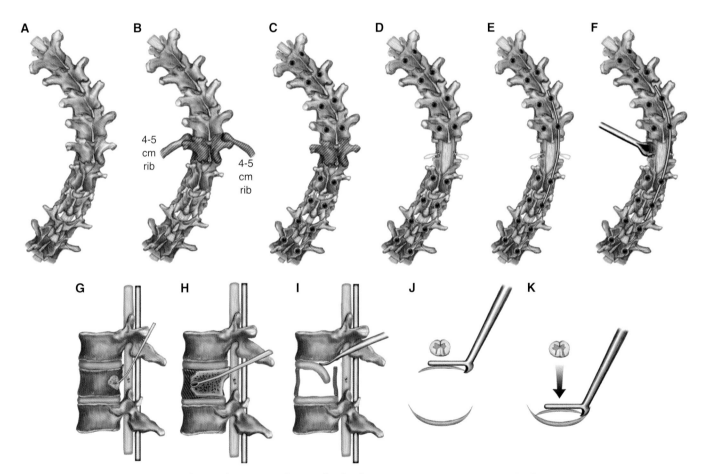

Fig. 40-3 Key steps in the performance of a vertebral column resection. **A,** Exposure. **B,** Costotransversectomy. **C,** Pedicle screw placement. **D,** Laminectomy. **E,** Placement of a temporary rod. **F,** Vertebral body exposure. **G,** Lateral vertebral body access. **H,** Vertebral body removal. **I,** Discectomy. **J,** Posterior vertebral body wall impactor placement. **K,** Impaction of the posterior wall.

Continued

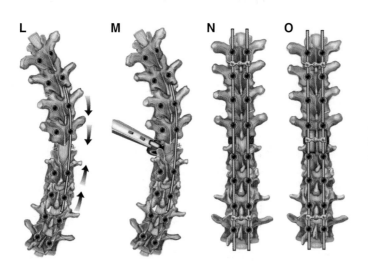

Fig. 40-3, cont'd **L,** Compression closure. **M,** Cage placement. **N,** Final correction. **O,** Rib bridge graft.

Several options exist to execute closure of the vertebral resection site. The closure always begins on the convexity with a compression force. Compression can be accomplished with an adjacent screw and a rod gripper, with an adjacent screw-to-screw technique, or with a construct-to-construct technique based on dominoes positioned at the apex of the deformity connecting the two halves of the vertebral column. Construct-to-construct closure is preferable, as it distributes forces across multiple segments rather than on a single screw (Fig. 40-3, *L*). Compression should be performed slowly, and the dura and the epidural spaces should be inspected carefully after each round of compression. When adequate compression and closure of the resection is complete, an appropriately sized interbody cage is inserted to act as a hinge for further correction and to prevent excessive shortening of the spinal canal (Fig. 40-3, *M*). A permanent rod is then placed on the contralateral side, and the temporary rod is replaced with a permanent rod (Fig. 40-3, *N*). An intraoperative radiograph is obtained, and this is followed by decortication and bone grafting. The laminectomy defect is covered with the previously harvested ribs or an allograft rib (Fig. 40-3, *O*). The rib graft is split in half longitudinally, with the cancellous surface placed along the entire laminectomy defect from the lamina above to the lamina below. This creates a bridge of bone that protects the dura and provides a posterior surface area for fusion. The rib grafts are secured with either Mersilene tape or 1-0 Vicryl sutures. Hemostasis is obtained, and the wound is closed in layers over two Hemovac drains (one subfascial and one suprafascial). The patient is then moved to a regular bed, and an intraoperative wake-up test is performed while the patient is still intubated.

POTENTIAL COMPLICATIONS AND MANAGEMENT

Even in the most experienced hands, the posterior VCR is a highly technical and challenging procedure. One of the most concerning events is the intraoperative loss of neuromonitoring motor data. This can occur at any stage of the procedure, and the surgeon and the operative team need to be well versed in troubleshooting and expeditiously making an accurate diagnosis. The patient's mean blood pressure should be kept at a minimum of 80 to 90 mm Hg when there is a loss of motor data. The surgeon should carefully inspect the surgical field to confirm that there is no epidural compression caused by scar tissue, bony or disc fragments, ligaments, or vertebral column subluxation. Typically a loss of data is associated with a corrective maneuver, so the reversal of any such maneuver should be performed by the surgeon. Spinal subluxation is not uncommon in these cases, and can cause ventral, dorsal, or lateral compression of the spinal cord. The use of multiaxial reduction screws at the apices of the deformity can be vital to reducing subluxation if it occurs. As previously discussed, placement of a temporary rod early during the bony resection is mandatory to prevent sudden subluxation. If the loss of data occurs as a result of overshortening, distracting the segment back open and placing a larger interbody cage can restore the appropriate anterior length to the spinal cord.

PATIENT EXAMPLE

This 54-year-old woman presented with severe lumbar collapsing kyphoscoliosis after having undergone neuroblastoma resection and radiation when she was a child. She had an L2 VCR with anterior spinal fusion from L1-3, transforaminal lumbar interbody fusions, and instrumented posterior spinal fusion from T8-sacrum/ilium. In Fig. 40-4 this patient is shown both preoperatively and postoperatively. At her 1-year follow-up visit, she was doing very well and had no complaints. She has marked correction of her severe deformity and states that she is very active. Her correction is well maintained, and she has good alignment and balance.

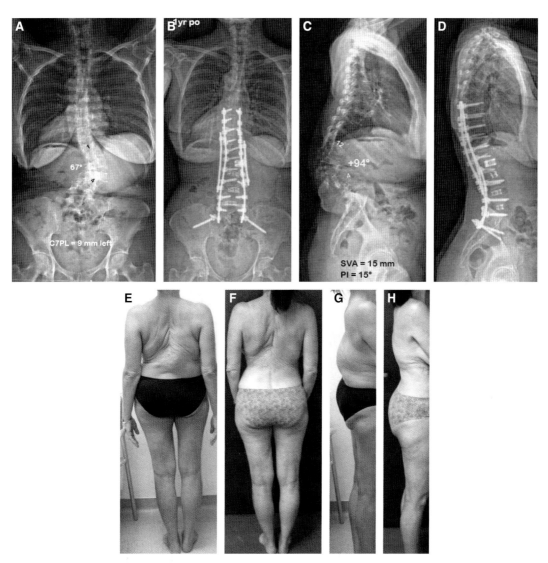

Fig. 40-4 **A-D,** Preoperative and postoperative radiographs, AP and lateral views. **E-H,** Preoperative and postoperative clinical photographs show the great improvement of this patient's deformity.

CONCLUSION

When it is properly executed, the posterior thoracic VCR provides complete resection of all vertebral elements, including 360 degrees neural decompression, and allows marked spinal column realignment.[2-7,10] This technically demanding yet powerful procedure can result in dramatic radiographic and clinical correction. At our institution, it has replaced separate anterior and posterior approaches for patients with severe and/or rigid spinal deformities.

REFERENCES

1. Cho KJ, Bridwell KH, Lenke LG, et al. Comparison of Smith-Petersen versus pedicle subtraction osteotomy for the correction of fixed sagittal imbalance. Spine 30:2030-2037, 2005.
2. Bradford DS. Vertebral column resection. Orthop Trans 11:502, 1987.
3. Boachie-Adjei O, Bradford DS. Vertebral column resection and arthrodesis for complex spinal deformities. J Spinal Disord 4:193-202, 1991.
4. Suk SI, Chung ER, Kim JH, et al. Posterior vertebral column resection for severe rigid scoliosis. Spine 30:1682-1687, 2005.
5. Lenke LG, Sides BA, Koester LA, et al. Vertebral column resection for the treatment of severe spinal deformity. Clin Orthop Relat Res 468:687-699, 2010.
6. Lenke LG, O'Leary PT, Bridwell KH, et al. Posterior vertebral column resection for severe pediatric deformity: minimum two-year follow-up of thirty-five consecutive patients. Spine 34:2213-2221, 2009.
7. Lenke LG, Newton PO, Sucato DJ, et al. Complications after 147 consecutive vertebral column resections for severe pediatric spinal deformity: a multicenter analysis. Spine 38:119-132, 2013.
8. Newton PO, Bastrom TP, Emans JB, et al. Antifibrinolytic agents reduce blood loss during pediatric vertebral column resection procedures. Spine 37:E1459-E1463, 2012.
9. Raynor BL, Bright JD, Lenke LG, et al. Significant change or loss of intraoperative monitoring data: a 25-year experience in 12,375 spinal surgeries. Spine 38:E101-E108, 2013.
10. Lenke LG. Posterior vertebral column resection (VCR), 2011. Available at *www.srs.org*.

41

Spinopelvic Fixation Techniques

Rishi Wadhwa ▪ *Hai V. Le* ▪ *Rajiv Saigal* ▪ *Praveen V. Mummaneni*

Long-instrumented spinal fusion extending from L2 or higher to the sacrum can exert significant biomechanical strain on S1 pedicle screws.[1,2] Sacral pedicle screw fixation in such long-segment cases is prone to a high incidence of screw pullout, pseudarthrosis, and failure.[3-6] To overcome this problem, spine surgeons often consider supplemental spinopelvic fixation to augment S1 pedicle screw fixation.

Today, the most commonly used spinopelvic fixation technique is iliac (pelvic) screw fixation. The addition of iliac screws has the biomechanical advantage of decreasing the lumbosacral range of motion and S1 screw-bending moments.[2] Iliac screw fixation in multilevel fusion (above L3 to S1) can help to reduce lumbosacral screw strain, which has been shown to decrease L5-S1 pseudarthrosis rates and sacral insufficiency fractures at S1-2.[1,7] Spinopelvic fixation serves as a temporary scaffolding to allow lumbosacral fusion to occur. Iliac fixation does not typically result in fusion across the sacroiliac joint.

In this chapter, we review common spinopelvic fixation techniques and detail the operative technique for iliac screw fixation, which has become the mainstay for supplemental spinopelvic fixation. Case examples are presented to highlight key concepts and principles.

INDICATIONS AND CONTRAINDICATIONS

The indications for spinopelvic fixation are summarized in Box 41-1.[1] The most common indications are grade II or higher L5-S1 spondylolisthesis and long-segment fusions to the sacrum (L2 or above to S1) for various spinal pathologies, including degenerative kyphoscoliosis and trauma.

Relative contraindications for long-segment spinal and spinopelvic fixation include severe osteoporosis and severe malnutrition, both of which can increase the rate of pseudarthrosis and complications.[8] Patients with poor bone quality or insufficient bony pelvic structures, for example, congenital caudal regression syndrome and prior iliac fracture with subsequent malunion or nonunion, may not be good candidates for spinopelvic fixation because of altered anatomy or poor bone quality that is insufficient for optimal screw purchase.[9]

PREOPERATIVE PLANNING

As with all preoperative planning, a thorough history is obtained and a physical examination is performed before surgery. Prior spinal surgical history is reviewed. Preoperative MRI is obtained to evaluate for spinal and foraminal stenosis. In addition, a CT scan is useful to assess bone quality, to plan screw sizes and trajectories, and for three-dimensional evaluation of all spinal deformity. A DEXA scan can be completed

---

BOX 41-1   Indications for Extension of Lumbosacral Fusions to the Ilium

- Grade II or higher L5-S1 spondylolisthesis
- Long-segment fusions to the sacrum (L2 or above to S1)
  - Spinal deformity (scoliosis or kyphosis)
  - Lumbar fractures
    - Trauma
    - Osteomyelitis
    - Neoplasm
- Lesions that destroy the sacrum
  - Neoplasm
  - Osteomyelitis
  - Fractures
- Treatment of L5-S1 pseudarthrosis

Adapted from Tumialan LM, Mummaneni PV. Long-segment spinal fixation using pelvic screws. Neurosurgery 63:183-190, 2008.

---

if indicated to assess for osteopenia and osteoporosis.[10] Medical comorbitities should be thoroughly evaluated and optimized before surgery.

Spinopelvic parameters (pelvic tilt, sacral slope, and pelvic incidence) are assessed on 36-inch, standing long-cassette radiographs. Cobb angles (coronal and sagittal), sagittal vertical axis, and coronal olisthesis are measured preoperatively. The degree of correctable deformity should be planned preoperatively. The surgical plan should ideally reestablish lumbar lordosis to within 10 degrees of the pelvic incidence. The sagittal vertical axis should be restored to within 5 cm of the posterior sacral endplate.

OVERVIEW OF SPINOPELVIC FIXATION TECHNIQUES

SACRAL ALAR SCREW FIXATION

Sacral alar screw fixation involves the unicortical placement of sacral alar screws anterolaterally toward the sacral wings. The screw entry point is 5 mm cephalad to the S1 foramen and midway between the distal aspect of the superior articular process and the S1 foramen. The screw is directed 30 to 40 degrees laterally and 25 degrees caudally. Sacral alar screw length typically averages 35 mm.[11,12] The screws can be integrated with a longitudinal connector. Placement of a sacral alar screw in a combination plate with an S1 screw can add up to 20% to 30% of cantilever force resistance.[13,14] Care must be taken to prevent damage to nearby structures, including the lumbosacral trunk, internal iliac vein, and sacroiliac joint[11,12] (see Fig. 41-1).

GALVESTON ILIAC FIXATION

Allen and Ferguson first described Galveston iliac fixation in 1982.[15] The technique was historically useful in cases of neuromuscular scoliosis. It requires placement of a contoured, L-shaped rod (L-rod) into each ilium. The entry point is the posterior superior iliac spine (PSIS). An L-rod is typically directed 20 to 25 degrees laterally from the PSIS and 30 to 35 degrees caudally.[16] It is extended between the inner and outer tables of the pelvis until it is positioned roughly 1.5 cm above the greater sciatic notch.[16-18] The L-rods are subsequently attached to the thoracolumbar fusion construct with sublaminar wires, pedicle screws, or hooks to achieve spinopelvic fixation.[19] L-rods offer great resistance against flexion and lateral bending but not axial pullout.[19] For this reason, kyphosing forces can cause distal fixation pullout and rod migration.[20,21] L-rods can be technically challenging to contour to the acceptable curvature, and rod bend points are prone to fracture.[22]

Jackson Intrasacral Rod Fixation

Jackson and McManus[23] introduced the concept of sacral buttressing and observed that the ilia and the sacroiliac ligaments supporting the posterolateral sacrum can serve as a buttress for rod insertion.[19] Intrasacral rod fixation involves the insertion of an S1 pedicle screw toward the sacral promontory. A 7 mm rod is then directed distally into the posterolateral sacrum inferior to the S1 screw.[24] The rods are attached to the segmental pedicle screws, starting at the S1 level and extending cephalad to achieve spinopelvic fixation.[19] Because this fixation is entirely intrasacral, the sacroiliac joint is not traversed, and the iliac crests are not compromised.[19,23] Intrasacral rod fixation is not recommended for patients with low bone quality, because the lateral sacral masses need to be strong enough for rod anchorage to prevent axial pullout.[19] The technique is relatively contraindicated in patients with congenital or acquired pathologies that disrupt the integrity of the proximal sacrum such as tumors and infections.[19,23,24]

Sacral Alar Iliac Fixation

Sacral alar iliac fixation involves the placement of screws from S2 into the ilia[25-27] (Fig. 41-1). The entry point for S2 alar iliac (S2AI) screws is 2 to 4 mm lateral and 4 to 8 mm distal to the S1 foramen. This deep entry point overcomes the problem of implant prominence often observed with iliac screw fixation.[28] Their medial entry point places the S2AI screws directly in line with the S1 pedicle screws, thus allowing longitudinal alignment with the lumbosacral rod. The rods can be connected directly to the bony anchors without the use of medial-to-lateral connectors or the need for multiple separate fascial incisions.[28,29] Ideally, a screw should be angled 40 degrees laterally in the transverse plane and 40 degrees caudally in the sagittal plane and aimed directly toward the anterior superior iliac spine.[30] Sacral alar iliac fixation provides greater pullout strength, because the screws cross the sacroiliac joint. Pullout strength is improved when the S2AI screw passes adjacent to the thick cortical bone immediately above the greater sciatic notch.[25-27] An AP fluoroscopic view and obturator outlet view are recommended in S2AI screw placement to better visualize the screw as it crosses the SI joint.[31,32] S2AI screw length is typically 80 to 100 mm, which is more than 20 mm longer than an average iliac screw length (65 to 80 mm). Typical screw diameters are 7 to 8 mm. A power drill may be needed to penetrate the thick cortical bone of the sacroiliac joint.

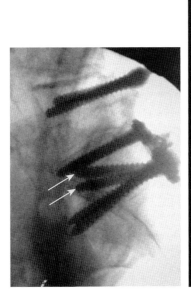 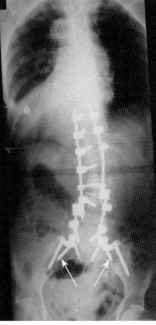

Fig. 41-1 Placement of sacral alar screw *(arrows)*.

ILIAC SCREW FIXATION

Iliac screw fixation involves the placement of iliac screws through the ilium to stabilize the lumbosacral junction for L5-S1 fusion (Fig. 41-2). Several authors[3,5] have previously described the steps for this technique, including Tumialan and Mummaneni[1] (Box 41-2). The patient is positioned prone. The paraspinal muscles are mobilized to expose the PSIS. The ideal entry point is 1 cm deep to the superficial edge of the PSIS and 1 cm proximal to the palpated inferior end of the PSIS.[1,19] Intraoperative fluoroscopy can help to identify the *teardrop* on the obturator outlet oblique view, which serves as the target for the iliac screw (Fig. 41-3). The bony cortex is decorticated using a high-speed burr or awl. Under fluoroscopy guidance, a gear-shift probe is used to create a pilot hole, aiming toward the anterior superior iliac spine. The screw path is then palpated with a ballpoint probe to verify that the cortical walls have not been violated. The screw length is measured, and the screw path is tapped. The iliac screw is finally inserted, angled 30 to 45 degrees downward in the axial plane and 30 to 45 degrees inferiorly in the coronal plane. The iliac screws are then connected to the lumbosacral rods. A typical iliac screw length is 65 to 80 mm.[19,33]

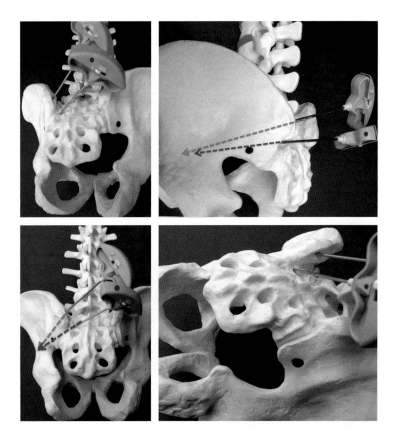

Fig. 41-2   The entry point and trajectory of an S2AI screw *(red)* and an iliac screw *(blue)* is shown in multiple views.

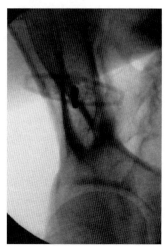

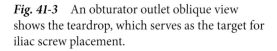

Fig. 41-3   An obturator outlet oblique view shows the teardrop, which serves as the target for iliac screw placement.

BOX 41-2   Steps in Pelvic Screw Fixation Technique

1. The posterior superior iliac spine is exposed.
2. The entry point for the pelvic screw (iliac screw) is located as follows:
   - 1 cm deep to the superficial edge of the posterior superior iliac spine
   - 1 cm proximal to the palpated inferior end of the posterior superior iliac spine
3. The entry point is decorticated with a drill or awl.
4. The pilot hole for the screw is created with a gearshift probe.
   - The target is the thick bone just above the greater sciatic notch.
   - The pilot hole is typically angled 30 to 45 degrees downward in the axial plane and 30 to 45 degrees inferiorly in the coronal plane.
   - The depth is usually 60 to 80 mm.
   - AP, pelvic inlet, and obturator outlet fluoroscopic views help to guide the trajectory.
   - Exposure of the superficial surface of ilium can be helpful to guide the screw trajectory in the axial plane.
5. A pilot hole is tapped with an undersized tap.
6. Probing is performed to detect cortical wall violation.
7. A pelvic screw is placed, with the head recessed into the posterior superior iliac spine.
8. The screw is connected to a lumbosacral rod inferior to the S1 level.
   - A connector can be used.

Adapted from Tumialan LM, Mummaneni PV. Long-segment spinal fixation using pelvic screws. Neurosurgery 63:183-190, 2008.

POTENTIAL COMPLICATIONS AND MANAGEMENT

Several complications are possible with iliac screw fixation, including damage to neurovascular structures within the greater sciatic notch (that is, the sciatic nerve and superior gluteal artery). Injury to the superior gluteal artery can lead to pelvic hematoma, which can be clinically undetectable temporarily. Intraoperative hypotension, serially decreasing hematocrit values, or pelvic pain/mass should raise suspicion. Endovascular embolization of this injury may be necessary, because the vessel can retract into the pelvis. Injury to the acetabulum occurs rarely if the screw is too long and the trajectory is too inferior. Violation of the lateral cortical surface of the pelvis is fairly common and can be prevented by angling the screw more medially. One obvious advantage of this technique is the ease of PSIS identification for screw placement. Another advantage is its modularity and ease of connection to the lumbosacral rods.[19,34] A common drawback of this technique is the high rate of implant prominence, which occurs if the surgeon does not use the deep entry point that we described. Prominent screw heads can be prevented by choosing an entry point that is slightly deep to the PSIS, along the medial aspect of the inner table of the ilium.[1,35,36]

Potential complications of iliac screw fixation include local irritation from the iliac screw head, pseudarthrosis of L5-S1, and infection. The iliac screw head can be seated well below the PSIS to minimize implant prominence especially in slender patients. To minimize the risk for lumbosacral pseudarthrosis, surgeons should consider incorporating interbody grafts at L5-S1.

PATIENT EXAMPLES

This 41-year-old woman presented with significant back pain. She had Harrington rods placed over a decade ago to treat a traumatic spinal fracture. She was neurologically intact. Preoperative 36-inch long-cassette radiographs revealed rods at L1-4, with a lumbar flat back and a 39-degree LL-PI mismatch. She also has 2.5 cm of coronal offset and a 17-degree scoliosis apex to the left (Fig. 41-4, *A* and *B*). We performed a two-stage surgery for correction. Initially, she underwent a two-level ALIF at L4-5 and L5-1. Two days later, Harrington rods were removed, and she had T11-pelvis fixation with an L3-4 TLIF and Smith-Petersen osteotomies at L1-4. On postoperative 36-inch long-cassette radiographs, her LL-PI mismatch is reduced to 10 degrees, with 6 degrees coronal scoliosis (Fig. 41-4, *C* and *D*). Her back pain is significantly improved.

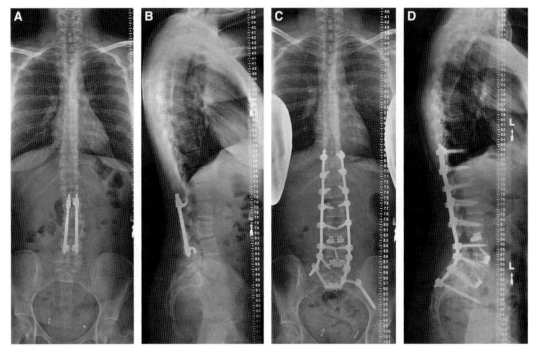

Fig. 41-4   **A** and **B,** This patient's preoperative scoliosis radiographs showed Harrington rods from L1-4 and a 39-degree LL-PI mismatch. She had 2.5 cm of coronal offset and a 17-degree scoliosis apex to the left. **C** and **D,** Postoperative scoliosis radiographs show an LL-PI mismatch of approximately 10 degrees, with 6 degrees coronal scoliosis.

This 64-year-old woman had severe back pain. Preoperative 36-inch long-cassette radiographs showed coronal and sagittal imbalance from a decompensated kyphoscoliosis. She had an LL-PI mismatch of 21 degrees and a lumbar coronal deformity with the apex at L3-4. Her coronal Cobb angle measured 35 degrees (Fig. 41-5, *A* and *B*). She underwent T10 to pelvis fixation with L1-S1 facet osteotomies and L4-5 and L5-S1 transforaminal lumbar interbody fusions. Postoperative 36-inch long-cassette radiographs show an LL-PI mismatch of 9 degrees and a coronal Cobb angle of 15 degrees (Fig. 41-5, *C* and *D*). Her pain is improved after surgery.

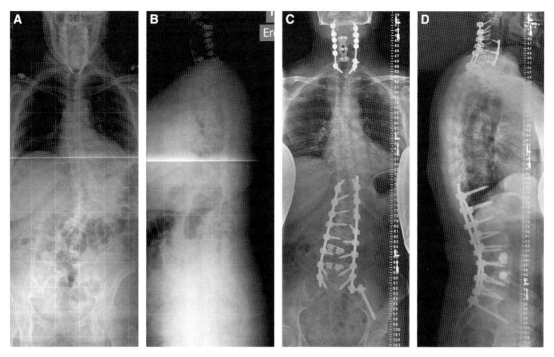

Fig. 41-5 **A** and **B,** This patient's preoperative scoliosis showed an LL-PI mismatch of 21 degrees and a lumbar coronal deformity with the apex at L3-4. The coronal Cobb angle measured 35 degrees. **C** and **D,** Postoperative scoliosis radiographs show an LL-PI mismatch of 9 degrees and a coronal Cobb angle of 15 degrees.

CONCLUSION

Spinopelvic fixation provides additional stabilization across the lumbosacral junction and improved L5-S1 fusion, compared with traditional lumbosacral fixation alone. Several spinopelvic fixation techniques have been described. Most spine surgeons prefer iliac screw fixation for S1 screw augmentation.

REFERENCES

1. Tumialan LM, Mummaneni PV. Long-segment spinal fixation using pelvic screws. Neurosurgery 63:183-190, 2008.
2. Mummaneni PV, Ondra SL, Haid RW. Principles of spinal deformity. II. Advances in the operative treatment of thoracolumbar deformity. Contemp Neurosurg 24:1-10, 2002.
3. Kuklo TR, Bridwell KH, Lewis SJ, et al. Minimum 2-year analysis of sacropelvic fixation and L5-S1 fusion using S1 and iliac screws. Spine 26:1976-1983, 2001.
4. Weistroffer JK, Perra JH, Lonstein JE, et al. Complications in long fusions to the sacrum for adult scoliosis: minimum five-year analysis of fifty patients. Spine 33:1478-1483, 2008.
5. Kostuik JP, Hall BB. Spinal fusions to the sacrum in adults with scoliosis. Spine 8:489-500, 1983.
6. Bridwell KH. Utilization of iliac screws and structural interbody grafting for revision spondylolisthesis surgery. Spine 30:S88-S96, 2005.
7. Tsuchiya K , Bridwell KH , Kuklo TR, et al. Minimum 5-year analysis of L5-S1 fusion using sacropelvic fixation (bilateral S1 and iliac screws) for spinal deformity. Spine 31:303-308, 2006.
8. Badlani N, Allen RT. Pelvic fixation. In Jandial R, McCormick PC, Black PM, eds. Core Techniques in Operative Neurosurgery. Philadelphia: Elsevier, 2011.
9. Saer E, Winter R, Lonstein J. Long scoliosis fusion to the sacrum in adults with nonparalytic scoliosis: an improved method. Spine 15:650-653, 1990.

10. Dabney K, Miller F, Lipton GE, et al. Correction of sagittal plane deformities with unit rod instrumentation in children with cerebral palsy. J Bone Joint Surg Am 86:156-168, 2004.

11. Kebaish K, Defrawy MH. Sacropelvic fixation. In Vacarro AR, Baron EM, eds. Spine Surgery: Operative Techniques, ed 2. Philadelphia: Elsevier, 2012.

12. Keeler KA, Kuklo TR. Sacropelvic instrumentation for disorders of the thoracolumbar spine. In Shen FH, Shaffrey CI, eds. Arthritis and Arthroplasty: The Spine. Philadelphia: Elsevier, 2010.

13. Leong JC, Lu WW, Zheng Y, et al. Comparison of the strengths of lumbosacral fixation achieved with techniques using one and two triangulated sacral screws. Spine 23:2289-2294, 1998.

14. McCord DH, Cunningham BW, Shono Y, et al. Biomechanical analysis of lumbosacral fixation. Spine 17(8 Suppl):S235-S243, 1992.

15. Allen BL Jr, Ferguson RL. The Galveston technique for L rod instrumentation of the scoliotic spine. Spine 7:276-284, 1982.

16. Shen FH, Mason JR, Shimer AL, et al. Pelvic fixation for adult scoliosis. Eur Spine J 22(Suppl 2):S265-S275, 2013.

17. Allen BL Jr, Ferguson RL. The Galveston technique of pelvic fixation with L-rod instrumentation of the spine. Spine 9:388-394, 1984.

18. Allen BL, Ferguson RL. A pictorial guide to the Galveston LRI pelvic fixation technique. Contemp Orthop 7:51-61, 1983.

19. Moshirfar Ali, Rand FF, Sponseller PD, et al. Pelvic fixation in spine surgery. Historical overview, indications, biomechanical relevance, and current techniques. J Bone Joint Surg Am 87:89-106, 2005.

20. Peelle MW, Lenke LG, Bridwell KH, et al. Comparison of pelvic fixation techniques in neuromuscular spinal deformity correction: Galveston rod versus iliac and lumbosacral screws. Spine 31:2392-2398, 2006.

21. Sink EL, Newton PO, Mubarak SJ, et al. Maintenance of sagittal plane alignment after surgical correction of spinal deformity in patients with cerebral palsy. Spine 28:1396-1403, 2003.

22. Early S, Mahar A, Oka R, et al. Biomechanical comparison of lumbosacral fixation using Luque-Galveston and Colorado II sacropelvic fixation: advantage of using locked proximal fixation. Spine 30:1396-1401, 2005.

23. Jackson RP, McManus AC. The iliac buttress. A computed tomographic study of sacral anatomy. Spine 18:1318-1328, 1993.

24. Jackson RP, Burton DC. Intrasacral (Jackson) and Galveston rod contouring and placement techniques. In Vaccaro AR, Albert TJ, eds. Spine Surgery: Tricks of the Trade, ed 2. New York: Thieme, 2009.

25. Sponseller P. The S2 portal to the ilium. Semin Spine Surg 2:83-87, 2007.

26. Mattei TA, Fassett DR. Low-profile pelvic fixation with sacral alar-iliac screws. Acta Neurochir 155:293-297, 2013.

27. Chang TL, Sponseller PD, Kebaish KM, et al. Low profile pelvic fixation: anatomic parameters for sacral alar-iliac fixation versus traditional iliac fixation. Spine 34:436-440, 2009.

28. Matteini LE, Kebaish KM, Volk WR, et al. An S-2 alar iliac pelvic fixation: technical note. Neurosurg Focus 28:E13-E16, 2010.

29. Dafrawy MH, Kebaish KM. Spinopelvic fixation techniques. In Eck JC, Vaccaro AR, eds. Surgical Atlas of Spinal Operations. New Delhi: Jaypee Brothers Medical Publishers, 2013.

30. Martin CT, Kebaish KM. Sacropelvic fixation techniques. In Rhee JM, Boden SD, Flynn JM, et al, eds. Operative Techniques in Spine Surgery. Philadelphia: Lippincott Williams & Wilkins, 2013.

31. O'Brien JR. Matteini L, Yu WD, et al. Feasibility of minimally invasive sacropelvic fixation: percutaneous S2 alar iliac fixation. Spine 35:460-464, 2010.

32. Martin CT, Witham TF, Kebaish KM. Sacropelvic fixation: two case reports of a new percutaneous technique. Spine 36:E618-E621, 2011.

33. Berry JL, Stahurski T, Asher MA. Morphometry of the supra sciatic notch intrailiac implant anchor passage. Spine 26:E143-E148, 2001.

34. Schwend RM, Sluyters R, Najdzionek J. The pylon concept of pelvic anchorage for spinal instrumentation in the human cadaver. Spine 28:542-547, 2003.

35. O'Brien MF. Sacropelvic fixation in spinal deformity. In DeWald RL, ed. Spinal Deformities: The Comprehensive Text. New York: Thieme, 2003.

36. Kuklo TR. Sacropelvic fixation options. In Mummaneni PV, Lenke LG, Haid RW, eds. Spinal Deformity: A Guide to Surgical Planning and Management. St Louis: Quality Medical Publishing, 2008.

42

Degenerative Sacral Fracture: Diagnosis and Treatment

Randall B. Graham ▪ *Tyler R. Koski*

Degenerative sacral fractures (also known as *sacral insufficiency fractures*) were first described in the early 1980s.[1] These fractures do not exhibit specific symptoms, and few epidemiologic data exist, so diagnosis is often delayed. They are considered a rare cause of low back pain, but their true occurrence is likely underreported. Nevertheless, the incidence of degenerative fractures of the sacrum and pelvis in patients with osteoporosis seems to be increasing, most likely because better imaging techniques are available.[2] Although the true incidence of these fractures is unknown, their potential prevalence has been estimated to be 1.8% in women older than 55 years presenting with low back pain.[3]

Degenerative fractures tend to occur in weakened bones under conditions of normal stress. Thus they are usually seen in older patients with osteoporosis, rheumatologic conditions, disorders of calcium metabolism, Paget's disease, or previous radiotherapy.[2] Rare cases have been described in younger patients, particularly military personnel and long-distance runners.[4] Degenerative fractures occurring during the final trimester of pregnancy and during the early postnatal period have also been reported.[5,6]

CLINICAL PRESENTATION

Symptoms of degenerative sacral fractures are variable and nonspecific. The most common complaint is acute intractable low back or pelvic pain that is rarely accompanied by pain in the legs, groin, or buttocks without a history of trauma. The pain is most often relieved by rest in a supine position and is exacerbated by weight-bearing activities. Neurologic deficits are rare but can be quite severe, occasionally presenting as acute cauda equina syndrome.[7]

Patients are typically tender over both the sacral area and the pubic symphysis, because up to 78% of cases are associated with pubic ramus fractures.[8] Other provocative maneuvers can be used, such as lateral sacral compression, the flexion-abduction-external-rotation (FABER) test, Gaenslen's test, and a squish test.[9]

LABORATORY FINDINGS

Although laboratory data are typically unremarkable, the presence of reversible causes of osteoporosis (such as osteomalacia, inflammatory arthritis, and parathyroid disorders) should be considered.[10] An appropriate laboratory workup should thus include levels of parathyroid hormone, calcium, phosphorous, vitamin D, urinary calcium, alkaline phosphatase, C-reactive protein, rheumatoid factor, and erythrocyte sedimentation rate.

PRETREATMENT IMAGING

Plain radiographs of the lumbar spine, sacrum, and pelvis are often the first imaging obtained, but they have limited sensitivity. Initially, these fractures can be shrouded by bowel gas, vascular calcifications, and fecal material. The fracture is then not seen until the healing process is underway. As mentioned previously, a concomitant fracture in the anterior pelvic ring in the setting of acute back pain without trauma is suspicious for a degenerative sacral fracture.

MRI is often considered the benchmark procedure for diagnosing these fractures.[2] They are typically observed as areas of T1 hypointensity and T2 hyperintensity with the higher signal of short tau inversion recovery (STIR) sequences. CT is a sensitive and specific alternative to MRI. CT scans can accurately localize fracture lines in multiple planes and are useful for determining various stages of healing by highlighting sclerotic changes.[9]

FRACTURE CLASSIFICATION

A classification system for sacral insufficiency fractures does not exist; however, the Denis classification system for traumatic sacral fractures can be used to predict potential neurologic and biomechanical complications. The Denis system subdivides the sacrum into three separate zones[11] (Fig. 42-1). Zone 1 involves the sacral ala, and fractures here are typically not complicated by neurologic symptoms. Zones 2 and 3 involve the foramina and the body and canal of the sacrum, respectively, and these are usually associated with lumbosacral radiculopathies and saddle anesthesia with loss of sphincter tone. Most sacral insufficiency fractures occur in the sacral ala (zone 1) and have an approximately vertical course in parallel with the sacroiliac joint. They are thus rarely associated with neurologic symptoms.

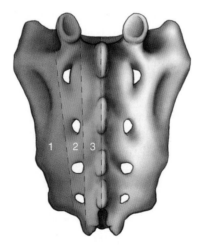

Fig. 42-1   The Denis classification of sacral zones 1, 2, and 3. Most insufficiency fractures occur in zone 1.

TREATMENT

MEDICAL THERAPIES

There is no established treatment for sacral insufficiency fractures, but the initial step is pain control. Centrally acting analgesics, such as opioids, should almost always be given to relieve the pain of these fractures. NSAIDs can block the activity of prostaglandins, thus preventing bone healing. They are associated with delayed union (or nonunion) of fractures and are not recommended in the treatment of sacral insufficiency fractures.[12]

Historically, degenerative sacral fractures were treated with bed rest for 3 to 6 months. Such prolonged immobilization causes multiple complications, including accelerated bone mineral density loss, venous thromboembolism, muscle atrophy, infections, pressure ulcers, cardiovascular deconditioning, and adverse psychological effects.[13] Early mobilization, on the other hand, has been proven to stimulate muscle tension and osteoblastic activity, resulting in increased bone formation. Early mobilization for stable fractures is thus typically recommended.

Many of the medical treatments for sacral insufficiency fractures focus on calcium and vitamin D metabolism. Because vitamin D deficiency is common in older patients, it should be suspected in patients with degenerative sacral fractures, and oral calcium and vitamin D supplements should be prescribed. Bisphosphonates act by inhibiting bone resorption and are effective in increasing bone mineral density, especially during the first few months of therapy. Concerns have been raised, however, about the potential oversuppression of bone turnover with long-term use of these agents, which can lead to an overall paradoxical suppression of bone formation.[14] Overuse of bisphosphonates can also lead to osteonecrosis of the jaw and hypermineralization, which causes brittle bones that are even more susceptible to fracture. Clinical trials have yet to prove the effectiveness of these agents in the management of stress fractures.[15] Calcitonin, which also decreases bone turnover, is approved for the prevention and treatment of postmenopausal osteoporosis. It has low potency compared with other agents but can increase bone mass and reduce the risk of vertebral fractures. Raloxifene, a selective estrogen receptor modulator, is also used for the treatment and prevention of postmenopausal osteoporosis. Although it is effective in reducing the risk of vertebral fractures, it is not considered first-line therapy because it increases the risk of venous thromboembolism. Strontium ranelate is both an antiresorptive and anabolic agent that protects and increases formation of osteoblasts. It has fewer side effects and is generally better tolerated by patients than bisphosphonates. Teriparatide, a recombinant form of human parathyroid hormone, is more of an anabolic agent and increases both trabecular and cortical bone formation, reducing fracture risk. It can only be used for 2 years, however, because it increases the risk of developing sarcoma.[16]

INTERVENTIONAL THERAPIES

Electrical and ultrasonic therapies were developed after observation that bone tissue carries electrical properties. Electric fields have been shown to induce reactions in bones, with electronegative regions inducing bone formation. Thus electrical stimulation devices have been used to enhance bone formation. Pulsed electromagnetic fields is an FDA-approved device that creates a magnetic field and secondary electric impulse, causing a release of calcium with subsequent upregulation of multiple bone growth factors.[17] Low-intensity pulsed ultrasound is another technique that stimulates osteoblastic activity through a direct effect on ion channels.[18]

Extracorporeal shock wave therapy uses high-energy acoustic waves that create a biologic response in various tissues. It enhances bone repair by increasing mesenchymal stem cell recruitment with proliferation and differentiation into osteoblasts. This type of treatment has been shown to promote fracture healing and increase local concentrations of bone-promoting growth factors in animal models.[19]

Vertebroplasty (sacroplasty) has recently been used to treat sacral stress fractures. Small quantities of poly-methylmethacrylate (PMMA) are injected directly into fracture lines. Patients are typically mobilized the same day (Fig. 42-2); pain scores are usually significantly improved within hours.[13] Although no complications have been recorded, long-term studies have not been reported regarding the duration of stabilization, the possible side effects from the exothermic reaction of PMMA with subsequent osteonecrosis, or nerve damage from the aberrant spread of cement.[2]

Surgical intervention is usually reserved for rare cases of instability, neurologic damage, or severe deformity of sacral alignment. Surgery typically consists of fixation and fusion with instrumentation across the sacropelvic apparatus using screws or hinges. The major caveat regarding such interventions is the high incidence of osteoporosis within the population of patients with degenerative sacral fracture, which can make fixation challenging. Furthermore, long-term studies have not been reported regarding the stability of these sacral constructs.[20] Degenerative sacral fracture differs from a fracture of the sacrum in a patient with a previous fusion to S1. Fractures below a fusion construct are often associated with instrumentation failure and can be a cause of a progressive kyphotic deformity and sagittal imbalance. These fractures are outside the scope of this chapter; however, management of these two similar fracture patterns is quite different.

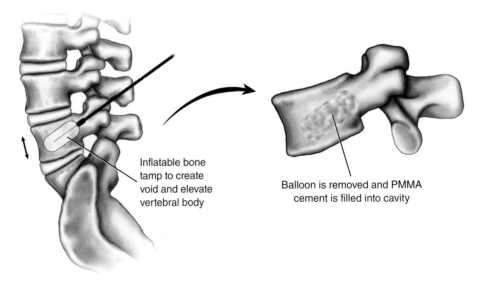

Inflatable bone tamp to create void and elevate vertebral body

Balloon is removed and PMMA cement is filled into cavity

Fig. 42-2   A typical procedure for cement augmentation of a vertebral segment. This procedure can be done through a variety of methods and may or may not use an initial step to create a void, which is then filled with bone cement.

PATIENT EXAMPLE

This 67-year-old woman had a previous L3-S1 fusion. She presented with progressive severe low back pain and sagittal imbalance and was diagnosed with a sacral fracture below the instrumentation, which healed in kyphosis. She was treated with sacral osteotomy for correction of sagittal imbalance. Six years postoperatively she has had a significant, durable improvement in pain, quality of life measures, and sagittal alignment.

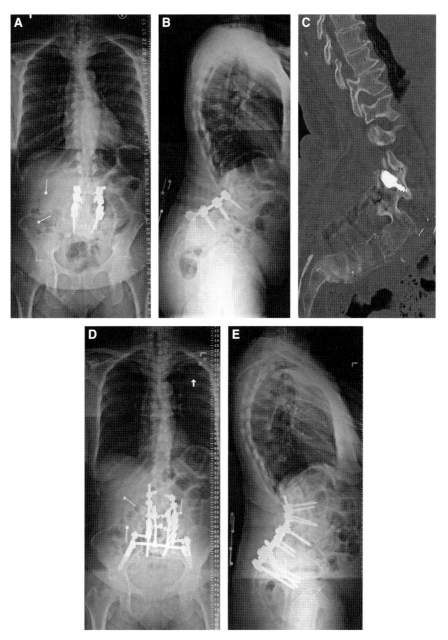

Fig. 42-3 **A** and **B,** Preoperative PA and lateral scoliosis radiographs showed L3-S1 fusion with a sacral fracture below the instrumentation. **C,** A sagittal CT reconstruction showed fracture and sacral kyphosis. **D** and **E,** Postoperative radiographs after sacral osteotomy and sacral pelvic reconstruction show significantly improved sagittal alignment as well as a normalization of her pelvic incidence/lumbar lordosis ratio.

CONCLUSION

Degenerative sacral fractures are an uncommon but likely underdiagnosed cause of low back pain that typically affects older patients with osteoporosis. These fractures should be suspected in an acute presentation of low back pain with no history of trauma. MRI and CT (especially when used together) are the best tests for establishing the diagnosis. Pain control and brief periods of rest with early immobilization are the mainstays of therapy, with medical therapies primarily focusing on calcium and vitamin D metabolism. Biophysical treatments are being used increasingly because they have few side effects. Sacroplasty and surgery can be performed in refractory or more severe cases, but their long-term effects have not been studied in detail.

REFERENCES

1. Lourie H. Spontaneous osteoporotic fracture of the sacrum. An unrecognized syndrome of the elderly. JAMA 248:715-717, 1982.
2. Longhino V, Bonora C, Sansone V. The management of sacral stress fractures: current concepts. Clin Cases Miner Bone Metab 8:19-23, 2011.
3. Weber M, Hasler P, Gerber H. Insufficiency fractures of the sacrum. Twenty cases and review of the literature. Spine 18:2507-2512, 1993.
4. Leroux JL, Denat B, Thomas E, et al. Sacral insufficiency fractures presenting as acute low-back pain. Biomechanical aspects. Spine 18:2502-2506, 1993.
5. Karatas M, Basaran C, Ozgul E, et al. Postpartum sacral stress fracture: an unusual case of low-back and buttock pain. Am J Phys Med Rehabil 87:418-422, 2008.
6. Celik EC, Oflouglu D, Arioglu PF. Postpartum bilateral stress fractures of the sacrum. Int J Gynaecol Obstet 121:178-179, 2013.
7. Muthukumar T, Butt SH, Cassar-Pullicino VN, et al. Cauda equina syndrome presentation of sacral insufficiency fractures. Skeletal Radiol 36:309-313, 2007.
8. Aretxabala I, Fraiz E, Pérez-Ruiz F, et al. Sacral insufficiency fractures. High association with pubic rami fractures. Clin Rheumatol 19:399-401, 2000.
9. Tsiridis E, Upadhyay N, Giannoudis PV. Sacral insufficiency fractures: current concepts of management. Osteoporos Int 17:1716-1725, 2006.
10. Schindler OS, Watura R, Cobby M. Sacral insufficiency fractures. J Orthop Surg (Hong Kong) 15:339-346, 2007.
11. Denis F, Davis S, Comfort T. Sacral fractures: an important problem. Retrospective analysis of 236 cases. Clin Orthop Rel Res 227:67-81, 1988.
12. Dimmen S, Nordsletten L, Engebretsen L, et al. Negative effect of parecoxib on bone mineral during fracture healing in rats. Acta Orthop 79:438-444, 2008.
13. Lever M, Lever E, Lever EG. Rethinking osteoporotic sacral fractures. Injury 40:466, 2009.
14. Compston J. Recent advances in the management of osteoporosis. Clin Med 9:565-569, 2009.
15. Shima Y, Engebretsen L, Iwasa J, et al. Use of bisphosphonates for the treatment of stress fractures in athletes. Knee Surg Sports Traumatol Arthrosc 17:542-550, 2009.
16. Mitchner NA, Harris ST. Current and emerging therapies for osteoporosis. J Fam Pract 58(7 Suppl Osteoporosis):S45-S49, 2009.
17. Gan JC, Glazer PA. Electrical stimulation therapies for spinal fusions: current concepts. Eur Spine J 15:1301-1311, 2006.
18. Massari L, Caruso G, Sollazzo V, et al. Pulsed electromagnetic fields and low intensity pulsed ultrasound in bone tissue. Clin Cases Miner Bone Metab 6:149-154, 2009.
19. Chen YJ, Wurtz T, Wang CJ, et al. Recruitment of mesenchymal stem cells and expression of TGF-beta 1 and VEGF in the early stage of shock wave-promoted bone regeneration of segmental defect in rats. J Orthop Res 22:526-534, 2004.
20. Tjardes T, Paffrath T, Baethis H, et al. Computer assisted percutaneous placement of augmented iliosacral screws: a reasonable alternative to sacroplasty. Spine 33:1497-1500, 2008.

PART VIII

Minimally Invasive Surgery: Considerations for Management of Spinal Deformity

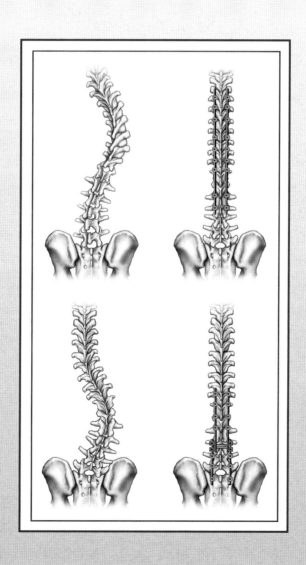

43

Minimally Invasive Surgery Instrumentation: A Review of Available Systems and Biomechanical Considerations

Daniel M. Mazzaferro ▪ *Sergey Mlyavykh* ▪ *D. Greg Anderson*

Minimally invasive surgery of the spine has become popular in recent years, because it results in decreased blood loss and a reduced infection rate. Patient interest in these approaches for spinal problems has increased. Minimally invasive instrumentation has a defined learning curve,[1] which is a major factor that limits adoption of these techniques. In addition, minimally invasive fusion techniques decrease a surgeon's ability to prepare and fuse the posterior column of the spine; thus in most cases anterior interbody fusion without a facet fusion is performed. Long-term outcome studies comparing the results of minimally invasive fusion with open fusion are lacking, although shorter-term studies show favorable results and cost efficiency for these techniques.[2]

The kinematic behavior of the natural spine is complex. Likewise, spinal loads and forces on the spinal joints are difficult to measure in vivo. To simplify the task of understanding spinal movements and forces, researchers often model spinal motions as occurring in three orthogonal planes (axial, sagittal, and coronal) and around three axes of rotation.[3] In vitro modeling of the spine is frequently performed with explanted spines placed in a supportive fixture. Movements are tracked in three-dimensional space, and forces are measured with attached strain gauges or through servohydraulic testing machines. Although this type of modeling has been extremely helpful to understand some properties of the human spine, to compare various spinal states (normal, posttraumatic, and postsurgical), and to analyze several types of spinal instrumentation, it is only a crude approximation of a normal spine. In particular, most of the biomechanical modeling that has been done fails to provide a realistic simulation of the muscular forces that are imparted by the intact soft tissue envelope of the spine.

Spinal instrumentation is performed for a variety of purposes. It can be employed to restore stability to a segment of the spine destabilized by trauma or surgical tissue removal, to improve the alignment of the spine in a setting of a spinal deformity, and to immobilize a section of the spine to improve the environment for bony arthrodesis. As with traditional surgery, surgeons who perform minimally invasive techniques will choose instrumentation to achieve one or more of these goals.

From a theoretical perspective, spinal instrumentation that provides the most anatomic reconstruction of the spine should achieve good load-sharing between the instrumentation and the host tissues (bone, ligaments, and muscles). When a spine is fused, the optimal constructs should transmit physiologic compressive forces along the anterior column and neutralize excessive tensile loads to the posterior column during postoperative activities. Ideally, instrumentation should minimize the transmission of nonphysiologic forces to the spinal segments adjacent to the fusion.[4]

In this chapter, we discuss the use of spinal instrumentation in minimally invasive surgeries and describe how surgeons have used instrumentation to achieve the goals of surgery in this setting.

HOW IS MINIMALLY INVASIVE SPINAL SURGERY DIFFERENT?

All minimally invasive surgeries have a common goal of limiting soft tissue disruption of the surgical approach. By lessening the detachment of muscles, tendons, and ligaments, the degree of spinal destabilization is theoretically reduced. This can in turn reduce the stresses transmitted to the instrumentation construct. In some cases, an intact musculoligamentous envelope can decrease the burden of instrumentation or allow surgeons to stop a construct at a high stress region such as the L1 level.

Minimally invasive application of pedicle screws is generally performed without detachment of the muscular elements, in particular the multifidus muscles. The multifidus has been shown to be an important segmental stabilizer of the spine.[5] An additional benefit of minimally invasive pedicle screw insertion is the reduced risk of transection of the medial branch of the dorsal ramus, which is the primary nerve supply to the multifidus.[6] When the function of the multifidus is maintained, dynamic stabilization of the spinal segments is achievable in the postoperative period, and load-sharing with the instrumentation can occur.

Minimally invasive spinal surgery in the setting of spinal deformity correction can result in less complete release of the deformity, compared with a traditional open surgical technique. The spinal deformity might thus be stiffer and require increased forces to obtain correction. These increased forces are transmitted to the bone implant interface during deformity correction.[7]

Table 43-1   Comparison of Minimally Invasive Instrumentation Systems

Manufacturer	Medtronic Sofamor Danek (Minneapolis, MN)	Stryker (Kalamazoo, MI)	K2M (Leesburg, VA)
MIS system	CD Horizon Longitude II	ES2	Everest
Pedicle Screws			
Available lengths (mm)	30-110	25 (in 4.5 mm only), 30, 35, 40, 45, 50, 55, 60, 65, 70, 75, 80, 85, 90	30-100
Available diameters (mm)	4.5-10.5	4.5, 5.5, 6.5, 7.5, 8.5	4.5-8.5
Thread pitch	Corticocancellous	Corticocancellous	2
Dual-lead thread form	Yes	No	Yes
Difference between the major and minor diameter of the screw (size of the screw thread) (mm)	4.5-3.4 5.5-3.85	Constant major thread outer diameter, tapered minor thread diameter (cylinder major thread, conical minor thread)	2

mm, Millimeter.

With good maintenance of the muscular envelope of the spine, the forces imparted to the adjacent segments may be more physiologic. The factors that lead to adjacent-segment degeneration are complex and poorly characterized. However, three potential causes of adjacent-segment degeneration that can be prevented with MIS include the following: injury to the facet capsule of the superjacent level, injury to the medial branch of the ramus, and loss of attachment of the multifidus tendons and infraspinous/supraspinous ligaments.[8]

MINIMALLY INVASIVE INSTRUMENTATION

Screw and rod constructs are the workhorse of minimally invasive surgical instrumentation, as they are with open spinal reconstructive surgery (Table 43-1). Most minimally invasive pedicle screws are cannulated, resulting in a small decrease in bending stiffness and strength, compared with noncannulated screws. In most cases, the quality of the bone-implant interface is the rate-limiting factor in determining the screw-rod construct pullout forces. The bone-implant interface is affected by bone density, the size of the pedicle screw relative to the pedicle, the length of the screw, the angle of the pedicle screw relative to the sagittal plane, and the thread form of the pedicle screw. To improve the quality of the bone-implant interface, surgeons can place a larger-diameter screw or a longer screw, use a more anatomic pedicle passage, or choose a screw with more surface area on the threads. V-shaped threads with an outer cylindrical and inner conical conformation have been shown to maximize pullout strength, regardless of bone density.[9] Some surgeons have reported on the use of bone cement to increase screw pullout resistance, even though it is not approved by the U.S. FDA. The distance between implants affects stiffness of the construct. When segmental fixation is achieved at every level, the stiffness of the overall construct is enhanced, and the resistance to pullout is increased by load sharing of multiple implants.[10]

DePuy (Warsaw, IN)	Globus Medical (Audubon, PA)	NuVasive (San Diego, CA)
Viper	Corridor	Precept
Pedicle Screws		
30-100	25-90	4.5 × 25-45 5.5 × 30-55 (5 mm increments) 6.5 × 30-55 (5 mm increments) 7.5 × 60-100 (10 mm increments) 8.5 × 35-55 (5 mm increments) 8.5 × 60-100 (10 mm increments)
4.35, 5, 6, 7.5, 8, 9	5.0, 5.5, 6.5, 7.5, 8.5	4.5, 5.5, 6.5, 7.5, 8.5
Corticocancellous	2 mm for all sizes except 8.5 mm, which is 2.5	2.75
Yes	Yes (except 8.5 mm)	Yes
3	5.0-3.8 5.5-4.0 6.5-5.0 7.5-6.0 8.5-6.5	4.7-3.1 5.5-3.9 6.5-4.5 7.5-5.3 8.5-6.3

Continued

Table 43-1 Comparison of Minimally Invasive Instrumentation Systems—cont'd

Manufacturer	Medtronic Sofamor Danek (Minneapolis, MN)	Stryker (Kalamazoo, MI)	K2M (Leesburg, VA)
MIS system	CD Horizon Longitude II	ES2	Everest
Pedicle Screws—cont'd			
Cortical threaded screw available	Yes	No	No
Screw self-tapping	No	Yes	No
Angulation of the screw head (degrees)	25 Options SAS (± 13)	25	35
Minimum distance the screw sits above the bone (mm)	17.04 (for 5.5/6.0 rod) and 14.8 (for 4.75 rod)	15.3	16
Size of the cannulation hole (mm)	1.59	1.4	1.5
Types of screws			
Locking mechanism	Break-off set screw	Buttress-thread set screw (blocker)	Set screw
Torque required (nm)	9-10.5 (for 4.75 rod) 10.5-12.5 (for 5.5/6.0 rod)	12	90 inch-pounds
How much rod reduction is built into the locking mechanism? (mm)	101	15	30
Rods			
Available rod diameter(s) (mm)	4.75, 5.5, 6.0	5.5, 6.0	5.5, 6.0
Available materials	TiCP, Ti alloy, CoCr, CoCr+	Ti alloy, CoCr	Ti alloy, CoCr, PEEK
Is the rod introduced through a separate incision?	Two options: yes and no	No	No
Does the instrument set provide a method of rod reduction?	Yes	Yes	Yes
Does the instrument set provide a mechanism of rod rotation?	Yes	Yes	Yes
Does the system have an option for MIS iliac bolt/screw fixation?	Yes	Yes	Yes
How would the system be linked to an open screw rod option from the same manufacture?	The platform is offered in cannulated and noncannulated options.	The screw uses the same diameters of rod as an open system, and multiple, different connectors can optimize rod-to-rod connection.	Side-to-side connectors

CoCR, Cobalt-chromium; *MIS*, minimally invasive surgery; *mm*, millimeter; *nm*, nanometer; *PEEK*, polyetheretherketone; *SAS*, sagittal adjusting screw.
Ti, titanium; *TiCP*, titanium-carbide particle.

DePuy (Warsaw, IN)	Globus Medical (Audubon, PA)	NuVasive (San Diego, CA)
Viper	Corridor	Precept
Pedicle Screws—cont'd		
Yes	No	No (It has no cutting flute, but the screw thread form is aggressive enough to be placed without a tap.)
No	Yes	Yes
30	30	30
14.5	17	15.5
1.77	1.8	1.6
Polyaxial Monoaxial Uniplanar X-tab		Polyaxial Iliac Reduction Modular
Square thread design	Nonthreaded locking cap	Helical flange
80 inch-pounds[2]	5.5	10.2 nm 90 inch-pounds
Only the X-tab: 10 and 25	The system offers 22 mm rod reduction capability. Most of the reduction is accomplished through the instrumentation, but the locking mechanism provides 2 mm of rod reduction.	12.5 through the reduction screws
Rods		
5.5	5.5	5.5
Ti alloy, CoCr, PEEK	Ti, CoCr	Ti alloy, CoCr
No	Two options: yes and no	No, can depend on the technique
Yes	Yes	Yes
Yes	Yes	Yes
Yes	No	Yes
It is compatible with the Expedium 5.5 system, and can be connected to an existing construct using the Expedium Universal Connector set.	It is compatible with the Revere 5.5 system.	It is compatible with the 5.5 mm open screw system.

When choosing an implant strategy for posterior rod and screw fixation, surgeons should consider the diameter and material composition of the rod. Larger-diameter rods are stiffer and stronger. In addition, some materials such as cobalt-chromium are stiffer, and particular forms of some materials can be considered to obtain the specific characteristics optimal for a construct. For example, titanium rods are often available in multiple forms with varying stiffness and strength. The most common rod options currently available include stainless steel, titanium alloys, cobalt-chromium, titanium-carbide particle, and polyetheretherketone. The most commonly available rod diameters range from 4.75 to 6.25 mm. A comparison of different rod systems should include evaluation of yield strength, stiffness, and fatigue life.[11] In deformity correction procedures, highly stiff rods may be more difficult to use, because they do not contour as easily and can have an increased risk of screw pullout during the persuasion maneuver.

Another factor to consider in designing an optimal construct is the quality of the anterior column support. Multiple minimally invasive surgical approaches are now available to achieve anterior column support and fusion. These include the transforaminal interbody fusion, posterior lumbar interbody fusion, direct lateral interbody fusion, extreme lateral interbody fusion, and anterior lumbar interbody fusion. Some approaches such as direct lateral interbody fusion allow surgeons to implant a graft with a very large surface area, which provides more stability to axial settling or collapse of the construct. Additionally, anterior column fusion procedures increase the rate and likelihood of fusion success. This reduces the longer-term risks to a construct that might occur in the setting of a delayed union or nonunion. The materials chosen for an interbody device can affect a construct. Materials that have a modulus of elasticity close to that of the vertebral body bone are theoretically preferred, because their use is less likely to result in endplate violation and settling. Particular materials (for example, titanium with porosity) are more conducive to bone formation in a fusion procedure.

Various types of screw-to-rod connections have been used in spinal surgery. The most common screw-to-rod connection currently is the tulip-head screw, which is available in fixed (monoaxial) and polyaxial forms. Although monoaxial screws theoretically provide a more stable base for deformity correction, they present a much more challenging connection to the rod, because the screw head does not adjust to accommodate small degrees of malalignment between adjacent screws within the construct. Most minimally invasive spinal fixation involves polyaxial screws, which provide an easier screw-to-rod attachment and are more forgiving of small malalignments between adjacent screws.[12]

Long constructs that extend to the pelvis place substantial loads on the lower construct pedicle screws and present a significant potential for screw loosening, breakage, or pseudarthrosis. In recent years, iliac fixation using a minimally invasive technique has become available and can use similar surgical techniques to what has become standard in open surgery. Various surgical strategies for iliac fixation have been described.[13,14]

Cross-links have traditionally been used in longer fusion constructs to provide additional rotational and lateral-bending stability. Unfortunately, the application of a cross-link generally requires a larger, open incision and removal of the midline structures. For this reason, they have not been employed as frequently in minimally invasive procedures. It is conceivable that the more common use of screws at most or all pedicle levels and maintenance of the dynamic and static soft tissue stabilizers makes up for some of the theoretical losses in construct rigidity, compared with traditional constructs that use no cross-links. No studies have adequately supported this statement to date.

CONCLUSION

Minimally invasive instrumentation can theoretically be performed for most thoracolumbar procedures, although the procedural difficulty inherent in deformity correction is substantial. Spinal surgeons should have substantial experience with both spinal deformity surgery and the use of minimally invasive instrumentation before tackling a major deformity with this instrumentation. Unfortunately, fusion of the posterior column of the spine remains the "weak link" of performing minimally invasive deformity surgery, because currently available fusion strategies for the posterior column of the spine do not seem to reproduce the quality of fusion bed preparation and application of bone graft that is feasible with open surgery. In contrast, minimally invasive fusion techniques tend to rely on anterior column fusion with or without facet fusion. Additional research comparing these techniques in patients with spinal deformity is necessary.

Reduced blood loss and a lower rate of complications such as surgical site infection are quite desirable and are the major driving factors for many surgeons to learn minimally invasive instrumentation strategies and to incorporate these techniques into their treatment of spinal deformity patients.

REFERENCES

1. Sclafani JA, Kim CW. Complications associated with the initial learning curve of minimally invasive spine surgery: a systematic review. Clin Orthop Relat Res 472:1711-1717, 2014.
2. Anderson GD, Wang P. Value analysis of minimally invasive spine surgery. Semin Spine Surg 26:52-55, 2014.
3. Marras WS. Biomechanics of the spine motion segment. In Herkowitz HN, Garfin SR, Eismont FJ, et al, eds. Biomechanics of the Spine Motion Segment. Rothman-Simeone: The Spine, ed 6. Philadelphia: Saunders Elsevier, 2011.
4. Welch W, Cheng BC, Awad TE, et al. Dynamic stabilization of the lumbar spine. In Quiñones-Hinojosa A, ed. Schmidek & Sweet Operative Neurosurgical Techniques: Indications, Methods, and Results, ed 6. Philadelphia: Saunders Elsevier, 2012.
5. Kim DY, Lee SH, Chung S, et al. Comparison of multifidus atrophy and trunk extension muscle strength: percutaneous versus open pedicle screw fixation. Spine 30:123-129, 2005.
6. Kim CW, Schwender KD, Foley K, et al. Minimally invasive posterior lumbar instrumentation. In Herkowitz HN, Garfin SR, Eismont FJ, et al, eds. Rothman-Simeone: The Spine, ed 6. Philadelphia: Saunders Elsevier, 2011.
7. Kim CW, Schwender KD, Foley K, et al. Minimally invasive posterior approaches to the spine. In Herkowitz HN, Garfin SR, Eismont FJ, et al, eds. Rothman-Simeone: The Spine, ed 6. Philadelphia: Saunders Elsevier, 2011.
8. Wilsa MS, Malveaux C, Sharan AD. Adjacent segment disease after lumbar spinal fusion: a systematic review of the current literature. Semin Spine Surg 23:266-274, 2011.
9. Kim YY, Choi WS, Rhyu KW. Assessment of pedicle screw pullout strength based on various screw designs and bone densities: an ex vivo biomechanical study. Spine J 12:164-168, 2012.
10. Cuartas E, Rasouli A, O'Brien M, et al. Use of all-pedicle-screw constructs in the treatment of adolescent idiopathic scoliosis. J Am Acad Orthop Surg 17:550-561, 2009.
11. Lubelski D, Healy AT, Mageswaran P, et al. Biomechanics of the lower thoracic spine after decompression and fusion: a cadaveric analysis. Spine J. 2014 Mar 22. [Epub ahead of print]
12. Haher TR, Valdevit A. Biomechanics of spinal instrumentation. In Errico TJ, Lonner BS, Moulton AW, eds. Surgical Management of Spinal Deformities. Philadelphia: Saunders Elsevier, 2009.
13. Martin CT, Witham TF, Kebaish KM. Sacropelvic fixation: two case reports of a new percutaneous technique. Spine 36:E618-E621, 2011.
14. Tsimpas A, Wang MY. Minimally invasive placement of iliac screws: a technical note. Open Spine J 2:24-28, 2010.

44

Mini-open Lateral Approach for Thoracolumbar Anterior Lumbar Interbody Fusion

William D. Smith ▪ *Juan S. Uribe*

The minimally disruptive lateral transpsoas approach for anterior lumbar interbody fusion (eXtreme lateral interbody fusion, XLIF, NuVasive, Inc. San Diego, CA) was developed in the late 1990s and early 2000s by Dr. Luiz Pimenta and introduced in the literature in 2006.[1] The procedure was developed as a less invasive alternative to direct anterior approaches for interbody fusion. It avoids many of the complications (vascular and visceral injury) associated with anterior approaches while preserving posterior bony, ligamentous, and muscular architecture. This minimizes infection risk while allowing for the placement of an interbody fusion device and many types of supplemental internal fixation without repositioning the patient. The procedure is performed either through a single lateral incision or with a second fascial incision to guide access into the retroperitoneal space. In addition, XLIF allows placement of an interbody graft whose footprint and endplate coverage are similar to those of a direct anterior interbody fusion, spanning the ring apophysis for resistance to subsidence and providing large cage apertures for a wide fusion area. In contrast to direct anterior approaches, XLIF preserves the anterior and posterior longitudinal ligaments to facilitate indirect decompression, the restoration of segmental alignment, and maintenance of cage position through ligamentotaxis. The mini-open lateral approach has been established for use in the lumbar spine and is increasingly applied for more advanced thoracolumbar and thoracic indications, including adult deformity, thoracic disc herniations, and corpectomy for fractures and tumors.[2-14]

ANATOMIC CONSIDERATIONS

LUMBAR REGION

The most relevant anatomic structures to a lateral approach in the lumbar spine are the nerves of the lumbar plexus.[15,16] These lie within and around the lateral disc space, within and on the psoas muscle, within the lateral retroperitoneal space, and within and between the superficial muscles of the abdominal cavity (Fig. 44-1). Advanced neuromonitoring techniques (NV M5, NuVasive, Inc.) integrated into the approach and procedural instrumentation are used to gain geographic (location and distance) information on neural proximity to the approach corridor.[15,17] Other structures that are important to the approach in the lumbar spine are the retropleural space, iliopsoas muscle, and vasculature (Fig. 44-2).

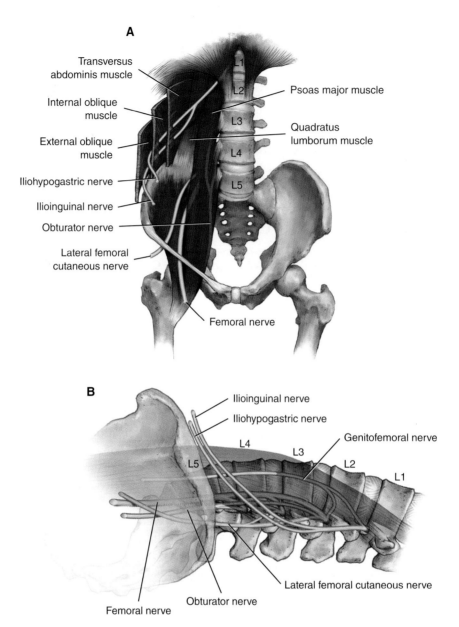

Fig. 44-1 **A,** The lumbar spine and surrounding structures, including the deep and superficial neural and muscular anatomy relevant to the lateral transpsoas approach. **B,** The deep muscles and superficial and deep neural anatomy of the lumbar spine in relation to the lateral transpsoas approach. (Courtesy of NuVasive, Inc.)

THORACOLUMBAR JUNCTION

At the thoracolumbar junction, the most relevant anatomic structures to a lateral approach are the diaphragm and the inferior border and aspect of the pleural sac (depending on the level treated).[5] Management of the diaphragm includes consideration for preservation at upper lumbar levels (L1 and L2) and deflection superiorly during exposure of the retroperitoneal cavity. At the thoracolumbar junction and lower thoracic levels, the diaphragm can be inadvertently violated during mobilization for adequate lateral disc space exposure. A transdiaphragmatic approach can be used, often with blunt dissection through the layer and without closure after the retractor is removed. The lower ribs are important structures to consider, although upper lumbar levels are generally approachable without rib resectioning, sometimes with

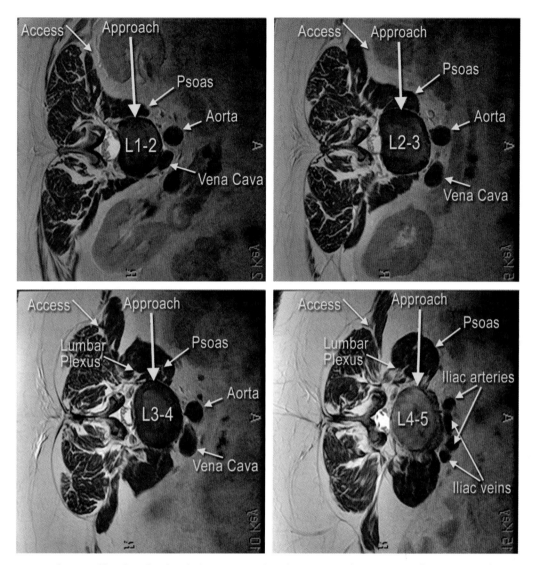

Fig. 44-2 Axial MRI of lumbar disc levels (L1-2 to L4-5) with anatomic designations of structures relevant to a lateral transpsoas approach for interbody fusion. (Courtesy of NuVasive, Inc.)

the assistance of angled procedural instruments. Alternatively, exposure can be obtained between the ribs using a split-blade retractor (MaXcess, NuVasive, Inc.).

THORACIC REGION

In the thoracic spine, the main anatomic structures relevant to the approach are the ribs and neurovascular bundle, the pleural cavity, and the rib head at the costal facet. The neurovascular bundle runs along the anteroinferior aspect of each rib. This should be preserved during the initial approach and when suturing. Once the superficial exposure has been completed, the pleural cavity can be managed through a transpleural or a retropleural approach.[13] A retropleural approach involves careful mobilization of the pleura from the chest wall and generally obviates the need for a chest tube postoperatively. Finally, each rib head is a landmark for a thoracic level. At each level treated, the posterior disc border, the pedicle, and the dural sheath need to be identified. Rib heads should be resected in most cases to gain adequate exposure to the lateral disc space, especially at upper thoracic levels.

INDICATIONS AND LIMITATIONS

Surgical indications for XLIF include any disease requiring interbody fusion in the thoracolumbar spine above the L5 level and below approximately T4. Access is rarely and only carefully obtained at other levels with this approach. Examples of specific applications include degenerative disc disease, degenerative spondylolisthesis (grade II or lower), degenerative scoliosis, pseudarthrosis, acute or chronic sequelae of discitis, revisions (for example, of prior fusions or total disc replacement), postlaminectomy instability, and adjacent-segment disease.

Relative limitations of the approach include pathologies at the L5-S1 level, where a lateral approach is typically limited by the position of the iliac crest and bifurcation of iliac vessels. At levels cranial to approximately T4, the heart, vascular anatomy, and position of the scapula limit access. In patients with a nonmobile L5-S1 motion segment and/or a deeply seated L4-5 motion segment, access may be difficult in the lower lumbar spine. Other relative limitations include prior bilateral retroperitoneal surgery, for example, prior bilateral kidney surgery; anomalous vascular anatomy that interferes with the lateral approach, which can occur in rotational deformities; and degenerative spondylolisthesis higher than grade II, which can result in a far-anterior position of exiting spinal nerves, limiting the area of lateral interbody access. Similarly, lateral access can be challenging in patients whose sacrum is lumbarized and L5-6 is a functional L4-5 segment, because the lumbar plexus can be more anterior and the iliac vessels more lateral.[18] Vascular and neural anatomic variations can present similar challenges in otherwise normal patients. The location of these structures relative to a lateral approach is often identified preoperatively during careful review of MRI.[18,19]

PREOPERATIVE PLANNING

In addition to a detailed history and physical examination, imaging modalities are a powerful tool for diagnosing patients, planning their treatment, and helping to ensure an optimal clinical outcome. Preoperative plain radiographs are a useful tool for initial evaluation and for assessing deformity and trauma. CT provides detail of the bony anatomy and neural tissues required for diagnosis. MRI is an excellent modality for studying the spinal cord and cauda equina.

Additionally, care is required for proper preoperative, intraoperative, and postoperative analgesia and anesthesia.[20] Preoperative administration of pregabalin or gabapentin helps to prophylactically attenuate the effects of intraoperative irritation of neural structures adjacent to the approach corridor. Dexamethasone can be given to dampen the inflammatory cascade after neural or muscular tissue trauma.[21]

Because intraoperative EMG is used throughout a case, limited muscle relaxants and paralytics are given, or preferably none at all. If these are needed for induction or other reasons, only short-lifespan varieties are delivered to prevent interference with EMG readings.

Specialized equipment required for minimally disruptive lateral interbody fusion includes a radiolucent surgical table that tilts in ventrodorsal and craniocaudal directions and has a bendable break. A fluoroscope (C-arm), an access system and peripherals (MaXcess, NuVasive, Inc.), general anterior and lateral procedural instruments, a neuromonitoring platform (NV M5), and bipolar electrocautery are also needed.

OPERATIVE TECHNIQUE

The following five steps are essential for an efficient and reproducible XLIF procedure[1,22,23]:
- Careful patient positioning
- Gentle retroperitoneal development and dissection
- Meticulous psoas passage using advanced neuromonitoring integrated into the approach and procedural instrumentation
- An adequate discectomy and proper endplate preparation
- Appropriate interbody implant sizing and placement

PATIENT POSITIONING AND FLUORORADIOGRAPHY

The operating room is organized so that the operating surgeon can view the monitor of the fluoroscope and the neuromonitoring monitor while having adequate room to place and articulate the C-arm. Before surgical exposure is performed, the EMG surface or needle electrodes are applied to the lower extremities and checked for correct impedance.

The patient is placed in a lateral decubitus position. The side for exposure is based on the pathology and/or surgeon's preference. The table break is between the greater trochanter and the iliac crest, so that the iliac crest is above the table break. The hips and knees are slightly flexed (approximately 30 degrees) to relax the iliopsoas muscle. Pressure points are properly protected. The patient is secured to the table with tape across the pelvis, along the lateral aspect of the upper and lower leg, and across the chest (Fig. 44-3).

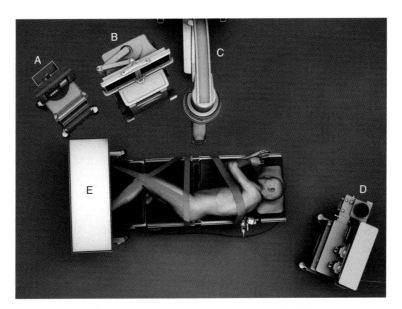

Fig. 44-3 Tape is placed to secure the patient to the operating room table. The operating room setup for a lateral transpsoas approach includes a neuromonitoring monitor *(A)*, a fluoroscopy monitor *(B)*, a C-arm *(C)*, anesthesia and/or suction *(D)*, electrocautery, lights, and a tray *(E)*. (Courtesy of NuVasive, Inc.)

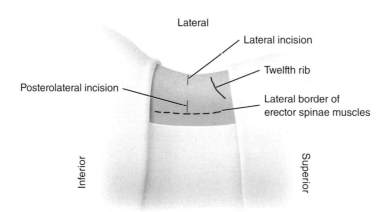

Fig. 44-4   A posterior view of externally identifiable anatomic landmarks for a lateral transpsoas approach to the lumbar spine. (Courtesy of NuVasive, Inc.)

To access the lower lumbar levels (L4-5), it is generally necessary to laterally flex the lumbar spine through a break and bend in the table of approximately 20 degrees. More or less bending is required, depending on each patient's needs and the surgeon's preference. Typically, the smallest-needed break is used to prevent pressure point problems and overtensioning of the iliopsoas muscle and lumbar plexus.[24] An approachable trajectory for a lateral approach should then be able to be developed from approximately L1 through L5 (bordered superiorly by the ribs and inferiorly by the iliac crest). Surface anatomy serving as landmarks for the approach includes the iliac crest, the lateral border of the dorsal lumbar musculature (erector spinae), and the twelfth rib (Fig. 44-4).

An essential part of the procedure that is needed to ensure reproducibility is the confirmation of a true lateral and AP orientation with respect to the direction of the surgical corridor and intraoperative fluororadiography. To obtain a true AP orientation on fluororadiography, the C-arm is placed in a cross-table (0-degree) position and oriented to be in-line with the lordosis of the level treated (Fig. 44-5, *A*). When the level is targeted, the left-right tilt function on the table is used to bring the segment into alignment. In a true AP view, the spinous process is visualized at the midline of the vertebral body, the pedicles are symmetrical and have a unified cortex, and the superior endplate is linear (Fig. 44-5, *B*). To obtain a true lateral view and orientation, the C-arm should remain in its place while the arm is rotated to be perpendicular to the floor (90-degree position). The table is then adjusted in the horizontal plane until a true lateral view is confirmed. With this orientation, the surgical corridor and intraoperative fluoroscopic visualization are orthogonal to the floor, providing true orthogonal access to the sagittal plane of the disc space. It also provides a safe trajectory between the endplates, away from sensitive contralateral anterior or posterior structures (vasculature and nerves) and helps to limit inadvertent ligamentous and endplate damage (Fig. 44-5, *C*).

Communication with anesthesia providers is essential for XLIF procedures, because the use of directional EMG requires a general anesthetic without muscle relaxation. An EMG twitch test is performed to evaluate the presence of residual muscle relaxants and to qualify the integrity of motor responses through EMG in the lower myotomes.

ACCESS

Each level to be treated is identified and confirmed individually. Before the surgical site is prepared in a standard aseptic fashion, the level location and lateral incision placement are confirmed and marked. The

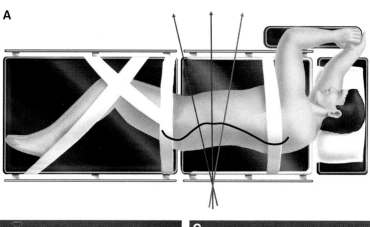

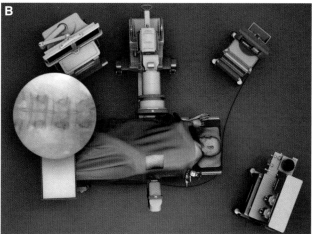
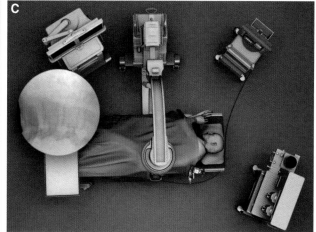

Fig. 44-5   **A,** Patient positioning, taping, and C-arm projections *(colored arrows)* for AP views. Each arrow indicates a specific segmental angle. **B,** Patient positioning and operating room setup for a true AP view during a lateral transpsoas approach. The *inset* shows an intraoperative fluororadiograph. **C,** Patient positioning and operating room setup for a true lateral view during a lateral transpsoas approach. The *inset* shows an intraoperative fluororadiograph. (Courtesy of NuVasive, Inc.)

skin is marked at the anterior and posterior borders of the level to be treated, the approximate docking target site, and the disc space, and all are confirmed under lateral fluororadiography (Fig. 44-6). A second incision is recommended on the posterolateral aspect of the spine (the border of the erector spinae) for blunt dissection of the retroperitoneal space. Skin is incised sharply for the posterolateral and lateral incisions. A careful finger-over-scissors technique is useful to separate subcutaneous tissues and muscular layers. With this two-incision approach, the posterolateral incision is made first. Blunt digital dissection is used to access the retroperitoneal space and release the peritoneal contents through development of the plane, through the retroperitoneal fat. Once the retroperitoneal plane has been adequately developed (typically mobilization of the peritoneal contents is palpable once release is achieved), the inserted digit can be used to palpate the interior wall of the lateral abdomen at the site of the incision. The same technique is applied to make a lateral incision. To prevent thermal injuries, monopolar electrocautery is not used, only bipolar or no cautery at all. After passage through the superficial musculature of the abdominal wall is completed, the finger is inserted through the posterolateral incision to guide approach instrumentation (dilators) to the lateral border of the psoas muscle. The finger protects the peritoneum by leading the initial dilator into the developed and confirmed retroperitoneal plane (Fig. 44-7, *A* and *B*). A target on the lateral disc space posterior to the midline, typically at the border between the posterior and middle thirds of the disc space, is confirmed on lateral fluoroscopy (Fig. 44-7, *C*).

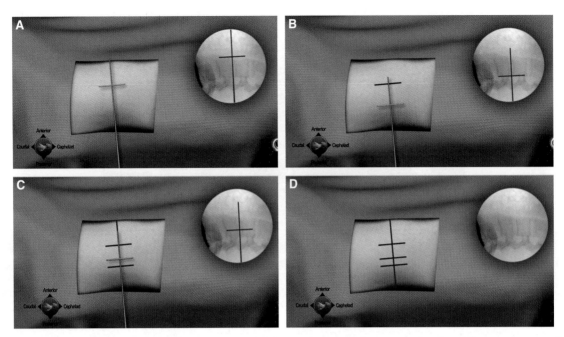

Fig. 44-6   Skin markings. Fluororadiography *(insets)* shows the targeted operative level. **A,** The anterior vertebral body border. **B,** The posterior vertebral body border. **C,** The disc space approach target. **D,** The position of the intersecting disc space. (Courtesy of NuVasive, Inc.)

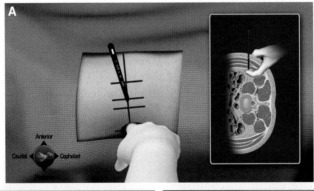

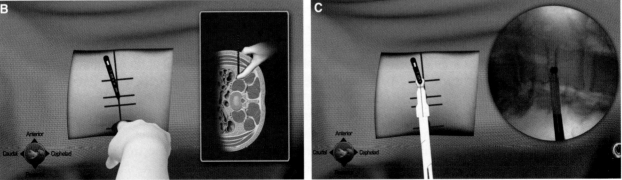

Fig. 44-7   **A,** Digital guidance (through the posterolateral incision) of the initial dilator (through the lateral incision) into the retroperitoneal space for a lateral transpsoas approach. **B,** Passage of the initial dilator to the lateral border of the iliopsoas muscle, guided by the surgeon's finger through the posterolateral incision. **C,** The dilator is positioned on the lateral aspect of the disc space. (Courtesy of NuVasive, Inc.)

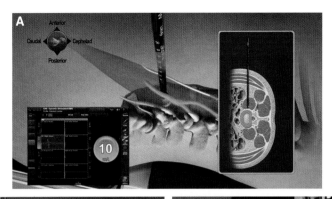

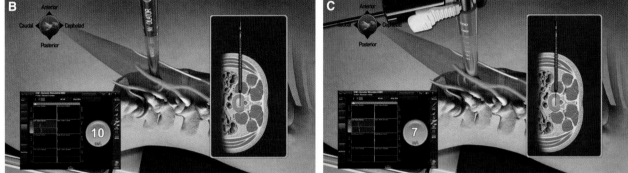

Fig. 44-8 **A,** A lateral transpsoas approach at L4-5. Directional EMG stimulation through the initial dilator and a discrete-threshold response *(bottom left)* provide information on the direction and distance of motor nerves with respect to the approach instrumentation. **B** and **C,** The second and third sequential dilators, respectively, are passed under stimulated EMG guidance to the lateral disc space in a lateral transpsoas approach. (The anatomy is not drawn to scale or morphology.) (Courtesy of NuVasive, Inc.)

Once the initial dilator is resting on the border of the psoas, dynamically evoked EMG (NV M5) is used to bluntly and carefully pass the dilator through the fibers of the muscle. The three sequential dilators have localized stimulating fields on their distal tips to stimulate directionally while the monitoring platform provides discrete-threshold EMG responses to indicate the relative distance of motor nerves from the approach instrumentation. For example, a lower response indicates closer proximity to the stimulating field. Thus, while the dilator is advanced through the substance of the psoas muscle, geographic information about the lumbar plexus is collected and can be interpreted to guide the approach. Because the lumbar plexus generally lies on the posterior aspect of the lateral disc space, lower-threshold EMG responses in the posterior direction and high EMG responses in the anterior direction suggest that the dilator is anterior to the lumbar plexus (the preferred location).[16,25,26] If low readings in the anterior direction are generated, it is generally advisable to remove the dilator and readjust the trajectory to avoid anterior neural structures, with guidance from EMG feedback. After the initial dilator is safely passed to and docked on the lateral aspect of the disc (Fig. 44-8, *A*), a K-wire is placed before two sequential dilators are passed in the same fashion (Fig. 44-8, *B* and *C*). After the third dilator is placed, a table-mounted, split-blade retractor is delivered over the final dilator. The retractor itself is fitted with the same EMG evaluating capabilities as the dilators, through only the posterior aspect of the center (posterior) blade (Fig. 44-9, *A* and *B*). The placement of the retractor on the lateral disc space is confirmed on AP and lateral fluororadiography. Next, the retractor is stabilized using a table-mounted articulating arm (Fig. 44-9, *C*).

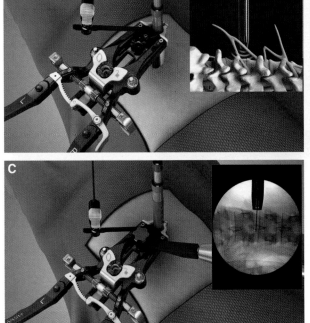

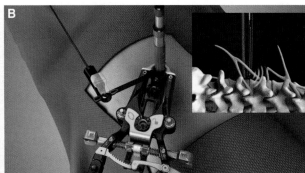

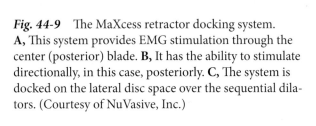

Fig. 44-9   The MaXcess retractor docking system. **A,** This system provides EMG stimulation through the center (posterior) blade. **B,** It has the ability to stimulate directionally, in this case, posteriorly. **C,** The system is docked on the lateral disc space over the sequential dilators. (Courtesy of NuVasive, Inc.)

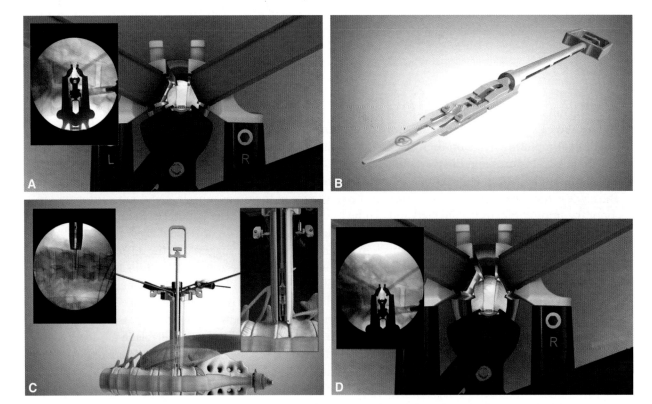

Fig. 44-10   **A,** The surgical view during a lateral transpsoas procedure. **B,** An intradiscal shim. **C,** The shim is delivered, securing the retractor system at the disc space. **D,** Isolated ventral retraction of the superior and inferior (anterior) retractor blades. (Courtesy of NuVasive, Inc.)

Once the retractor is placed and secured using the table-mounted arm, a light source is introduced along the cranial and caudal retractor blades to illuminate the disc space. A ball-tipped EMG probe is useful to determine if the surgical exposure is free of motor nerves and to probe posterior to the center blade to positively confirm the location of the plexus. Next, an intradiscal shim is placed in the center blade to secure the retractor at the surgical site and prevent tissue creep through the distal end of the retractor (Fig. 44-10, *A* through *C*). The K-wire is then removed, and the final position is confirmed with lateral fluororadiography (Fig. 44-10, *D*).

The disc space can be exposed independently in cranial, caudal, ventral, or dorsal directions. However, because the center blade is shimmed to the disc space, ventral expansion is typically performed to prevent irritation or injury to the lumbar plexus posteriorly, either by posterior retraction or compression against the transverse process through the substance of the psoas muscle.

Disc Space Preparation and Implantation

The disc space is prepared with standard techniques and instrumentation. An annulotomy on the lateral disc space is made to the approximate size of the subsequent intervertebral implant. The nucleus and remaining disc material needed to advance the implant are then removed. The contralateral annulus is released to allow parallel distraction, which is particularly important in the correction of coronal deformities. The cartilaginous endplate is carefully removed and prepared for fusion. Care should be taken to preserve the endplates, particularly the cortical bone of the apophyseal ring, to decrease the risk of intervertebral cage subsidence. Graft material is delivered at the discretion of the operating surgeon, though the use of supraphysiologic bone graft material has been associated in the lateral approach with elevated postoperative neural injury rates.[27]

Once the disc space is adequately developed for interbody fusion, implant trials can be introduced for appropriate sizing (Fig. 44-11, *A*). An appropriate and physiologic implant is selected and delivered into the space with slides that guide it and protect the endplates from violation during implantation (Fig. 44-11, *B*). The final position of the implant is confirmed with lateral and AP fluororadiography (Fig. 44-11, *C* and *D*).

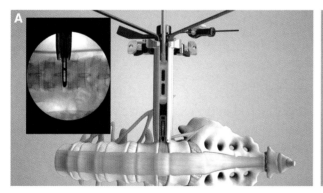 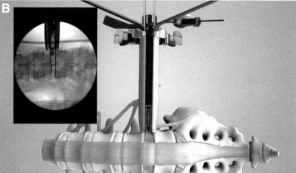

Fig. 44-11 **A,** Intervertebral implants are trialed to determine an appropriate cage size for lateral transpsoas interbody fusion. **B,** An intervertebral implant is delivered using endplate-protecting slides.

Continued

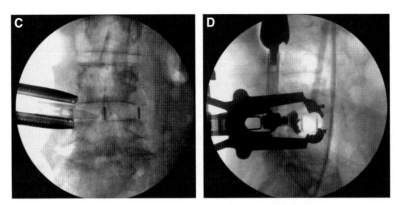

Fig. 44-11, cont'd   **C** and **D,** AP and lateral intraoperative fluororadiographs show final placement of the intervertebral cage in XLIF. (Courtesy of NuVasive, Inc.)

FIXATION AND CLOSURE

Supplemental fixation can be applied through a variety of methods. Anterolateral plating can be used for a single-incision interbody fusion and supplemental internal fixation. In addition, several fixation types can be applied without patient repositioning, including bilateral transpedicular facet fixation, spinous process plating, and unilateral (sometimes bilateral) pedicle screw and rod fixation. Avoidance of patient repositioning maximizes surgical efficiency and decreases anesthesia risks.

If anterolateral plating is not applied, the intradiscal shim and retractor can be carefully removed after the intervertebral spacer is placed. Although substantial bleeding generally does not occur with this procedure, hemostasis at the surgical site and the surrounding tissue (particularly the psoas muscle) is required (with bipolar cautery and hemostatic agents) and confirmed to decrease the possibility of painful hematomata. Some surgeons apply 2 to 3 ml of 0.25% Marcaine onto the psoas muscle and infiltrate the skin, subcutaneous, and muscular tissues of the lateral body wall to assist in managing early postoperative pain. In most cases, the muscles of the lateral body wall do not require direct repair, though abdominal wall muscles and/or fascia can be sutured to protect against postoperative hernias. Subcutaneous tissue is approximated with absorbable suture, and the skin is closed with the surgeon's method of choice.

POSTOPERATIVE CARE

Patients are encouraged to ambulate within hours of surgery to aid in the recovery of psoas function and to minimize risk of postsurgical complications from inactivity such as atelectasis, venous thrombosis, and ileus. Patients are typically discharged within 24 hours of surgery. This is determined on a case-by-case basis.[22,28,29]

POTENTIAL COMPLICATIONS AND MANAGEMENT

Mini-open lateral approaches have risks and challenges. A 90-degree off-midline lateral approach and lateral development of the retroperitoneal space are generally not taught as part of conventional spine surgery training; therefore the anatomy might be relatively unfamiliar. Passage through the substance of the psoas major requires identification and avoidance of the nerves of the lumbar plexus, with trunks and roots posterior and the genitofemoral nerve at lower lumbar levels anterior to the exposure corridor. Advanced neuromonitoring is required to localize neural anatomy.

Postoperative side effects of XLIF include transient discomfort and/or weakness with active hip flexion and/or postoperative sensory disturbances on the operative-side groin, leg, or thigh. Transient postoperative hip flexion weakness is thought to be related to psoas muscle dissection and atonia. Sensory disturbances are likely the result of irritation to sensory nerves relevant to the approach. Careful attention to the extent and duration of retraction can mitigate such side effects, highlighting the need for surgical efficiency during the procedure.[17]

Complication rates after XLIF vary, though most have generally favorable and acceptable findings, compared with conventional surgery, and are at least equivalent to alternative, less-invasive approaches for a variety of surgical indications.[7,21,28-33] Complications include injury to the lumbar plexus (distal motor weakness and/or significantly adverse sensory changes); graft subsidence; subpsoas, intrapsoas, or retroperitoneal hematoma; and graft migration typically after inadvertent anterior longitudinal ligament release.[17,22,34-37] A wide range of lumbar plexus injuries manifesting as distal weakness are reported in the literature. The best available evidence is from a prospective, multicenter, IRB-approved study of 102 XLIF cases at L3-4 and/or L4-5.[17] The authors reported a 2.9% rate of new distal weakness (two in the quadriceps and one in the tibialis anterior), all of which had resolved by 6 months postoperatively. They also observed a rate of 28% for hip flexion weakness on the approach side and a rate of 18% for mild thigh sensory changes, which all resolved in the early postoperative period without intervention. Similarly, in a large series study of 600 consecutive XLIF cases, Rodgers et al[21] reported an overall perioperative complication rate of 6.2%, with a 0.7% (4/600) rate of new distal weakness.

Complication avoidance techniques include careful preoperative review of imaging (particularly axial MRI) to evaluate anatomy at each level to be treated, adherence to intraoperative neuromonitoring feedback, and diligent adherence to surgical technique. Graft subsidence is best prevented by careful attention to intraoperative endplate integrity and consideration of supplementation with bilateral pedicle screw and rod fixation in the case of identified intraoperative endplate violation. Additionally, the relationship between cage subsidence and the use of supraphysiologic bone graft material is not well understood, but should be considered, especially in patients with diminished bone quality. With respect to hematomata, confirmation of site and approach corridor is important. Finally, graft migration typically occurs after inadvertent anterior longitudinal ligament release. This complication can be prevented by intraoperative attention to the integrity of the ligament, noting audible or palpable evidence of release and sudden looseness of the cage or trial in the intervertebral space. If this is identified, an internally fixated intervertebral cage should be placed.

Clinical and radiographic outcomes after XLIF have been reported in a variety of publications and show broad efficacy over mid- and long-term time points.[10,38-41] Direct comparisons show that outcomes are at least equivalent to those of conventional approaches.

PATIENT EXAMPLE

This patient presented with L4-5 degenerative disc disease with modic changes and slight retrolisthesis (Fig. 44-12, *A*). A single-position XLIF was performed at L4-5 with transpedicular facet fixation. The patient is shown postoperatively with good maintenance of disc height, alignment, and evidence of fusion (Fig. 44-12, *B* and *C*).

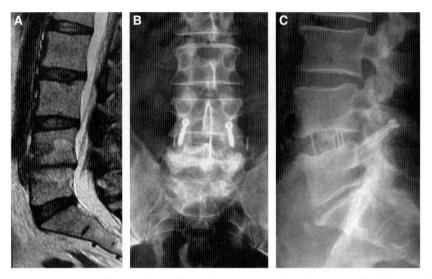

Fig. 44-12   **A,** Preoperative sagittal MRI showed L4-5 degenerative disc disease with slight retrolisthesis. **B** and **C,** Postoperative radiographs after XLIF with fixation.

CONCLUSION

A lateral approach to treat thoracolumbar pathology allows for efficient delivery of a minimally disruptive interbody fusion that decreases associated surgical morbidity, in general. This approach has been shown to provide favorable outcomes in the perioperative through long-term postoperative period. However, careful preoperative planning, attention to surgical technique, and adherence to intraoperative neuromonitoring are needed for a reproducibly efficient procedure.

REFERENCES

1. Ozgur BM, Aryan HE, Pimenta L, et al. Extreme Lateral Interbody Fusion (XLIF): a novel surgical technique for anterior lumbar interbody fusion. Spine J 6:435-443, 2006.
2. Baaj AA, Dakwar E, Le TV, Smith WD, Uribe JS, et al. Complications of the mini-open anterolateral approach to the thoracolumbar spine. J Clin Neurosci 19:1265-1267, 2012.
3. Berjano P, Damilano M, Lamartina C. Sagittal alignment correction and reconstruction of lumbar post-traumatic kyphosis via MIS lateral approach. Eur Spine J 21:2718-2720, 2012.
4. Dakwar E, Smith WD, Malone KT, Uribe JS. Minimally invasive lateral extracavitary resection of foraminal neurofibromas. J Clin Neurosci 18:1510-1512, 2011.
5. Dakwar E, Ahmadian A, Uribe JS. The anatomical relationship of the diaphragm to the thoracolumbar junction during the minimally invasive lateral extracoelomic (retropleural/retroperitoneal) approach. J Neurosurg Spine 16:359-364, 2012.

6. Deviren V, Kuelling FA, Poulter G, et al. Minimal invasive anterolateral transthoracic transpleural approach: a novel technique for thoracic disc herniation. A review of the literature, description of a new surgical technique and experience with first 12 consecutive patients. J Spinal Disord Tech 24:E40-E48, 2011.

7. Isaacs RE, Hyde J, Goodrich JA, et al. A prospective, nonrandomized, multicenter evaluation of extreme lateral interbody fusion for the treatment of adult degenerative scoliosis: perioperative outcomes and complications. Spine 35(26 Suppl):S322-S330, 2010.

8. Karikari IO, Nimjee SM, Hardin CA, et al. Extreme lateral interbody fusion approach for isolated thoracic and thoracolumbar spine diseases: initial clinical experience and early outcomes. J Spinal Disord Tech 24:368-375, 2011.

9. Nacar OA, Ulu MO, Pekmezci M, et al. Surgical treatment of thoracic disc disease via minimally invasive lateral transthoracic trans/retropleural approach: analysis of 33 patients. Neurosurg Rev 36:455-465, 2013.

10. Phillips FM, Isaacs RE, Rodgers WB, et al. Adult degenerative scoliosis treated with XLIF: clinical and radiographic results of a prospective multicenter study with 24-month follow-up. Spine 38:1853-1861, 2013.

11. Smith WD, Dakwar E, Le TV, Uribe JS. Minimally invasive surgery for traumatic spinal pathologies: a mini-open, lateral approach in the thoracic and lumbar spine. Spine 35(26 Suppl):S338-S346, 2010.

12. Uribe JS, Dakwar E, Le TV, Smith WD, et al. Minimally invasive surgery treatment for thoracic spine tumor removal: a mini-open, lateral approach. Spine 35(26 Suppl):S347-S354, 2010.

13. Uribe JS, Dakwar E, Cardona RF, et al. Minimally invasive lateral retropleural thoracolumbar approach: cadaveric feasibility study and report of 4 clinical cases. Neurosurgery 68:32-39, 2011.

14. Uribe JS, Smith WD, Pimenta L, et al. Minimally invasive lateral approach for symptomatic thoracic disc herniation: initial multicenter clinical experience. J Neurosurg Spine 16:264-279, 2012.

15. Uribe JS, Vale FL, Dakwar E. Electromyographic monitoring and its anatomical implications in minimally invasive spine surgery. Spine 35(26 Suppl):S368-S374, 2010.

16. Uribe JS, Arredondo N, Dakwar E, et al. Defining the safe working zones using the minimally invasive lateral retroperitoneal transpsoas approach: an anatomical study. J Neurosurg Spine 13:260-266, 2010.

17. Tohmeh AG, Rodgers WB, Peterson MD. Dynamically evoked, discrete-threshold electromyography in the extreme lateral interbody fusion approach. J Neurosurg Spine 14:31-37, 2011.

18. Smith WD, Youssef JA, Christian G, et al. Lumbarized sacrum as a relative contraindication for lateral transpsoas interbody fusion at L5-6. J Spinal Disord Tech 25:285-291, 2012.

19. Rasanen P, Ohman J, Sintonen H, et al. Cost-utility analysis of routine neurosurgical spinal surgery. J Neurosurg Spine 5:204-209, 2006.

20. Buvanendran A, Thillainathan V. Preoperative and postoperative anesthetic and analgesic techniques for minimally invasive surgery of the spine. Spine 35:S274-S280, 2010.

21. Rodgers WB, Gerber EJ, Patterson J. Intraoperative and early postoperative complications in extreme lateral interbody fusion: an analysis of 600 cases. Spine 36:26-32, 2011.

22. Peterson MD, Youssef JA. Extreme lateral interbody fusion (XLIF®): lumbar surgical technique. In Goodrich JA, Volcan IJ, eds. Extreme Lateral Interbody Fusion (XLIF®). St Louis: Quality Medical Publishing, 2013.

23. Rodgers WB, Cox CS, Gerber EJ. Experience and early results with a minimally invasive technique for anterior column support through eXtreme Lateral Interbody Fusion (XLIF). US Musculoskelet Rev 2:28-32, 2007.

24. Dakwar E, Rifkin SI, Volcan IJ, Uribe JS, et al. Rhabdomyolysis and acute renal failure following minimally invasive spine surgery: report of 5 cases. J Neurosurg Spine 14:785-788, 2011.

25. Park DK, Lee MJ, Lin EL, et al. The relationship of intrapsoas nerves during a transpsoas approach to the lumbar spine: anatomic study. J Spinal Disord Tech 23:223-228, 2010.

26. Regev GJ, Chen L, Dhawan M, et al. Morphometric analysis of the ventral nerve roots and retroperitoneal vessels with respect to the minimally invasive lateral approach in normal and deformed spines. Spine 34:1330-1335, 2009.

27. Lykissas MG, Aichmair A, Sama AA, et al. Nerve injury and recovery after lateral lumbar interbody fusion with and without bone morphogenetic protein-2 augmentation: a cohort-controlled study. Spine J 14:217-224, 2014.

28. Lucio JC, VanConia RB, Deluzio KJ, et al. Economics of less invasive spinal surgery: an analysis of hospital cost differences between open and minimally invasive instrumented spinal fusion procedures during the perioperative period. Risk Manag Healthc Policy 5:65-74, 2012.

29. Smith WD, Christian G, Serrano S, Malone KT. A comparison of perioperative charges and outcome between open and mini-open approaches for anterior lumbar discectomy and fusion. J Clin Neurosci 19:673-680, 2012.

30. Le TV, Smith DA, Greenberg MS, Uribe JS, et al. Complications of lateral plating in the minimally invasive lateral transpsoas approach. J Neurosurg Spine 16:302-307, 2012.

31. Rodgers WB, Cox CS, Gerber EJ. Early complications of extreme lateral interbody fusion in the obese. J Spinal Disord Tech 23:393-397, 2010.

32. Rodgers WB, Gerber EJ, Rodgers JA. Lumbar fusion in octogenarians: the promise of minimally invasive surgery. Spine 35(26 Suppl):S355-S360, 2010.

33. Arnold PM, Anderson KK, McGuire RA Jr. The lateral transpsoas approach to the lumbar and thoracic spine: a review. Surg Neurol Int 3(Suppl 3):S198-S215, 2012.

34. Daffner SD, Wang JC. Migrated XLIF cage: case report and discussion of surgical technique. Orthopedics 33:518, 2010.

35. Le TV, Baaj AA, Dakwar E, et al. Subsidence of polyetheretherketone intervertebral cages in minimally invasive lateral retroperitoneal transpsoas lumbar interbody fusion. Spine 37:1268-1273, 2012.

36. Le TV, Burkett CJ, Deukmedjian AR, Uribe JS. Postoperative lumbar plexus injury after lumbar retroperitoneal transpsoas minimally invasive lateral interbody fusion. Spine 38:E13-E20, 2013.

37. Marchi L, Abdala N, Oliveira L, et al. Radiographic and clinical evaluation of cage subsidence after stand-alone lateral interbody fusion. J Neurosurg Spine 19:110-118, 2013.

38. Kotwal S, Kawaguchi S, Lebl D, et al. Minimally invasive lateral lumbar interbody fusion: clinical and radiographic outcome at a minimum 2-year follow-up. J Spinal Disord Tech. 2012 Sep 6. [Epub ahead of print]

39. Rodgers JA, Gerber EJ, Lehmen JA, et al. Clinical and radiographic outcome in less invasive lumbar fusion: XLIF at two year follow-up. J Spine Neurosurg 2:1-6, 2013.

40. Rodgers WB, Gerber EJ, Patterson JR. Fusion after minimally disruptive anterior lumbar interbody fusion: analysis of extreme lateral interbody fusion by computed tomography. SAS J 4:63-66, 2010.

41. Rodgers WB, Gerber EJ, Rodgers JA. Clinical and radiographic outcomes of extreme lateral approach to interbody fusion with β-tricalcium phosphate and hydroxyapatite composite for lumbar degenerative conditions. Int J Spine Surg 6:24-28, 2012.

45

Minimally Invasive Surgical Treatment of Spondylolisthesis

Michael S. Park ▪ *Mark D. Peterson* ▪ *Juan S. Uribe*

Axial back pain with radiculopathy, neurogenic claudication, and instability associated with lumbar spondylolisthesis are indications for surgical intervention. Spondylolisthesis has traditionally been classified by cause as dysplastic, isthmic (which is subclassified into spondylolytic, pars elongation, and acute traumatic pars fracture), degenerative, traumatic, and pathologic.[1] Treatment options have ranged from limited decompression with anterior and/or posterior fusion with or without listhesis correction to multilevel fusion for deformity correction.[2,3] In patients with spondylolisthesis and related neurologic symptoms, radiographic and clinical outcomes have been shown to be superior after spinal fusion, compared with conservative treatment and decompression alone.[4-8] Traditional posterior approaches in combination with anterior arthrodesis have been routinely performed for spinal fusion with satisfactory results in this population.[9-10] However, posterior approaches necessitate relatively extensive muscle dissection and removal of posterior elements, which can further compromise spinal stability. Such approach-related risks and complications should be considered before a particular surgical technique is chosen.[11-14]

Minimally invasive surgery has been developed to potentially mitigate approach-related risks and surgical morbidity.[15-18] Minimally invasive transforaminal lumbar interbody fusion, mini-open transforaminal lumbar interbody fusion/posterior lumbar interbody fusion, and anterior lumbar interbody fusion are common and effective techniques that allow direct decompression of neural elements, interbody fusion, and deformity correction through a single approach. However, these procedures involve a degree of ligamentous and/or facet disruption.

Lateral retroperitoneal transpsoas minimally invasive surgery–lumbar interbody fusion (MIS-LIF) has become an increasingly popular means of fusion, because it does not disrupt the posterior stabilizing elements of the spine, provides indirect foraminal decompression, and allows placement of a larger interbody implant with satisfactory fusion rates.[16,19-21] In this chapter, we review the indications, contraindications, surgical technique, and outcomes for minimally invasive surgical treatment of spondylolisthesis with retroperitoneal transpsoas lumbar interbody fusion with percutaneous pedicle screw instrumentation.

TREATMENT OPTIONS

Nonsurgical and surgical options are available for the treatment of spondylolisthesis. Physical therapy and rehabilitative exercises can be helpful to strengthen core muscles and improve aerobic conditioning and, along with weight loss and obesity reduction, can help to prevent disease progression. Medications that are frequently used for treating symptoms of spondylolisthesis include nonsteroidal antiinflammatory medications, short-term glucocorticoids, and narcotic-based analgesics. Low-dose antidepressants, gabapentin, and pregabalin can be given to treat neuropathic pain. Interventional pain management techniques include epidural steroid injections, facet injections, and rhizotomy.[22]

In the presence of neurologic deficits and/or pain refractory to nonoperative measures, surgical intervention is warranted. For degenerative spondylolisthesis, the Spine Patient Outcomes Research Trial (SPORT) demonstrated superior clinical outcomes after fusion, compared with nonoperative care,[23,24] and long-term (4-year) greater cost effectiveness of instrumented fusion, compared with simple decompression.[24,25] Glassman et al[26] showed that decompression and posterolateral fusion had the best outcomes with regard to pain improvement and quality of life at 1 and 2 years postoperatively when performed for degenerative spondylolisthesis versus other degenerative pathology.[26] However, data showed a decreased risk of failure with instrumented versus noninstrumented fusion.[5,27]

Given these considerations, we believe the best surgical option for the treatment of lumbar spondylolisthesis is interbody fusion with bilateral pedicle screw instrumentation. Compared with other interbody fusion methods, a lateral retroperitoneal transpsoas approach prevents approach-related morbidity from anterior or posterior, including mobilization of critical vascular structures, disruption of the anterior longitudinal ligament, the risk of retrograde ejaculation in males, and disruption of the posterior ligamentous structures. A lateral approach, as with anterior lumbar interbody fusion, allows placement of a large interbody cage for greater restoration of disc height and fusion rates, compared with posterior lumbar interbody fusion or transforaminal lumbar interbody fusion cages. It also provides indirect decompression and restoration of anatomic alignment without disruption of the anterior longitudinal ligament, the posterior longitudinal ligament, or posterior ligamentous structures.

INDICATIONS AND CONTRAINDICATIONS

Indications for lateral retroperitoneal transpsoas lumbar interbody fusion for degenerative spondylolisthesis include Meyerding[28] grade I or II spondylolisthesis. For higher grades of listhesis, a lateral approach for lumbar interbody fusion is generally not recommended, because the working window is effectively closed by the anterior migration of neural structures. Posterior element insufficiency, demonstrated by a pars defect or by an intact pars with mobility on dynamic radiographs, warrants instrumented fusion. Relative contraindications to transpsoas approaches are generally limited to prior abdominal or especially retroperitoneal surgery and aberrant vascular anatomy on the side of the planned approach, although the procedure may possibly be safely performed from the other side.

PREOPERATIVE EVALUATION AND PLANNING

Preoperative evaluation starts by obtaining a patient's history and performing a physical examination. In particular, prior surgical intervention is reviewed, especially laminectomy, facetectomy, or instrumentation and fusion, and abdominal or retroperitoneal procedures, because this may dictate the side of a chosen approach or preclude a lateral approach altogether. Unlike transforaminal lumbar interbody fusion, in which the side of approach is dictated by symptomatology, the side of approach for a lateral retroperitoneal transpsoas interbody fusion is most often determined by the side of more favorable local anatomy. Lumbar spine radiographs with dynamic flexion-extension films are routinely obtained to assess mobility of the listhesis and to confirm the degree of listhesis. Prone MRI has a tendency to diminish the degree of listhesis; therefore dynamic plain films are especially important if positional MRI (which is not routinely used) is not obtained.

Many patients will have already obtained an MRI of the lumbar spine, which can be used to determine the degree of canal and neuroforaminal stenosis. If MRI is precluded (for example, because of the presence of a non-MRI-compatible cardiac pacemaker or defibrillator), then CT myelography can provide these data. The presence of a pars interarticularis defect can be detected on MRI, but this is better demonstrated on CT. Particularly in the setting of prior lumbar surgery, CT is useful for surgical planning to determine the presence of laminectomy, instrumentation, and the status of the facet joints. We routinely obtain a CT for such planning and to accurately measure pedicle screw diameters and lengths. The configuration of the psoas musculature and the major vascular anatomy (for example, the aorta, inferior vena cava, and iliac vessels) need to be identified for a planned lateral approach, along with the relative location of the segmentary vessels in relation to the disc space if possible, because injury to these vessels has been observed during contralateral annulus release. Finally, we obtain standing 36-inch scoliosis films to assess global spinal alignment, although this is less of a consideration for a one-level spondylolisthesis.

OPERATIVE TECHNIQUE: MINIMALLY INVASIVE LATERAL TRANSPSOAS LUMBAR INTERBODY FUSION

In 2006 Ozgur et al[16] originally described the anterolateral (or direct lateral) transpsoas approach for placement of a large interbody cage. The patient is given general endotracheal anesthesia and positioned in a true lateral decubitus position. In many cases, much of the listhesis will correct when the patient is placed in a lateral position. We believe that this occurs because the anteroposterior shearing forces are eliminated. Conversely, when a patient is placed in a prone or supine position, gravity can supply these shearing forces.

Proper orthogonal visualization is confirmed by cross-table AP and lateral films. The skin is marked with fluoroscopic guidance and then incised. The retroperitoneal space is entered in a blunt fashion after gentle splitting of the abdominal wall muscles and transversalis fascia. After the retroperitoneal space is entered, the surgeon uses his or her finger to sweep the peritoneum anteriorly and palpate down to the psoas muscle (Fig. 45-1, A). The anteroposterior midpoint of the psoas muscle is approximated by palpating for the greatest bulk of the psoas muscle. This serves as a suitable initial entry point for the first dilator, which is introduced to the surface of the psoas muscle, while the index finger guides the dilator safely to the desired location. This is confirmed on a lateral fluoroscopic image.

The fibers of the psoas muscle are gently dissected using a dilator, with directional EMG monitoring to assess the proximity of the lumbar plexus nerve roots. Serial dilators are passed over the initial dilator, provided that EMG readings are safe, and an expandable tubular retractor such as MaXcess (NuVasive, San Diego, CA) is passed over the largest dilator and attached to a table-mounted system (Fig. 45-1, B).

With the retractor in place, a discectomy can be performed with a combination of curettes, rongeurs, rasps, and broaches. The contralateral annulus is released with a Cobb elevator to accommodate a long (that is, wide) implant that can rest on both lateral margins of the epiphyseal ring, maximizing endplate support. Interbody distraction and implant placement in an anterior and bilateral epiphyseal location restores disc height and corrects sagittal and coronal plane imbalance.

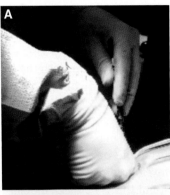

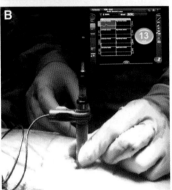

Fig. 45-1   A minimally invasive lateral approach. **A,** Blunt finger dissection is performed after the retroperitoneal space has been entered. **B,** Serial directional EMG dilators are placed. A sample directional EMG reading is shown in the *inset.*

In the setting of spondylolisthesis, several technical considerations are particularly important. The retractor will often be placed more anterior on the posterior level of the spondylolisthesis than usual, to prevent placement of the shim posterior to the posterior longitudinal ligament. In higher-grade (grade II) spondylolisthesis and/or at L4-5, surgeons should pay special attention to the EMG readings and the location of the lumbar plexus, particularly the femoral nerve; these migrate anteriorly because of the anterolisthesis. Once the lateral disc space is exposed, the working window may be smaller than that encountered in patients without spondylolisthesis, requiring the initial discectomy to be started in a limited area. As disc material is removed, the segment will relax. An incrementally larger disc area is exposed, facilitating subsequent discectomy and endplate preparation. Because of the listhesis, every effort should be made to ensure the integrity of the anterior and posterior longitudinal ligaments, which are essential for ligamentotaxis and its effects on realignment and indirect decompression. If these structures are disrupted, the interbody cage should be fixated to the adjacent vertebral body with posterior pedicle screw instrumentation.[22]

Selection of an appropriate implant is critical. One of the advantages of lateral retroperitoneal transpsoas interbody fusion is the ability to place a larger implant for greater cross-sectional area and rates of fusion. However, an excessively large cage can undergo retropulsion when the listhesis is reduced. Furthermore, an oversized implant can prevent further deformity reduction with the use of pedicle screws (for example, with in situ bending) if necessary. An unduly large cage increases the risk of subsidence and loss of indirect decompression. For these reasons we often place a 22 mm long (anterior to posterior) cage and do not use 26 mm cages.

Finally, we recommend posterior bilateral pedicle screw instrumentation for supplemental internal fixation. This can be performed in a percutaneous, minimally invasive fashion. As opposed to lateral plating (which has the advantage of providing interbody fusion and internal fixation through a single incision and approach, is weakest in flexion and extension, and may not provide adequate support for generally unaccounted-for anteroposterior shearing forces), pedicle screw instrumentation provides three-column fixation and is the optimal construct for spondylolisthesis.[29]

OUTCOMES

Several reports have been published on the results of lateral retroperitoneal transpsoas MIS-LIF for spondylolisthesis. Ahmadian et al[30] reported on a series of 26 patients with grade I and 5 patients with grade II spondylolisthesis, all at L4-5, who had MIS-LIF with bilateral percutaneous pedicle screw instrumentation. None had posterior element manipulation. The mean follow-up was 18 months. No weakness or motor deficit was reported postoperatively. This was a significant finding, given the increased concern for lumbar plexus injury with transpsoas approaches at this level. All patients had improvement in their listhesis, and only 4 (12.9%) had residual postoperative listhesis. Transient anterior thigh numbness was noted in 22.9% of patients in this series, all of which resolved by 3 months. No hardware failures or pseudarthroses occurred. Mean ODI, SF-36, and VAS scores improved significantly postoperatively.[30]

In a report of transpsoas MIS-LIF for grade II spondylolisthesis, 97% of which were at L4-5, Rodgers et al[31] presented a series of 63 patients who were followed for 1 year. No permanent neurologic deficits, infections, or pseudarthroses were noted. The mean slip corrected from 11.1 mm preoperatively to 3.0 mm postoperatively and to 3.6 mm at 1 year ($p < 0.001$). The disc height was nearly doubled 1 year postoperatively ($p < 0.001$). Mean pain VAS scores improved from 8.6 preoperatively to 2.2 at 1 year. Satisfaction rates were nearly 90%. Internal fixation was performed with pedicle screws in 98% of patients in this series. Two complications were reported: one postoperative ileus and one broken screw 14 months postoperatively, which occurred in a motor vehicle accident.

In another series, stand-alone transpsoas MIS-LIF was performed in 52 patients with grade I or II stable degenerative spondylolisthesis.[32] Patients were followed for a minimum of 24 months. Nineteen percent of patients had hip flexion weakness, and 9.6% had anterior thigh numbness, although these effects resolved within 6 weeks. The authors relied on only ligamentotaxis and indirect decompression. They reported a 55% increase in disc height and an 87% fusion rate, with improvement of 54.5% ($p = 0.001$) and 60% ($p < 0.001$) in the ODI and VAS scores, respectively. No pseudarthroses occurred; therefore no patients required reoperation for this indication. Listhesis improved from a mean of 15.1% preoperatively to 7.1% at 24 months ($p < 0.001$). Cage subsidence occurred in 9 of 52 cases (17.3%). Seven patients required reoperation: 5 for recurrent stenosis after cage subsidence and 2 for inadequate decompression. It can be argued that restenosis from subsidence might have been avoided with the placement of supplemental internal fixation.

These reports compare favorably with results for PLIF and transforaminal lumbar interbody fusion in the setting of degenerative spondylolisthesis. In a series of 251 patients undergoing posterior lumbar interbody fusion (82% for spondylolisthesis), 10.3% had surgical complications.[33] In particular, neurologic complications occurred in 8.3% of patients, 90% of which included motor deficits; 21% of these were permanent and 47% were severe. Reported complication rates for transforaminal lumbar interbody fusion in patients with spondylolisthesis are 33%[34] to 34%[35]; the former series had a greater improvement in VAS and ODI scores in younger compared with older patients, whereas the latter series reported that 64% of 24 patients had improved back pain after the procedure.

PATIENT EXAMPLE

This 34-year-old man presented with a 2-year history of lower back pain and neurogenic claudication. His preoperative MRI revealed a grade I anterolisthesis at L4-5, and dynamic radiographs showed 3 to 4 mm of translation (Fig. 45-2, *A* through *D*). Left-sided lateral retroperitoneal transpsoas lumbar interbody fusion was performed at L4-5, with percutaneous pedicle screw instrumentation. The patient is shown postoperatively with his spondylolisthesis nearly fully reduced (Fig. 45-2, *E* and *F*). He reports complete resolution of his symptoms, as demonstrated on his VAS responses (Fig. 45-2, *G* and *H*). His wounds have healed nicely (Fig. 45-2, *I*).

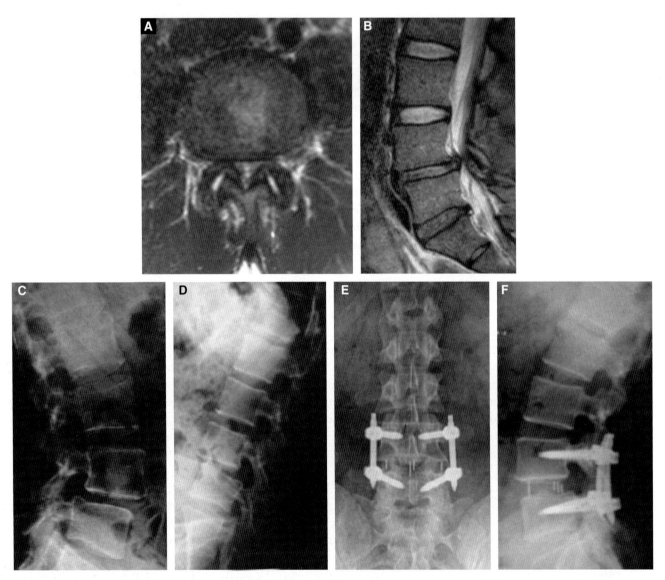

Fig. 45-2   **A** and **B,** Preoperative T2-weighted MRI. **C** and **D,** Preoperative extension and flexion radiographs. **E** and **F,** Postoperative AP and lateral radiographs.

G

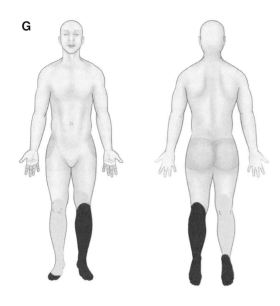

PREOP VAS Pain Scale Questions

11. On a scale from 0 to 10, mark the intensity of your <u>back pain</u> during the past week, with 0 being "None" and 10 being "Unbearable pain." *(Mark only one.)*

0 1 2 3 4 5 6 7 8 9 10
None I-O-O-O-O-O-O-O-O-O-●-O-I Unbearable

12. On a scale from 0 to 10, mark the intensity of your <u>left leg pain</u> during the past week, with 0 being "None" and 10 being "Unbearable pain." *(Mark only one.)*

0 1 2 3 4 5 6 7 8 9 10
None I-O-O-O-O-O-O-O-O-O-●-O-I Unbearable

13. On a scale from 0 to 10, mark the intensity of your <u>right leg pain</u> during the past week, with 0 being "None" and 10 being "Unbearable pain." *(Mark only one.)*

0 1 2 3 4 5 6 7 8 9 10
None I-O-O-O-O-O-O-O-O-O-●-O-I Unbearable

H

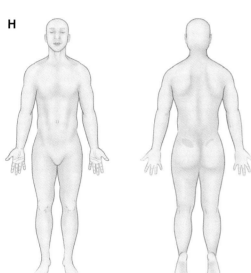

POSTOP VAS Pain Scale Questions

11. On a scale from 0 to 10, mark the intensity of your <u>back pain</u> during the past week, with 0 being "None" and 10 being "Unbearable pain." *(Mark only one.)*

0 1 2 3 4 5 6 7 8 9 10
None I-O-O-●-O-O-O-O-O-O-O-O-I Unbearable

12. On a scale from 0 to 10, mark the intensity of your <u>left leg pain</u> during the past week, with 0 being "None" and 10 being "Unbearable pain." *(Mark only one.)*

0 1 2 3 4 5 6 7 8 9 10
None I-●-O-O-O-O-O-O-O-O-O-O-I Unbearable

13. On a scale from 0 to 10, mark the intensity of your <u>right leg pain</u> during the past week, with 0 being "None" and 10 being "Unbearable pain." *(Mark only one.)*

0 1 2 3 4 5 6 7 8 9 10
None I-●-O-O-O-O-O-O-O-O-O-O-I Unbearable

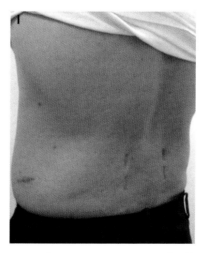

Fig. 45-2, cont'd   **G** and **H,** Preoperative and postoperative VAS and self-reported data. **I,** Lateral and posterior minimally invasive surgical incisions.

CONCLUSION

Minimally invasive retroperitoneal transpsoas interbody fusion, in conjunction with bilateral pedicle screw instrumentation, can be performed to successfully treat grade I or II lumbar spondylolisthesis. Placement of a large interbody cage can provide indirect decompression and restore anatomic alignment. By performing this from a lateral retroperitoneal transpsoas approach, the morbidity and posterior ligamentous disruption that occurs with more traditional posterior approaches are prevented. Internal fixation and further reduction of the spondylolisthesis are required, bilateral pedicle screw instrumentation is recommended.

REFERENCES

1. Wiltse LL, Newman PH, Macnab I. Classification of spondylolisis and spondylolisthesis. Clin Orthop Relat Res 117:23-29, 1976.
2. Mardjetko SM, Connelly PJ, Shott S. Degenerative lumbar spondylolisthesis. A meta-analysis of literature 1970-1993. Spine 19(20 Suppl):S2256-S2265, 1994.
3. Rousseau MA, Lazennec JY, Bass EC, et al. Predictors of outcomes after posterior decompression and fusion in degenerative spondylolisthesis. Eur Spine J 14:55-60, 2005.
4. Gibson JN, Waddell G. Surgery for degenerative lumbar spondylosis. Cochrane Database Syst Rev 4:CD001352, 2005.
5. Martin CR, Gruszczynski AT, Braunsfurth HA, et al. The surgical management of degenerative lumbar spondylolisthesis: a systematic review. Spine 32:1791-1798, 2007.
6. Turner JA, Ersek M, Herron L, et al. Surgery for lumbar spinal stenosis. Attempted meta-analysis of the literature. Spine 17:1-8, 1992.
7. Weinstein JN, Lurie JD, Tosteson TD, et al. Surgical compared with nonoperative treatment for lumbar degenerative spondylolisthesis: four-year results in the Spine Patient Outcomes Research Trial (SPORT) randomized and observational cohorts. J Bone Joint Surg Am 91:1295-1304, 2009.
8. Zagra A, Giudici F, Minoia L, et al. Long-term results of pediculo-body fixation and posterolateral fusion for lumbar spondylolisthesis. Eur Spine J 18(Suppl 1):S151-S155, 2009.
9. Gill GG, Manning JG, White HL. Surgical treatment of spondylolisthesis without spine fusion: excision of the loose lamina with decompression of the nerve roots. J Bone Joint Surg Am 37:493-520, 1955.
10. Yan DL, Pei FX, Li J, et al. Comparative study of PLIF and TLIF treatment in adult degenerative spondylolisthesis. Eur Spine J 17:1311-1316, 2008.
11. Asha MJ, Choksey MS, Shad A, et al. The role of the vascular surgeon in anterior lumbar spine surgery. Br J Neurosurg 26:499-503, 2012.
12. Lee P, Fessler RG. Perioperative and postoperative complications of single-level minimally invasive transforaminal lumbar interbody fusion in elderly adults. J Clin Neurosci 19:111-114, 2012.
13. Mehta VA, McGirt MJ, Garcés Ambrossi GL, et al. Trans-foraminal versus posterior lumbar interbody fusion: comparison of surgical morbidity. Neurol Res 33:38-42, 2011.
14. Than KD, Wang AC, Rahman SU, et al. Complication avoidance and management in anterior lumbar interbody fusion. Neurosurg Focus 31:E6, 2011.
15. Adogwa O, Parker SL, Bydon A, et al. Comparative effectiveness of minimally invasive versus open transforaminal lumbar interbody fusion: 2-year assessment of narcotic use, return to work, disability, and quality of life. J Spinal Disord Tech 24:479-484, 2011.
16. Ozgur BM, Aryan HE, Pimena L, et al. Extreme Lateral Interbody Fusion (XLIF): a novel surgical technique for anterior lumbar interbody fusion. Spine J 6:435-443, 2006.
17. Pelton MA, Phillips FM, Singh K. A comparison of perioperative costs and outcomes in patients with and without workers' compensation claims treated with minimally invasive or open transforaminal lumbar interbody fusion. Spine 37:1914-1919, 2012.
18. Rodgers WB, Gerber EJ, Rodgers JA. Lumbar fusion in octogenarians: the promise of minimally invasive surgery. Spine 35(26 Suppl):S355-S360, 2010.
19. Benglis DM, Elhammady MS, Levy AD, et al. Minimally invasive anterolateral approaches for the treatment of back pain and adult degenerative deformity. Neurosurg 63(3 Suppl):S191-S196, 2008.

20. Eck JC, Hodges S, Humphreys SC. Minimally invasive lumbar spinal fusion. J Am Acad Orthop Surg 15:321-329, 2007.

21. Pimenta L, Oliveira L, Schaffa T, et al. Lumbar total disc replacement from an extreme lateral approach: clinical experience with a minimum of 2-years' follow-up. J Neurosurg Spine 14:38-45, 2011.

22. Khajavi K, Peterson MD, Shen AY, et al. XLIF for degenerative spondylolisthesis. In Goodrich JA, Volcan IJ, eds. eXtreme Lateral Interbody Fusion (XLIF), ed 2. St Louis: Quality Medical Publishing, 2013.

23. Weinstein JN, Lurie JD, Tosteson TD, et al. Surgical versus nonsurgical treatment for lumbar degenerative spondylolisthesis. N Engl J Med 356:2257-2270, 2007.

24. Tosteson AN, Lurie JD, Tosteson TD, et al. Surgical treatment of spinal stenosis with and without degenerative spondylolisthesis: cost-effectiveness after 2 years. Ann Intern Med 149:845-853, 2008.

25. Tosteson AN, Tosteson TD, Lurie JD, et al. Comparative effectiveness evidence from the spine patient outcomes research trial: surgical versus nonoperative care for spinal stenosis, degenerative spondylolisthesis, and intervertebral disc herniation. Spine 36:2061-2068, 2011.

26. Glassman SD, Carreon LY, Djurasovic M, et al. Lumbar fusion outcomes stratified by specific diagnostic indication. Spine J 9:13-21, 2009.

27. Watters WC III, Bono CM, Gilbert TJ, et al. An evidence-based clinical guideline for the diagnosis and treatment of degenerative lumbar spondylolisthesis. Spine J 9:609-614, 2009.

28. Meyerding HW. Spondylolisthesis; surgical fusion of lumbosacral portion of spinal column and interarticular facets; use of autogenous bone grafts for relief of disabling backache. J Int Coll Surg 26:566-591, 1956.

29. Cappuccino A, Cornwall GB, Turner AW, et al. Biomechanical analysis and review of lateral lumbar fusion constructs. Spine 35(26 Suppl):S361-S367, 2010.

30. Ahmadian A, Verma S, Mundis GM Jr, et al. Minimally invasive lateral retroperitoneal transpsoas interbody fusion for L4-5 spondylolisthesis: clinical outcomes. J Neurosurg Spine 19:314-320, 2013.

31. Rodgers WB, Lehmen JA, Gerber EJ, et al. Grade 2 spondylolisthesis at L4-5 treated by XLIF: safety and midterm results in the "worst case scenario." ScientificWorldJournal 2012:356712, 2012.

32. Marchi L, Abdala N, Oliveira L, et al. Stand-alone lateral interbody fusion for the treatment of low-grade degenerative spondylolisthesis. ScientificWorldJournal 2012:456346, 2012.

33. Okuda S, Miyauchi A, Oda T, et al. Surgical complications of posterior lumbar interbody fusion with total facetectomy in 251 patients. J Neurosurg Spine 4:304-309, 2006.

34. Park Y, Ha JW, Lee YT, et al. Surgical outcomes of minimally invasive transforaminal lumbar interbody fusion for the treatment of spondylolisthesis and degenerative segmental instability. Asian Spine J 5:228-236, 2011.

35. Takahashi T, Hanakita J, Minami M, et al. Clinical outcomes and adverse events following transforaminal interbody fusion for lumbar degenerative spondylolisthesis in elderly patients. Neurol Med Chir (Tokyo) 51:829-835, 2011.

46

Minimally Disruptive Treatment of Degenerative Disc Disease

William D. Smith

The appropriate treatment of chronic low back pain, often associated with degenerative disc disease (DDD), is one of the main challenges of primary care providers and spine surgeons today. Because DDD primarily manifests with low back pain, the two are inextricably linked when the best treatment course and prognosis are considered. Low back pain has a significant societal impact on health, quality of life, and productivity. The lifetime prevalence of low back pain is estimated to be 80% to 90% of all people in the United States, and low back pain is the most common musculoskeletal condition as well as the fifth most common reason for physician visits.[1-3] The burden of low back pain and DDD to society is substantial. It is estimated that direct and indirect costs of low back pain in the United States total approximately $100 billion (2007 dollars) per year, of which two thirds is from lost work and productivity.[1-3]

The disease and symptoms are relatively challenging to reproducibly treat for many reasons. Intervertebral disc degeneration is a natural process of aging whereby water content of the disc nucleus is slowly lost, altering the motion of the disc and resistance to compression. Most people have some amount of disc degeneration asymptomatically or without chronic symptoms (3 months or longer of continual symptoms[4,5]). DDD, as described by Adams and Roughley,[6] is caused by a combination of changes in cell function, metabolism, and healing ability in the disc, in parallel with functional alterations of the disc, often accompanied by annular defects, disc prolapse, and endplate (Modic) changes in response to functional changes. These changes can ultimately lead to internal disc disruption, disc narrowing, formation of osteophytes, segmental instability, facet disruption, and discogenic pain. Because this cascade is a function of age, the societal problem is exacerbated by both increasing rates of life expectancy and a fast-expanding elderly population, led by maturation of the baby boomers in the United States. This is coupled with increased physical and quality of life requirements of the elderly, including longer working lives, elevated expectations for higher-impact activity later in life, and increased demand for efficient and effective medical treatment. Appropriate and effective treatment of this broad and rapidly growing population will truly be the future of spinal surgery.

DEFINITION OF THE PROBLEM

Conservative management is the primary course of care for patients with chronic low back pain. However, in some patients with severe and intractable pain secondary to DDD, surgical intervention is an option. Evidence-based medicine in support of surgical intervention (for example, spinal fusion) for chronic low back pain without radiculopathy is challenged by various publications that show mixed results with respect to functional outcome in patients who are treated surgically and those treated conservatively.[7-10] This variability can be explained by differences in the type and relative quality of surgical and conservative treatment modalities studied, the types of study design used, and the parameters measured.[11,12] For example, posterolateral fusion (PLF)–alone for DDD, a common procedure for spinal fusion, treats segmental instability, but it likely will not treat discogenic pain, because the disc is avoided. Conversely, unstructured, conservative management protocols likely underestimate the value of such care. With respect to study designs, challenges in evidence-based medicine for DDD are largely artifacts of poorly designed or clinically irrelevant historical randomized controlled trials on the topic (a fusion procedure versus conservative care for patients with DDD and chronic low back pain); nonrandomized studies or studies with randomization to other surgical options such as total disc replacement (TDR) have been considered in decision-making only more recently.[5] The larger body of available evidence for surgical intervention for DDD shows that fusion procedures are much more effective than is commonly understood.[5] Despite recent improvements in understanding of the surgical management of DDD, the reported historical variability has led to broad denials of spinal fusion for DDD by insurance companies in the United States. A more adversarial relationship between payers and providers has resulted. This is further complicated, because most medical devices used in fusion procedures (for example, intervertebral spacers) are cleared by the U.S. FDA only for treatment of DDD or DDD with up to grade I spondylolisthesis, based on clinical evidence. Thus the indication for which the FDA has cleared the use of spinal fusion devices is one of the most challenging surgical indications to have approved by private insurance companies. This situation leads to off-label use or less effective, alternative treatments. However, a more modern understanding of the disease and the availability of a wider variety of targeted treatment options may lead to improved outcomes that challenge these historical results. In the future, reproducibility of surgical outcomes may be more influenced by proper patient *and* procedural selection, rather than by arguments (by payers) that inappropriate or unnecessary care is being delivered.

For example, in 2009 Glassman et al[13] examined outcomes 1 and 2 years after PLF, based on diagnostic stratification. Spondylolisthesis was one of the most responsive indications in terms of symptom resolution, and DDD was one of the least responsive. In this study, 71% of patients with spondylolisthesis met the minimum clinical important difference (MCID) threshold for disability, based on ODI results 2 years postoperatively, whereas 57.6% of patients in the DDD group met the MCID. Thus more than 40% of patients with DDD did not improve sufficiently after PLF surgery to perceive a difference in their level of disability. These results show that PLF is more effective in limiting sagittal plane instability in spondylolisthesis than it is in treating discogenic disease, as mentioned previously. Unfortunately, this study has largely driven current thinking toward accepting the diminished impact of surgical treatment for DDD.

Recent findings replicating the efforts of Glassman et al[13] suggest that the type of fusion procedure performed can be a salient factor in improving outcomes after spinal fusion in patients with DDD. Khajavi et al[14] examined outcomes stratified by preoperative diagnosis in patients treated with eXtreme lateral interbody fusion (XLIF, NuVasive, Inc., San Diego, CA), which is a minimally disruptive, lateral transpsoas approach to the lumbar spine. The authors posited that an approach that directly treats the pathology (DDD) with more favorable construct biomechanics and minimal morbidity may improve outcomes, compared with historical results. The authors found far less difference in clinical outcome between surgical indications (for example, DDD compared with degenerative spondylolisthesis) and, in general, a larger magnitude of clinical improvement in a larger number of patients. A comparison of the XLIF DDD cohort of Khajavi et al[14] and the PLF cohort of Glassman et al[13] shows the following results: a net disability improvement of 18.2 (ODI) (XLIF DDD cohort) versus 16.7 (PLF DDD cohort), a net low back pain improvement of 3.7 points (VAS) (XLIF DDD) versus 2.7 points (PLF DDD cohort), and a net improvement in quality of life (SF-36 physical component score) of 11.5 (XLIF DDD cohort) versus 7.9 (PLF DDD cohort). In the XLIF DDD patients, 69.2% had *substantial* clinical benefit, a higher threshold of improvement compared with MCID, whereas only 57.6% of PLF DDD patients met the MCID. These findings may be the result of more direct treatment of the pathologic site, improved segmental stability with the anterior column supported, and/or the preservation of healthy surrounding soft and bony tissue. Regardless of the reason or reasons, these results are promising in helping to better understand the role of modern procedures in treating patients with clinical challenges. The rest of this chapter focuses on the use of XLIF in the treatment of DDD.

EVOLUTION OF THE TECHNIQUE

Luiz Pimenta developed the XLIF surgical technique in the late 1990s and early 2000s, and it was introduced in the literature in 2006 as a less invasive and more efficient (no need for an access surgeon) alternative to direct anterior lumbar interbody fusion.[15] Since that time, the approach has been used for an increasing number of expanded and complex indications, including degenerative deformity, trauma, tumor, and thoracic disc herniations.[16-19] However, XLIF was initially used for basic degenerative conditions above the L5-S1 level, which is not generally approachable because of the position of the iliac crest; therefore it is regularly performed to treat patients with symptomatic DDD and collapsed discs.

ADVANTAGES AND DISADVANTAGES

Advantages of XLIF include access to the spine for anterior lumbar interbody fusion through a 90-degree lateral approach using blunt dissection through the retroperitoneal space, without the need for an access surgeon. After the lateral aspect of the spine is accessed through the iliopsoas muscle, the disc is removed in the standard fashion, preserving the anterior and posterior longitudinal ligaments. These ligaments allow realignment of the segment and loading of the intervertebral spacer through ligamentotaxis. With an anterior column approach, a large-footprint intervertebral spacer can be placed that spans the ring apophysis to resist subsidence and provide more robust construct stiffness. The spacer has large apertures through which improved bony growth occurs. For DDD patients with discogenic pain (either present or suspected) and segmental instability, this procedure is one of the most targeted and efficient surgical options with minimal morbidity.

The procedure, however, is not without risk. Although the primary risks of ALIF (great vessel and visceral injury) are largely avoided in XLIF, passage through the psoas muscle risks injury to the lumbar plexus, which is a serious concern. Thus an XLIF approach requires the integration of advanced neuromonitoring into procedural instrumentation to identify and avoid nerves of the lumbar plexus in real time.[20,21]

INDICATIONS AND CONTRAINDICATIONS

Surgical intervention is considered for patients who present with severe clinical symptoms and have failed an appropriate course of nonoperative therapy of at least 6 months' duration. In patients with DDD and chronic low back pain without radiculopathy, MRI should corroborate clinical symptoms as much as possible, although this is not always straightforward in the treatment of DDD. There are no direct pathologic contraindications to the treatment of DDD with spinal fusion; however, relative limitations to an XLIF approach include any limitations that might challenge or prevent the procedure itself, such as lumbarized sacra with unfavorable neural anatomy and variant vascular anatomy. Individual patient anatomy and pathologic morphology should be reviewed preoperatively with respect to the specific procedure to be performed and a surgical plan developed accordingly.

PREOPERATIVE PLANNING

PHYSICAL EXAMINATION

Patient selection in the surgical treatment of DDD is of utmost importance. Patients may present with various complaints, but nearly all have low back pain. While pain location, type, and intensity vary, dull aching with bandlike pressure on the lower back is commonly reported. Radicular symptoms can be present and should be consistent with pathologic levels during localization of pain generators. Vascular claudication is ruled out in patients with claudication symptoms. Some patients have hip and groin pain. Objective pain (VAS), disability (ODI), and quality of life (SF-36) measures are useful to understand the extent of the effects of symptoms more objectively.

Physical examination is performed according to standard protocol and typically includes motor, sensory, and reflex evaluations. Abnormalities in any of these areas are compared with results of imaging and other diagnostic studies. Other preoperative examinations in the diagnosis of DDD can include provocative or anesthetic discography. Localization of the pain generator or generators is one of the primary challenges in diagnosing and treating DDD. Provocative discography is a diagnostic technique in which the disc is targeted with a needle, and saline is injected into the nucleus to pressurize the space in an attempt to elicit a painful response. Generally, this procedure is performed at multiple levels to obtain pain response information on control levels. This technique is controversial, because it is subjective in interpretation and can theoretically damage discs and annular material in suspected pathologic and control levels. An alternative to provocative discography is anesthetic discography, which involves the same procedure, but an anesthetic is injected instead of saline. In cases of suspected discogenic pain, attenuation or resolution of symptoms with anesthetic delivery suggests that the target area is the pain generator. Discography in either form should be used judiciously. It is performed only if a patient's symptoms are severe enough to warrant surgical intervention and a mismatch is obvious between imaging or physical examination results and symptomatology, or if other clinical questions remain in diagnosing the patient. I use discography selectively, and I have them performed only by experienced discographers with trusted interpretations.

Radiographic Workup and Preoperative Imaging

Standard preoperative imaging studies (plain neutral and dynamic radiographs, MRI, and CT) are helpful to evaluate the relationship between radiographic signs and clinical symptoms. Characteristic radiographic signs of DDD or degenerative arthritis of the disc include the presence of subchondral cysts, sclerosis, disc collapse, and/or marginal vertebral osteophytes. Disc height loss and listhesis are the most apparent features on lateral radiographs, though DDD can present without disc height collapse. In severe cases with fully collapsed spaces, vacuum discs can be present and should be evaluated on dynamic (particularly extension) imaging to determine the segmental mobility before surgical intervention.[22]

MR imaging is essential in the evaluation of disc integrity and endplate changes in DDD cases. Several features on MRI are important in diagnosing DDD. First, the characteristic black disc, which appears as a hypointense region on T2-weighted images, will highlight the relative lack of water content of the nucleus and may present with decreased height with respect to neighboring discs. Disc bulging with disc height loss and/or annular defects is most common in the posterior disc. It is easily visualized on sagittal and axial MRI in order to determine the relative impact of bulging or herniation on the central canal or neural foramen. Although MRI is the best modality for evaluation of soft tissue structures, one of the most important elements for visualization and assessment of DDD pathology is the integrity of the vertebral bodies on MRI, indicated by the presence of Modic changes. Modic changes are changes to the bone marrow within the vertebral bodies surrounding the changing disc (Fig. 46-1). They occur after alterations in the motion of the segment, which results from disc degeneration. When abnormal motion occurs because of a loss of disc integrity, the endplates and vertebral bodies will react and remodel accordingly. Three types of Modic changes exist. Type I is characterized by decreased T1 and increased T2 signal and typically suggests an acute process. Type II is most common in DDD and is characterized by increased T1 signal with a slightly hyperintense or isointense T2 signal. This is more typically associated with chronic processes. It represents endplate disruption and replacement with yellow marrow in response to chronic changes in the mechanics of the segment. Type I typically converts to type II, which is a stable state. Type III Modic changes include both decreased T1 and T2 signals and represent sclerotic bone without the presence of marrow. The presence of Modic changes in a patient with chronic low back pain and disc pathology consistent with DDD is a sensitive diagnostic combination.

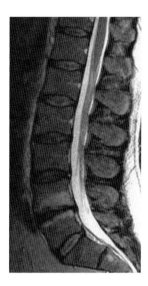

Fig. 46-1   Sagittal MRI shows degenerative disc disease and type II Modic changes at the L4-5 level.

CT can be useful in the evaluation of DDD patients, though it is not sensitive to soft tissue changes in the disc. However, annular fissures, bony abnormalities (for example, osteophytes), and Modic changes can be well visualized. Often, CT is performed as a secondary modality to MRI in the diagnosis of DDD.

SPINAL MEASUREMENTS

I believe that the evaluation and consideration of spinopelvic parameters in all spinal surgical cases is important. The broader balance measures common to the treatment of spinal deformities may not be as essential in effective treatment and outcome for DDD patients, especially when only a single level is pathologic. Surgical planning for radiographic goals should include the evaluation of segmental and lumbar lordosis to determine the physiologic goal of correction.

OPERATIVE TECHNIQUE

The operative technique for XLIF has been previously described in detail by others in the published literature[15,23] and in this book.[24] Therefore this chapter presents an abbreviated version of the surgical technique.

The XLIF procedure is performed with the patient in a lateral decubitus position, reversed (from head to toe) from the standard position, on a radiolucent table that rotates on several axes and has a break (Jackson table; Mizuho OSI, Union City, CA). The table break should be located at approximately the downside iliac crest. The patient is secured in this position with tape in several locations (Fig. 46-2, *A*). Next, each level to be treated is oriented with respect to the surgical corridor, the floor, and the fluoroscopy unit. A true AP and lateral orientation of each level to be treated is confirmed, with the lateral projection orthogonal to the floor (Fig. 46-2, *B* and *C*). This ensures that the working trajectory is perpendicular to the floor and parallel with the frontal plane of the disc space, which decreases risk of instrumentation migration anteriorly or posteriorly, especially on the contralateral side. Once the patient is positioned and the surgical orientations confirmed, the level or levels to be treated are targeted and marked. An incision is made at the 90-degree lateral mark, where the procedural approach will take place. Another incision is made in a posterolateral location, where a separate fascial exposure is made, through which the initial dilator will be inserted and guided into the retroperitoneal space to the lateral border of the iliopsoas muscle (Fig. 46-2, *D*).

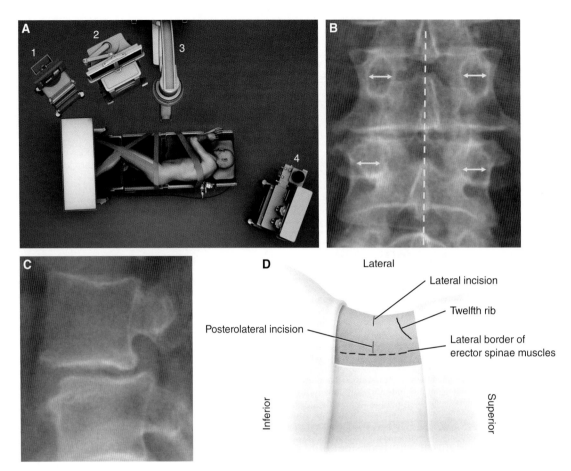

Fig. 46-2   A, Patient taping and the operating room setup for a lateral transpsoas approach, including a neuromonitoring device *(1),* a fluororadiography monitor *(2),* a C-arm *(3),* and an anesthesia table *(4).* **B** and **C,** Intraoperative AP and lateral fluororadiography show true AP and lateral views that are used in performing eXtreme lateral interbody fusion. **D,** A posterior view shows externally identifiable anatomic landmarks for a lateral transpsoas approach to the lumbar spine, including marks for the lateral and posterolateral incisions. (**A** and **D,** Courtesy of NuVasive, Inc.)

Once the initial dilator is on the lateral border of the psoas muscle, blunt passage through the muscle is guided by advanced intraoperative neuromonitoring, avoiding nerves of the lumbar plexus. In general, the border between the posterior thirds of the lateral disc space serve as the target point for the approach and procedure. Sequential dilators and, last, a specialized retractor (MaXcess, NuVasive, Inc.) are placed (Fig. 46-3, *A*). Once the lateral disc space has been exposed with the retractor, discectomy is performed and the disc space is prepared with standard surgical techniques and standard instrumentation. The anterior and posterior longitudinal ligaments are preserved. Implant trialing is performed to determine the appropriate implant size (Fig. 46-3, *B*), and an intervertebral spacer is delivered (Figs. 46-3, *C* through *E*).

Because the procedure preserves all of the posterior elements, a variety of supplemental internal fixation can be delivered, including lateral plating through the same incision, unilateral pedicle screws, interspinous plating, bilateral transpedicular facet fixation with the patient in the lateral decubitus position, and bilateral pedicle screw fixation after the patient is repositioned. (Alternatively, this can be performed with the patient in a lateral position, with special considerations.)

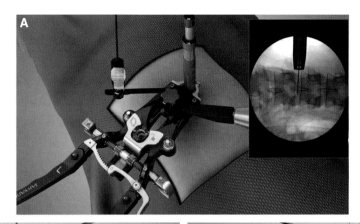

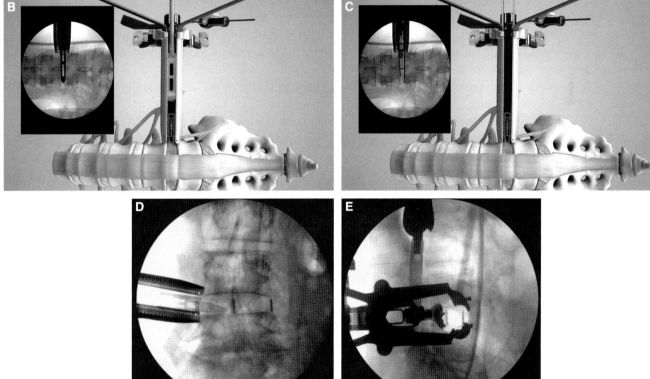

Fig. 46-3 **A,** A lateral view and an AP intraoperative fluororadiograph *(inset)* show a MaXcess retractor system docked on the lateral disc space over sequential dilators. **B,** An anterior image and AP intraoperative fluororadiograph *(inset)* show trialing of intervertebral implants in lateral transpsoas interbody fusion to determine appropriate cage dimensions. **C,** An anterior image and AP intraoperative fluororadiography *(inset)* demonstrate the delivery of intervertebral implants in lateral transpsoas interbody fusion. **D** and **E,** AP and lateral intraoperative fluororadiographs indicate final placement of the intervertebral cage in eXtreme lateral interbody fusion. (Courtesy of NuVasive, Inc.)

POTENTIAL COMPLICATIONS AND MANAGEMENT

XLIF has risks and potential complications, regardless of the pathologic condition it is performed to treat. The most apparent cause of complications is passage through the psoas muscle, adjacent to the lumbar plexus, to expose the lateral disc space. These neural structures travel within or on the superficial surface of the psoas muscle and may not be visually identifiable. Therefore advanced neuromonitoring is needed to locate and avoid these structures. Advanced neuromonitoring (evoked and free-run EMG) is used as part of a surgeon-directed, real-time neuromonitoring platform (NV M5, NuVasive, Inc.) integrated into the approach and procedural instrumentation. It provides discrete-threshold EMG responses in directional orientations to locate the relative position and distance of motor nerves from procedural instrumentation. This allows the approach corridor to be as posterior (on the lateral aspect of the spine) as possible to maximize the alignment, stability, and loading characteristics of the primary load-bearing column of the anterior spine (posterior to the lateral midline).

Along with intraoperative evaluation with neuromonitoring, one of the most important neural complication avoidance techniques in XLIF is the preoperative use of axial MRI to carefully plan each level to be treated.[25] In addition to standard operative planning, XLIF requires preoperative evaluation of the size, shape, and location of the psoas muscle at each level to be treated. This provides important information on the anatomic corridor for the approach. A more anterior and/or anteriorly elongated psoas muscle at the L4-5 level may signify the presence of a fully or partially lumbarized sacrum, or transitional anatomy, with an L5-6 segment acting as a functional L4-5 (Fig. 46-4). In these cases, it is likely that the muscular and neural anatomy resemble the anatomy at L5-S1, which has a far more anteriorly located lumbar plexus. This presents a great challenge with a lateral approach.

Other postoperative complications that can occur in the treatment of DDD with XLIF pertain to intervertebral cage-related implants, specifically, cage subsidence into the endplate or endplates and/or cage migration. Cage subsidence can be largely prevented through the use of wider-footprint intervertebral spacers, which span the ring apophysis and have more cage-endplate contact area.[26] In addition, the use of supraphysiologic biologic materials with substantial inflammatory periods may need to be avoided, especially in patients with less than ideal bone quality (for example, patients with lower bone mineral density). Cages migrate primarily after inadvertent rupture of the anterior longitudinal ligament (ALL), which can occur with trialing or implantation of implants that are taller than physiologic conditions allow. Placement of appropriate-sized implants helps to preserve the anterior longitudinal ligament and prevent anterior migration of the implant and iatrogenic endplate violation, which can lead to postoperative cage subsidence. In this case of ALL disruption, an implant with integrated fixation should be used to prevent migration.

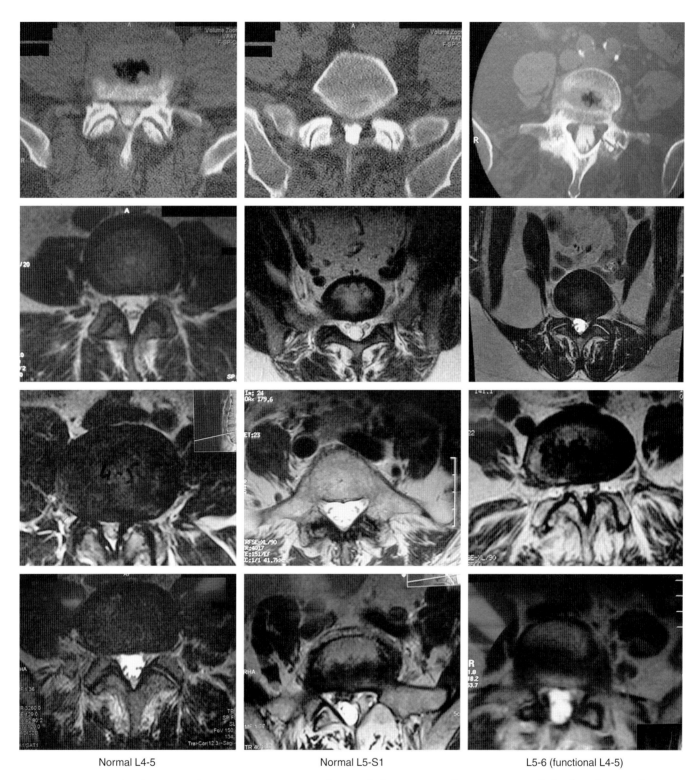

Normal L4-5　　　　　　　　Normal L5-S1　　　　　　　　L5-6 (functional L4-5)

Fig. 46-4 Axial imaging shows various psoas muscle morphology in normal L4-5 segments *(left column),* normal L5-S1 segments *(center column),* and lumbarized sacrum (L5-6 segments) *(right column).*

PATIENT EXAMPLE

This 58 year-old man presented with a 5-year history of progressively increasing low back pain without radicular symptoms or a precipitating event. He had undergone several rounds of physical therapy without resolution and was taking high-dose narcotics for pain management. He was no longer able to work and was on disability. The patient reported that his low back pain intensity was 8/10 (VAS), his disability (ODI) was 56%, and his quality of life (SF-36) score was 45. MRI revealed a severely degenerated L4-5 disc with type II Modic changes (Fig. 46-5, *A*). After consultation with the patient, an L4-5 XLIF with bilateral transpedicular facet fixation was performed, with the XLIF and posterior supplemental internal fixation delivered with the patient in a lateral decubitus position (Fig. 46-5, *B* and *C*). Operative time was 65 minutes and intraoperative blood loss was less than 25 ml (Fig. 46-5, *D*). No intraoperative or postoperative complications were reported, though hip flexion weakness (4/5) on the side ipsilateral to the XLIF approach was present for approximately 3 weeks postoperatively. Hip flexion weakness after XLIF is common and believed to be caused by muscular trauma during the transpsoas approach. One year postoperatively the patient reports back pain of 2/10, his ODI is 22%, and his SF-36 score is 65. He is very satisfied with his outcome.

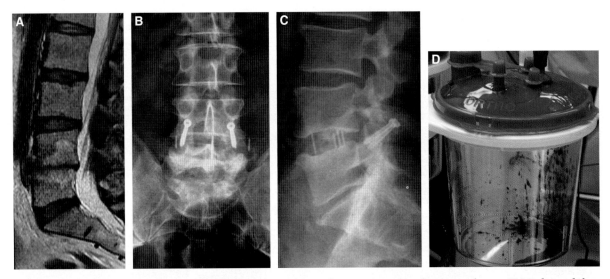

Fig. 46-5   **A,** Preoperative sagittal lumbar MRI showed L4-5 degenerative disc disease with type II Modic endplate changes. **B** and **C,** Postoperative radiographs after treatment with eXtreme lateral interbody fusion and transpedicular facet fixation. **D,** Intraoperative blood loss was less than 25 ml.

CONCLUSION

While appropriate patient selection in the surgical treatment of DDD remains a clinical challenge, when properly indicated, treatment with XLIF represents a strong, minimally disruptive alternative to conventional procedures to directly treat discal pathology and allow for a favorable biomechanic construct for long-term maintenance of correction.

REFERENCES

1. Katz JN, Losina E. Cost-effectiveness of spine surgery: the jury is out. Ann Intern Med 149:901-903, 2008.

2. Katz JN. Lumbar disc disorders and low-back pain: socioeconomic factors and consequences. J Bone Joint Surg Am 88(Suppl 2):S21-S24, 2006.

3. Katz JN. Lumbar spinal fusion. Surgical rates, costs, and complications. Spine 20(24 Suppl):S78-S83, 1995.

4. Fourney DR, Andersson G, Arnold PM, et al. Chronic low back pain: a heterogeneous condition with challenges for an evidence-based approach. Spine 36(21 Suppl):S1-S9, 2011.

5. Phillips FM, Slosar PJ, Youssef JA, et al. Lumbar spine fusion for chronic low back pain due to degenerative disc disease: a systematic review. Spine 38:E409-E422, 2013.

6. Adams MA, Roughley PJ. What is intervertebral disc degeneration, and what causes it? Spine 31:2151-2161, 2006.

7. Deyo RA, Mirza SK, Martin BI. Back pain prevalence and visit rates: estimates from U.S. national surveys, 2002. Spine 31:2724-2727, 2006.

8. Deyo RA, Ciol MA, Cherkin DC, et al. Lumbar spinal fusion. A cohort study of complications, reoperations, and resource use in the Medicare population. Spine 18:1463-1470, 1993.

9. Deyo RA, Mirza SK, Turner JA, et al. Overtreating chronic back pain: time to back off? J Am Board Fam Med 22:62-68, 2009.

10. Deyo RA, Gray DT, Kreuter W, et al. United States trends in lumbar fusion surgery for degenerative conditions. Spine 30:1441-1445, 2005.

11. Deyo RA, Andersson G, Bombardier C, et al. Outcome measures for studying patients with low back pain. Spine 19(18 Suppl):S2032-S2036, 1994.

12. Deyo RA, Haselkorn J, Hoffman R, et al. Designing studies of diagnostic tests for low back pain or radiculopathy. Spine 19(18 Suppl):S2057-S2065, 1994.

13. Glassman SD, Carreon LY, Djurasovic M, et al. Lumbar fusion outcomes stratified by specific diagnostic indication. Spine J 9:13-21, 2009.

14. Khajavi K, Shen AY, Lagina M, et al. Comparison of clinical outcomes following minimally invasive lateral interbody fusion stratified by preoperative diagnosis. Presented at the Thirtieth Annual Meeting of the AANS/CNS Joint Section on Disorders of the Spine and Peripheral Nerves, Orlando, FL, March 2014.

15. Ozgur BM, Aryan HE, Pimenta L, et al. Extreme Lateral Interbody Fusion (XLIF): a novel surgical technique for anterior lumbar interbody fusion. Spine J 6:435-443, 2006.

16. Dakwar E, Cardona RF, Smith DA, et al. Early outcomes and safety of the minimally invasive, lateral retroperitoneal transpsoas approach for adult degenerative scoliosis. Neurosurg Focus 28:E8, 2010.

17. Deukmedjian AR, Le TV, Baaj AA, et al. Anterior longitudinal ligament release using the minimally invasive lateral retroperitoneal transpsoas approach: a cadaveric feasibility study and report of 4 clinical cases. J Neurosurg Spine 17:530-539, 2012.

18. Smith WD, Dakwar E, Le TV, et al. Minimally invasive surgery for traumatic spinal pathologies: a mini-open, lateral approach in the thoracic and lumbar spine. Spine 35(26 Suppl):S338-S346, 2010.

19. Uribe JS, Smith WD, Pimenta L, et al. Minimally invasive lateral approach for symptomatic thoracic disc herniation: initial multicenter clinical experience. J Neurosurg Spine 16:264-279, 2012.

20. Tohmeh AG, Rodgers WB, Peterson MD. Dynamically evoked, discrete-threshold electromyography in the extreme lateral interbody fusion approach. J Neurosurg Spine 14:31-37, 2100.

21. Uribe JS, Vale FL, Dakwar E. Electromyographic monitoring and its anatomical implications in minimally invasive spine surgery. Spine 35(26 Suppl):S368-S374, 2010.

22. Malcolm JR, Hyde JA, Malcolm JG, et al. XLIF for degenerated/collapsed disc. In Goodrich JA, Volcan IJ, eds. eXtreme Lateral Interbody Fusion (XLIF), ed 2. St Louis: Quality Medical Publishing, 2013.

23. Peterson MD, Youssef JA. eXtreme Lateral Interbody Fusion (XLIF): lumbar surgical technique. In Goodrich JA, Volcan IJ, eds. eXtreme Lateral Interbody Fusion (XLIF), ed 2. St Louis: Quality Medical Publishing, 2013.

24. Smith WD, Uribe JS. Mini-open lateral approach for thoracolumbar anterior lumbar interbody fusion. In Haid RW Jr, Shaffrey CI, Youssef JA, et al, eds. Global Spinal Alignment: Principles, Pathologies, and Procedures. St Louis: Quality Medical Publishing, 2015.

25. Smith WD, Youssef JA, Christian G, et al. Lumbarized sacrum as a relative contraindication for lateral transpsoas interbody fusion at L5-6. J Spinal Disord Tech 25:285-291, 2012.

26. Le TV, Baaj AA, Dakwar E, et al. Subsidence of polyetheretherketone intervertebral cages in minimally invasive lateral retroperitoneal transpsoas lumbar interbody fusion. Spine 37:1268-1273, 2012.

47

Minimally Invasive Surgical Treatment of Idiopathic Scoliosis

Firoz Miyanji

The prevalence of adolescent idiopathic scoliosis (AIS) is reported to be 2% to 3%, and approximately less than 0.1% of all adolescents have curves larger than 40 degrees.[1,2] The goals of surgical treatment in this setting are threefold:
1. To prevent progression of the deformity by obtaining a solid arthrodesis
2. To limit the extent of the fusion
3. To obtain a three-dimensional correction of the deformity to achieve a balanced spine in all three planes

To date, surgical options include open posterior instrumented fusion, open anterior instrumented fusion, and thoracoscopic techniques. Although the goals of AIS treatment are achieved with these techniques, each with its own reported advantages and disadvantages, any emphasis on approach-related morbidity with these conventional procedures is minimal. The rationale of minimally invasive surgery (MIS) of the spine for patients with AIS is to minimize the approach-related morbidity inherent in the current available techniques. This chapter discusses the indications, technique, early results, and some of the limitations of MIS in adolescent deformity, and stresses the importance of longer-term follow-up of MIS in the setting of AIS.

The primary debate between anterior and posterior surgery for AIS is centered around concerns of the crankshaft phenomenon for very young patients, the distal extent of the fusion, the ability to restore and maintain the sagittal plane, and appropriate treatment for severe, rigid deformities. More favorable postoperative lung function has been reported with thoracoscopic techniques, compared with open anterior thoracotomies[3-5]; however, the perioperative morbidity with single-lung ventilation should not be overlooked.[6,7] In addition, anterior thoracoscopic instrumented fusions rely on a single anterior rod, with most surgeons favoring a postoperative bracing protocol because of reports of significant pseudarthrosis rates in some studies.[6-8]

Conventional open spine procedures for AIS are often associated with significant blood loss, soft tissue disruption, prolonged recovery, and postsurgical pain. Many authors have reported on significant soft tissue and muscle morbidity of standard open spine procedures, which can lead to increased perioperative morbidity and long-term pain.[8-26] The motivation for MIS in the setting of AIS is therefore to minimize approach-related morbidity inherent in the current available surgical options for this patient population.

INDICATIONS

Surgical indications for AIS include a thoracic curve reaching 50 degrees or more in skeletally mature patients because of the risk of progression into adulthood. In patients with thoracolumbar/lumbar scoliotic curves, a magnitude of 40 to 45 degrees is generally an indication for surgical stabilization. Patient factors are as important as established curve characteristics in guiding surgical intervention for patients with AIS. Once the decision to perform surgery is made, the indications for MIS rely heavily on curve magnitude, flexibility, and patient factors. Generally, curves smaller than 70 degrees that correct to less than 30 to 35 degrees on side-bending films can be considered for MIS. The Lenke curve type or the extent of the fusion is not a contraindication for MIS. Patient factors that suggest poor protoplasm, factors that affect fusion such as smoking, and compliance issues with the slow, graduated postoperative return to activity protocol should be very carefully evaluated before MIS is considered.

PREOPERATIVE PLANNING

Patients considered as surgical candidates for AIS should have a thorough physical examination and appropriate preoperative imaging. Physical examination is helpful to evaluate coronal and sagittal balance (trunk shift and C7-S1 plumb line, hyperkyphosis or hypokyphosis, and positive or negative sagittal balance) and shoulder, waist, and pelvic asymmetry to help guide structurality of curves. A scoliometer is used to measure rib and/or lumbar prominences on forward bend (Fig. 47-1). A detailed neurologic examination, specifically, abdominal reflexes, and assessment of the patient's integument for evidence of spinal dysraphism are very important to confirm a diagnosis of *idiopathic* scoliosis, which should always be considered a diagnosis of exclusion. Preoperative imaging includes standing PA and lateral full-length scoliosis radiographs, AP radiographs of the pelvis to assess Risser grade and triradiate closure, and bending films to evaluate curve structure and flexibility. Traction films are considered to assess curve flexibility preoperatively. Preoperative radiographs are useful for documenting the Cobb angles of all curves, and bending films help to determine those that are structural according to Lenke criteria. Lateral radiographs are needed to assess T5-12 kyphosis and T2-5 and T10-L1 measurements. They are equally important for determining the proximal and distal extent of fusion. Pelvic incidence should be evaluated; however, its role in preoperative decision-making for AIS is not yet confirmed.

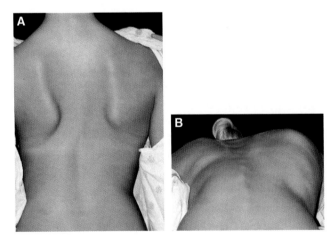

Fig. 47-1   **A,** Preoperative assessment of trunk shift and C7-S1 plumb line. **B,** Preoperative shoulder and waist asymmetry and rib and lumbar prominences are evident on forward bend.

OPERATIVE TECHNIQUE

Three separate midline skin incisions are planned using fluoroscopy (Fig. 47-2, *A*). In our practice, fluoroscopy is limited to preoperative planning of the incisions. The skin is then undermined laterally to make paramedian fascial incisions approximately one fingerbreadth from midline (Fig. 47-2, *B*). A blunt muscle-sparing approach is used down to the facet joints, which are visualized with the aid of handheld retractors. Wide facetectomies are performed, and the pedicles are cannulated using a freehand technique (Fig. 47-2, *C*). The pedicles remain localized by placement of guide wires or cannulated bone pegs. This facilitates *bilateral* facetectomies without committing to passage of a single rod before fully mobilizing the spinal column. The facet joints are then meticulously decorticated with a high-speed burr. Bone graft comprising autograft and freeze-dried allograft is placed before screw insertion to help augment fusion (Fig. 47-2, *D* and *E*). An appropriate-sized pedicle screw is inserted, and the guide wire is removed.

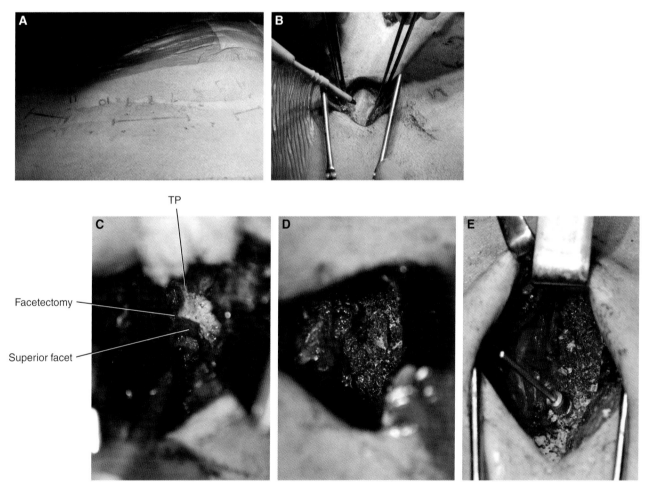

Fig. 47-2 **A,** Skin incisions are marked using fluoroscopic guidance. **B,** Paramedian fascial incisions. **C,** Facetectomy and pedicle screw cannulation. **D** and **E,** Morselized bone graft and a bone peg are placed, and the pedicle is localized. (*TP,* transverse process.)

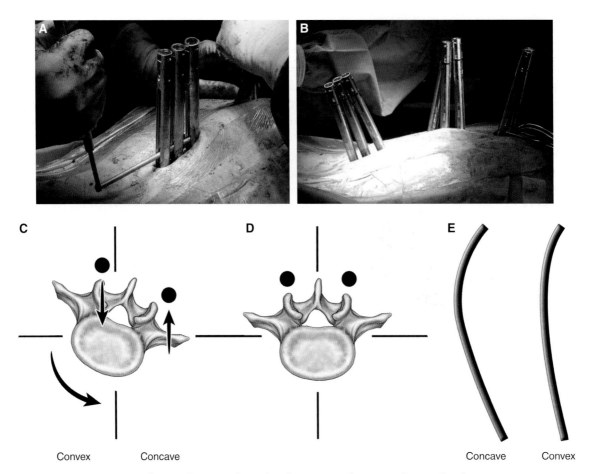

Fig. 47-3   **A** and **B,** Rod passage from distal to proximal. **C-E,** Differential rod contouring.

Once the screws are placed at all levels, a rod of appropriate length that is contoured to the correct sagittal profile is introduced. The rod is passed from distal to proximal below the soft tissues and under the skin bridges to be captured within the tulips of the pedicle screws (Fig. 47-3, *A* and *B*). The cylinders are made collinear to allow most of the deformity to be corrected before placement of the rod. The rod is reduced to the pedicle screws using the reduction instruments and secured using set screws. Further correction is obtained with rod derotation into the appropriate sagittal plane. Before placement of the second rod, en bloc direct vertebral apical derotation can be performed using available instruments. The second convex rod is then undercontoured in the sagittal plane and placed from distal to proximal. Undercontouring of this rod allows further deformity correction in the axial plane (Fig. 47-3, *C* through *E*). Uniaxial screws are primarily used.

OUTCOMES

Current data are limited regarding outcomes of MIS techniques in AIS. Anand et al[27] reported on a series of 12 adult patients with degenerative scoliosis who had an average of 3.64 segments fused. They reported a feasibility study in which patients underwent a lateral retroperitoneal approach followed by percutaneous pedicle screw placement. Functional or long-term data were not available in this series. Similarly, Hsieh et al[28] have described MIS procedures on a heterogeneous group of patients with complex spine disorders, but only one patient was treated for deformity. Samdani et al[29] retrospectively reviewed their experience with MIS in 15 patients. The average preoperative major Cobb angle was 54 degrees. This corrected to 18 degrees, resulting in a 67% correction. The average blood loss in their series was 254 ml, and average operative time was 470 minutes.

We recently prospectively compared MIS and open standard posterior techniques in the setting of AIS, with the goal of comparing curve correction and perioperative variables.[30] The study revealed near-equivalent curve correction between the two groups (63% in the open group and 68% in the MIS group). The advantages of MIS over open posterior procedures were significantly lower average blood loss and decreased length of hospital stay. However, the operative time was considerably longer in patients treated with MIS. This may be the effect of the learning curve for this new technique. However, it may be a potential limitation of MIS in the setting of deformity.

COMPLICATIONS AND MANAGEMENT

INFECTION

Infection remains a concern and is one of the most frequently reported complications after spine surgery. Some authors claim that MIS techniques can reduce the rate of spinal infection; however, this was not true in our experience. In 3 of our 28 AIS patients who had MIS procedures, chronic infection presented more than 1 year after the index procedure. *Propionibacterium acnes* was isolated in all 3 cases and treated with hardware removal (either partial or complete) and 6 weeks of IV antibiotics. All infections were successfully eradicated (Fig. 47-4).

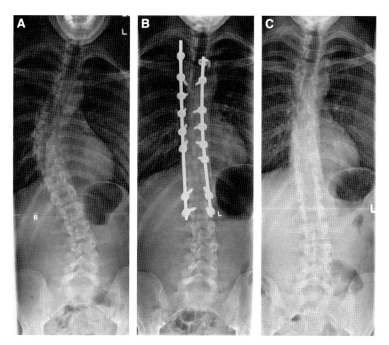

Fig. 47-4　**A** and **B,** Preoperative and postoperative radiographs of a 17-year-old male who was treated with an MIS technique and developed *P. acnes* infection 14 months postoperatively. **C,** He was treated successfully with hardware removal and IV antibiotics.

PSEUDARTHROSIS

Pseudarthrosis is a significant concern with MIS procedures, specifically in adolescent deformity. Limited periosteal stripping, reduced surface area for fusion, and reliance strictly on facet fusions can potentially increase the pseudarthrosis risk. Patient factors that increase this risk include smoking and poor compliance with postoperative, graduated return to activities. Pseudarthrosis in the setting of MIS can be treated through traditional open techniques (Fig. 47-5).

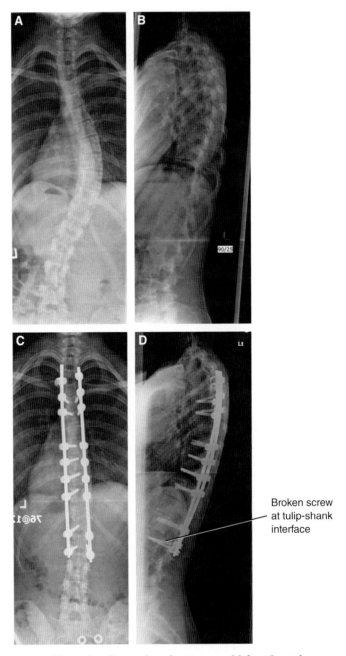

Broken screw at tulip-shank interface

Fig. 47-5   **A** and **B,** Preoperative PA and lateral radiographs of a 16-year-old female with progressive adolescent idiopathic scoliosis. **C** and **D,** Fifteen-month postoperative radiographs confirm broken hardware at the tulip-shank interface of the screw. Revision surgery confirmed pseudarthrosis at the distal L1-2 level, with similar failure of all four distal pedicle screws.

PATIENT EXAMPLES

This 17-year-old female presented with progressive adolescent idiopathic scoliosis. Her right main thoracic curve measured 54 degrees preoperatively, and her sagittal T5-12 profile was 45 degrees (Fig. 47-6, *A* and *B*). Her bending films confirmed a Lenke 1A+ curve pattern. She underwent an MIS T4-T12 posterior instrumented fusion with curve correction to 11 degrees. Her hyperkyphosis is restored to 26 degrees postoperatively (Fig. 47-6, *C* and *D*).

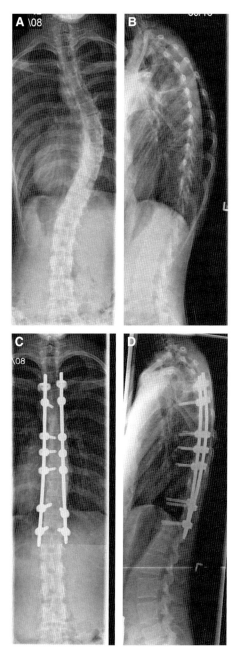

Fig. 47-6 **A** and **B,** Preoperative PA and lateral radiographs of a 17-year-old female who presented with progressive adolescent idiopathic scoliosis. **C** and **D,** Four years after an MIS T4-T12 posterior instrumented fusion.

This 11-year-old healthy female presented with a curvature of her spine (Fig. 47-7, *A* and *B*). Her history, physical examination, and imaging confirmed AIS. The patient was a Jehovah's Witness; therefore either autologous or allogenic blood and/or blood product transfusions were contraindicated. Her curve had progressed to 54 degrees, and her Risser grade was 1. The patient's lateral profile showed significant hypokyphosis with a T5-12 angle of 5 degrees. She underwent a T4-12 posterior instrumented fusion through an MIS technique to help minimize blood loss, which was 250 ml. Her main thoracic curve was reduced to 20 degrees, and her T5-12 sagittal profile improved to 20 degrees (Fig. 47-7, *C* and *D*).

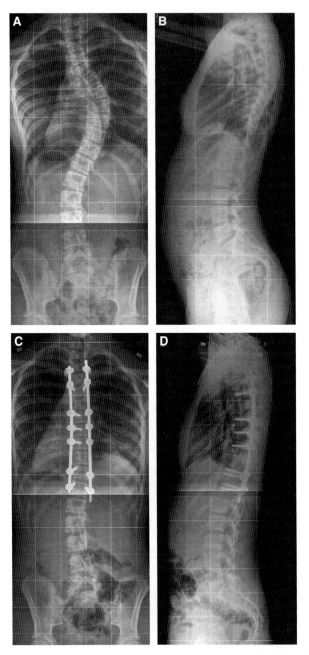

Fig. 47-7   **A** and **B,** Preoperative PA and lateral radiographs of an 11-year-old female with adolescent idiopathic scoliosis. She underwent a T4-12 posterior instrumented fusion through an MIS technique. **C** and **D,** Eighteen-month postoperative PA and lateral radiographs.

This 18-year-old ballerina had progression of her right main thoracic curve to 58 degrees (Fig. 47-8, *A* and *B*). Preoperative bending films confirmed the proximal thoracic curve to be structural; hence she had a Lenke 2AN curve pattern. Her T5-12 preoperative sagittal profile was 17 degrees, with a T2-5 hyperkyphotic profile of 24 degrees. She underwent a T2-L2 posterior instrumented fusion through an MIS technique to improve her coronal decompensation and sagittal profile. Her main thoracic curve is improved to 11 degrees, and her T5-12 postoperative sagittal Cobb measurement is 32 degrees (Fig. 47-8, *C* and *D*).

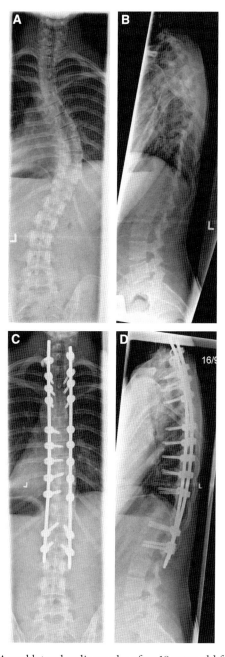

Fig. 47-8 **A** and **B,** Preoperative PA and lateral radiographs of an 18-year-old female with a Lenke 2AN curve pattern. She underwent a T2-L2 posterior instrumented fusion through an MIS technique. **C** and **D,** Three-year PA and lateral radiographs confirm improvement of her sagittal profile from 17 degrees to 32 degrees. Her main thoracic curve is improved from 58 degrees to 11 degrees.

This 14-year-old female presented with AIS. A structural right main thoracic curve resulted in right-sided trunk shift, elevation of her right shoulder, and right rib prominence accentuated on forward bend (Fig. 47-9, *A* and *B*). She underwent a T4-T12 posterior instrumented fusion through an MIS technique. Postoperatively the patient has a nice clinical result with restoration of her coronal balance and significant reduction of her rib prominence (Fig. 47-9, *C* and *D*). Her three midline skin incisions show minimal scarring.

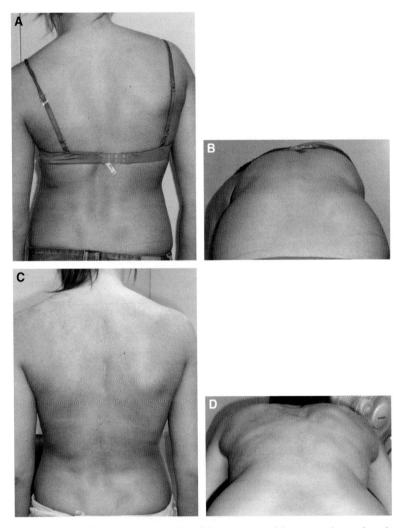

Fig. 47-9   **A** and **B,** Preoperative clinical photographs of this 14-year-old patient showed scoliotic deformity and a rib-hump deformity. **C** and **D,** Eighteen months after an MIS procedure, clinical images show good alignment and correction of the rib hump.

LIMITATIONS AND FUTURE TRENDS

Curve correction, fusion, rod passage, and length of operative time are theoretical concerns with MIS. Although a number of deformity correction techniques exist for open procedures, not all are applicable in the setting of MIS. Greater emphasis is placed on rod rotation, deferential rod contouring, distraction, compression, and intraoperative traction with MIS cases.

The fusion model in pediatric patients is different than in adults and appears to be more favorable.[31,32] However, fusion rates and/or time to fusion have not been reported for AIS patients treated with MIS techniques. This should be the focus of much-needed prospective longer-term follow-up studies to demonstrate the true clinical benefits of MIS in the setting of adolescent deformity.

The evolution of MIS as an effort to decrease the rate of approach-related morbidity associated with conventional open procedures has shown potential for AIS, at least in the short term. It provides surgeons and patients with additional options when planning surgical treatment for AIS.

REFERENCES

1. Kane WJ. Scoliosis prevalence: a call for a statement of terms. Clin Orthop 126:43-46, 1977.
2. Miller NH. Cause and natural history of adolescent idiopathic scoliosis. Orthop Clin North Am 30:343-352, 1999.
3. Kishan S, Bastrom T, Betz RR, et al. Thoracoscopic scoliosis surgery affects pulmonary function less than thoracotomy at 2 years postsurgery. Spine 32:453-458, 2007.
4. Lonner BS, Auerbach JD, Estreicher MB, et al. Pulmonary function changes after various anterior approaches in the treatment of AIS. J Spinal Disord Tech 22:551-558, 2009.
5. Newton PO, Perry A, Bastrom TP, et al. Predictors of change in postoperative pulmonary function in adolescent idiopathic scoliosis: a prospective study of 254 patients. Spine 32:1875-1882, 2007.
6. Reddi V, Clarke DV Jr, Arlet V. Anterior thoracoscopic instrumentation in adolescent idiopathic scoliosis: a systematic review. Spine 33:1985-1994, 2008.
7. Wong HK, Hee HT, Yu Z, et al. Results of thoracoscopic instrumentation and fusion versus conventional posterior instrumented fusion in AIS undergoing selective thoracic fusion. Spine 29:2031-2038, 2004.
8. Newton PO, Upasani VV, Lhamby J, et al. Surgical treatment of main thoracic scoliosis with thoracoscopic anterior instrumentation. A five-year follow-up study. J Bone Joint Surg Am 90:2007-2089, 2008.
9. German JW, Adamo MA, Hoppenot RG, et al. Perioperative results following lumbar discectomy: comparison of minimally invasive discectomy and standard microdiscectomy. Neurosurg Focus 25:E20, 2008.
10. Ryang YM, Oertel MF, Mayfrank L, et al. Standard open microdiscectomy versus minimal access trocar microdiscectomy: result of a prospective randomized study. Neurosurgery 62:174-181, 2008.
11. Righesso O, Falavigna S, Avanzi O, et al. Comparison of open discectomy with microscopic discectomy in lumbar disc herniations: results of a randomized controlled trial. Neurosurgery 61:545-549, 2007.
12. Peng CW, Yue WM, Poh SY, et al. Clinical and radiographic outcomes of minimally invasive versus open transforaminal lumbar interbody fusion. Spine 34:1385-1389, 2009.
13. Katayama Y, Matsuyama Y, Yoshishara H, et al. Comparison of surgical outcomes between macro discectomy and micro discectomy for lumbar disc herniation: a prospective randomized study with surgery performed by the same spine surgeon. J Spinal Disord Tech 19:344-347, 2006.
14. Rampersaud YR, Annand N, Dekutoski MB. Use of minimally invasive surgical techniques in the management of thoracolumbar trauma: current concepts. Spine 31(11 Suppl):S96-S104, 2006.
15. Smith JS, Ogden AT, Fessler RG. Minimally invasive posterior thoracic fusion. Neurosurg Focus 25:E9, 2008.
16. Kawaguchi Y, Matsui H, Tsuji H. Back muscle injury after posterior lumbar spine surgery. A histologic and enzymatic analysis. Spine 21:941-944, 1996.
17. Kawaguchi Y, Matsui H, Tsuji H. Back muscle injury after posterior lumbar spine surgery. I. Histologic and histochemical analyses in rats. Spine 19:2590-2597, 1994.
18. Kawaguchi Y, Matsui H, Tsuji H. Back muscle injury after posterior lumbar spine surgery. II. Histologic and histochemical analyses in humans. Spine 19:2598-2602, 1994.
19. Kawaguchi Y, Yakubi S, Styf J, et al. Back muscle injury after posterior lumbar spine surgery. Topographic evaluation of intramuscular pressure and blood flow in the porcine back muscle during surgery. Spine 21:2683-2688, 1996.
20. Kim DY, Lee SH, Chung SK, et al. Comparison of multifidus muscle atrophy and trunk extension muscle strength: percutaneous versus open pedicle screw fixation. Spine 30:123-129, 2005.
21. Macnab I, Cuthbert H, Godfrey CM. The incidence of denervation of the sacrospinales muscle following spinal surgery. Spine 2:294-298, 1977.

22. Mayer TG, Vanharanta H, Gatchel RJ, et al. Comparison of CT scan muscle measurements and isokinetic trunk strength in postoperative patients. Spine 14:33-36, 1989.

23. Rantanen J, Hurme M, Falck B, et al. The lumbar multifidus muscle five years after surgery for a lumbar intervertebral disc herniation. Spine 18:568-574, 1993.

24. Sihvonen T, Herno A, Paljärvi L, et al. A local denervation atrophy of paraspinal muscles in postoperative failed back syndrome. Spine 18:575-581, 1993.

25. Styf JR, Willén J. The effects of external compression by three different retractors on pressure in the erector spine muscles during and after posterior lumbar spine surgery in humans. Spine 23:354-358, 1998.

26. Weber BR, Grob D, Dvorák J, et al. Posterior surgical approach to the lumbar spine and its effect on the multifidus muscle. Spine 22:1765-1772, 1997.

27. Anand N, Baron EM, Thaiyananthan G, et al. Minimally invasive multilevel percutaneous correction and fusion for adult lumbar degenerative scoliosis: a technique and feasibility study. J Spinal Disord Tech 21:459-467, 2008.

28. Hsieh PC, Koski TR, Sciubba DM, et al. Maximizing the potential of minimally invasive spine surgery in complex spinal disorders. Neurosurg Focus 25:E19, 2008.

29. Samdani AF, Asghar J, Miyanji F, et al. Minimally invasive treatment of pediatric spinal deformity. Semin Spine Surg 23:72-75, 2011.

30. Miyanji F, Samdani AF, Marks M, et al. Minimally invasive surgery for AIS: an early prospective comparison with standard open posterior surgery. J Spine S5:001, 2013.

31. Cahill PJ, Marvil S, Cuddihy L, et al. Autofusion in the immature spine treated with growing rods. Spine 35:E1199-E1203, 2010.

32. Betz RR, Petrizzo AM, Kerner PJ, et al. Allograft versus no graft with a posterior multisegmented hook system for the treatment of idiopathic scoliosis. Spine 31:121-127, 2006.

48

Minimally Invasive Surgical Treatment of Adult Spinal Deformity

Vedat Deviren ▪ *Murat Pekmezci*

The goals of surgical treatment of adult degenerative scoliosis are to decompress the neural elements, correct the deformity, and maintain the correction with arthrodesis.[1] These goals can be obtained through several approaches (anterior, posterior, or combined). Posterior approaches are most commonly used in adult deformity surgery. They allow direct decompression of the canal through excision of the redundant ligamentum flavum, decompression of the foramen by undercutting of the facet joints and achieve arthrodesis when bone graft is laid between the transverse processes. However, in the setting of severe loss of disc height, up-down stenosis at the foramen cannot be corrected unless the disc height is restored through an interbody fusion. As degenerative changes in the anterior structures (disc-osteophyte complexes) increase the rigidity of the curves, the deformity correction via a posterior approach might be limited.

An anterior approach has three major advantages. It restores lost disc space height through decompression of the foramina and the spinal canal by tensioning and eliminating the buckling of the ligamentum flavum. This reduces the need for secondary decompressive maneuvers such as laminectomy. Second, depending on the technique used, the cage helps to correct sagittal and coronal balance. Finally, because the anterior column has better vascularity and increased surface area for fusion, the rate of successful arthrodesis is higher. Interbody fusion can be achieved with direct anterior lumbar interbody fusion (ALIF) or lateral lumbar interbody fusion (LLIF) or by indirect posterior lumbar interbody fusion (PLIF) or transforaminal lumbar interbody fusion (TLIF).

For adult degenerative scoliosis, deformity correction and indirect decompression of the neural elements are superior with direct anterior approaches. The interbody devices are larger and can better engage the periphery of the endplate, with a lower risk of subsidence. This results in a more reliable restoration and maintenance of the disc height, providing excellent decompression and deformity correction.[2] Because of the limited exposure, posterior cages are much smaller and inevitably engage the central, weaker portion of the endplate. Furthermore, preparation of the disc space and insertion of the interbody device require extensive nerve and dural manipulation during posterior approaches, which may lead to neurologic deficits and dural tears. In addition, a posterior approach requires removal of most of the posterior elements (including the lamina and all or part of the facet joint) to decompress the neural elements; only the transverse processes remain to achieve arthrodesis and may result in lower fusion rates.

Anterior approaches are not risk free, however. First, many spine surgeons are less familiar with anterior exposures and may require an approach surgeon. Conventional anterior approaches involve excessive dissection, causing potential intraabdominal and abdominal wall morbidity.[3] Ileus and bowel injury are common postoperative complications[4] Although vascular injuries are rare, they can be life threatening. During exposure of L5-S1, injury to the hypogastric plexus can result in retrograde ejaculation, a cause of significant morbidity, especially in younger patients.[5,6]

Although it is possible to treat adult spinal deformity with an anterior-only approach, the common practice is to combine anterior and posterior approaches. An anterior procedure allows restoration of disc height, deformity correction, and solid arthrodesis; a posterior procedure permits more directed decompression and additional stability to maintain correction and prevent subsidence. However, combined approaches expose patients to multiple surgical procedures, further increasing the risk of complications. The solution is in less invasive techniques that achieve the same results with fewer complications and less morbidity to the patient.

Pimenta and colleagues[7,8] described the lateral transpsoas approach in 2001. Their goal was to develop a less invasive anterior approach that maintained the benefits of anterior column support while limiting the associated morbidity. In the lumbar spine, this is a true anterior retroperitoneal approach from L1-5 through the psoas muscle. Because it eliminates the need to mobilize the vessels, an approach surgeon is not required. At higher levels, it allows access up to T5 through a retropleural or transthoracic approach. This technique provides the necessary access to treat the anterior column, because it allows an extensive discectomy and reduces the main deforming forces by releasing the annulus on the lateral aspect of the disc. Two key technical features make this approach superior to conventional ALIF. First, it preserves the anterior longitudinal ligament. This allows deformity correction through ligamentotaxis and stability, because the interbody cage is kept in place by the tightened anterior and posterior longitudinal ligaments. Second, because the interbody cage is inserted in a lateral approach, it can span the ring apophysis with a larger-footprint cage, which decreases the risk of subsidence and increases the likelihood of successful fusion.[9] The minimally invasive nature of this approach decreases operative time and blood loss.

Lateral Lumbar Interbody Fusion

INDICATIONS AND CONTRAINDICATIONS

Indications for LLIF in adult deformity surgery are similar to those of any interbody fusion between L1 and L5 and include adjacent-segment degeneration, pseudarthrosis, and primary degenerative scoliosis with or without sagittal balance. Adjacent-segment degeneration is ideal for stand-alone techniques.

The incidence of *adjacent-segment degeneration* after lumbar surgery is as high as 35%.[10] It is most often corrected through a posterior approach, with the classic associated risks and limitations. Posterior approaches are associated with more blood loss, increased risk of infection, dural tear, and pseudarthroses. LLIF is an attractive alternative, because the pathology can be addressed directly through a separate approach in a virgin territory. It allows restoration of the height of the collapsed or slipped disc, thus providing indirect decompression of the neural foramen.[11] LLIF can be accompanied by anterior instrumentation to increase the chance of fusion and decrease the risk of subsidence. Klopfenstein et al[10] performed LLIF on 14 patients to treat a variety of pathologies, including spondylolisthesis, postlaminectomy instability, and adjacent-segment disease. All patients achieved union, and 71% had improved radicular symptoms.

Stand-alone LLIF is commonly performed to treat adjacent-segment disease, but it can also be appropriate in select patients with degenerative scoliosis.[12] The main advantage is that the lack of supplemental fixation decreases surgical time and retraction on the psoas, potentially decreasing the risk of injury to the lumbar plexus. A recent biomechanical study found that when a cage with a big footprint is fit between the tensioned anterior and posterior ligaments, flexion-extension and lateral-bending motion decrease by 70% at the instrumented site.[13] Placement of a lateral plate or a pedicle screw decreased the motion by an additional 10% to 15%. As the arthritic changes in the facet joints progress parallel to the degenerative cascade, the ROM at the affected segment is further limited. When an anterior cage is implanted, the treated segment will hypothetically have adequate rigidity to achieve fusion. Marchi et al[12] reported an 87% union rate with this technique; however, the rate of high-grade subsidence was 17%, half of which required additional procedures to achieve a rigid fixation. Therefore adherence to appropriate surgical technique is essential to decrease the risk of this complication. Preservation of the endplates is critical, as is placement of an appropriately sized implant to maximize biomechanical spread of force. In addition, a thorough preoperative screening to identify patients with poor bone quality can possibly decrease the chance of subsidence. DXA helps to determine overall bone quality; a CT scan is routinely performed to evaluate the endplates and facet joints. The senior author (V.D.) uses the following criteria to identify candidates for this procedure: a primary degenerative pathology, no radiographic evidence of significant adult degenerative scoliosis or kyphosis, minimal motion on side-bending radiographs, a bone density result with T-score greater than −1.5, and radiographic evidence of facet hypertrophy confirmed with preoperative CT.

In a review of five patients with an average age of 79.2 years and a mean DXA T-score of 1.1, three patients had four-level (L1-5) and two patients had three-level (L2-5) stand-alone LLIF. At a mean 1.1-year follow-up, all patients had full union, and the rate of grade 2 to 3 subsidence was 17%. One patient with grade 3 subsidence required kyphoplasty. The ODI score improved from a mean of 39.2 (range 28 to 58) to 21 (range 14 to 32) at the final follow-up. In summary, a stand-alone lateral retroperitoneal transpsoas approach can be safely performed in select patients with degenerative spine disease requiring multilevel (more than three) lumbar fusion when strict selection criteria are used.

Complex deformity and degenerative scoliosis is another indication for which LLIF offers several advantages over more traditional techniques. LLIF corrects deformity through several methods. It straightens and derotates the spine through bilateral annular release, and insertion of a large implant across the disc space spanning the ring apophysis results in ligamentotaxis. Segmental interbody implants realign the endplates to a horizontal position, restore disc and foraminal heights, and indirectly decompress the neural elements.[11] Lordotic or nonlordotic implants placed in the anterior disc space correct and maintain sagittal balance. Isaacs et al[14] studied 107 patients with adult degenerative scoliosis who were treated with eXtreme lateral interbody fusion (XLIF); the overall complication rate was 12.1%, which was lower than the rate in previous reports of open techniques.[15,16] Keshavarzi et al[17] found that most correction in both the coronal and sagittal plane was achieved during the initial LLIF procedure. In addition, the interbody space provides a superior environment for fusion, compared with the posterolateral gutter used for posterior approaches. The interbody space is commonly used as the first stage of a combined approach. Staging the second posterior approach a couple days after the LLIF allows time to reevaluate the patient to determine the need for posterior decompression. Often, indirect decompression provided by LLIF eliminates the need to perform additional posterior decompression. In a CT study, Kepler et al[18] found that LLIF resulted in a 64% increase in foraminal height and a 35% increase in foraminal area. In a study of TLIF and PLIF, maximum foraminal height restoration was 30%.[19] Anterior release through LLIF may not sufficiently treat the deformity in patients with severe sagittal imbalance, which can require aggressive posterior osteotomy techniques. However, LLIF has an adjunctive role of decreasing the pseudarthrosis rates by providing interbody fusion. The best example is a pedicle subtraction osteotomy in a de novo scoliosis patient who has not had previous anterior interbody fusion.[20] Side-bending radiographs should be carefully scrutinized for flexibility of the curve. In the presence of a rigid fractional curve, correction of the main curve may lead to coronal decompensation after an LLIF procedure. This can be corrected during the posterior procedure; however, awareness of this potential complication is important and should be discussed with the patient before the procedure.[17]

Anterior column realignment (ACR) is the most extreme application of LLIF. This technique involves release of the anterior longitudinal ligament and anterior annulus in addition to a discectomy, followed by insertion of a special interbody cage with up to 30 degrees of lordosis. ACR is often combined with a posterior Smith-Petersen osteotomy. Akbarnia et al[21] reported 28 degrees of correction with ACR and an additional 7 degrees with posterior osteotomy, for a total correction of 35 degrees. This is comparable to the correction achieved with a pedicle subtraction osteotomy, with the advantage of less morbidity to the patient, because the anterior part of the procedure is a separate stage with minimal morbidity. The preliminary results in the 17 patients studied are promising; however, careful case selection is essential.

I (V.D.) performed ACR on 10 patients whose mean age was 65.8 years (range 49 to 78 years). All patients but one had a type 1 posterior-approach osteotomy. One patient with severe sagittal imbalance required a type 3 posterior osteotomy. Perioperative complications included ileus (n = 1), thigh pain (n = 3), transient psoas weakness (all patients), and proximal junctional failure (n = 1). At a mean follow-up of 14.8 months (range 12 to 21 months), the mean preoperative ODI improved from 60 (range 40 to 80) to 36 (range 12 to 52). In summary, ACR provided significant acute correction and was best suited for patients with acute kyphotic deformity at the disc level, who did not have posterior instrumentation spanning the target segment.[22]

Limitations for ACR are similar to those of any interbody fusion surgery, such as infection or a previous anterior approach. Another limitation specific to this procedure is its limited use in the L5-S1 disc space, this area is not reproducibly accessible because of the location of the iliac crest. Complex deformity procedures often include L5-S1 as part of the construct; thus the best treatment solution for L5-S1 often is to perform the interbody procedure during supplemental posterior fixation through either ALIF or TLIF. High-grade spondylolisthesis, particularly at L4-5, can also be challenging because of migration of the lumbar plexus anteriorly with the deformity. Obesity is not as challenging as it may be in ALIF, because lateral decubitus positioning of the patient allows the abdominal contents and adipose tissue to fall forward out of the surgical field.

PREOPERATIVE PLANNING

Evaluation consists of a thorough history, a physical examination, and necessary radiographic studies. Radiographic studies specific to preparing for LLIF include the following.

Standing radiographs are always important for evaluation of disc height and coronal and sagittal alignment. Assessment of the curve direction and the coronal alignment is important, because in some cases correction of the main curve can result in decompensation in the coronal plane, which may require additional measures during the posterior stage. Radiographs provide information on the accessibility of the L4-5 disc space and help to determine the appropriate side for incision. Deciding from which side to approach the spine is a critical step in preoperative planning. Surgical approach from the concavity of the scoliosis is beneficial, because it provides access to multiple levels though a single skin incision. The fractional curve at the lumbosacral junction places the L4-5 disc in the convex side of the fractional curve and in the concave side of the main curve. This provides a reliable approach to L4-5, where the iliac crest typically obstructs access from the convex side of the main curve. On the convex side of the curve the lumbar plexus will already be draped over the curve and under tension. Further traction by the retractors during the procedure would place the lumbar plexus at higher risk for injury. However, on the concave side of the curve, the lumbar plexus is relaxed, and this risk is theoretically decreased. In addition, the soft tissues and bridging osteophytes are more prominent on the concave side. Direct release of these structures allows better curve correction, restoration of foraminal height, and indirect neural decompression. Side-bending views provide information on the flexibility of the curve. A rigid major curve allows a surgeon to perform a stand-alone procedure if the other selection criteria are met. A rigid fractional curve might require coronal decompensation after the initial anterior approach, particularly if the patient had an imbalance toward the concave side of the fractional curve. In this case, as the main curve is corrected, the rigid fractional curve does not correct, and further decompensation occurs.

Although MRI is excellent for visualizing the disc and stenosis, it is often done while the patient is recumbent and thus overestimates the intervertebral disc height. Radiographs provide a more accurate disc height measurement and are critical in evaluating the need for height restoration in the anterior column.

CT myelography can be used in place of MRI in patients who have had prior surgery with metal implants. Furthermore, CT myelography can better detail sclerosis of the endplates and the degree of facet arthritis, which are important parameters to evaluate when considering the use of stand-alone constructs. If bone density is a concern, DXA is warranted.

OPERATIVE TECHNIQUE

The keys to performing LLIF successfully and with minimal complications include careful patient selection, proper positioning, and meticulous surgical technique. The patient is placed in a lateral decubitus position; an axillary roll helps to minimize the risk of axillary nerve neuropraxia.

Intraoperative monitoring is useful to prevent lumbosacral plexus injury. Fluoroscopy is essential for viewing the spine in real time. Good-quality AP and lateral projections should be obtained before the procedure is performed. The disc space of interest is marked on the lateral fluoroscopic view. The fluoroscope is positioned at 90 degrees to the patient at all times, and the table is rotated or tilted to obtain a true lateral view of the disc. This helps to maintain a straight up-down orientation and lateral trajectory of all instruments being passed in and out of the disc. Failure to maintain a strict up-down orientation can result in serious vascular or neurologic injuries caused by inappropriate trajectory. The direct lateral incision can be an oblique incision running parallel to the fibers of the external abdominal oblique musculature. A second posterior incision is made lateral to the border of the erector spinae musculature to introduce a finger bluntly into the retroperitoneal space, to open the space, and to guide the initial dilators safely to the surface of the psoas muscle (Fig. 48-1, A). The dilator is advanced through the psoas muscle using dynamically triggered EMG to identify the direction and proximity of spinal nerves relative to the distal end of the dilator. Once the dilator is safely through the psoas muscle, its location is confirmed with lateral fluoroscopy before a K-wire is placed into the disc space (Fig. 48-1, B and C). Subsequent dilators are ad-

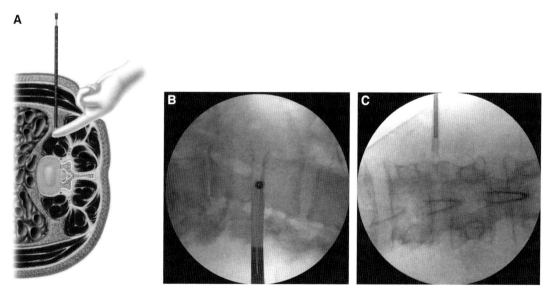

Fig. 48-1 **A,** The first dilator is guided onto the psoas in the retroperitoneal space through a second posterior incision. **B,** The first dilator is docked on the posterior half of the targeted disc space on the lateral view. **C,** The dilator should be flush with the disc on an AP view.

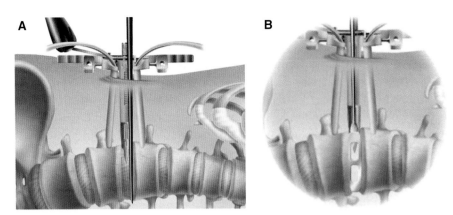

Fig. 48-2   **A,** A Cobb elevator is advanced under AP fluoroscopic guidance over the endplate to the contralateral annulus. The elevator is rotated to release attachment. **B,** Trials are inserted into the disc space to determine the ideal cage size (width, depth, and height). (Images courtesy of NuVasive, Inc.)

vanced over the first to separate muscle fibers and widen the exposure, each guided by dynamically triggered EMG. A retractor is then placed, and a lateral fluoroscopic image is obtained to ensure that it is in the proper AP location. It is critical that the working zone is not too anterior; it should lie between the posterior and middle thirds of the lateral disc space. The retractor is opened minimally, and the area is stimulated with a triggered EMG probe to identify all traversing neural elements. If a nerve is seen in the field, it is gently moved with a Penfield dissector and positioned posteriorly behind the retractor. The retractor can be widened independently in the AP and cranial-caudal directions; care should be taken to limit exposure to minimize trauma to the psoas muscle. Once the retractor is expanded, the location of the anterior vertebral body is defined by identifying the anterior fiber of the anterior longitudinal ligament. This helps to minimize the risks of vascular injury and of anterior graft placement and dislodgment. The location of the ALL should be assessed throughout the discectomy procedure.

An ipsilateral discectomy is performed using a disc knife to excise the annulus. With gentle tapping, a Cobb elevator is passed across the disc space beyond the contralateral annulus under fluoroscopic guidance (Fig. 48-2, *A*). After the elevator passes through the opposite annulus, it is rotated to release the contralateral endplate attachment. This allows the cage to engage with the contralateral ring apophysis, allowing for restoration of disc height and helping with deformity correction.

Meticulous technique is required to prevent endplate violation. Fluoroscopy should be used when spinal instruments such as curettes, rasps, and Cobb elevators are passed into the disc space. Trials are then introduced serially into the disc space, with care taken not to oversize the graft (Fig. 48-2, *B*). A wide implant is generally placed to take advantage of the biomechanical strength of the dense ring apophysis.

ACR differs from the standard technique, because it includes excision of the anterior annulus and anterior longitudinal ligament. The interval between the anterior longitudinal ligament, the anterior annulus, and the aorta is exposed through blunt dissection, and a special retractor blade is inserted anteriorly. The ipsilateral anterior annulus and anterior longitudinal ligament are released with a disc knife under direct vision. The contralateral structures are usually released indirectly through insertion of serial trials. Although this technique allows better sagittal plane correction, it decreases the stability of the cage in the disc space, because the anterior tension band is removed. Therefore special cages with built-in holes for screw fixation should be implanted. Usually, fixation to one vertebral body provides adequate stability, and leaving the other vertebral body uninstrumented allows further deformity correction if a posterior osteotomy is performed.

Autologous iliac crest bone graft or a bone graft replacement can be placed within the spacer before it is implanted into the disc space. An understanding of the anatomy, vigilant monitoring of the surrounding neurologic structures, a meticulous and thorough discectomy, and appropriate implant placement can minimize complications.

POTENTIAL COMPLICATIONS AND MANAGEMENT

Complications associated with lateral transpsoas approaches are related to the specific approach and can be categorized as neural, visceral, or vascular. Several neurologic structures are at risk of damage during the approach, including the nerves of the lumbar plexus running within the psoas muscle and the nerves over the psoas and on the abdominal wall. Iliohypogastric, ilioinguinal, and lateral femoral cutaneous nerves run on the inner surface of the abdominal muscles and can be easily injured during dissection of the muscle layers. Thus it is essential to perform blunt rather than Bovie dissection through the abdominal muscles to minimize injury to these structures. The path of the genitofemoral nerve varies considerably. It courses in a tangential manner and pierces the psoas near L3-4, and it is susceptible to injury over the psoas.[23] The lateral transpsoas approach requires placement of a retractor through the psoas muscle, where the lumbosacral plexus lies. These lumbosacral plexus nerves run within and around the psoas and are not easily visible; therefore they are *indirectly* monitored and protected through a special neuromonitoring system. It is essential for a surgeon to study the position of these nerves at each level. Above L4-5 they lie at the posterior quarter of the vertebral body, whereas at L4-5 they cross more anteriorly into the middle-posterior quarter of the vertebral body.[24] In the setting of spondylolisthesis, the cephalic segment moves the plexus farther anteriorly; thus this translation can be increased. In addition, anatomic anomalies are seen in up to 20% of patients.[4] With such possible variability in the course of these nerves, complications are possible, and prevention is based on proper neuromonitoring with free-run and triggered EMG.[25,26] The most common complication after a transpsoas approach is transient hip flexor weakness (up to 27.5%), which is believed to be a consequence of trauma to the psoas muscle itself, rather than a neural injury.[25] Distal motor deficits (such as quadriceps weakness) has been reported at an incidence of 0.7% to 3%.[25,27] Meticulous surgical technique with an excellent knowledge of the local anatomy is essential to decrease the potential neurologic complications. Limited mobilization of the peritoneal contents and vascular structures decreases the risk of injury to visceral and vascular structures significantly, compared with a direct anterior approach but does not eliminate it; iliac vein and bowel injury have been reported, although the incidence in the larger population is uncertain.[28] A single-incision technique with dissection of the retroperitoneal space under direct vision may help to decrease potential injuries and is my (V.D.) preferred method.

PATIENT EXAMPLES

ADJACENT-SEGMENT DISEASE

This 55-year-old man presented with back pain and right lower extremity radiculopathy that was nonresponsive to conservative treatment. He had a previous L4-S1 fusion. His evaluation revealed adjacent-segment disease (Fig. 48-3, *A* through *C*). An L3-4 XLIF procedure was performed that relieved his leg pain and improved his back pain (Fig. 48-3, *D* and *E*).

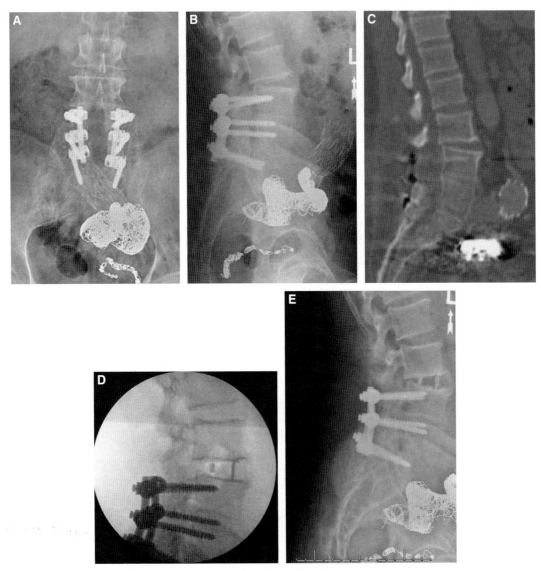

Fig. 48-3 **A-C,** Preoperative radiographs and CT showed previous L4-S1 fusion and adjacent-segment disease. **D** and **E,** Postoperative radiographs after a stand-alone L3-4 eXtreme lateral interbody fusion procedure show indirect decompression.

Degenerative Scoliosis

This 79-year-old man presented with back and bilateral leg pain. Radiographs showed degenerative scoliosis (Fig. 48-4, *A* and *B*). CT was performed to evaluate the endplate and revealed sclerosis (Fig. 48-4, *C*). A stand-alone XLIF was performed at L1-5 (Fig. 48-4, *D* and *E*). One year after surgery, the patient has continued resolution of symptoms.

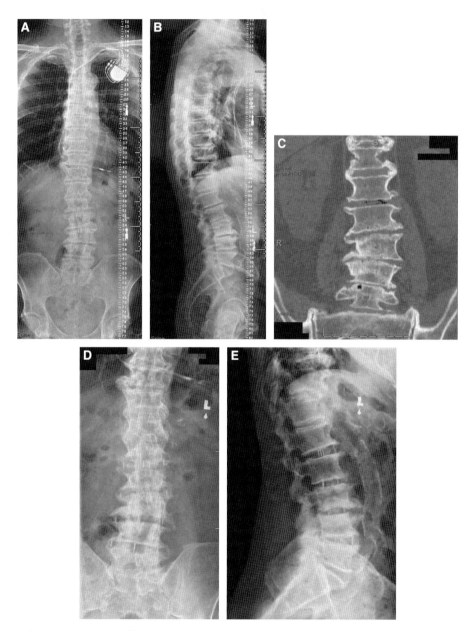

Fig. 48-4   **A** and **B,** Preoperative radiographs showed degenerative scoliosis. **C,** CT revealed endplate sclerosis. **D** and **E,** Postoperative radiographs after stand-alone eXtreme lateral interbody fusion at L1-5 show resolution of symptoms.

Complex Deformity and Degenerative Scoliosis

This 69-year-old woman presented with low back, bilateral hip, and left leg pain. Preoperative radiographs showed decompensation away from the convexity of her structural lumbar curve in the coronal plane (Fig. 48-5, *A* and *B*). After treatment of the anterior column, the patient's pain was immediately reduced, and radiographs showed improved coronal alignment (Fig. 48-5, *C* and *D*). Two days after the anterior portion of the procedure, posterior fusion was performed to further improve sagittal balance and coronal alignment (Fig. 48-5, *E* and *F*). One year after surgery the patient is able to walk several blocks and has increased her lifting abilities to meet her needs for daily living.

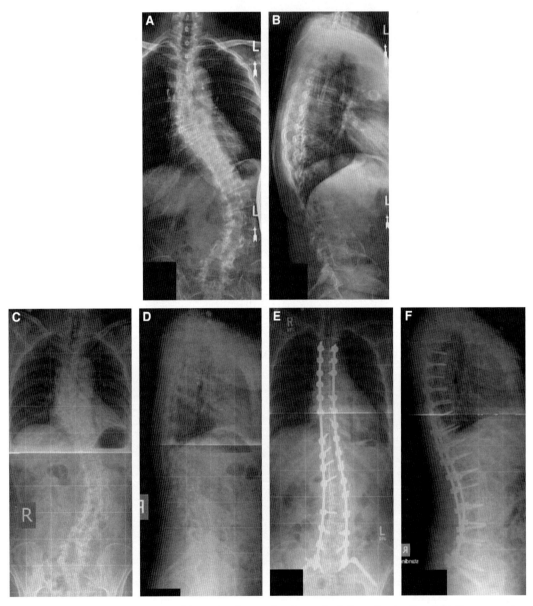

Fig. 48-5   **A** and **B,** Preoperative AP and lateral radiographs showed adult scoliosis. **C** and **D,** Postoperative radiographs showed improved coronal alignment after first-stage multilevel lateral interbody fusions. **E** and **F,** Postoperative radiographs after second-stage posterior fusion show further improved sagittal balance and coronal alignment.

DEGENERATIVE SCOLIOSIS WITH FLAT-BACK SYNDROME

This 58-year-old woman presented with worsening back pain and right lower extremity radiculopathy. The preoperative imaging studies showed adult degenerative scoliosis with flat-back syndrome (Fig. 48-6, *A*). A three-level ACR was performed followed by T10-ilium posterior instrumentation fusion with L5-S1 TLIF (Fig. 48-6, *B* and *E*). She had excellent coronal and sagittal balance that was maintained at her 1-year follow-up (Fig. 48-6, *C* and *F*).

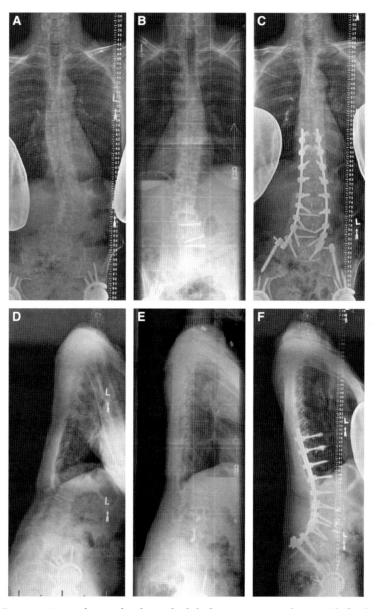

Fig. 48-6 **A** and **D,** Preoperative radiographs showed adult degenerative scoliosis with flat-back syndrome. **B** and **E,** Postoperative radiographs after a three-level anterior column realignment. **C** and **F,** One-year postoperative radiographs after T10-ilium posterior instrumentation fusion with L5-S1 transforaminal lumbar interbody fusion show excellent coronal and sagittal balance.

CORONAL AND SAGITTAL PLANE DEFORMITY WITH SPINAL STENOSIS

This 75-year-old woman presented with back pain and bilateral leg pain and was required to use a cane. Preoperative imaging showed mild coronal and sagittal plane deformity with spinal stenosis (Fig. 48-7, *A* through *C*). She underwent a staged anterior L2-4 XLIF followed by posterior percutaneous L2-ilium instrumentation, L5-S1 TLIF, and an L4 laminectomy through a mini-midline exposure. Her lumbar lordosis improved from 31 to 52 degrees (Fig. 48-7, *D* and *E*). Six months after surgery, her back and leg pain are improved significantly, and she is ambulating without assistance.

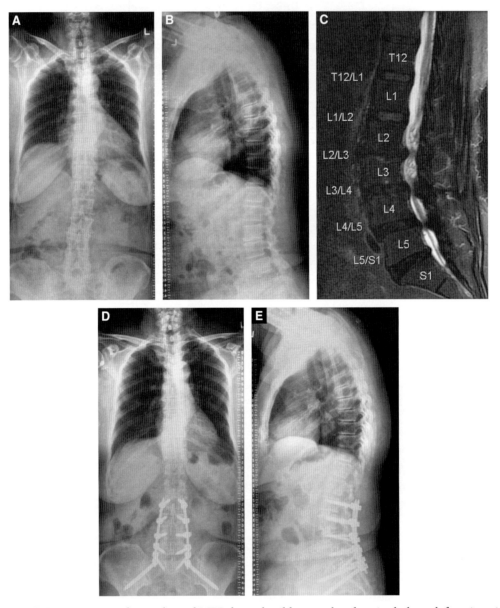

Fig. 48-7   **A-C,** Preoperative radiographs and MRI showed mild coronal and sagittal plane deformity with spinal stenosis. **D** and **E,** Postoperative radiographs after a staged anterior L2-4 eXtreme lateral interbody fusion followed by posterior percutaneous L2-ilium instrumentation, L5-S1 TLIF, and an L4 laminectomy through a mini-midline exposure show improved lumbar lordosis.

Minimally Invasive Posterior Approaches

As instrumentation systems are becoming more advanced, minimally invasive posterior approaches are gaining popularity. Initially, these approaches were designed to perform simple decompressions such as microdiscectomy for disc herniations and one- to two-level percutaneous TLIFs for simple degenerative cases.[29,30] As surgeons become more proficient, the number of levels instrumented through a posterior percutaneous approach has increased. This has led to its use in thoracolumbar trauma and adult deformity cases.[31,32] The main advantage of posterior percutaneous instrumentation is the limited soft tissue dissection, which in turn decreases blood loss and narcotic medication use and results in rapid mobilization.[33] All of these factors potentially limit perioperative complications such as cardiac events, pneumonia, venous thromboembolic events, delirium, and prolonged immobilization. Although benefits of minimally invasive posterior instrumentation have been shown for degenerative cases, the value of this approach for deformity cases has not been well documented. Anand et al[32] reported their initial experience with 12 patients in whom minimally invasive surgery (MIS) techniques were used and suggested that MIS allows deformity correction with less blood loss and morbidity, compared with open techniques. The International Spine Study Group reviewed 118 patients with a minimum 2-year follow-up and showed that MIS can be applied effectively to augment an open operation hybrid (HYB) or be used circumferentially to treat adult spinal deformity.[34] We have demonstrated the sustainability of these results at the 2-year follow-up, with satisfactory improvement in health-related quality of life (HRQOL) and radiographic parameters. Complications and reoperation rates are comparable with those of traditional techniques with no significant impact on HRQOL.

Percutaneous pedicle screw insertion is the mainstay of posterior instrumentation. Because of the rotation and the malalignment of the spine, cannulation of the pedicles may be more challenging, compared with nondeformity pathologies. Pedicle screw insertion can be performed with either simple biplanar fluoroscopy or three-dimensional fluoroscopy and CT-based navigation systems. Although the latter systems are more expensive, they increase accuracy and decrease the radiation exposure to the surgeon. On the other hand, biplanar fluoroscopy is available at most hospitals and is quite accurate. Heintel et al[35] reviewed 502 screws; 98% were graded as being in an excellent or good position. One screw was revised because of medial placement with a subsequent neurologic deficit. Park et al[31] reported on 172 screws in a trauma population and found an 82% accuracy (no violation) rate; only 2.9% had a breach larger than 2 mm. Idler et al[36] reported a very low (1.5%) breach rate in a retrospective study of 326 pedicle screws placed in the lumbar spine using guidance technology. Shin et al[37] compared fluoroscopy-based navigation with O-arm–based navigation and found accuracy rates of 88% and 92%, respectively.

Placement of rods through long segments and performing the correction maneuver through the MIS incision are additional disadvantages. As the number of segments involved increases, ensuring the passage of the rod through each tulip becomes more difficult, because the tactile feedback becomes less reliable. Some instrumentation systems have an open design instead of towers, allowing surgeons to visually confirm the rod placement. A midline skin incision and extension of the dissection over the fascia bilaterally decreases the effective thickness of the soft tissue envelope a surgeon works through and facilitates passage of the rod. No space is available for in situ benders; therefore rods should have the final contour on insertion. This further complicates the deformity correction, because a surgeon must estimate the appropriate bends in the rod and cannot know whether the angle is correct until after the rod has been inserted and reduced into the tulips. Although rod derotation is possible, it is impossible to perform cantilever techniques unless part of the spine is exposed to perform a minimally invasive corpectomy or osteotomy. Another limitation is that any osteotomy other than type 1 may require soft dissection similar to open techniques and potentially take longer because of the limited visibility. Therefore, ideally, most of the deformity correction should be obtained through the anterior approach, and the posterior instrumentation should be applied mainly for the maintenance of the correction. Initial LLIF for deformity correction followed by posterior percutaneous instrumentation appears to be the best minimally invasive combination to correct adult spinal deformity. Even with this technique, sagittal plane correction can be limited. Wang and Mummaneni[38] reported on 23 patients in whom the mean coronal deformity correction was 20 degrees but sagittal plane correction was only 8 degrees. Acosta et al[39] reported on 35 patients treated with lateral MIS who had a similar result: a mean coronal plane correction of 12 degrees but only 4 degrees of sagittal plane correction. Finally, Karikari et al[40] reported on 22 patients with thoracic and thoracolumbar pathologies, who obtained a mean of only 5 degrees of correction in the sagittal plane. These data indicate a higher risk of inadequate sagittal and coronal plane correction after minimally invasive posterior techniques; therefore this method should be reserved for patients with minimal deformity.

Another challenge of minimally invasive posterior approaches is extension of fusion to the sacrum and pelvis, which is common in adult spinal deformity. The classic iliac screw insertion is not in line with the S1 screws and requires an offset connector to be connected to the rod, which necessitates wider exposure and precludes minimally invasive techniques. Several authors have described techniques that allow placement of regular iliac screws in MIS so that the fusion can be extended to the pelvis. Wang et al[41] described percutaneous insertion of iliac screws in a series of 10 adult deformity patients, which further expanded the indications for posterior MIS. Another development is S2-alar screws that start from S2 and enter the iliac wing by crossing through the sacroiliac joint. This screw better aligns with the S1 screw and can be attached to the rod without an offset connector. In a cadaver study, O'Brien et al[42] found that this screw can be inserted accurately under fluoroscopic guidance. Martin et al[43] reported on two patients in whom pelvic fixation was obtained with this technique. Either a posterior percutaneous TLIF or ALIF can achieve the L5-S1 anterior fusion.

Finally, because percutaneous posterior instrumentation eliminates exposure of the posterior bony structures, the area for posterior fusion is minimal, and usually the facet joints are the only feasible target for posterior fusion. Therefore this technique relies mainly on the anterior fusion and hence creates a potentially higher risk for pseudarthrosis. Wang and Mummaneni[38] reported on 23 patients who had no pseudarthrosis at the 13-month follow-up. The International Spine Study Group performed a review comparing 118 patients who had all-open, hybrid (anterior MIS with posterior open surgery), or all-MIS techniques to treat spinal deformity.[34] The minimum follow-up was 2 years. The rate of revision surgery was not significantly different between the groups ($p = 0.196$): 15.8% for MIS (6 of 38), 31.6% for hybrid techniques (12 of 38), and 31.6% for open techniques (12 of 38). The most common reason for reoperation in the open group was neurologic deficit (10.5%), followed by proximal junctional kyphosis (PJK; 7.9%). The most common cause of reoperation in the hybrid group was proximal junctional kyphosis (13.2%), followed by infection (7.9%). The most common reason in the MIS group was pseudarthrosis (7.9%). Although reoperation rates were not statistically different between the MIS, hybrid, and open groups, the incidence was twice as high in the hybrid and open groups. In a similar study, the International Spine Study Group reviewed 114 patients for proximal junctional kyphosis.[44] The minimum follow-up was 2 years. MIS pedicle screw fixation resulted in a similar rate of radiographic proximal junctional kyphosis in patients who were propensity matched for sagittal vertical axis (less than 5 cm), pelvic incidence minus lumbar lordosis mismatch (10 to 20 degrees), and levels fused. MIS cases required less reoperation for proximal junctional kyphosis.

As surgeons become comfortable with minimally invasive techniques, the variety of procedures that can be performed with MIS is expanding. Wang and Madhavan[45] described a minimally invasive pedicle subtraction osteotomy. The cranial and caudal fixation was performed through percutaneous instrumentation that was followed by a pedicle subtraction osteotomy through a limited incision. Deformity was corrected through cantilever forces, and the rods were connected at the osteotomy site with side-to-side connectors. The sagittal balance was improved to 20 mm from 95 mm, and the blood loss was 900 ml. In summary, posterior minimally invasive instrumentations are gaining popularity in adult deformity surgery. As with all MIS techniques, a surgeon should be comfortable with the open procedure before attempting the minimally invasive version.

INDICATIONS AND CONTRAINDICATIONS

Although any adult patient with deformity is a potential candidate for minimally invasive posterior techniques, awareness of the limitations of this approach and careful patient selection are essential for success. Early results in the literature suggest that sagittal plane correction with any minimally invasive approach is limited, and patients with significant sagittal imbalance may not be the best candidates for posterior MIS. Overall, the role of posterior percutaneous instrumentation is to supplement the anterior intervention rather than serving as the primary intervention, and an ideal patient has a flexible, short thoracolumbar and lumbar curve with minimal sagittal plane deformity.

PREOPERATIVE PLANNING

The magnitude and flexibility of the deformity is first evaluated on full-standing scoliosis and side-bending radiographs. An ideal patient has a moderate, flexible curve, which allows most of the correction to be performed through the initial anterior approach. More severe, rigid curves likely require extensive soft tissue releases or major osteotomies, even when performed as open surgery. An attempt to achieve the same goal with MIS in these patients will only result in inadequate correction of the deformity. Radiographs to evaluate spine anatomy for pedicle screw placement are then obtained. CT aids in evaluating the diameter and orientation of the pedicles. This allows a surgeon to plan for appropriately sized screws and obtain navigation assistance for safe screw placement in patients with complex anatomy. MRI is useful for evaluating the degree and location of stenosis and for planning the decompression maneuvers.

OPERATIVE TECHNIQUE

The patient is positioned prone on a Jackson table (Mizuho OSI, Union City, CA) with a four-post frame. Simple biplanar fluoroscopy can be used to guide insertion of the screws. For short-segment instrumentations (two levels), bilateral paramidline incisions are made for each pedicle screw. For longer instrumentations, a midline incision is preferred. The dissection is extended bilaterally over the fascia, and separate fascial incisions are made for each screw. This results in a better-looking scar and decreases the overall thickness of the soft tissue envelope (the distance from the posterior elements to the surface), facilitating passage of the rod. The incision for each screw should be made slightly lateral to the pedicle image (Fig. 48-8). A Jamshidi needle is then inserted and docked on the lateral edge of the pedicle image. An average

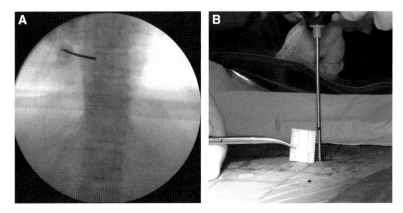

Fig. 48-8 Minimally invasive posterior approach. **A,** The entry site of the Jamshidi needle should be just on the lateral border of the pedicle, based on an AP view. **B,** The average pedicle length, 20 mm, is marked on the needle.

Continued

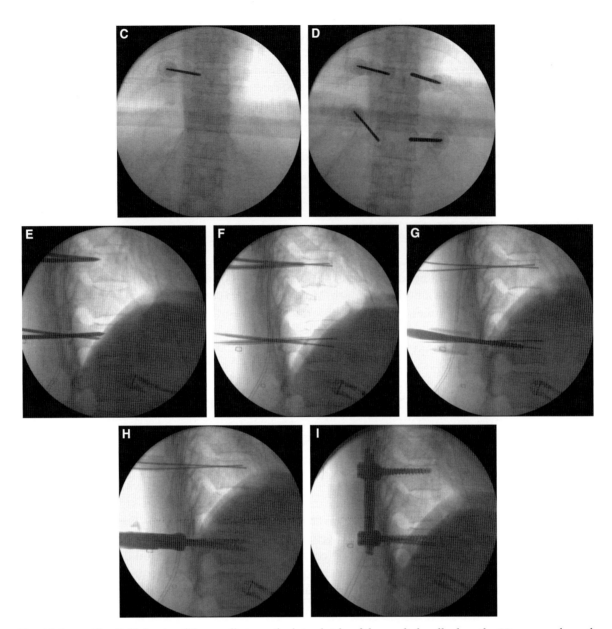

Fig. 48-8, cont'd **C,** If the tip of the needle is on the lateral side of the medial wall when the 20 mm mark on the needle reaches the skin, the needle placement is safe. **D,** Needles can be placed in an AP view and confirmed in a lateral view. **E,** If the tip of the needle is anterior to the posterior wall, the needle is beyond the pedicle. **F,** Guide wires are introduced against the anterior wall, and the needles are removed. **G,** The pedicle is tapped. **H,** The screw is placed with the assistance of a lateral view. **I,** All screws and rods can be placed with a lateral view.

pedicle length of 20 mm should be marked on the needle, and the needle is advanced to this mark under AP fluoroscopic guidance. When the mark is reached, the tip of the needle should be lateral to the medial wall of the pedicle. If the needle tip reaches the medial wall before the 20 mm mark is reached, the needle should be retrieved and a new path developed. This technique allows insertion of multiple screws with minimal C-arm manipulation. A small-caliber needle can flex if it encounters the medial wall and is preferable over a larger-caliber needle.

Lateral fluoroscopy is used to confirm that the tip of the needle is anterior to the posterior wall of the vertebral body, and the stylet of the needle is removed. A guide wire is inserted until it contacts the anterior wall of the vertebral body. The needle is removed while the guide wire is retained, and dilators are introduced to develop a plane in the paraspinal muscles. The path is tapped, and a preselected screw is inserted under fluoroscopic guidance. During these two stages, the guide wire may bind to the tap or the screw and be inadvertently advanced; frequent fluoroscopic images are essential to monitor for this potential complication. The screw is driven until it is snug, and its position is monitored on a lateral view. The positions of the successive screws are also monitored to ensure that all of the screw tulips are at the same level, unless spondylolisthesis is present. If the tulips remain different heights, subsequent rod passing is challenging and places excessive stress on the screws as the set screws are inserted. The screw position is confirmed by AP fluoroscopy. Once all of the screws are inserted, a soft tissue path is developed with special dissectors to connect the tulips. The iliac screws or S2-alar screws can be inserted with the help of an obturator outlet view.[41,43] S2-alar screws provide a significant advantage, because they require a more medial starting point; therefore they do not require an offset connector to connect to the rod. An appropriately contoured rod is inserted, appropriate correction maneuvers are carried out, and final tightening is performed.

POTENTIAL COMPLICATIONS AND MANAGEMENT

Pedicle screw malposition is one of the most important complications of minimally invasive posterior approaches. A detailed preoperative preparation with appropriate imaging studies and strict adherence to the surgical technique are essential to prevent this complication. Although accuracy of biplanar fluoroscopy is high, advanced navigation systems decrease the radiation exposure to the surgeon and have better accuracy rates. Another potential complication is inadequate correction of the deformity; careful patient selection prevents this problem. Risk of wound dehiscence, deep infection, and postoperative hematoma is greatly decreased with posterior minimally invasive techniques because of decreased soft tissue stripping.

CONCLUSION

LLIF has many applications in the treatment of complex adult spinal deformity. It is a useful alternative to traditional interbody fusion techniques, with expanded indications in stand-alone constructs and ACR. Although its use has limitations and inherent risks, adherence to indications and meticulous surgical technique make it reproducible and safe, with excellent clinical outcomes. Posterior percutaneous instrumentation offers significant advantages such as decreased soft tissue stripping and decreased wound complications; however, it should be reserved for select patients because of its limited capacity for deformity correction.

REFERENCES

1. Tanaka N, An HS, Lim TH, et al. The relationship between disc degeneration and flexibility of the lumbar spine. Spine J 1:47-56, 2001.
2. Lund T, Oxland TR, Jost B, et al. Interbody cage stabilization in the lumbar spine: biomechanical evaluation of cage design, posterior instrumentaion and bone density. J Bone Joint Surg Br 80:351-359, 1998.
3. Kim YB, Lenke LG, Kim YJ, et al. The morbidity of an anterior thoracolumbar approach: adult spinal deformity patients with greater than five-year follow-up. Spine 34:822-826, 2009.
4. Samudrala S, Khoo LT, Rhim SC. Complication during anterior surgery of the lumbar spine: an anatomically based study and review. Neurosurg Focus 7:e9, 1999.
5. Rajaraman V, Vingan R, Roth P. Visceral and vascular complications resulting from anterior lumbar interbody fusions. J Neurosurg 91(1 Suppl):S60-S64, 1999.
6. Quraishi NA, Konig M, Booker SJ, et al. Access related complications in anterior lumbar surgery performed by spinal surgeons. Eur Spine J 22(Suppl 1):S16-S20, 2013.
7. Pimenta L. Lateral endoscopic transpsoas retroperitoneal approach for lumbar spine surgery. Presented at the Eighth Annual Brazilian Spine Society Meeting, Belo Horizonte, Minas Gerais, Brazil, May 2001.

8. Ozgur BM, Aryan HE, Pimenta L, et al. Extreme lateral interbody fusion (XLIF): a novel surgical technique for anterior lumbar interbody fusion. Spine J 6:435-443, 2006.

9. Pekmezci M, McDonald E, Kennedy A, et al. Can a novel rectangular footplate provide higher resistance to subsidence than circular footplates? An ex vivo biomechanical study. Spine 37:E1177-E1181, 2012.

10. Klopfenstein JD, Kim LJ, Feiz-Erfan I, et al. Retroperitoneal approach for lumbar interbody fusion with anterolateral instrumentation for treatment of spondylolisthesis and degenerative foraminal stenosis. Surg Neurol 65:111-116; discussion 116, 2006.

11. Oliveira L, Marchi L, Coutinho E, et al. A radiographic assessment of the ability of the extreme lateral interbody fusion procedure to indirectly decompress the neural elements. Spine 35(26 Suppl):S331-S337, 2010.

12. Marchi L, Abdala N, Oliveira L, et al. Stand-alone lateral interbody fusion for the treatment of low-grade degenerative spondylolisthesis. ScientificWorldJournal 2012:456346, 2012.

13. Cappuccino A, Cornwall GB, Turner AW, et al. Biomechanical analysis and review of lateral lumbar fusion constructs. Spine 35(26 Suppl):S361-S367, 2010.

14. Isaacs RE, Hyde J, Goodrich A, et al. A prospective, nonrandomized, multicenter evaluation of extreme lateral interbody fusion for the treatment of adult degenerative scoliosis. Spine 35:S322-S330, 2010.

15. Fujita T, Kostuik JP, Huckell CB, et al. Complications of spinal fusion in adult patients more than 60 years of age. Orthop Clin North Am 29:669-678, 1998.

16. Cho KJ, Suk SI, Park SR, et al. Complications in posterior fusion and instrumentation for degenerative lumbar scoliosis. Spine 32:2232-2237, 2007.

17. Keshavarzi S, Mundis G, Pekmezci M, et al. The utility and limitations of XLIF in adult scoliosis. In Proceedings of the Fourth Annual SOLAS (Society of Lateral Access Surgery) Research Meeting. San Diego: The Society, March-April 2011.

18. Kepler CK, Sharma AK, Huang RC, et al. Indirect foraminal decompression after lateral transpsoas interbody fusion. J Neurosurg Spine 16:329-333, 2012.

19. Groth AT, Kuklo TR, Klemme WR, et al. Comparison of sagittal contour and posterior disc height following interbody fusion: threaded cylindrical cages versus structural allograft versus vertical cages. J Spinal Disord Tech 18:332-336, 2005.

20. Deviren V, Tang JA, Scheer JK, et al. Construct rigidity after fatigue loading in pedicle subtraction osteotomy with or without adjacent interbody structural cages. Global Spine J 2:213-220, 2012.

21. Akbarnia BA, Mundis GM Jr, Moazzaz P, et al. Anterior column realignment (ACR) for focal kyphotic spinal deformity using a lateral transpsoas approach and ALL release. J Spinal Disord Tech 27:29-39, 2013.

22. Demirkian G, Theologis AA, Pekmezci M, Ames CP, Deviren V. Anterior column release for complex adult spinal deformity correction: is this the end of the pedicle subtraction osteotomy? Presented at the Seventh Annual SOLAS Research Meeting, Miami Beach, FL, April 2014.

23. Bergey DL, Villavicencio AT, Goldstein T. Endoscopic lateral transpsoas approach to the lumbar spine. Spine 29:1681-1688, 2004.

24. Moro T, Kikuchi S, Konno S. An anatomic study of the lumbar plexus with respect to retroperitoneal endoscopic surgery. Spine 28:423-428, 2003.

25. Tohmeh TG, Rodgers WB, Peterson MD. Dynamically evoked, discrete-threshold electromyography in the extreme lateral interbody fusion approach. J Neurosurg Spine 14:31-37, 2011.

26. Uribe JS, Vale FL, Dakwar E. Electromyographic monitoring and its anatomical implications in minimally invasive spine surgery. Spine 35(26 Suppl):S368-S374, 2010.

27. Rodgers WB, Gerber EJ, Patterson J. Intraoperative and early postoperative complications in extreme lateral interbody fusion: an analysis of 600 cases. Spine 36:26-33, 2011.

28. Tormenti MJ, Maserati MB, Bonfield CM. Complications and radiographic correction in adult scoliosis following combined transpsoas extreme lateral interbody fusion and posterior pedicle screw instrumentation. Neurosurg Focus 28:E7, 2010.

29. Adogwa O, Parker SL, Bydon A, et al. Comparative effectiveness of minimally invasive versus open transforaminal lumbar interbody fusion: 2-year assessment of narcotic use, return to work, disability, and quality of life. J Spinal Disord Tech 24:479-484, 2011.

30. Rahman M, Summers LE, Richter B, et al. Comparison of techniques for decompressive lumbar laminectomy: the minimally invasive versus the "classic" open approach. Minim Invasive Neurosurg 51:100-105, 2008.

31. Park DK, Thomas AO, St Clair S, et al. Percutaneous lumbar and thoracic pedicle screws: a trauma experience. J Spinal Disord Tech. 2012 Mar 27. [Epub ahead of print]

32. Anand N, Baron EM, Thaiyananthan G, et al. Minimally invasive multilevel percutaneous correction and fusion for adult lumbar degenerative scoliosis: a technique and feasibility study. J Spinal Disord Tech 21:459-467, 2008.

33. Kim CW. Scientific basis of minimally invasive spine surgery: prevention of multifidus muscle injury during posterior lumbar surgery. Spine 35(26 Suppl):S281-S286, 2010.

34. Mundis GM, Akbarnia BA, Mummaneni PV, Kanter AS, Okonkwo DO, Park P, Uribe JS, Deviren V, et al. Adult spinal deformity treated with minimally invasive techniques: two-year multicenter clinical and radiographic outcomes study comparing circumferential MIS and hybrid surgery. Presented at the International Spine Study Group Annual Meeting, Valencia, Spain, 2014.

35. Heintel TM, Berglehner A, Meffert R. Accuracy of percutaneous pedicle screws for thoracic and lumbar spine fractures: a prospective trial. Eur Spine J 22:495-502, 2013.

36. Idler C, Rolfe KW, Gorek JE. Accuracy of percutaneous lumbar pedicle screw placement using the oblique or "owl's-eye" view and novel guidance technology. J Neurosurg Spine 13:509-515, 2010.

37. Shin MH, Hur JW, Ryu KS, et al. Prospective comparison study between the fluoroscopy guided and navigation coupled with O-arm® guided pedicle screw placement in the thoracic and lumbosacral spines. J Spinal Disord Tech. 2013 Nov 6. [Epub ahead of print]

38. Wang MY, Mummaneni PV. Minimally invasive surgery for thoracolumbar spinal deformity: initial clinical experience with clinical and radiographic outcomes. Neurosurg Focus 28:E9, 2010.

39. Acosta FL, Liu J, Slimack N, et al. Changes in coronal and sagittal plane alignment following minimally invasive direct lateral interbody fusion for the treatment of degenerative lumbar disease in adults: a radiographic study. J Neurosurg Spine 15:92-96, 2011.

40. Karikari IO, Nimjee SM, Hardin CA, et al. Extreme lateral interbody fusion approach for isolated thoracic and thoracolumbar spine diseases: initial clinical experience and early outcomes. J Spinal Disord Tech 24:368-375, 2011.

41. Wang MY, Ludwig SC, Anderson DG, et al. Percutaneous iliac screw placement: description of a new minimally invasive technique. Neurosurg Focus 25:E17, 2008.

42. O'Brien JR, Matteini L, Yu WD, et al. Feasibility of minimally invasive sacropelvic fixation: percutaneous S2 alar iliac fixation. Spine 35:460-464, 2010.

43. Martin CT, Witham TF, Kebaish KM. Sacropelvic fixation: two case reports of a new percutaneous technique. Spine 36:E618-E621, 2011.

44. Park P, Mummaneni PV, Mundis GM, Anand N, Nunley PD, Uribe JS, Wang MY, Kanter AS, Okonkwo DO, Fessler RG, Deviren V, et al. Does the use of minimally invasive pedicle screw fixation lower the rate of PJK? Presented at the IMAST Annual Meeting, Valencia, Spain, 2014.

45. Wang MY, Madhavan K. Mini-open pedicle subtraction osteotomy: surgical technique. World Neurosurg 81:843, e11-e14, 2012.

49

Minimally Invasive Surgical Treatment of Adjacent-Segment Pathology: Hybrid Techniques

Jim A. Youssef ▪ *Douglas G. Orndorff* ▪ *Morgan Scott*
Rachel Eve Ebner ▪ *Elisa R. Mullikin*

Adjacent-segment pathology (ASP) is a diagnosis referring to any type of deterioration at motion segments proximal or less commonly distal to the location of an earlier spinal fusion.[1] It can manifest as several separate or related diagnoses, including stenosis, degenerative disc degeneration or breakdown, and spondylolisthesis or retrolisthesis.[2,3] Previous research focused on how biomechanical fusion causes one area of the spine to be more rigid, especially when augmented with instrumentation, increasing motion and facet load at adjacent levels to partially compensate for the reduced area of motion. The amount of force redistributed is directly related to the number of segments fused.[4] Although the exact cause of ASP is unknown, the additional adjacent-level stress may be implicit in accelerating degenerative changes at such levels. Newer research, however, indicates that some patients may be predisposed to further spinal degeneration and deformity.[5-7] Other factors have been found to increase risk for ASP, including smoking status, age, obesity, comorbidities such as diabetes and Parkinson's disease, and preexisting lumbar degenerative disease and sagittal and coronal alignment. Patients who have abnormal sacral inclination or retrolisthesis are at higher risk and should undergo extended follow-up after spinal surgery to assess for degenerative changes.[8] ASP can manifest as a radiographic finding, without associated clinical symptoms; therefore clinical correlation is required. ASP symptoms vary from patient to patient but commonly include axial pain, radiculopathy, neurogenic claudication, and back pain from stenosis, arthritis, spondylolisthesis with or without instability, and disc herniation. Loss in function with weakness can occur. Whereas proximal ASP is most common, a small but significant number of patients develop distal ASP.[3,9] For patients receiving lumbar spinal fusion, research indicates that 41% develop alterations at adjacent levels after surgery, and approximately 90% of affected levels are proximal to the original fusion.[3,10]

ASP can be challenging for patients and surgeons, because no hard and fast rules exist for treating symptoms or associated deformity. Although revision surgery poses a higher rate of risks, including pseudarthrosis, infection, cerebrospinal fluid leakage, instrumentation failure, and further ASP, the severity of the symptoms may prompt a surgical recommendation when nonoperative treatments fail to control clinical symptoms.[11] Treatment options vary depending on the number of adjacent levels involved, the location of the degenerative levels in relation to the thoracolumbar junction and/or lumbosacral junction, and the overall global spinal alignment. Surgical decision-making requires consideration of all sagittal and coronal alignment parameters, the health status and bone quality of the patient, and the need for decompressive surgery. Fused segments can affect surgical recommendation because of the presence of sagittal malalignment or flat-back syndrome. Proper preoperative evaluation is required. Initial medical optimization for each patient is strongly suggested. Treatment of underlying nutritional deficits such as vitamin D deficiency or metabolic bone disease can aid in achieving a better clinical and surgical outcome.[12] A complete radiographic analysis, including a standing AP and lateral scoliosis series, flexion and extension radiographs, and other diagnostic imaging studies, is required for appropriate preoperative planning. Identification of the presence of pseudarthrosis or hardware failure is imperative. Obtaining old surgical records and implant records aids in surgical preparation and helps to determine surgical options for extending the fusion to adjacent levels. Further understanding of how a patient responded to the initial surgical intervention is important. Postoperative infection at the time of the index procedure is important for planning subsequent surgical intervention. Once all of these steps have been accomplished in the preoperative planning process, a surgeon should have several available surgical options to maximize the outcome for patients with ASP. In addition to treating the adjacent level and clinical complaints, surgeons need a global understanding of each patient's clinical and radiographic coronal and sagittal alignment. Treatment of only the adjacent level in isolation places other adjacent levels at risk for future degeneration. Appropriate preoperative planning is critical to attempt to reduce such iatrogenic problems.

Surgical decision-making can include hardware removal, osteotomy planning, vertebral column resection, and simple extension of decompression and fusion to the adjacent level. In all circumstances, proper surgical planning reduces the potential for intraoperative limitations or inability to effectively correct the global spinal alignment of the patient. Historically, the surgical approach to ASP involved removal of old pedicle screws and rods with either instrumented or noninstrumented posterolateral fusions after decompression. Pedicle subtraction osteotomies and reinstrumentation with new pedicle screws and rods inclusive of the adjacent levels being treated is a common surgical treatment for such deformities. Furthermore, to help achieve such sagittal corrections and improve fusion rates, anterior lumbar, thoracolumbar, and lumbosacral fusion techniques can supplement the surgical treatment of ASP. Anterior interbody fusion is a proven treatment for achieving fusion and sagittal correction; however, when performed in an open fashion, it can add to the surgical morbidity of an already challenging surgical problem.[13-15] Results for such surgical intervention are varied, and clinical and radiographic results are less promising than those of initial fusions.[14] Although clinical and functional results of revision surgery are similar to those of index deformity surgery, the surgical treatment of ASP using standard open techniques increases operating time, blood loss, and neurologic deficit and lengthens hospital stays.[16]

With the evolution of minimally invasive surgery (MIS) techniques, surgeons are able to minimize patient risk by reducing blood loss, hospital stay, operating room time, and complication rates.[17] Not all diagnoses can be treated with MIS alone; however, the indications for employing such techniques in treating ASP are expanding. In patients who are appropriate candidates for surgical treatment of a breakdown at an adjacent level, MIS hybrid (HYB) techniques may improve patient-reported outcomes. These techniques may not be appropriate for all patients, and they should not be performed as an alternative when traditional open techniques are indicated.

When an appropriate ASP diagnosis is made and clinical conditions are met, a HYB technique can be employed as a newer surgical option. Literature on this technique is limited. It involves an anterior and a posterior approach to an adjacent level. In the case of anterior interbody fusion, a lateral transpsoas approach (XLIF; NuVasive, Inc., San Diego, CA) is performed in conjunction with a posterior spinal fusion with instrumentation connecting to the existing hardware and posterior arthrodesis. The surgical goals of this technique are to restore global sagittal alignment, correct the areas of compressive stenosis, and extend the fusion segments, with shorter operative times, reduced estimated blood loss, shortened hospital stays, less narcotic usage, and rapid recovery times.[18] Soft tissue and muscle damage are minimized, while spinal deformity can be maximally corrected without removal of previous hardware, with combined lateral and posterior access. Instrumentation is completed either as a rod-to-rod extension of the previous fusion or by removal and reinstrumentation of only the rods and extension through the new fusion area.

Despite all of the advantages of a HYB technique, shortcomings do exist. For instance, because previous instrumentation is not removed in its entirety, sagittal alignment cannot be completely corrected in all cases. Furthermore, XLIF cannot be performed at L5-S1, and occasionally L4-5 is not accessible with this technique.

INDICATIONS AND CONTRAINDICATIONS

Not all patients who have a diagnosis of ASP are candidates for a MIS lateral approach. Patients require surgical intervention if they are symptomatic and have unsuccessfully completed nonoperative treatment. Many patients who have radiographic evidence of ASP do not require treatment at the time of diagnosis.[2,19] Approximately 2% to 15% of patients who have adjacent-level problems will have a second procedure after an initial fusion.[19,20] Patients should attempt conservative therapy for at least 6 months before operative care is indicated.[21] MIS HYB techniques should be considered for patients whose pathology is in the thoracolumbar spine between T4 and L5, who have had a previous spinal fusion (anterior, posterior, or both), with or without posterior instrumentation consisting of pedicle screws and connecting rods spaced adequately to allow rod-to-rod extension or removal of preexisting rods and extension.

The patient in Fig. 49-1 presented with L2-3 adjacent-level stenosis to a previous L3-5 remote fusion, disc degeneration, severe low back pain, bilateral radicular features, and neurologic deficit. Conservative care was unsuccessful. AP, lateral, and flexion-extension views of her lumbar spine revealed significant disc space collapse at L2-3 and solid arthrodesis at L3-5. She later had her fusion extended with rod-to-rod connectors through an MIS hybrid technique.

Contraindications for this novel technique include all of the contraindications for XLIF; such as spinal fracture, deformity, including anatomy that precludes the approach, prior lateral retroperitoneal approaches that caused scarring, and tumors. A patient who has adjacent-level disease with previous anterior-posterior fusion might not be a good candidate if the symptomatic level is not accessible through a lateral approach, if significant deformity limits access to the intended disc level or levels, or if spondylolisthesis of grade II

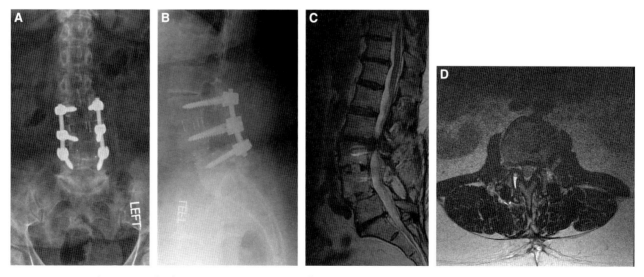

Fig. 49-1 This patient had a previous extension and reinstrumentation and is a candidate for revision with an MIS hybrid fusion. **A** and **B,** AP and lateral radiographs. **C** and **D,** MRI demonstrates previous fusion at L3-5 and adjacent-segment pathology at L2-3 with stenosis and disc space collapse.

or higher is present. General surgical contraindications consist of smoking, specific psychological conditions, infection, malignancy, and metabolic conditions affecting bone, such as osteoporosis with major loss of disc space height.[22] Placement of an intervertebral cage in these patients increases risk for vertebral body or endplate fracture or subsidence postoperatively. Generally, patients who are appropriate candidates for XLIF fusion can be considered for MIS hybrid techniques if symptomatic levels can be accessed from a lateral approach. Access is possible only if anatomy is favorable for the MIS portion of the procedure.[17,22-25]

PREOPERATIVE PLANNING

Approximately 5.2% to 18.5% of patients who have an initial lumbar surgery have developed a symptomatic adjacent-segment disease by 45 to 164 months postoperatively.[2] Although ASP is common, patients present for a variety of problems that might not be related to the previous fusion. To make a differential diagnosis before surgical planning, a surgeon needs to perform a standard set of assessments. First, all patients should complete a detailed health history before the initial visit. This allows practitioners the opportunity to assess prior conservative and surgical care, symptoms, comorbidities, and overall health and to construct a timeline of events related to a patient's disorder, which helps to determine whether a complaint is new or related to previous concerns. Second, a complete physical examination, as well as radiographic assessment for the presence of osteoporosis are essential in the workup of a patient. A DEXA scan will reveal the extent of osteopenia or osteoporosis. Typically, the prevalence of osteoporosis is higher in patients who develop proximal junctional kyphosis, compared with those who do not (20.4% versus 9.8%).[26]

PHYSICAL EXAMINATION

A physical examination is an important part of the diagnostic process. For example, previous incisions are examined for location, evidence of infection and proper healing are checked. A neurologic evaluation should include sensory, motor, and reflex assessment. Hip and knee flexion contractures, gait abnormality unrelated to the existing spinal condition, and the presence of other physical limitations must be assessed. Global coronal and sagittal alignment, pelvic obliquity, and leg-length discrepancies should be noted.[22,27-29] Prior records should be collected, if possible, to note a patient's presurgical diagnosis and operative details, including approach, instrumentation type, implants, and response to the index surgery, which can influence diagnosis and future surgical planning.

Assessment of a patient for ASP can be complicated. The location of ASP, the number of levels involved, the presence of both proximal and distal pathology, and overall patient health status are paramount to appropriate preoperative planning. The desired surgical outcomes depend on patient assessment and an operative plan.

RADIOGRAPHIC WORKUP AND PREOPERATIVE IMAGING

Patients are asked to undergo a radiographic workup to facilitate assessment of instability or flexibility of the deformity. This includes AP and lateral radiographs, dynamic standing flexion-extension images, and full-length standing AP and lateral scoliosis views. Spinopelvic parameters are calculated from the standing radiographs. Pelvic incidence is a constant spinopelvic parameter that is independent of the position of the pelvis. Pelvic tilt and sacral slope are dependent on the pelvic position. Methods for calculating these parameters are discussed in other chapters. Spinopelvic parameters are imperative for appropriate preoperative planning, understanding of sagittal balance, and achieving desired correction with surgical intervention. Further imaging studies include CT to assess previous fusion, retained hardware, and bony integrity and MRI to evaluate disc integrity, stenosis, and facet degeneration. New radiographs are compared with older films to identify deterioration or other changes in condition.

OPERATIVE TECHNIQUE: MINIMALLY INVASIVE LATERAL FUSION

PATIENT POSITIONING

Patient positioning is a critical part of a surgical process. XLIF is the first step of the procedure. Patients are placed in a 90-degree lateral position, most often with the right side down. However, right-sided approaches may be more common for HYB techniques, because the anatomy favors such access. Tape is placed to maintain the lateral position. Tape is secured over the thoracic region; over the hips (just below the iliac crest), from the iliac crest to the knee, then to the table, and from the table back to the knee; and past the ankle and to the table. All bony prominences are well padded to prevent skin and nerve injury. The use of a fluoroscope, also known as a *C-arm*, helps to confirm 90-degree positioning (Fig. 49-2). The table is flexed slightly to increase the distance between the iliac crest and the rib cage. Real-time neural monitoring and fluoroscopy are required for the procedure.

ANTERIOR HYBRID LATERAL APPROACH

After a patient is taped and prepared for surgery, K-wires and lateral imaging are used to identify the lumbar disc's midposition. This position is marked on the patient's lateral side, indicating the incision site and location of the disc space to be accessed by the tissue dilators and an expandable retractor. The retractor will be used to create the working portal for access to the spine. The anterior border of the vertebral body is also marked to help identify the front of the disc space and the anterior longitudinal ligament. The location of the vasculature needs to be considered.

When a two-incision technique is performed for an XLIF procedure, an additional marking is made posterior to the first mark, at the anatomic border between the erector spinae muscles and the abdominal obliques. The second mark is approximately 2 cm long and is intended to allow passage of the surgeon's index finger anteriorly to part the muscle layers for identification of the proper retroperitoneal space. Blunt dissection scissors can be used to spread the muscle fibers to facilitate this process. When the retroperitoneal space is identified, the peritoneum is carefully swept aside with an index finger, with care to prevent

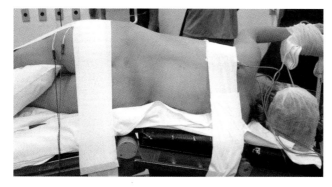
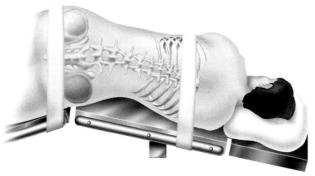

Fig. 49-2   Typical patient positioning for an XLIF anterior HYB procedure. Once the patient is properly taped to the table, appropriate break in the table facilitates surgical access and anatomic imaging. (Courtesy of NuVasive, Inc.)

perforation, and advanced to the psoas muscle (Fig. 49-3, *A*). From the psoas muscle, the surgeon sweeps the finger up to the direct lateral target mark, indicating where the next incision should be made for insertion of the initial dilator (Fig. 49-3, *B* and *C*). With the index finger, the dilator is guided to the top of the psoas (Fig. 49-3, *D*). Imaging is then used to confirm that the dilator is placed exactly over the index level disc space (Fig. 49-3, *E*). Care is critical to minimize trauma when separating the fibers between the middle and anterior third of the psoas muscle. Staying toward the central, anterior portion of the muscle helps to prevent damage to the nerves of the lumbar plexus. The genitofemoral nerve, in particular, should be noted and avoided while approaching the disc space. Neuromonitoring with directional EMG helps to limit iatrogenic nerve injury by indicating the proximity to nerve roots near the advancing dilator.

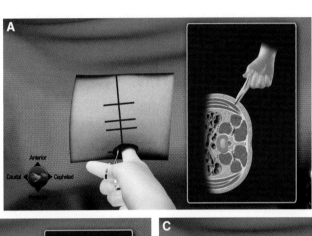

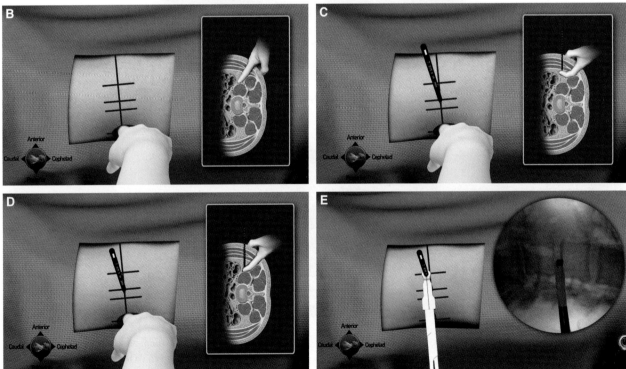

Fig. 49-3   **A,** A finger-over-scissors approach is performed to access the retroperitoneal space through the posterolateral incision using the two-incision technique. **B,** The retroperitoneal space is accessed, and the lateral border of the psoas muscle is palpated through the posterolateral incision. **C,** The initial dilator is guided with a finger into the retroperitoneal space through the posterolateral incision. **D,** The initial dilator is guided through the posterolateral incision to the lateral border of the psoas muscle. **E,** The dilator is positioned on the lateral aspect of the disc space. (Courtesy of NuVasive, Inc.)

A K-wire is then lowered into the space (Fig. 49-4, *A*). Subsequent dilators are introduced to gradually dilate the psoas muscles to facilitate retractor insertion over the largest dilator in a careful fashion (Fig. 49-4, *B* and *C*). A rigid articulating arm is attached to the retractor and the surgical table, allowing customizable retraction throughout the procedure. It is critical to use directional EMG neuromonitoring to safely map the positions of the nerve before disc preparation. All parts of the lumbosacral plexus should be posterior to the retractor. Once the disc is gently exposed, a thorough discectomy is completed using standard instruments, including rongeurs, scrapers, and broaches (Fig. 49-4, *D* through *F*). The posterior annulus is left intact, and the contralateral annulus is released using a Cobb dissector in conjunction with fluoroscopy to prevent endplate damage. This allows placement of a wide implant (22 to 26 mm) that aids in disc height restoration and correction of sagittal and coronal alignment. If sagittal balance is not corrected, overall long-term outcomes can be adversely affected.[30] In some patients in whom anterior column correction is required, but an osteotomy at the original surgical site is undesirable, release of the anterior longitudinal ligament should be considered. This is a highly challenging technique that requires extensive

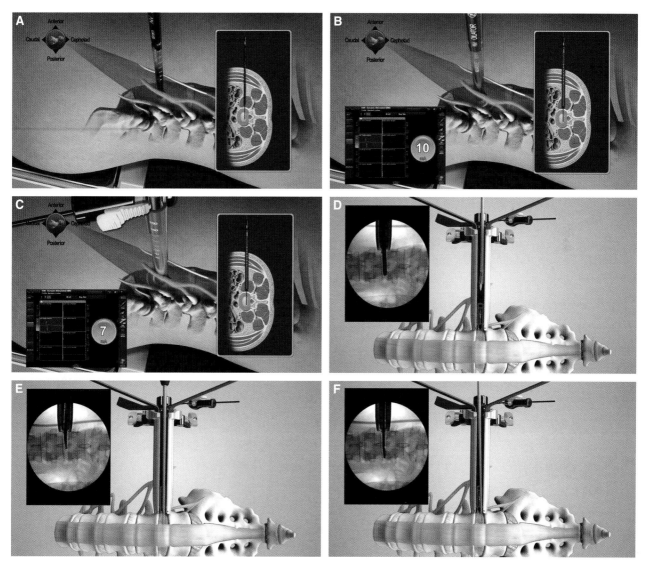

Fig. 49-4 **A,** A K-wire is placed through the initial dilator. (Anatomy is not drawn to scale or morphology.) **B** and **C,** Passage of the second and third sequential dilators with the use of stimulated EMG to determine the relative position of motor nerves. **D,** Discectomy and disc space preparation. **E** and **F,** A curette and a rasp, respectively, are passed through the MaXcess retractor (NuVasive, Inc.). (Courtesy of NuVasive, Inc.)

experience with anterior thoracolumbar surgery, a practice dedicated to deformity-correction surgery, and a fundamental understanding of the inherent anatomy in these regions. Anterior column realignment has been found to improve the mean motion segment angle from 9 degrees preoperatively to −19 degrees postoperatively.[30] Specific tabbed cages with fixation screws are used in anterior longitudinal ligament–release anterior thoracolumbar fusion to prevent cage migration during positioning for the posterior portion of the procedure and to enhance fusion at the operative level.

If the index level is part of the thoracolumbar junction, from approximately T11 to L2, then the XLIF approach will pass through an area of variable anatomy, including the diaphragm, pleura, ribs, and associated neurovascular bundles. The diaphragm is a musculotendinous plane between the peritoneum and pleura, attached to the sternum, costal cartilages, and lumbar vertebrae. Posteriorly, the right and left crura can be mobilized around the thoracolumbar junction to provide inferior or superior disc exposure to circumvent the diaphragm. The diaphragm can also be avoided when using an angled approach and procedural instrumentation. Unlike the diaphragm, ribs cannot be avoided when surgery is performed on upper lumbar and thoracic levels. For single-level procedures, access is determined by aligning the incision between ribs, with retractors positioned posteriorly or anteriorly at 90 degrees or in line with the ribs at 45 degrees.[31] If more than one level will be fused, then resection of the ribs will be required for adequate access. It may be necessary to resect the rib head for access to the lateral aspect of the disc space. Access to T4-9 requires a right-sided approach, because the vascular anatomy in this area includes the aorta's downward path on the anterior aspect of the spine. Great vessels and segmental arteries also supply portions of the spinal cord within the thoracic spine, increasing risk with the wide lateral exposure of XLIF. To decrease risk of devascularizing the neural axis in the intercostal spaces, these vessels should not be ligated.

After implant and graft placement, the exposed area is irrigated, hemostasis is obtained, and the retractors are removed slowly. While deliberately removing the retractor, the surgeon pays close attention to the rebounding of the psoas muscle and to iatrogenic bleeding to reduce the risk of postoperative hematoma. Meticulous hemostasis is required to prevent postoperative hematoma formation. Both surgical sites are closed using the usual fashion in layers. The table is leveled and appropriate intraoperative imaging obtained in the AP and lateral planes (Fig. 49-5). Once the surgeon is comfortable with the cage placement, correction of the sagittal deformity, and disc height restoration, the posterior portion of the procedure begins.

Posterior Spinal Fusion

Posterior spinal fusion is conducted under the same anesthetic unless clinical reasons exist for staging the procedures such as hemodynamic instability, concern for intraoperative cardiopulmonary problems, or an undesired prolonged anesthetic. If none of these issues exist, the patient is positioned prone on a Jackson frame (Mizuho OSI, Union City, CA) using a radiolucent table. The posterior fusion can be completed in a mini-open or an open procedure, depending on the patient's anatomic and surgical considerations. Radiographs are obtained after the patient is positioned to confirm that none of the cages has shifted.

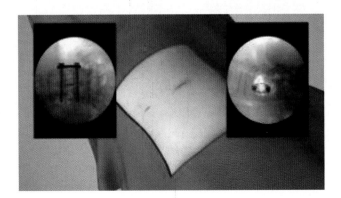

Fig. 49-5   Incision closures and AP and lateral images of an L4-5 XLIF with anterolateral plating. (Courtesy of NuVasive, Inc.)

For mini-open procedures, bilateral Wiltse incisions are centered over the surgical levels for a paraspinal muscle-splitting approach. The levels are located, and two longitudinal incisions are made over the lateral border of the pedicles. Sharp dissection is carried through the subcutaneous tissue to identify the fascia tissue. The next step can be conducted as a mini-open or fully open procedure. As a fully open procedure, bilateral paraspinal muscles are dissected subperiosteally to expose the spinous process, interlaminar space, and lamina laterally to the facet joints.[32] Dissection is continued ventrally, following the contour of the superior articulating facet; the transverse process can then be palpated and exposed. The dissection is limited in a mini-open procedure to exposure of the mammillary process and transverse process for percutaneous pedicle screw insertion through soft tissue dilation and cannulated screw placement.

For percutaneous screw placement, a small stab incision is made in the skin over the desired pedicle, and a cannulated Jamshidi needle is inserted and directed into the desired vertebral bodies through the respective pedicle. The guide wire is placed through the Jamshidi needle and carefully placed within but not beyond the anterior third of the vertebral body using biplanar fluoroscopy. This is performed under EMG guidance to ensure that the pedicle is not breached during placement of the Jamshidi needle. Tissue over the pedicle is sequentially dilated. The pedicle is then tapped and measured, and an appropriate-sized pedicle screw is placed over the guide wire and into the vertebral body. Once the pedicle screw has entered the posterior third of the vertebral body, the guide wire is removed. This prevents migration of the guide wire beyond the confines of the vertebral body. Great care is needed to prevent guide wire migration throughout this process. Direct EMG stimulation can then be performed through the attached towers to ensure that the screw does not breach and impinge an exiting nerve root. This only applies to motor nerves in the lumbar region (L1-S1). Fig. 49-6 shows pedicle screw placement at each vertebral body involved in the adjacent-level correction.

During the procedure proper radiographic imaging is employed to manage placement of the pedicle screws. C-arm fluoroscopy can help to identify the relevant bony anatomy and ensure proper positioning of screws. Before screws are inserted, imaging such as preoperative MRI and planning should be reviewed to identify anatomic landmarks and assess osseous abnormalities. Once pedicle screws have been placed at the adjacent levels, decompression can begin. This can be accomplished using the same mini-open or standard open techniques. In less invasive approaches, further tissue dilation and special retractors can help to identify the associated adjacent anatomy, including the facet joints, lamina, and pars intraarticularis. Facetectomies and laminoforaminotomies can be completed, and compressive anatomic structures such as the ligamentum flavum can be resected under direct visualization. Contralateral decompression can also be performed through the same approach by removing the ligamentum flavum and performing an adequate foraminotomy to allow the passage of a ball-tip probe along the contralateral nerve root or roots. Once decompression is adequate, the wound is inspected and irrigated appropriately, and attention is turned to rod placement and compression or distraction to facilitate further correction of the deformity.

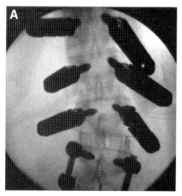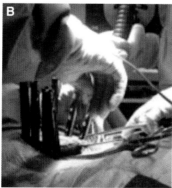

Fig. 49-6 Intraoperative placement of percutaneous pedicle screws during posterior lumbar fusion.

Connection of the rods is the next step in this HYB technique. Proper preoperative planning techniques can facilitate measuring the distance between the two cephaladmost screws in the construct. This may require using the rod between the next two caudal screws in the existing construct if the allowable distance between the most cephalad screws is insufficient to accommodate a rod-to-rod connector. To facilitate HYB rod-to-rod technique, the distance between the most proximal (cephalad) screws is measured on preoperative CT images. A minimum distance is required to accommodate a rod-to-rod connector. The soft tissue is removed without disturbing the existing fusion mass. Each pedicle screw system has its own rod-to-rod connector, but universal systems are readily available. Once rod-to-rod connectors are applied to the existing rod, the extension rod is connected to the newly placed pedicle screws. Compressive and distraction techniques can be applied to further facilitate correction of the deformity. All nuts and rod-to-rod connectors are torque tightened. Intraoperative AP and lateral radiographs are obtained to visualize the correction and newly placed instrumentation.

Posterolateral fusion is the next step. Through the incision used for screw placement and associated decompression maneuvers, the transverse processes are reexposed with Cobb elevators and appropriate retractors. The bone over the lateral pars, transverse processes, and facet joints are decorticated. Bone graft material (autograft and/or allograft) is placed along the posterolateral gutters between the intervening transverse processes and down to the previous fusion mass.

ASP can occur on the cephalad or caudal aspects of the previous fusion. The previously described technique explains the cephalad correction and placement of pedicle screw and rod-to-rod fixation systems. Treatment options for caudal degeneration have similar requirements and include restoration of sagittal balance. HYB techniques performed caudal to existing fusion constructs at the lumbosacral junction require an anterior lumbar interbody fusion procedure and a posterior extension possibly to the pelvis for fixation. Similar preoperative planning is required to identify an adequate rod distance between the most caudal existing screws. Iliac fixation is usually the preferred method to facilitate fusion across the L5-S1 segment. If appropriate sagittal realignment cannot be achieved with anterior lumbar interbody fusion alone, a posterior interbody fusion with an interbody cage and bone graft placement within the L5-S1 intervertebral space is an option. This can be combined with a pedicle subtraction osteotomy to restore sagittal balance and shorten the posterior column, extending fusion to the sacrum.[33] Fig. 49-7 shows the final rod-to-rod construct for treatment of ASP.

Subfascial and subcutaneous drains can be placed to reduce the chance of postoperative hematoma formation. The subcutaneous tissue and skin are then closed in a routine manner. Box 49-1 presents the pearls and pitfalls of this technique.

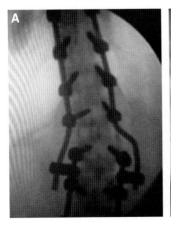
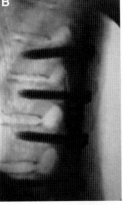

Fig. 49-7   Intraoperative radiographs show pedicle screw placement and the final rod-to-rod connection using blocking nuts.

BOX 49-1   Pearls and Pitfalls of the Minimally Invasive Hybrid Technique

- Candidates for consideration include those with pathology in the thoracolumbar spine between T4 and L5 in combination with a previous spinal fusion (anterior, posterior, or both), with or without posterior instrumentation, consisting of pedicle screws and connecting rods spaced adequately to allow rod-to-rod extension or removal of preexisting rods and extension.
- Knowledge of a patient's anatomy based on MRI visualization preoperatively is needed.
- Because previous instrumentation is not removed in its entirety, sagittal alignment cannot be completely corrected in all cases.
- XLIF cannot be performed at L5-S1, and occasionally L4-5 is not accessible with this technique.
- Benefits of minimally invasive procedures include reduced operation time, blood loss, and length of hospital stay.
- Appropriate patient selection is essential to successful fusion.

COMPLICATIONS AND MANAGEMENT

Surgery is complex, and inevitably complications occur regardless of procedure or approach, often because of anatomic variations, unavoidable surgical intricacies, or a patient's comorbidities.[34] Surgery requires assessment of benefit versus risk. In spine surgery, the increasing development of minimally invasive and hybrid techniques has largely reduced but not completely eliminated the comorbidities that occur with standard open-exposure techniques. The average complication rate for in-hospital noncardiac procedures is 6.9%, which suggests that baseline complications occur regardless of avoidance practices.[35] Many of these complications can be mitigated by preoperative planning and intraoperative monitoring.[36] Information about hybrid techniques is sparse, specifically posterior rod-to-rod extension of a previous fusion and MIS XLIF for placement of an interbody cage. An assessment of complications associated with HYB procedures involves evaluation of anterior and posterior procedures separately.

Conventional surgical approaches for lumbar fusion, despite long-term efficacy, are associated with high morbidities and complications that can offset the overall benefits of a procedure.[37] Although posterior open procedures allow single-incision access for an interbody fusion, direct decompression, placement of posterior fusion instrumentation, retraction of the cauda equina in PLIF, and proximity to the nerve root during a TLIF do increase the risk of neurologic deficits.[38] Mobbs et al[39] reported on a cohort of 82 patients divided into two groups: 41 had an MIS procedure, and 41 had an open procedure. Complication rates were 5.4% for the MIS group and 33.3% for the open procedure group. Major complications with open procedures included infection (6.7%), nonunion (6.7%), and paralytic ileus (10%). In TLIF procedures, Goldstein et al[40] conducted a systematic review of the complications and cost benefits of MIS and open procedures. Compared with patients who had open posterior lumbar procedures, MIS patients had a lower estimated blood loss, a generally shorter length of hospital stay, and a tendency toward lower surgical and medical complications. However, patient-reported outcomes were equivalent between the two groups.

XLIF has many benefits; however, no surgery is without complications. Studies have been conducted to assess the risk of complications associated with specific comorbidities such as obesity. Rodgers et al[36] reported on a cohort of 432 patients; 10 patients in the obese category reported complications and 17 in the nonobese group reported complications. The nonobese patients had more complications associated with gastrointestinal concerns; however, the difference between the complication rates was not statistically significant. In large series studies, XLIF has had favorable complication rates and treatment variables. Rodgers et al[41] reported on an analysis of 600 patients, and the treatment of 741 levels. Supplemental internal fixation was performed in 99.2%, and 83.2% included pedicle screw instrumentation. An overall incidence of perioperative complications was 6.2%, with 1.5% related to in-hospital events and 2.8% related to in-hospital medical events. The rate of out-of-hospital events was 1%, and the rate of out-of-hospital medical events was 5%. The rate of transient postoperative neurologic deficits was 0.7%. They reported no wound infections, vascular injuries, or intraoperative visceral injuries. Tohmeh et al[42] reported on 200 patients who received an XLIF at L3-4 or L4-5. EMG threshold values were recorded at the surface of the psoas muscle, at the mid-psoas, and on the spine. The resultant data showed that no significant long-lasting neural deficits were identified. New iliopsoas/hip flexion weakness was reported in 27.5%, and upper medial thigh sensory loss was reported in 17.6%. Transient motor deficits were identified in three patients and had resolved by the 6-month follow-up visit.

The literature is inconsistent regarding reported postoperative leg deficits after XLIF. We gathered internal outcome data on 10 patients after undergoing XLIF from 2011 to 2013. In our unpublished analysis, we reviewed postoperative leg deficits and associated intraoperative retraction times and assessed three categories based on the deficit: category 1 included patients with isolated numbness/dysesthesia without pain or weakness; category 2 patients had numbness plus pain on contraction, resulting in poor effort but not weakness; and category 3 patients had numbness and/or weakness, including psoas weakness with motor symptoms. Retraction times were compared in those who had postoperative leg pain and/or dysesthesia. At the 6-week follow-up, 4.1% of patients reported category 1 symptoms, 2.0% presented category 2 symptoms, and 8.2% reported category 3 symptoms. All of the symptoms were considered transient and had resolved by the 1-year follow-up.

Furthermore, preliminary results from a prospective, multi-center study have shown that prolonged retraction time and increasing evoked EMG thresholds throughout retraction are predictors of declining nerve integrity. Of the initial 318 patients, 283 had complete motor exams and intraoperative data. Motor weakness on the approach side was found in 4.6% (N = 13) of the patients. Consequently, patients with postoperative neuropraxia had a significantly longer retraction time compared to those without neuropraxia (32 versus 23 minutes, $p = 0.031$). Yet, initial center blade reading ($p = 0.600$), retraction size in both the cranial/caudal ($p = 0.551$), and anterior/posterior ($p = 0.419$) direction were not significantly different in patients with or without postoperative motor weakness. In addition, step-wise logistic regression analysis demonstrated that postoperative nerve injury, total retraction time ($p < 0.001$), and change in center blade thresholds ($p < 0.001$) are significantly related. Thus, the greater the retraction time or EMG threshold, the more likely postoperative nerve injury will occur. These data suggest that in order to reduce the occurrence of postoperative motor weakness, retraction time should be kept to a minimum and EMG thresholds should be consistently monitored during surgery.[43] Approach-related complications, specifically postoperative deficits, need to be investigated further to elucidate the cause and duration of these deficits (after XLIF surgery).

COMPLICATION MANAGEMENT

Surgeons have several ways of mitigating risks and complications during and after surgery. Preoperative planning is crucial in decreasing the number of complications. This includes a review of imaging to verify the abnormal anatomy that can limit the efficacy of the XLIF or posterior spinal fusion procedures. This topic is discussed in detail in other chapters. Perioperative techniques include specific positioning for the XLIF portion of a procedure. Correct patient positioning with adequate padding of pressure points and a sufficient table break to access the index level is important for two reasons. First, it can prevent rhabdomyolysis and ensuing renal failure, a rare occurrence resulting from inadequate padding.[41] Second, lateral flexion increases tightening of the psoas muscle and nerves in the lumbar plexus, which can increase neural complications. As spine surgery technology progresses, more techniques and equipment are available to reduce the occurrence of intraoperative complications. Uribe et al[44] conducted a literature review examining applications of intraoperative EMG neurophysiologic monitoring methods in minimally invasive procedures. They concluded that much of this monitoring is performed to assist with insertion of pedicle screws; EMG neuromonitoring has also been reported to be used for other types of MIS procedures. The addition of EMG to MIS procedures has decreased the overall complication rate from 30% to less than 1%.[44]

RESULTS

PERSONAL EXPERIENCE

We compiled internal outcome data retrospectively, identifying all patients who had a minimally invasive hybrid procedure from 2010 to 2012. All patients underwent both an anterior and an extension of posterior instrumentation. Anterior instrumentation included interbody implants without internal fixation. Posterior spinal fusion was performed through an open technique for proper decompression and extension of the previous surgery. Both anterior and posterior fusions were grafted using bone morphogenic protein (Infuse, Medtronic Sofamor Danek, Memphis, TN) in conjunction with allograft.

Variables collected in the chart review included baseline comorbidities, operative time, estimated blood loss, length of hospital stay, and incidence of complications. Approximately 1 year after the surgical procedure, CT, AP, lateral neutral, and lateral flexion-extension radiographs were reviewed to assess fusion. Approximately 2 years after the surgical procedure, additional diagnoses, additional surgeries, and VAS scores were assessed.

OUTCOMES

A total of 10 patients underwent an MIS HYB technique for ASP from 2010 to 2012. All patients were diagnosed with ASP above their previous lumbar spinal fusion. Patients presented with an ASP diagnosis in one to two levels and an average of 1.5 levels with symptomatic disease. ASP was diagnosed after previous multilevel (50%) and single-level (50%) fusions. The average patient age was 68.5 years; 90% of the patient cohort was female. Mean estimated blood loss was 327.5 ml (range 25 to 500 ml), and no additional transfusions were required. Operative time averaged 241.6 minutes (range 185 to 334 minutes). The mean length of hospital stay was 3 days (range 2-4 days). Two patients (20%) had postoperative complications: one developed a postoperative superficial wound infection, and the second had an epidural hematoma that was evacuated. Five patients (50%) had postoperative adjacent-level degeneration.

At the 1-year follow-up (11.5 months; range 7 to 16 months), all patients had solid arthrodesis, as confirmed on CT and dynamic radiography. Additional operations were reported in 5 patients (50%); secondary procedures were performed at 26 months (average) postoperatively. All secondary procedures were conducted for an additional ASP diagnosis. These patients had one or more of the following comorbidities: cervical degenerative disc disease, diabetes, and arthritis. Patients without additional surgeries did not report continued leg or back pain at the 2-year follow-up. The average back and leg pain VAS scores at 2 years had improved over preoperative scores, from 68 to 50. The average back and leg pain VAS score for patients without an additional ASP diagnosis improved from 70 to 45.

PATIENT EXAMPLE

This 70-year-old woman with minimal baseline comorbidities inclusive of arthritis and high blood pressure presented with neurogenic claudication, radicular symptoms down her left lower extremity to the foot, and right-sided buttock pain. Preoperative imaging revealed severe stenosis at L2-5, degenerative disc disease at L2-4, degenerative spondylolisthesis at L4-5, and a mild scoliotic curve (Fig. 49-8, *A* and *B*). A left-sided XLIF procedure was performed at L2-3 and L3-4, with posterior spinal fusion from L2 to L5 on the same day. Bilateral decompressive laminectomy with complete facetectomies was performed on levels L2-5, with autologous bone graft, bone morphogenic protein, and allograft bone. Bone morphogenic

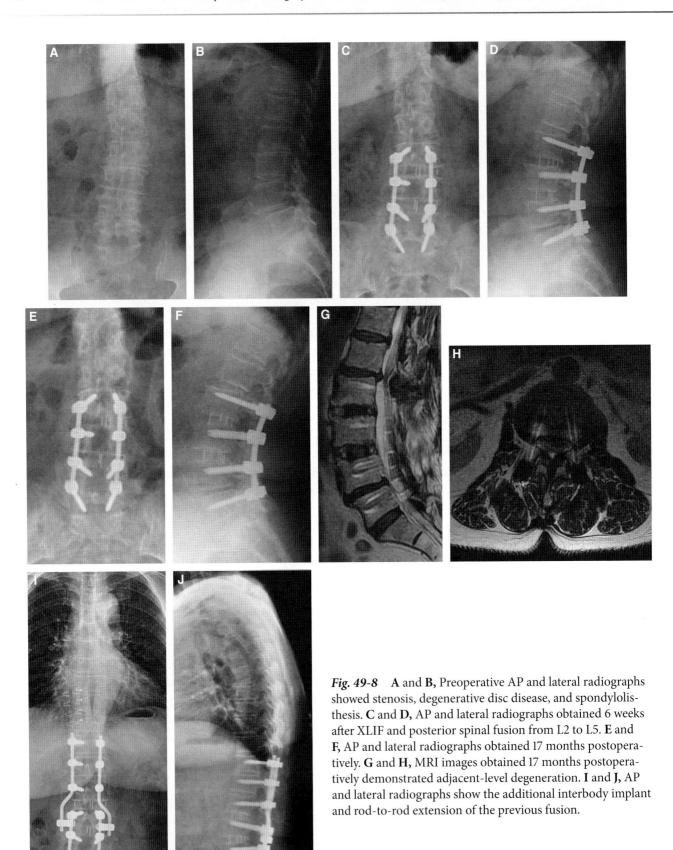

Fig. 49-8   **A** and **B,** Preoperative AP and lateral radiographs showed stenosis, degenerative disc disease, and spondylolisthesis. **C** and **D,** AP and lateral radiographs obtained 6 weeks after XLIF and posterior spinal fusion from L2 to L5. **E** and **F,** AP and lateral radiographs obtained 17 months postoperatively. **G** and **H,** MRI images obtained 17 months postoperatively demonstrated adjacent-level degeneration. **I** and **J,** AP and lateral radiographs show the additional interbody implant and rod-to-rod extension of the previous fusion.

protein was placed in the posterolateral gutters to augment fusion, because the patient smoked. Postoperative imaging demonstrated the interbody application and posterior spinal fusion (Fig. 49-8, *C* and *D*)

One year postoperatively the patient continued to have numbness in her lower extremities; however, her strength and pain had improved. She received a secondary diagnosis of bilateral sacroiliac joint dysfunction and greater trochanteric bursitis. The patient was seen 17 months postoperatively with increased pain, difficulty walking, and intermittent loss of leg control. Imaging showed adjacent-level degeneration superior to the spinal fusion, at L1-2, with clumping of nerve roots at L4-5 from arachnoiditis; degenerative disc disease; and facet arthroplasty superior and inferior to the spinal fusion, most prominent at the L1-2 level, with spinal stenosis and cauda equina nerve root entrapment (Fig. 49-8, *E* through *H*).

The patient underwent a secondary hybrid procedure. This consisted of an MIS left-sided anterior interbody fusion at L1-2, followed on the same day by open posterior decompressive laminectomy at L1-2 with extension of the previous fusion to the T10 level percutaneously and posterolateral fusion from T10 to L2 with rod-to-rod connectors to the existing hardware. Postoperative imaging showed the additional cage placement and extension of the previous fusion (Fig. 49-8, *I* and *J*). Ten months after the HYB procedure, the patient is independently ambulatory without pain, and her leg numbness is decreased. She has been following a regimen of vitamins and supplements to treat ongoing numbness in her lower extremities. The patient is well balanced sagittally and is happy with her recovery.

CONCLUSION

Numerous techniques have been performed to treat patients who have ASP. The minimally invasive hybrid techniques provide the biomechanical and surgical benefits of minimally invasive XLIF and the stabilization and access of the posterior spinal fusion. Further investigation of HYB techniques is warranted to establish the clinical and radiographic efficacy of such procedures. Clearly, with advancing technologies emerging in spine surgery, the opportunity to reduce morbidity without limiting the surgical correction is becoming more common. Although the use of these techniques is tempting, only select patients will meet criteria for such HYB procedures until we can demonstrate appropriate evidence and outcome to support their routine application.

REFERENCES

1. Anderson PA, Andersson GB, Arnold PM, et al. Terminology. Spine 37(22 Suppl):S8-S9, 2012.
2. Park P, Garton HJ, Gala VC, et al. Adjacent segment disease after lumbar or lumbosacral fusion: review of the literature. Spine 29:1938-1944, 2004.
3. Celestre PC, Montgomery SR, Kupperman, et al. Lumbar clinical adjacent segment pathology: predilection for proximal levels. Spine 39:172-176, 2014.
4. Weinhoffer SL, Guyer RD, Herbert M, et al. Intradiscal pressure measurements above an instrumented fusion. A cadaveric study. Spine 20:526-531, 1995.
5. Hilibrand AS, Robbins M. Adjacent segment degeneration and adjacent segment disease: the consequences of spinal fusion? Spine J 4(6 Suppl):190S-194S, 2004.
6. Ekman P, Möller H, Shalabi A, et al. A prospective randomised study on the long-term effect of lumbar fusion on adjacent disc degeneration. Eur Spine J 18:1175-1186, 2009.
7. Radcliff K, Curry P, Hilibrand A, et al. Risk for adjacent segment and same segment reoperation after surgery for lumbar stenosis: a subgroup analysis of the Spine Patient Outcomes Research Trial (SPORT). Spine 38:531-539, 2013.
8. Kumar M, Baklanov A, Chopin D. Correlation between sagittal plane changes and adjacent segment degeneration following lumbar spine fusion. Eur Spine J 10:314-319, 2001.
9. Harrop JS, Youssef JA, Maltenfort M, et al. Lumbar adjacent segment degeneration and disease after arthrodesis and total disc arthroplasty. Spine 33:1701-1707, 2008.

10. Gillet P. The fate of the adjacent motion segments after lumbar fusion. J Spinal Disord Tech 16:338-345, 2003.

11. Cho SK, Bridwell KH, Lenke LG, et al. Comparative analysis of clinical outcome and complications in primary versus revision adult scoliosis surgery. Spine 37:393-401, 2012.

12. Stoker GE, Buchowski JM, Bridwell KH, et al. Preoperative vitamin D status of adults undergoing surgical spinal fusion. Spine 38:507-515, 2013.

13. Whitecloud TS III, Davis JM, Olive PM. Operative treatment of the degenerated segment adjacent to a lumbar fusion. Spine 19:531-536, 1994.

14. Chen WJ, Lai PL, Niu CC, et al. Surgical treatment of adjacent instability after lumbar spine fusion. Spine 26:E519-E524, 2001.

15. Hsieh PC, Koski TR, O'Shaughnessy BA, et al. Anterior lumbar interbody fusion in comparison with transforaminal lumbar interbody fusion: implications for the restoration of foraminal height, local disc angle, lumbar lordosis, and sagittal balance. J Neurosurg Spine 7:379-386, 2007.

16. Hassanzadeh H, Jain A, El Dafrawy MH, et al. Clinical results and functional outcomes of primary and revision spinal deformity surgery in adults. J Bone Joint Surg 95:1413-1419, 2013.

17. Youssef JA, McAfee PC, Patty CA, et al. Minimally invasive surgery: lateral approach interbody fusion: results and review. Spine 35(26 Suppl):S302-S311, 2010.

18. Rodgers WB, Cox CS, Gerber EJ. Minimally invasive treatment (XLIF) of adjacent segment disease after prior lumbar fusions. Internet J Minimally Invasive Spinal Technol 3, 2009.

19. Lehmann TR, Spratt KF, Tozzi JE, et al. Long-term follow-up of lower lumbar fusion patients. Spine 12:97-104, 1987.

20. Ghiselli G, Wang JC, Bhatia NN, et al. Adjacent segment degeneration in the lumbar spine. J Bone Joint Surg Am 86:1497-1503, 2004.

21. Boden SD, Davis DO, Dina TS. Abnormal magnetic resonance scans of the lumbar spine in asymptomatic subjects: a prospective investigation. J Bone Joint Surg Am 72:403-408, 1990.

22. Bederman SS, Le VH, Pahlavan S, et al. Use of lateral access in the treatment of the revision spine patient. ScientificWorldJournal 308209, 2012.

23. Daubs MD. Anterior lumbar interbody fusion. In Vaccaro AR, Baron EM, eds. Operative Techniques: Spine Surgery. Philadelphia: Elsevier, 2008.

24. Crock HV. Anterior lumbar interbody fusion: indications for its use and notes on surgical technique. Clin Orthop Relat Res 165:157-163, 1982.

25. Le TV, Baaj AA, Dakwar E, et al. Subsidence of polyetheretherketone intervertebral cages in minimally invasive lateral retroperitoneal transpsoas lumbar interbody fusion. Spine 37:1268-1273, 2012.

26. Kim HJ, Bridwell KH, Lenke LG, Proximal junctional kyphosis results in inferior SRS pain subscores in adult deformity patients. Spine 38:896-901, 2013.

27. Ames CP, Smith JS, Scheer JK, et al. Impact of spinopelvic alignment on decision making in deformity surgery in adults: a review. J Neurosurg Spine 16:547-564, 2012.

28. Ozgur BM, Aryan HE, Pimenta L, et al. Extreme Lateral Interbody Fusion (XLIF): a novel surgical technique for anterior lumbar interbody fusion. Spine J 6:435-443, 2006.

29. Crock HV, Bedbrook GM. Practice of Spinal Surgery, ed 2. Wien: Springer-Verlag, 1993.

30. Akbarnia BA, Mundis GM Jr, Moazzaz P, et al. Anterior Column Realignment (ACR) for focal kyphotic spinal deformity using a lateral transpsoas approach and ALL release. J Spinal Disord Tech 27:29-39, 2014.

31. Goodrich JA, Volcan IJ, eds. eXtreme Lateral Interbody Fusion. St Louis: Quality Medical Publishing, 2013.

32. Warren A, Prasad V, Thomas M, et al. Pre-operative planning when using the Wiltse approach to the lumbar spine. Ann R Coll Surg Engl 92:74-75, 2010.

33. Kwon BK, Elgafy H, Keynan O, et al. Progressive junctional kyphosis at the caudal end of lumbar instrumented fusion: etiology, predictors, and treatment. Spine 31:1943-1951, 2006.

34. Andersson GB, Chapman JR, Dekutoski MB, et al. Do no harm: the balance of "beneficence" and "non-maleficence." Spine 35(9 Suppl):S2-S8, 2010.

35. Khan NA, Quan H, Bugar JM, et al. Association of postoperative complications with hospital costs and length of stay in a tertiary care center. J Gen Intern Med 21:177-180, 2006.

36. Rodgers WB, Cox CS, Gerber EJ. Early complications of extreme lateral interbody fusion in the obese. J Spinal Disord Tech 23:393-397, 2010.

37. Deyo RA, Ciol MA, Cherkin DC, et al. Lumbar spinal fusion: a cohort study of complications, reoperations, and resource use in the Medicare population. Spine 18:1463-1470, 1993.

38. Mroz TE, Wang JC, Hashimoto R, et al. Complications related to osteobiologics use in spine surgery: a systematic review. Spine 35(9 Suppl):S86-S104, 2010.

39. Mobbs RJ, Sivabalan P, Li J. Minimally invasive surgery compared to open spinal fusion for the treatment of degenerative lumbar spine pathologies. J Clin Neurosci 19:829-835, 2012.

40. Goldstein CL, Macwan K, Sundararajan K, et al. Comparative outcomes of minimally invasive surgery for posterior lumbar fusion: a systematic review. Clin Orthop Relat Res 472:1-11, 2014.

41. Rodgers WB, Gerber EJ, Patterson J. Intraoperative and early postoperative complications in extreme lateral interbody fusion. Spine 36:26-33, 2011.

42. Tohmeh AG, Rodgers WB, Peterson MD. Dynamically evoked, discrete-threshold electromyography in the extreme lateral interbody fusion approach: clinical article. J Neurosurg Spine 14:31-37, 2011.

43. Isaacs R, Youssef J, Uribe J. Evoked electromyography (EMG) throughout retraction to monitor nerve integrity during the XLIF® procedure. Preliminary results from a prospective, multi-center study. NASS Annual Meeting, San Francisco, CA, Nov 2014.

44. Uribe JS, Vale FL, Dakwar E. Electromyographic monitoring and its anatomical implications in minimally invasive spine surgery. Spine 35(26 Suppl):S368-S374, 2010.

50

Minimally Invasive Hybrid Treatment of Multilevel Degenerative Lumbar Deformity

Michael Y. Wang

Contemporary minimally invasive surgery (MIS) techniques are relatively successful at achieving the goals necessary for managing straightforward degenerative disease of the spine.[1] Neural decompression is carried out using keyhole approaches to remove offending disc, osteophyte, or ligamentous structures, and indirect decompression is possible with disc height restoration; solid fusion is achieved with interbody or posterolateral grafting; and stabilization can now be accomplished with a host of percutaneous bony fixation methods.[2-5]

During the past two decades, a tremendous wealth of knowledge has been amassed to guide the treatment of adult spinal deformities (ASD). In particular, the importance of regional and global balance has been increasingly recognized.[6-9] The treatment of regional deformities such as low-grade lumbar scoliosis and spondylolisthesis has been successfully managed with MIS surgery, and most methods for correction rely primarily on interbody distraction with cages to restore normal disc height and realign the spinal column.[10,11] These efforts have been undertaken in part because of the high morbidity and complication rates associated with open deformity surgery. For example, Pateder et al[12] presented a series of 361 patients, in whom the mortality rate from surgery was 2.4%. More recent reports from the Scoliosis Research Society, the French Study Group on Scoliosis, and the Twin Cities Group showed that even in expert centers, patients had complications at a rate of 29%, 39%, and 42%, respectively.[8,13,14]

Contemporary MIS methods have been shown to result in good corrections of moderate coronal malalignment.[15-20] A lateral interbody fusion or a multilevel MIS transforaminal lumbar interbody fusion can result in a Cobb curve correction of up to 30 degrees. However, the correction of more significant deformities was more difficult. This typically required a hybrid procedure in which posterior osteotomies were performed to mobilize the rigid spine and allow manipulation of the vertebral bodies.

Despite these advancements, contemporary MIS techniques have been very limited in improving sagittal balance. Typically, these techniques provide no additional lumbar lordosis for patients with abnormal sagittal parameters. In cases in which lordosis is desired, specific techniques using expandable cages or advanced lateral osteotomies can be employed. However, these methods are technically challenging, have had limited adoption, and are limited to relatively mild cases of sagittal imbalance.[21,22] In a recent study, Wang et al[23] (the International Spine Study Group) identified ceiling effects associated with specific MIS approaches. Hybrid surgeries were more effective than lateral interbody fusion and multilevel MIS transforaminal lumbar interbody fusion (Fig. 50-1).

Surgeons who prefer to perform MIS methods to treat severe, rigid ASD will likely have to employ hybrid techniques to achieve proper coronal and sagittal balance. Satisfactory thoracolumbar kyhposcoliosis correction will be achieved only by using osteotomies in combination with rigid polysegmental fixation. We now perform a mini-open pedicle subtraction osteotomy (PSO) technique that is a hybrid MIS method for treating thoracolumbar kyhposcoliosis.[24]

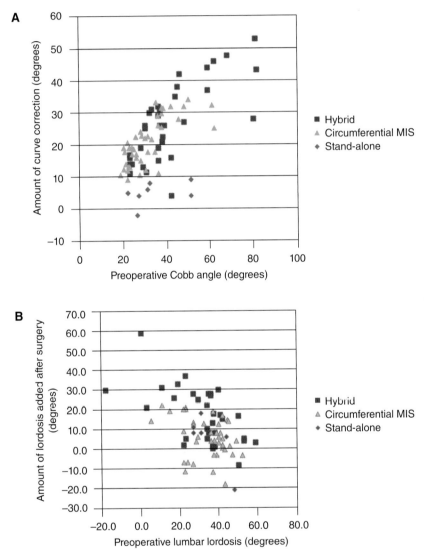

Fig. 50-1 These scatter diagrams present data from the Minimally Invasive Surgery–International Spine Study Group. They compare results from the following three minimally invasive surgery *(MIS)* methods for treating patients with adult spinal deformity: a stand-alone lateral interbody fusion, circumferential minimally invasive surgery methods such as minimally invasive transforaminal lumbar interbody fusion or lateral interbody fusion with percutaneous pedicle screws, and hybrid minimally invasive techniques. **A,** Correction of the Cobb angle. **B,** Improvement in lumbar lordosis.

INDICATIONS AND CONTRAINDICATIONS

The indications for hybrid MIS deformity surgery are the same as those for open surgery. Patients can have symptoms caused by neural compression, arthritic disease of the discs and facets, and/or global spinal imbalance. They may have had rapid and predictable progression of a deformity in the setting of less severe symptoms, noted with serial imaging.

Candidates have to be fit and able to undergo surgery in a prone position for 5 to 7 hours. Osteoporosis is common in these patients and can be a relative contraindication, because reduced bone quality increases the risk of immediate and delayed fixation problems. A strict contraindication is the presence of previous long-segment posterior fixation, which requires explantation in an open approach. In these cases, a more traditional open operation is more appropriate. Short (one- to two-segment) pedicle screw fixation at the site of the intended osteotomy is acceptable, however.

PATIENT PROFILES

Patients who are ideal candidates for an MIS hybrid deformity correction are considered to be high risk for the open surgical options. Examples include those with advanced age, immunosuppression, and a predisposition for soft tissue healing problems. In these settings, surgical risks are increased because of baseline comorbidities. However, if soft tissue envelope disruption is minimized, the risk of specific complications such as wound infection and transfusion-related hemodynamic problems will be reduced. Similarly, patients without a severe deformity may be candidates for even less invasive operations such as a multilevel MIS transforaminal lumbar interbody fusion or an MIS lateral interbody fusion. An ideal patient has a thoracolumbar scoliosis Cobb angle between 30 and 70 degrees and/or requires 20 to 35 degrees of additional lumbar lordosis.

PREOPERATIVE PLANNING

As with open surgery, 36-inch AP and lateral standing films, fine-cut reconstructed CT scans, and MRI are standard for preoperative evaluation. In addition, significant preoperative counseling is needed to inform the patient of the risks, benefits, pitfalls, and recovery process of such surgeries. Because most of these patients are elderly, preoperative counseling with the patient's family, including his or her adult children, is essential to answer questions, provide instructions, and temper expectations. Given the variability in patient factors, the wide variety of spinal pathologies, the diversity of treatments, and the profound level of misunderstanding regarding ASD, we will typically see patients two to five times in the clinic before scheduling surgery, even if they are crippled from ASD at the time of the first visit.

PHYSICAL EXAMINATION

Surgeons should be careful to diagnose all sacroiliac joint pain, hip arthritis, and leg length discrepancies before surgery. These conditions can confound the recovery process and will not likely be positively affected by spinal surgery for ASD.

OPERATIVE TECHNIQUE

PATIENT POSITIONING

The patient is positioned prone, as with open surgery. A Jackson table is useful for extending the lumbar spine and enhancing lordosis. Careful padding of dependent areas is critical if the surgery is prolonged. Concomitant cervical stenosis is highly prevalent and care should be taken to position the neck in a neutral, nonextended position. An arterial line is placed in all cases to ensure that blood specimens can be withdrawn while the patient is prone and to enhance blood pressure maintenance.

INCISION PLACEMENT

We make a long midline skin incision in all cases. The length of the construct is opened, but the fascia is not violated. The skin is reflected suprafascially so that all subsequent steps are performed through the superficial fascia. This is done for the following reasons:

- Most patients have already had a previous lumbar incision in the midline.
- Stab incisions have a tendency to bleed uncontrollably, contributing to blood loss.
- A single incision may not be longer than the combined lengths of multiple, combined, minimally invasive cuts.
- Handling the skin only at the beginning and end of the operation improves workflow and efficiency.
- Midline scars are less visible than flank or paramedian scars.
- Most elderly ASD patients are not very concerned with cosmesis.

DISSECTION AND EXPOSURE

After a dorsal midline skin incision is made and lateral subcutaneous dissection is completed, the muscle fascia is exposed so that all of the remaining steps are performed through the fascia. The spinal levels are confirmed radiographically with a fluoroscope to identify the PSO site (usually L2 or L3). Bilateral subperiosteal dissection is then taken laterally at the level of the intended PSO to fully expose the transverse processes at that segment. The total bony exposure will include the pedicle above and below. Typically this is the amount of exposure needed for a two-level open laminectomy and fusion. In addition, if interbody fusion below the level of the PSO is desired, then a unilateral subperiosteal exposure of the facet joints is undertaken at these levels to allow MIS transforaminal lumbar interbody fusions.

PEDICLE SUBTRACTION OSTEOTOMY

At the site of the PSO (for example, L3), the spinous process, lamina, and facets are removed with a rongeur. The exiting L3 nerve roots are fully exposed, and the annulus of the L2-3 disc is cauterized with bipolar electrocautery and incised with a No. 15 blade to create an extended PSO. The L3 pedicles are removed entirely using rongeurs and a high-speed drill. A bilateral decancellation osteotomy is then performed at L3 using a series of enlarging curettes to remove two cones of cancellous bone from the vertebral body. Central bone is removed with a curved curette, and the decancellation is extended superiorly into the L2-3 disc space. Cottonoids are then employed to dissect and secure the lateral vertebral wall and its associated vasculature. The lateral vertebral body wall is removed bilaterally with a Leksell rongeur in a wedge-shaped pattern to match the decancellation (Fig. 50-2).

Percutaneous pedicle screws are placed at least three levels above and below the PSO site to control the spine. A primarily AP-based fluoroscopic technique is helpful to compensate for axial rotation of the vertebral bodies, particularly in patients with complex ASD. The pedicles are cannulated with the use of Jamshidi needles under AP fluoroscopic guidance. The technique involves docking the needle tip at the junction of the transverse process and lateral facet joint. The needle is driven into the bone a distance of 2 cm

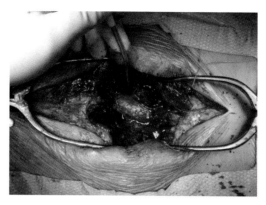

Fig. 50-2 The thecal sac is exposed, and decancellation is performed at the site of the pedicle subtraction osteotomy.

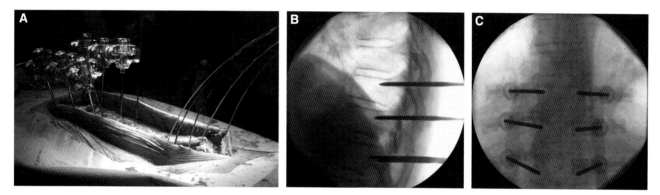

Fig. 50-3 **A,** Percutaneous fixation initiated with Jamhidi needles and K-wires. **B,** Lateral and **C,** AP radiographs showing the needles in 2 cm without passing the medial wall of the pedicle, indicating proper placement.

with a mallet, without passing the medial wall of the pedicle. This is confirmed on AP radiographs. Iliac screws are placed using an obturator outlet view for percutaneous cannulation, as previously described.[25] A window is made in the posterior superior iliac spine to prevent screw head prominence. Each needle is then exchanged for a K-wire. An insulating sheath protects the soft tissues while an awl and tap are used to create the path for the pedicle screw and final screw placement. The use of pedicle screw extensions prevents catastrophic vertebral translation during completion of the osteotomy (Fig. 50-3). The posterior vertebral body wall and posterior longitudinal ligament are removed by retraction of the thecal sac medially on each side successively.

No ventral bone or ligament should impinge on the thecal sac. This is conformed with direct visual inspection and palpation of the thecal sac. The osteotomy is then closed. A total of four rods are bent to the same degree of lordotic curvature (approximately 35 degrees). Each rod is passed through each set of screw heads above and below the PSO. It is impossible to pass a lordotic rod below the fascia in a kyphotic region of the spine. A rod-to-rod connector is placed on the end of each rod at the PSO site where the tip is exposed. Set screws are then used to loosely attach each of the four rods to its respective set of screws. Each of the four rod holders are held and forced toward each other to create a greenstick fracture at the osteotomy site and to place the spine in lordosis (Fig. 50-4). The four rod-to-rod connectors are used to rigidly attach the cranial rod to the caudal rod on the same side. The set screws are fastened tightly, and all articulations are tightened.

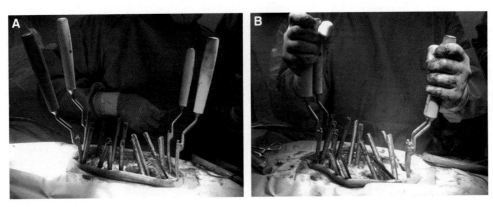

Fig. 50-4 **A,** Four rods are inserted. **B,** A cantilever technique is used to close the osteotomy site in a controlled and deliberate fashion.

BOX 50-1   Tips, Tricks, and Special Maneuvers

- Decancellation of the PSO site is improved with the use of serially enlarging curettes, both straight and angled, to remove the vertebral body bone.
- Rod passage should be subfascial to prevent pressure on the surrounding musculature when mating the rods to the screws.
- Rod connection is facilitated with an assistant surgeon to allow rotation of the cranial and caudal rods along their long axis to bring the rod ends together in the coronal and sagittal planes.
- Iliac screw mating to the caudal rod should be accomplished first to place a minimal amount of rod past the screw head, thus minimizing hardware prominence.
- Posterolateral facet fusion can be accomplished by drilling the facets with a burr after the screw tract is tapped and before hardware is inserted. Osteobiologic adjuvants are placed before screws are inserted to position the bone graft at the facet joint surface.

Adapted from Tumialan LM, Mummaneni PV. Long-segment spinal fixation using pelvic screws. Neurosurgery 63:183-190, 2008.

CLOSURE

The L3 nerve roots and thecal sac are inspected to ensure that no neural compression is present. Bleeding is controlled with powdered collagen matrix. A small subperiosteal exposure is then made on one side at the top of the construct, and an interlaminar fusion is created between the top three vertebral segments using autograft bone. The wound is closed over suction drainage in standard fashion. Box 50-1 highlights tips, tricks, and special maneuvers for performing this procedure.

POTENTIAL COMPLICATIONS AND MANAGEMENT

Screw misplacement can result from axial rotation of the spine and atrophic pedicles in scoliotic patients. Misplacement rates can be reduced using AP-guided cannulation, biplanar fluoroscopy, neuronavigation, and intraoperative three-dimensional imaging. Additionally, bleeding from cancellous bone at the PSO site can be reduced using powdered Gelfoam to occlude the open marrow spaces. Elevation of the skin can lead to seroma formation in the dead space. A suprafascial drain should be placed in all patients and the wound suctioned during the entire period of hospitalization.

PATIENT EXAMPLE

This 58-year-old white woman presented with a history of intractable back and left leg pain. The symptoms had been progressive over a 1-year period and were associated with a decreased ability to ambulate three blocks. She had begun to use an assistive device. The symptoms were exacerbated with standing and walking and were almost completely relieved with sitting or lying down. She had minimal right-sided leg pain, and her radicular symptoms were in the L3 and L4 distribution. Her leg and back pain were rated with numeric pain scores of 6 and 10, respectively. Her baseline ODI score was 62. Numerous conservative measures were unsuccessful, including physical therapy, injections, bracing, and pain medications. Her spinopelvic parameters included a pelvic incidence of 46 degrees, lumbar lordosis of 33 degrees, and pelvic tilt of 24 degrees (Fig. 50-5, A and C).

A hybrid MIS surgery was performed to decompress the neural elements and to correct her coronal and sagittal deformities. The plan was as follows:
- T10-S1 percutaneous instrumentation and fusion
- L3 mini-open PSO
- L3-4, L4-5, and L5-S1 MIS transforaminal lumbar interbody fusion

The patient lost 450 cc of blood over a period of 320 minutes. One year postoperatively all parameters are improved over preoperative measurements as follows (Fig. 50-5, B and D):
- Her Cobb angle is decreased from 61 to 13 degrees.
- Coronal alignment is improved from −10.9 to +3 mm.
- Lumbar lordosis is improved from 33 to 51 degrees.
- Her sagittal vertical axis is reduced from 3 to 0 cm.
- Pelvic tilt is decreased from 24 to 15 degrees.

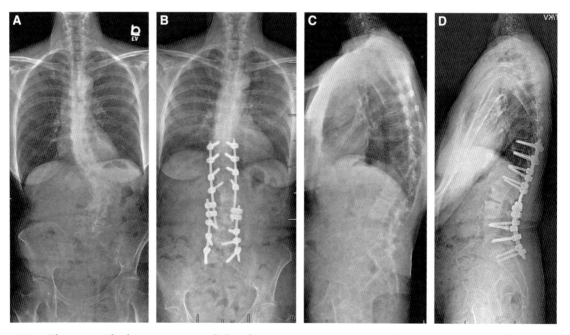

Fig. 50-5   This patient had a mini-open pedicle subtraction osteotomy. **A** and **C**, Preoperative AP and lateral standing 36-inch radiographs. The patient had a Cobb angle of 61 degrees, coronal alignment of −10.9 mm, lumbar lordosis of 33 degrees, a sagittal vertical axis of 3 cm, pelvic tilt of 24 degrees, and pelvic incidence of 46 degrees. **B** and **D,** One year postoperatively, AP and lateral radiographs show the following improvements: a Cobb angle of 13 degrees, coronal alignment of +3 mm, lumbar lordosis of 51 degrees, a sagittal vertical axis of 0 cm, pelvic tilt of 15 degrees, and pelvic incidence of 46 degrees.

CONCLUSION

Significant innovations have occurred during the past two decades in the fields of MIS and open deformity surgery. Because the ASD population is at high risk for developing complications from corrective surgery, less morbid methods for achieving surgical correction are highly desirable. Such techniques will be widely applied if the results are reproducible and found to satisfy the goals of traditional open surgeries. Advances for treating patients with ASD are occurring regularly, and it is likely that less and less invasive methods will be tolerated in the future.

REFERENCES

1. Jaikumar S, Kim DH, Kam AC. History of minimally invasive surgery. Neurosurgery 51(5 Suppl):S1-S14, 2002.

2. Wang MY, Cummock MD, Yu Y, et al. An analysis of the differences in the acute hospitalization charges following minimally invasive versus open posterior lumbar interbody fusion. J Neurosurg Spine 12:694-699, 2010.

3. McGirt MJ, Parker SL, Lerner J, et al. Comparative analysis of perioperative surgical site infection after minimally invasive versus open posterior/transforaminal lumbar interbody fusion: analysis of hospital billing and discharge data from 5170 patients. J Neurosurg Spine 14:771-778, 2011.

4. Wang MY, Lerner J, Lesko J, et al. Acute hospital costs after minimally invasive versus open lumbar interbody fusion: data from a US national database with 6106 patients. J Spinal Disord Tech 25:324-328, 2012.

5. Elowitz EH, Yanni DS, Chwajol M, et al. Evaluation of indirect decompression of the lumbar spinal canal following minimally invasive lateral transpsoas interbody fusion: radiographic and outcome analysis. Minim Invasive Neurosurg 54(5-6):201-206, 2011.

6. Bess S, Boachie-Adjei O, Burton D, et al. Pain and disability determine treatment modality for older patients with adult scoliosis, while deformity guides treatment for younger patients. Spine 34:2186-2190, 2009.

7. Smith JS, Shaffrey CI, Berven S, et al. Improvement of back pain with operative and nonoperative treatment in adults with scoliosis. Neurosurgery 65:86-93, 2009.

8. Smith JS, Shaffrey CI, Glassman SD, et al. Risk-benefit assessment of surgery for adult scoliosis. Spine 36:817-824, 2011.

9. Fu KM, Rhagavan P, Shaffrey CI, et al. Prevalence, severity, and impact of foraminal and canal stenosis among adults with degenerative scoliosis. Neurosurgery 69:1181-1187, 2011.

10. Schwender J, Holly L, Rouben D, et al. Minimally invasive transforaminal lumbar interbody fusion (TLIF): technical feasibility and initial results. J Spinal Disord Tech 18(Suppl):S1-S6, 2005.

11. Fessler RG. Minimally invasive percutaneous posterior lumbar interbody fusion. Neurosurgery 52:1512, 2003.

12. Pateder DB, Gonzales RA, Kebaish KM, et al. Short-term mortality and its association with independent risk factors in adult spinal deformity surgery. Spine 33:1224-1228, 2008.

13. Charosky S, Guigui P, Blamoutier A, et al. Complications and risk factors of primary adult scoliosis surgery: a multicenter study of 306 patients. Spine 37:693-700, 2012.

14. Weistroffer JK, Perra JH, Lonstein JE, et al. Complications in long fusions to the sacrum for adult scoliosis: minimum five-year analysis of fifty patients. Spine 33:1478-1483, 2008.

15. Scheufler KM, Cyron D, Dohmen H, et al. Less invasive surgical correction of adult degenerative scoliosis. I. Technique and radiographic results. Neurosurgery 67:696-710, 2010.

16. Anand N, Baron EM, Thaiyananthan G, et al. Minimally invasive multilevel percutaneous correction and fusion for adult lumbar degenerative scoliosis: a technique and feasibility study. J Spinal Disord Tech 21:459-467, 2008.

17. Wang MY, Mummaneni PV. Minimally invasive surgery for thoracolumbar spinal deformity: initial clinical experience with clinical and radiographic outcomes. Neurosurg Focus 28:E9, 2010.

18. Lonner B. Emerging minimally invasive technologies for the management of scoliosis. Orthop Clin N Am 38:431-440, 2007.

19. Hsieh PC, Koski TR, Sciubba DM, et al. Maximizing the potential of minimally invasive spine surgery in complex spinal disorders. Neurosurg Focus 25:E19, 2008.

20. Foley KT, Gupta SK. Percutaneous pedicle screw fixation in the lumbar spine: preliminary clinical results. J Neurosurg 97(1 Suppl):S7-S12, 2002.

21. Manwaring JC, Bach K, Ahmadian AA, et al. Management of sagittal balance in adult spinal deformity with minimally invasive anterolateral lumbar interbody fusion: a preliminary radiographic study. J Neurosurg Spine 20:515-522, 2014.

22. Wang MY. Improvement of sagittal balance and lumbar lordosis following less invasive adult spinal deformity surgery with expandable cages and percutaneous instrumentation. J Neurosurg Spine 18:4-12, 2013.

23. Wang MY, Mummaneni PV, Fu KM, et al; Minimally Invasive Surgery Section of the International Spine Study Group. Less invasive surgery for treating adult spinal deformities: ceiling effects for deformity correction with three different techniques. Neurosurg Focus 36:E12, 2014.

24. Wang MY, Madhavan K. Mini-open pedicle subtraction osteotomy: surgical technique. World Neurosurg. 2012 Oct 5. [Epub ahead of print]

25. Wang MY, Ludwig SC, Anderson DG, et al. Percutaneous iliac screw placement: description of a new minimally invasive technique. Neurosurg Focus 25:E17, 2008.

Index